AF322858

MEDICAL RADIOLOGY

Diagnostic Imaging and Radiation Oncology

Editorial Board

Founding Editors: L.W. Brady · M.W. Donner[†] · H.-P. Heilmann
F.H.W. Heuck

Current Editors: A.L. Baert, Leuven · L.W. Brady, Philadelphia
H.-P. Heilmann, Hamburg · F.H.W. Heuck, Stuttgart
J.E. Youker, Milwaukee

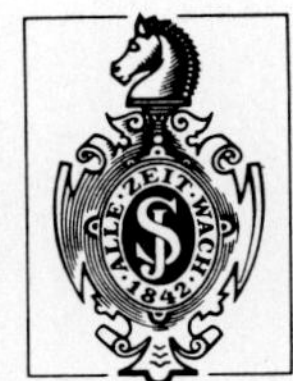

Radiation Therapy in Pediatric Oncology

Contributors

K.K. Ang · J.A. Belli. · A.L. Billet · J.R. Cassady · S.S. Donaldson
P.J. Eifel · R.G. Evans · K.W. Harter · J.J. Hutter · L.E. Kun
R.B. Marcus · K.L. McClain · P.S. Meltzer · N.P. Mendenhall
S.E. Sallan · B. Stea · P.S. Swift · A.J. van der Kogel
E. van der Schueren · M.D. Wharam

Edited by
J. Robert Cassady

Foreword by
Luther W. Brady and Hans-Peter Heilmann

With 77 Figures and 94 Tables

Springer-Verlag
Berlin Heidelberg New York
London Paris Tokyo
Hong Kong Barcelona
Budapest

J. Robert Cassady, M.D.

Professor, Department of Radiation Oncology
College of Medicine
The University of Arizona
Health Science Center
1501 North Campbell Ave.
Tucson, AZ 85724
USA

MEDICAL RADIOLOGY · Diagnostic Imaging and Radiation Oncology

Continuation of
Handbuch der medizinischen Radiologie
Encyclopedia of Medical Radiology

ISBN 3-540-54105-5 Springer-Verlag Berlin Heidelberg New York
ISBN 0-387-54105-5 Springer-Verlag New York Berlin Heidelberg

Library of Congress Cataloging-in-Publication Data. Radiation therapy in pediatric oncology / with contributions by K. Kian Ang ... [et al.]; edited by J. Robert Cassady; with a foreword by Luther W. Brady and Hans-Peter Heilmann.   p.   cm. – (Medical radiology) Includes bibliographical references and index.ISBN 0-387-54105. – ISBN 3-540-54105-5 1. Tumors in children – Radiotherapy. I. Ang, K.K. (K.Kian) II. Cassady, J. Robert (James Robert), 1938-   . III. Series. [DNLM: 1. Neoplasms – in infancy & childhood. 2. Neoplasms-radiotherapy. QZ 269 R 1284 1994] R C281. C4R23 1994 618.92′ 9920642 – dc20 DNLM/DLC for Library of Congress 94-2790

This work is subject to copyright. All rights are reserved, whether the whole or part of the material is concerned, specifically the rights of translation, reprinting, reuse of illustrations, recitation, broadcasting, reproduction on microfilm or in any other way, and storage in data banks. Duplication of this publication or parts thereof is permitted only under the provisions of the German Copyright Law of September 9, 1965, in its current version, and permission for use must always be obtained from Springer-Verlag. Violations are liable for prosecution under the German Copyright Law.

© Springer-Verlag Berlin Heidelberg 1994
Printed in Germany

The use of general descriptive names, registered, trademarks, etc. in this publications does not imply, even in the absence of a specific statement, that such names are exempt from the relevant protective laws and regulations and therefore free for general use.

Product liability: The publishers cannot guarantee the accuracy of any information about dosage and application contained in this book. In every individual case the user must check such information by consulting the relevant literature.

Typesetting: Thomson Press (India) Ltd., New Delhi

SPIN:10042321   21/3130/SPS – 5 4 3 2 1 0 – printed on acid-free paper

Foreword

The diagnosis of cancer in a child is a devastating finding not only to the parents but often to the child. Even though the situation is relatively easy to accept among adults, it is difficult to accept among children because of their general helpless state.

The advances that have been made in the management of a child with cancer in the last 20 years have been dramatic in character. These have occurred not only by virtue of the contributions from early diagnosis and more precise staging but also from the contributions made by surgery, radiation therapy, and the more widespread utilization of chemotherapy regimens. This volume by J. Robert Cassady sets forth the position of radiation oncology in the management of the child with cancer. Radiation therapy remains an important and significant part of the treatment of this group of diseases. The book presents the basic knowledge with regards to pediatric oncology and how it relates to radiation therapy. It gives a timely overview on the topic and is essential for all radiation oncologists involved in the management of children with cancer.

Hamburg/Philadelphia, June 1994

H.-P. HEILMANN
LUTHER W. BRADY

Preface

This book provides a thorough review of the role that radiation therapy currently plays in the management of most childhood tumors. Extensively augmented with figures and tables where appropriate, it also provides a concise review of current diagnostic and therapeutic approaches for major childhood malignancies. Extensive and up-to-date reference lists are an added benefit.

Chapters on principles of pediatric radiation therapy, etiology of childhood tumors, and newer, molecular approaches in pediatric oncology are provided.

Authors include leaders in the field writing on their particular areas of interest and expertise, providing a diversity of approach useful to the reader.

Many people have been responsible for this book. Primary thanks must go to our many childhood patients and their parents who have allowed us the privilege of treating them. Appreciation and thanks are due to my many teachers and particular role models, HENRY S. KAPLAN, M.D., ROBERT SAGERMAN, M.D., JOHN KIRKPATRICK, M.D., and SAMUEL HELLMAN, M.D.

Thanks are also due to my residents over the years, who have provided continuing stimulation.

Finally, thanks are due to my parents, who initiated my training in medicine, and most particularly to my wife, DEBORAH, without whose continuing intellectual challenge, stimulation, and support, this work would not have been possible.

Thanks also to CHARLOTTE RAMSEY for her skillful assistance in the preparation of this book.

Tucson, June 1994   J. ROBERT CASSADY

Contents

1 Pediatric Radiation Therapy: Introduction
   J. Robert Cassady 1

2 Etiology, Clinical Associations, and the Possibility of Prevention of
   Childhood Malignancies
   J. Robert Cassady 7

3 Acute and Chronic Normal Tissue Effects and Potential Modification
   in Pediatric Radiation Therapy
   Patricia J. Eifel 13

4 Molecular Biology and Genetic Advances in Childhood Malignancies
   Paul S. Meltzer 55

5 Principles of Damage Interactions Between Radiation and
   Chemotherapeutic Agents
   James A. Belli 75

6 Acute Lymphoblastic Leukemia
   Amy Louise Billet and Stephen E. Sallan 87

7 Acute Nonlymphocytic Leukemia
   Baldassarre Stea 99

8 Biologic and Physical Principles of Total Body Irradiation for
   Allogeneic and Autologous Bone Marrow Transplantation in
   Children with Leukemia and Lymphoma
   Richard G. Evans 115

9 Role of Radiation Therapy in Non-Hodgkin's Lymphoma in the Child
   Sarah S. Donaldson 123

10 Effects of Therapy on Central Nervous System Functions in Children
    K. Kian Ang, Albert J. Van Der Kogel, and
    Emmanuel Van Der Schueren 133

11 Hodgkin's Disease
    Nancy Price Mendenhall 151

12 Neuroblastoma
    J. Robert Cassady 175

13   Malignant Brain Tumors Including Medulloblastoma,
     Embryonal Neuroectodermal Tumors, and Tumors of the Pineal Region,
     with a Special Discussion of the Management of Brain Tumors in Children
     of 3 Years and Younger
     LARRY E. KUN 197

14   Brain Stem Gliomas in Children
     PATRICK S. SWIFT 215

15   Gliomas of the Supratentorium, Ventricular System, and Visual Pathways,
     and Tumors of the Sellar Region
     PATRICK S. SWIFT 221

16   Tumors of the Spinal Cord in Children
     PATRICK S. SWIFT 239

17   Wilms Tumor
     MOODY D. WHARAM, JR. 251

18   Ewing's Sarcoma
     ROBERT B. MARCUS JR. 265

19   Rhabdomyosarcoma
     J. ROBERT CASSADY 281

20   Osteosarcoma and the Less Common Sarcomas of Childhood
     K. WILLIAM HARTER 305

21   Retinoblastoma
     J. ROBERT CASSADY 319

22   Langerhans Cell Histiocytosis
     KENNETH L. McCLAIN, JOHN J. HUTTER, and
     J. ROBERT CASSADY 337

23   Epithelial Carcinomas in the Child
     WILLIAM K. HARTER 351

24   Unusual Neoplasms of Childhood
     J. ROBERT CASSADY 369

25   Future Prospects in Childhood Cancer
     J. ROBERT CASSADY 379

Subject Index 381

List of Contributors 387

1 Pediatric Radiation Therapy: Introduction

J. Robert Cassady

CONTENTS

1.1 Principles of Pediatric Radiation Therapy 1
1.2 Radiation Technique 5
    References 6

Major changes have occurred in the practice of pediatric radiation oncology in the past two to three decades. Common practices of the 1960s and 1970s, such as routine postoperative tumor bed irradiation for Wilms' tumor and irradiation of stage II neuroblastoma, are no longer indicated. Many factors, including improved systemic therapy, improved knowledge of the natural history of these tumors, and better risk-group analyses, have led to these changes. A curative goal at first presentation, even in the face of established metastatic disease, has been adopted more frequently in the child. Advances in the treatment of Wilms' tumor and osteosarcoma illustrate this fact, as does the nearly routine use of adjuvant systemic treatment as salvage of children who have developed metastases is often less effective.

Children may present with no systemic disease or, at the other extreme, with an overt metastasis(es). Between these two extremes, assuming normal distribution, lie children with very few (200 or less) or many (10^8) systemic tumor cells. Even when only modest sensitivity exists to available agents, prompt systemic or even regional (i.e., treatment of the lungs in Ewing's tumor, osteosarcoma, or Wilms' tumor) treatment may eliminate development of metastases in a substantial percentage. Fortunately, many childhood malignancies exhibit considerable sensitivity to available agents. Cure rates of childhood cancer have thus improved and, with this improvement, the radiation oncologist is now participating

J. Robert Cassady, M.D., Professor and Head, Department of Radiation Oncology, The University of Arizona, Health Sciences Center, 1501 North Campbell Ave., Tucson, AZ 85724, USA

in potentially curative treatment strategies in many disease settings previously considered palliative. In certain disease groups such as CNS tumors, although radiation therapy continues to be a mainstay of treatment, multimodal approaches are now being investigated in an attempt to improve both the quantity of survivors and their quality of life (Cassady 1991).

Thus, although the disease settings vary from the past, the pediatric radiation oncologist continues to play an important role in analysis and treatment of this rewarding group of children.

1.1 Principles of Pediatric Radiation Therapy

It is beyond the scope (and goals) of this text to provide a thorough review of basic radiation biology, physics, and treatment planning. Many excellent reviews exist which accomplish this purpose (Steel et al. 1983; Meyn and Withers 1980; Lodish et al. 1986; Perez and Brady 1987; Hall 1978). However, it is important to address certain aspects of pediatric radiation treatment which differ from adult practice owing to unique aspects presented by the child. Certain principles are critically important for all age groups. Perhaps the most important of these is the nature of a typical radiation dose-response curve. Figure 1.1a shows two important features of this curve. The first is that even a relatively low dose of irradiation will produce *some* effect (either tumor control or, perhaps, normal tissue injury); the second is that even a small reduction in dose at higher levels can produce a marked decrease in response (either undesirable normal tissue effects or tumor cell death) (Hellman 1989). Holthusen (1936) graphically showed these two relationships as the separation between two competing dose-response curves with the tumor control curve (hopefully) lying to the left of the normal tissue damage curve (Fig. 1.1a).

The pediatric therapist must constantly consider these relationships and balance the dose of

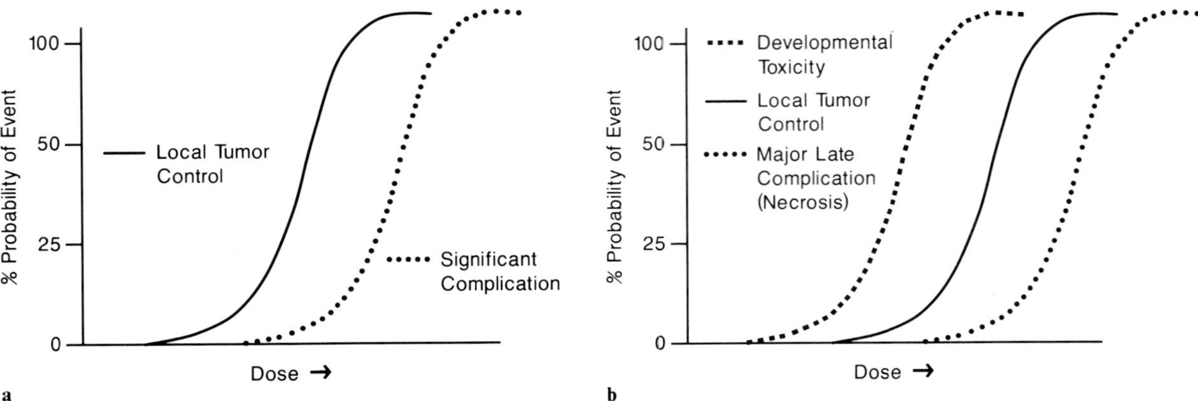

Fig. 1.1. a Holthusen dose-response curve demonstrating potential overlap between tumor control and late complications depending on dose chosen and likelihood of tumor control desired. Note also the rapid increase in tumor control (or complications) achieved by relatively small incremental increases in dose. The exact relationship between local tumor control and the complication being considered varies considerably with the clinical setting. **b** Similar dose-response diagram incorporating the concept of developmental toxicity. Of note is the placement of the developmental toxicity curve to the left (i.e., developmental toxicity occurs with lower dose) of the tumor control curve, in keeping with the modest dose of radiation required to produce some degree of growth arrest (muscle, bone, etc.) or other developmental toxicity

irradiation necessary for a high probability of local/regional control with that dose which unnecessarily injures normal, developing tissue (BLOOMER and HELLMAN 1975). Similar considerations regarding volume to be treated must also be made.

Many of these same considerations also have to be confronted when a decision must be made as to the best treatment plan in a child with a malignancy. As an example, when high-dose treatment is to be given to the adult pelvis, a relatively equally weighted four-field plan is usually desirable when compared to two-field or rotational options because of the shielding of normal tissue that can be accomplished (especially of small bowel) as well as the reduction in subcutaneous tissue dose that occurs. In the child, the dose that such an equally weighted plan delivers to the proximal femurs and pelvis may cause unacceptable bony growth alterations. However, when the nature of the dose-response relationship is understood and normal tissue/effect curves are known, both goals (reduction in subcutaneous tissue and bowel dose and minimal, if any, growth alteration) may be accomplished by a reduction in the usual lateral dose component so that critical skeletal tissues receive a dose that only minimally affects growth potential and the corresponding slight decrease in small bowel dose near or at the sharp inflection point of the toxicity curve markedly reduces the incidence of late bowel or subcutaneous tissue damage.

A second critical principle is that of immobilization. Clearly, the need for immobilization applies to

both children and adults to permit accuracy and precision in treatment delivery and thereby ensure that normal tissues will be spared and tumors fully irradiated. In contrast to most adults, children are frequently unable and/or unwilling to accept the degree of immobility necessary for optimum treatment. It is therefore desirable that the child be introduced to the personnel and equipment and rooms they will be treated in *prior* to the initiation of actual treatment if there exists any question or concern regarding immobilization. This approach has greatest value for the child of 3 1/2–10 years but may also be valuable for older children as well. In this way, considerable anxiety can be relieved and, where appropriate, through the use of closed-circuit television monitors, the treatment (*and immobilization and cooperation*) of other patients observed. It may also be appropriate, where possible, to delay placement of painful tattoos as permanent marks until the confidence of the child has been gained. Where such a delay is not possible, its performance by individuals *other than* the team that will be routinely treating the child has merit. In this way, a measure of trust may be obtained and the child become less fearful and hence more cooperative.

In younger children, sedation or, more frequently, general anesthesia is often necessary, at least initially (MURRAY 1989). This observer has not been impressed with the ability of various immobilization devices to hold the uncooperative child sufficiently quiet for ideal treatment. Some degree of patient motion exists with all such devices and it may be considerable in children older than 1 1/2–2 years, who frequently have remarkable strength relative to an adult. Exceptions may exist (i.e., the child of less than 1 year); however, for precision treatment (i.e., patient motion of less than a few millimeters), anesthesia is often imperative or desirable.

The potential consequences of inadequate immobilization are illustrated by two reports from the literature (JEREB et al. 1984; McCORMICK et al. 1988). The first of these demonstrated an unacceptably high rate of cribriform plate failures in children treated for medulloblastoma, which is easily understood if patient motion and dose-response relationships are considered relative to lens and orbit shielding (JEREB et al. 1984). The second report presented both a high rate of normal tissue damage (cataract formation) and a correspondingly high tumor failure rate when unanesthetized children were treated with a technically demanding plan for retinoblastoma (McCORMICK et al. 1988).

The lack of availability in many hospitals and free-standing facilities of an on-site expert pediatric anesthesia team used to dealing with children being irradiation is one of many compelling reasons for referral of children to an appropriate regional center for optimal treatment.

A large number of effective, rapid-acting anesthetic agents are currently available and the ability to anesthetize children on a daily (or even twice daily) basis with these agents for many weeks has been amply demonstrated (MENACHE et al. 1990).

Perhaps the most important structural and cosmetic principle to consider in irradiation of the child is that of symmetry. Many quite considerable growth alterations created by necessary irradiation in the growing child can be effectively masked if they are symmetrical. This has been the guiding principle behind the routine advocacy of homogeneous irradiation of the spine in order to prevent unequal growth and thus scoliosis, but it can be equally applied to lower extremity and/or facial treatment should such treatment lead to uncorrected leg-length discrepancy or facial asymmetry. It is particularly important to keep this principle in mind when irradiation of the very young child is necessary (e.g., for neuroblastoma) or when the young child with Hodgkin's disease is to receive combined modality treatment with low-dose "involved field" irradiation. In this latter example, it is usually preferable to treat both sides of the neck or deliver equally symmetrical treatment volumes rather than treat one such region unilaterally as asymmetry will become increasingly noticeable as the child matures.

Another importance difference between pediatric and adult cancer patients is the difference in normal tissue turnover and recovery rates. In general, children will manifest acute tissue damage reactions of rapid-response tissues (e.g., mucositis) more promptly than their more elderly counterparts, and such reactions are frequently enhanced by the use of nearly routine concomitant systemic treatment. However, the child will correspondingly recover more promptly than the adult and will usually be able to tolerate an intensity of treatment greater than that tolerated by even a young adult.

A factor contributing to the enhanced ability of children to recover from acute treatment effects is the lack of or limited exposure to smoking, alcohol, and other environmental pollutants that frequently compromise adult treatment. Children also rarely have significant comorbid diseases (e.g., atherosclerosis) affecting critical organs such as the heart, lungs, kidneys, blood vessels, and gastrointestinal tract that regularly are seen in the older adult population with cancer.

The ability of children to tolerate, with adequate support and monitoring, extremely aggressive treatment approaches has contributed to the higher rate of successful treatment seen in children.

Almost all children who are being irradiated have received or are being treated with systemic cytotoxic agents. Although this is increasingly reflected in adult practice, the frequency of concurrent treatment and the chemotherapeutic agents being used are often different in the childhood setting from those in adult practice, and many unfamiliar and/or novel drug–radiation interactions occur in the child. This necessitates careful and frequent observation and monitoring of the child during treatment and further supports the importance of experience for therapists conducting childhood treatment.

Also impressive are the interactions between acute tissue reactions such as mucositis and parameters such as the absolute white blood cell count. Frequently, a mucositis will rapidly become markedly worse when the white cell count decreases precipitously with drug administration and, correspondingly, a nearly confluent mucositis may entirely recover within 36–48 h of white blood cell count recovery. Whether this is a direct effect of neutropenia or simply a manifestation of similar effects on two acute-reacting tissues is not known.

As concurrent radiation and chemotherapy treatment is relatively common, unexpected, unusual interactions may develop. An example of this has been noted in the treatment of Wilms' tumor wherein radiation treatment affects the pharmacokinetics of drug metabolism. Two of the most effective systemic agents for Wilms' tumor are actinomycin D and vincristine. Both agents are detoxified in the liver. Thus, when a surgical hepatic insult or radiation hepatic injury occurs through necessary treatment of a large hepatic volume, decreased hepatic clearance of drug(s) takes place, leading to enhanced normal tissue effects and toxicity at a drug dose usually considered safe (CASSADY et al. 1979).

A difference between child and adult which can result in dramatic consequences is that of reserve. It has been noted that children are able to tolerate more intensive treatment and recover more promptly than their adult counterparts. However, children, especially when very young, usually have low fat or other nutritional reserve stores. Total blood pool and fluid/electrolyte reserves are also smaller. Therefore, use of central lines for fluid and electrolyte replacement as well as hyperalimentation approaches for nutrition are routine and important in intensive, combined modality treatment schemes with children. Because of decreased nutritional and/or fluid reserve, fluid loss and/or dehydration-weight loss that may be relatively trivial in the adult can have serious consequences in the young child.

Monitoring of the side-effects of treatment must be carried out more frequently than for the adult and more vigorous replacement policies utilized if one is to avoid preventable toxic effects of treatment.

Our ability to accurately monitor with increasing efficacy nutritional intake, fluids, blood, temperature, electrolytes, etc. in the past two decades and, where necessary, to rapidly correct abnormalities as they develop has been one of the major features that have contributed to improved pediatric cancer care. Other than the intrinsic ability of the child to withstand toxic insults discussed previously, it has been these monitoring approaches which have permitted our current intensive multimodal treatment approaches.

A frequently made but mistaken assumption has been to consider the child as a miniature adult. Nothing could be further from the truth. Different organ systems in the child mature at different rates and this difference in maturation and development can translate to marked differences in children's ability to withstand treatment. Two examples illustrates this point. Although the brain and CNS develop early in relation to the musculoskeletal system, complete myelinization of the CNS does not occur before age 3–4 years. Therefore, if irradiation can be withheld until after this time, consequences for function

will be reduced substantially. Similarly, renal development is not complete at birth and continued maturation and growth continue into early childhood. Apparent decreases in renal function have been noted in infants at radiation doses that have no discernible effect even in a child of 2 or 3 years (PESCHEL et al. 1981). Toxic effects of chemotherapeutic agents may also be differentially expressed depending on the age of the patient. Doxorubicin appears to produce a higher rate of cardiac dysfunction in very young children (especially those less than 1 year old) than in adults at equivalent total doses, suggesting a difference in susceptibility (LIPSHULTZ et al. 1991).

Age differences in maturation, growth, and development of normal tissues such as the brain and kidney have been noted. Similarly, the radiation dose which produces a 50% or 60% reduction in ultimate organ size or cell number varies as a function of tissue type and age when treatment is delivered. For all tissues, this dose is nearly always considerably less than the dose which will produce a significant frequency of *late* toxicity and necrosis, which thus limits treatment for many adult tumors. Thus, the concept of *developmental toxicity* must be introduced in childhood cancer treatment and represents a unique problem for the pediatric therapist. Knowledge of these maturation and dose differences and their timing on the part of the pediatric radiation oncologist is essential and may impose limitations in pediatric treatment that do not exist in adult treatment.

Radiation may also potentiate the toxicity of certain systemic agents through apparent direct effects either on cell membranes or perhaps on vascular permeability. Thus, methotrexate at certain concentrations may be administered intravenously with relative safety to brain tissue. However, if substantial prior radiation has been delivered to a limited volume (e.g., brain stem) or the entire brain, severe neurotoxicity may ensue after subsequent intravenous methotrexate administration. The sequence of administration of anticancer agents and modalities may therefore be very important.

Similarly, "recall" of radiation normal tissue reactions first described following actinomycin D administration to previously irradiated children may occur with a variety of agents, including actinomycin D, doxorubicin, and methotrexate (D'ANGIO et al. 1959; CASSADY et al. 1975; DONALDSON et al. 1974).

Because of the frequency of joint treatment of the child with chemotherapy and irradiation, most of the interactions here noted have been observed initially in the child.

1.2 Radiation Technique

Differences between acute and subacute radiation toxicity and the much more serious late necrosis that may occur following radiation treatment are well recognized by radiation oncologists. We have earlier introduced the concept of developmental toxicity separate from late necrosis as a phenomenon generally unique to the child. Three examples illustrate this point. A total radiation dose to a given bone of approximately 30 Gy will produce nearly complete cessation of future bony growth except for a small amount to which the bone was "committed" prior to treatment. Thus, even after delivery of 50–55 Gy in combination with cytotoxic drugs in the treatment of Ewing's sarcoma, some (~ 1–1.5 cm) growth can be measured. However, 30 Gy is less than half the radiation dose necessary to produce radiation osteoradionecrosis. Similarly, total radiation doses of 25–30 Gy will produce substantial muscle and soft tissue developmental "failure" (*not* atrophy) when children with Wilms' tumor or neuroblastoma are treated. However, again, this dose is less than one-half that which will very rarely produce soft tissue *necrosis.*

Finally, radiation-induced brain necrosis is an un-common occurrence and, when conventional fractionation is utilized, is rarely noted even following radiation doses of 60–65 Gy. However, much smaller doses, when delivered to certain areas of the brain of a young child (especially < 5 years), will produce intellectual and learning disabilities. Similar examples are available for many normal tissues and illustrate the importance conceptually of differentiating *developmental* toxicity from late radiation necrosis (Fig. 1.1b).

The cause of this "developmental toxicity" appears, in many cases, to be a cohort of cells which are transiently sensitive to radiation as they divide and/or expand. Sensitivity is lost when maturation/development is completed. This transient sensitivity may extend to tumor development as well in certain of these tissues. Thus, breast development can be markedly reduced by radiation doses of less than 15–18 Gy in childhood. Similarly, radiation to the breast(s) of a young girl can significantly increase the rate of breast cancer development in later life; however, after age 30–35, this risk markedly diminishes. Similar considerations apply to the thyroid gland.

Too often, in setting radiation dose limits for childhood treatment, differences between the toxicities of late necrosis and development are confused. Many "schedules" that have been published or utilized in the child which differentially proscribe tumor doses by age exhibit this difficulty as almost all dose levels in such schemes are usually well above the developmentally toxic dose.

In weighing the benefits and risks of radiation treatment and ultimately deciding on a treatment plan, these several toxicities must be carefully considered and separated. An example reported in the literature illustrates this point (Kiel and Suit 1984). In this report, a 10-year-old child with multiply recurrent desmoid tumor involving the entire forearm (including the ulna and radius) was referred for radiation therapy. Contrary to usual practice for adults with this tumor (55–60 Gy), total dose in this child was limited to 24 Gy and prompt recurrence developed (with unstated consequences for the arm) following treatment. We know of no data that confirm that late radiation necrosis of soft tissue is more common at a given dose in the child than in the adult. In fact, the absence of atherosclerosis, smoking, and other detrimental factors combined with tissue reserves may decrease this risk in the child. The total dose chosen (24 Gy) in this case ensured substantial ultimate bone and muscle growth arrest. Thus, to gain at most a modest increase in growth, dose was decreased by more than half and, given dose-response considerations illustrated in Fig. 1.1a and b, development of recurrence was not surprising. In all likelihood, function was lost in this attempt.

The goal of reduced normal tissue toxicity through radiation dose reduction is admirable. In the development of studies attempting to achieve this goal, especially in the multi-institutional group study format, a clear statement of expected gains from such dose reductions needs to be made and assessed as an end point to justify the potential risks inherent in such reductions.

Many alterations in typical radiation therapy practice have occurred in the past decade that have relevance for the child and may contribute significantly to both improved treatment efficacy and reduced normal tissue morbidity.

Childhood tumors are usually rapidly proliferating lesions in which clonogenic tumor cells have rapid doubling times. Withers, Fowler, and others have demonstrated the theoretical advantage in these settings of altered fractionation approaches—especially hyperfractionation techniques (Withers and Mason 1974; Van Der Schueren et al. 1983).

This approach has shown apparent benefit in at least four childhood tumor settings: Burkitt's lymphoma, brain stem gliomas, locally advanced rhabdomyosarcoma, and total body irradiation for bone marrow transplantation (NORIN and ONYANGO 1977; FREEMAN 1991; PACKER 1990; MANDELL et al. 1990; THOMAS et al. 1982). It may be of particular importance for the child because of the normal tissue protection it may provide in addition to the potential for improvements in tumor response and control.

Stereotaxic radiosurgery and intraoperative radiation therapy may also provide particular benefits for the child by permitting significant normal tissue sparing while correspondingly allowing delivery of larger effective doses to tumor-bearing tissue. Broadening stereotaxic approaches to non-CNS settings holds promise for the future. Similar examples of "targeting" of radiation to tumor sites with normal tissue sparing which have proved beneficial in pediatric practice include use of sophisticated brachytherapy approaches in the treatment of pediatric rhabdomyosarcoma and ^{125}I$^-$ or ^{131}I-MIBG treatment of advanced neuroblastoma.

These and many similar examples illustrate how pediatric oncology and pediatric radiation therapy must continue to be at the forefront of technical innovation and understanding of cancer. Only if this leading role is maintained in future decades will we successfully "put ourselves out of business" (HELLMAN S., personal communication, ASCO presidential speech).

References

Bloomer WD, Hellman S (1975) Normal tissue responses to radiation therapy. N Engl J Med 293: 8083

Cassady JR (1991) Keynote address: Contributions of pediatric oncology: examples derived from advances made in the treatment of rhabdomyosarcoma and neuroblastoma. Int J Radiat Oncol Biol Phys 20: 1177–1182

Cassady JR, Richter MP, Piro AJ et al. (1975) Radiation–adriamycin interactions: preliminary clinical observations. Cancer 36: 946–949

Cassady JR, Carabell SC, Jaffe N (1979) Chemotherapy–irradiation related hepatic dysfunction in patients with Wilms' tumor. Front Radiat Ther Oncol 13: 147–160

D'Angio GJ, Farber S, Maddock CL (1959) Potentiation of x-ray effects by actinomycin-D. Radiology 73: 175–177

Donaldson SS, Glick JM, Wilbur JR (1974) Adriamycin activating a recall phenomenon after radiation therapy. Ann Intern Med 81: 407–408

Freeman CR (1991) Hyperfractionated radiation therapy in brainstem tumors. Cancer 68: 474–481

Hall EJ (1978) Radiobiology for the radiologist, 2nd edn. Harper & Row, Hagerstown, Md.

Hellman S (1989) Principles of radiation therapy. In: DaVita VT, Hellman S, Rosenberg SA (eds) Cancer; principles and practice of oncology, 3rd edn. J.B. Lippincott, Philadelphia, pp 247–275

Holthusen H (1936) Erfahrungen über die Verträglichkeitsgrenze für Röntgenstrahler und deren Nutzanwendung zur Verhütung von Schäden. Strahlentherapie 57: 254–269

Jereb B, Krishnaswami S, Reid A, Allen JC (1984) Radiation for medulloblastoma adjusted to prevent recurrences to the cribriform plate region. Cancer 54: 602–604

Johns HE, Cunningham JR (eds) (1977) The physics of radiology. Charles C. Thomas, Springfield, Ill

Kiel KD, Suit HD (1984) Radiation therapy in the treatment of aggressive fibromatoses (desmoid tumors). Cancer 54: 2041–2055

Lipshultz SE, Colan SD, Gelber RD, Perez–Atayde AR, Sallan SE, Saunders SP (1991) Late cardiac effects of doxorubicin therapy for acute lymphoblastic leukemia in childhood. N Engl J Med 324: 808–815

Lodish H, Darnell J, Baltimore D (eds) (1986) Molecular cell biology. Scientific American Books, New York

Mandell L, Ghavimi F, LaQuaglia M (1990) Alternating chemotherapy (CT) and hyperfractionated (HF) radiotherapy (RT) in advanced rhabdomyosarcoma (RMS): an update (abstract C-1157). Prac Am Soc Clin Oncol 9:298

McCormick B, Ellsworth R, Abramson D et al. (1988) Radiation therapy for retinoblastoma: comparison of results with lens-sparing versus lateral beam techniques. Int J Radiat Oncol Biol Phys 15: 567–574

Menache L, Eifel PJ, Kennamer DL, Belli JA (1990) Twice daily anesthesia in infants receiving hyperfractionated irradiation. Int J Radiat Oncol Biol Phys 18: 625–629

Meyn RE, Withers HR (eds) (1980) Radiation biology in cancer research. Raven, New York

Murray WJ (1989) Anesthesia for external beam radiotherapy. In: Pediatric radiation oncology. Raven, New York, pp 399–407

Norin T, Onyango J (1977) Radiotherapy in Burkitt's lymphoma. Int J Radiat Oncol Biol Phys 2: 399–406

Packer RJ (1990) Hyperfractionated radiotherapy for children with brainstem gliomas: a pilot study using 7,200 cGy. Ann Neurol 27: 167–173

Perez CA, Brady LW (eds) (1987) Principles and practice of radiation oncology. J.B. Lippincott, Philadelphia

Peschel RE, Chen M, Seashore J (1981) The treatment of massive hepatomegaly in stage IV–S neuroblastoma. Int J Radiat Oncol Biol Phys 7: 549–553

Steel GG, Adams GE, Peckham MJ (eds) (1983) The biological basis of radiotherapy. Elsevier, Amsterdam

Thomas ED, Clift RA, Hersman J et al. (1982) Marrow transplantation for acute non-lymphoblastic leukemia in first remission using fractionated or single-dose irradiation. Int J Radiat Oncol Biol Phys 8: 817–821

Van der Schueren E, Van der Bogaert W, Aug KK (1983) Radiotherapy with multiple fractions per day. In: Steel GG, Adams GE, Peckham MJ (eds) The biological basis of radiotherapy. Elsevier Scientific, Amsterdam, pp 195–210

Withers HR, Mason KA (1974) The kinetics of recovery in irradiated colonic mucosa of the mouse. Cancer 34: 896–903

2 Etiology, Clinical Associations, and the Possibility of Prevention of Childhood Malignancies

J. Robert Cassady

CONTENTS

2.1   Introduction 7
2.2   Geographic and Ethnic Variation 8
2.3   Environmental Factors 8
2.3.1 Radiation 8
2.3.2 Drug Exposure..................... 8
2.3.3 Ultraviolet Light..................... 9
2.4   Conditions Known to Predispose the
       Child to Development of a Malignancy 9
2.4.1 Neurofibromatosis 9
2.4.2 Retinoblastoma 9
2.4.3 Beckwith-Wiedemann Syndrome 10
2.4.4 Immunodeficiency Syndromes............. 10
2.4.5 Down's Syndrome (Trisomy 21) 10
2.4.6 Klinefelter's Syndrome (47, XXY) and
       Turner's Syndrome (45, XY or 45, XO) 10
2.4.7 Fanconi's Anemia, Bloom's Syndrome,
       and Ataxia Telangiectasia 10
2.4.8 von Hippel-Lindau Disease............... 10
2.4.9 Congenital Anomalies 10
       References......................... 10

2.1 Introduction

Prevention consistently represents the most cost-effective, function-preserving, and numerically successful approach to control of a disease. Successful prevention approaches, however, require an intimate knowledge of disease causation. Unlike many adult malignancies where environmental toxins have been shown to be etiologically important, most childhood malignancies appear to be associated with consistent chromosomal abnormalities which place the child at increased risk for specific malignancies. Mulvihill (1992) has urged that the term *ecogenetics* be used in considering causation of tumors in the young. He argues that cancer in a child or adult is likely the product of many determinants and that to consider *only* environment or genetics is an oversimplification Mulvihill 1980).

J. Robert Cassady, M.D., Professor and Head, Department of Radiation Oncology, The University of Arizona, Health Sciences Center, 1501 North Campbell Ave., Tucson, AZ 85724, USA

In addition, a number of nonmalignant conditions predispose the child to ultimate development of a malignancy [e.g., von Reck linghausen's disease (Mulvihill et al. 1990), Wiskott-Aldrich syndrome (Hoover 1977), and Fanconi's anemia (Johnson et al. 1972; McCaughan et al. 1985)]. Primarily environmentally related childhood malignancies are thought to represent only a tiny fraction of childhood tumors, and thus measures which, if implemented, would markedly reduce the incidence of many adult tumors (e.g., elimination of cigarette smoking) will have relatively little impact on the incidence of childhood cancer.

Our knowledge of causation of childhood tumors has experienced explosive growth in the past decade coincident with our increased knowledge of molecular genetics and our enhanced ability to examine increasingly minute abnormalities in chromosome structure and function. Although the absolute rarity of any individual childhood tumor represents and additional economic barrier to potentially effective prevention approaches, it is hoped that with increasingly sophisticated understanding of the molecular events necessary for tumor production, we will be able to interdict progression and thereby accomplish prevention, at least in those children known to be especially susceptible. It is also possible that increased skill and understanding in gentic manipulation, utilizing procedures such as amniocentesis, will permit identification of a substantially larger cohort of "at risk" children than currently exists and might also allow successful early intervention.

At this point, however, "prevention" in children in fact comprises approaches for early diagnosis in tumors such as neuroblastoma (see Chap. 12), Wilms' tumor (with periodic surveillance of children with significant predisposition, e.g., those with hemihypertrophy and aniridia: Miller et al. 1964; Riccardi et al. 1978), and retinoblastoma (with regular retinal examination at birth and frequently thereafter in "at risk" children).

Childhood tumors differ in many respects from their adult counterparts. Carcinomas, which

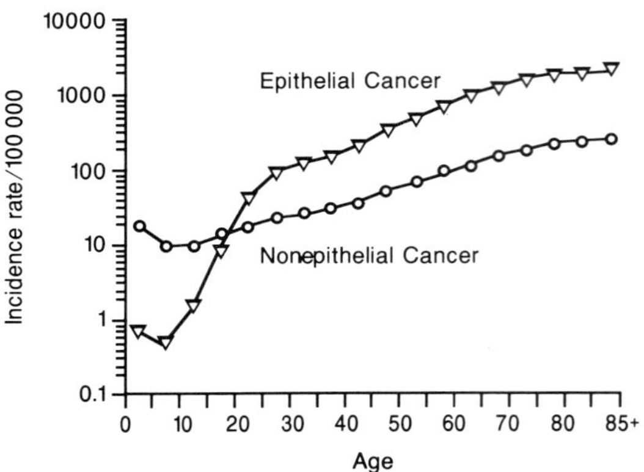

Fig. 2.1. Incidence of epithelial and nonepithelial cancer per 100 000 as a function of age. The relative rarity of epithelial tumors prior to age 15–20 years is notable. (Adapted from MILLER and MYERS 1983)

overwhelmingly predominate in the adult clinic, are rare in children, representing fewer than 10%–15% of all cases (Fig. 2.1) (MILLER and MYERS 1983). Leukemias and lymphomas also differ. Relatively common childhood malignancies such as T-cell lymphoblastic leukemia and Burkitt's lymphoma are rare or not seen in adults. Nodular lymphoma, relatively common in the adult, is almost never diagnosed in the child. Even Hodgkin's disease differs, at least in the United States, in that the lymphocyte-predominant subtype is more frequent in the child whereas the lymphocyte-depletion type is very rare (MAUCH et al. 1983).

Conditions known to predispose the child to malignancy will be discussed in Sect. 2.4.

2.2 Geographic and Ethnic Variation

Although certain tumors, such as Wilms' tumor, occur with relatively consistent frequency in many areas of the world (INNIS 1972), many pediatric malignancies vary considerably in frequency from country to country or between ethnic groups. Thus, retinoblastoma is extremely common in Central East Africa (Tanzania, Sudan) and certain parts of Arabia (Yemen), India, and Central America (JENSEN and MILLER 1987). Burkitt's lymphoma is diagnosed with much greater frequency in Central Africa, where it was first described, than in other parts of the world (BURKITT 1958). Similarly, Japanese children have a striking incidence of pineal tumors (KOIDE et al. 1980). In the United States, Ewing's tumor has long been recognized to be exceedingly rare in black children and leukemias are also less frequently diag-

nosed in black children, although prognostically more serious (MILLER 1989).

2.3 Environmental Factors

2.3.1 Radiation

A higher than expected incidence of leukemia has been noted following exposure of Japanese children to the Hiroshima and Nagasaki atomic bomb blasts (ICHIMARU et al. 1986; DARBY et al. 1985; BEEBE 1979). Although the findings are controversial, exposure of the fetus to prenatal (diagnostic) radiation has been correlated with a higher than expected incidence of many tumors; such a correlation was not, however, noted in exposed Japanese (BITHELL and STEWART 1975; MILLER 1979; JABLON and KATO 1970; MAC MAHON 1985).

Children exposed in the past to low doses of radiation for supposed enlarged tonsils, adenoids, and thymus glands have been noted to have an increase over the expected incidence of thyroid cancer, salivary gland tumors, and other neoplasms (DUFFY and FITZGERALD 1950; SHORE et al. 1985; HEMPELMANN et al. 1975). Children receiving low doses of radiation for ringworm of the scalp (tinea capitis) have also been noted to have an enhanced risk of schwannomas, meningiomas, and cortical gliomas (RON and MODAN 1984; MODAN et al. 1977).

Finally, children, especially those with genetic conditions such as retinoblastoma, are well known to have an increased risk of *second* malignancies. Following radiation treatment those that appear in the irradiation field apparently have a shorter latent period than do second tumors in other parts of the body (SAGERMAN et al. 1969; ABRAMSON et al. 1988).

However, despite abundant evidence attesting to the neoplastic potential of radiation, cosmic and background radiation is not felt to be a major causative factor in the vast majority of newly diagnosed childhood tumors.

2.3.2 Drug Exposure

In utero exposure to a variety of agents taken by the mother, including alcohol, steroid hormones, phenytoin, and diethylstilbestrol, has been recognized to increase the probability of certain malignancies, including neuroblastoma, clear cell carcinoma of the vagina, hepatoblastoma, and adrenal cancers (KINNEY et al. 1980; PENDERGRASS and HANSON 1976;

SHERMAN and ROIZEN 1976; HERBST et al. 1971; MELNICH et al. 1987; LI et al. 1975; SEELER et al. 1979; OTTEN et al. 1977). Interestingly, tumors noted to be more frequent in children with the fetal alcohol syndrome are those seen with increased frequency in children with hemihypertrophy (MILLER et al. 1964; FRAUMENI et al. 1968).

2.3.3 Ultraviolet Light

Although recognized to increase the incidence of skin tumors, including melanoma, squamous cell carcinoma, and basal cell tumors, sun exposure, except in high-risk individuals (albinism, xeroderma pigmentosum), rarely increases the incidence of these malignancies in the pediatric or young adult age group as the latent period is usually several decades. However, in populations where these predisposing factors are relatively common, a significant excess in incidence may occur (OKORO 1975; MILLER 1977).

2.4 Conditions Known to Predispose the Child to Development of a Malignancy

In the past two decades, the frequent association of certain childhood tumors with consistent chromosomal abnormalities has been recognized. Both loss (deletions) and gain (gene amplification) of genetic material as well as genetic rearrangements are now well recognized in many childhood tumors. In addition, the type and the location of the genetic abnormality are associated with a certain tumor or tumors. Chapter 4 will discuss this exciting area in depth; however, many childhood diseases, congenital anomalies, and syndromes which are known or presumed to have a genetic basis are also recognized to be associated with an increased frequency of childhood tumors.

2.4.1 Neurofibromatosis

Neurofibromatosis (NF), a relatively common inherited condition, is well recognized to predispose children and adults to development of both benign and malignant tumors. Perhaps the most interesting aspect of tumor predilection in children with NF is the variety of tumor types that are seen with increased frequency in affected children.

In the past decade, explosive growth in our knowledge of this fascinating condition has occurred. We now know that there are at least two specific conditions: NF1, characterized by café au lait maculae, neurofibroma(s), axillary or inguinal freckling, Lisch retinal nodules, bone dysplasia (e.g., sphenoid dysplasia), and tumor development including optic glioma, astrocytomas, leukemia, and Wilms' tumor, and NF2, characterized by bilateral (or rarely unilateral) acoustic neuromas, posterior subcapsular cataract formation, and development of other tumors including meningioma, schwannoma, and spinal cord ependymoma (MULVIHILL et al. 1990).

NF1 is regularly associated with an abnormality of the NF1 gene located on the 17th chromosome (17q11.2). This gene has been sequenced and a 360 amino acid sequence has been noted to be similar to a yeast product (IRA1) with homology to mammalian GAP (GTPase-activating protein) (MULVIHILL et al. 1990; LISTERNICK and CHARROW 1990).

In contrast, NF-2 has been localized to chromosome 22 (22q11.2). Sequencing studies are being pursued vigorously (MULVIHILL et al. 1990; LISTERNICK and CHARROW 1990). In addition to these "classic" forms of NF, various intermediate or atypical forms have also been described [e.g., the Proteus syndrome, thought to be the condition affecting John Merrick, "the Elephant Man," and a neurofibromatosis–Noonan's syndrome combination (NFNS)], and it is not known at this time whether these conditions involve different genetic abnormalities (LISTERNICK and CHARROW 1990).

In addition to malignant "degeneration" of long-standing neurofibromas into highly lethal neurofibrosarcomas (usually occurring after the pediatric age period has passed), children with NF are recognized to have an increased risk of rhabdomyosarcoma (MCKEEN et al. 1978), acute leukemia (usually lymphoblastic) (BADER and MILLER 1978), Wilms' tumor (STAY and VAWTER 1977), and neuroblastoma (WITZLEBEN and LINDY 1974; KNUDSON and AMROMIN 1966). Thus tumors of mesenchymal origin, in addition to neuroectodermally derived tumors, are enhanced in frequency.

2.4.2 Retinoblastoma

In addition to ocular tumors, children with retinoblastoma (RB) who have a known family history and/or bilateral disease have an enhanced frequency of many tumors both within and outside any field of irradiation (SAGERMAN et al. 1969; ABRAMSON et al. 1988). Osteosarcoma has been most frequently noted; however, melanoma, soft tissue sarcomas, and pineal tumors have also occurred in conjunction with RB (ROARTZ et al. 1988; TRABONLSI et al. 1988; DRAPER et al. 1986; BADER et al. 1982; JAKOBIEC et al. 1977). Great attention is currently being given to the significance of the absent RB tumor suppressor gene in the etiology of certain adult tumors, including adenocarcinoma of the colon and certain lung tumors. Approximately 5% of children with bilateral disease will, at some point, develop a highly malignant primitive neuroectodermal tumor of the pineal region first described by JAKOBIEC et al. (1977), which has been reported with increasing frequency and which has been uniformly fatal to date.

2.4.3 Beckwith-Wiedemann Syndrome

Beckwith-Wiedemann Syndrome is a rare childhood symptom complex (omphalocele, macroglossia, visceromegaly with hypoglycemia) that is recognized to be associated with childhood tumors. Approximately one in ten children with this condition have had a malignancy diagnosed, most frequently intra-abdominal in location. Thus, adrenal carcinoma, Wilms' tumor, neuroblastoma, and hepatoblastoma have all been described (SOTELO-AVILA and GOOCH 1976; MULVIHILL 1989).

2.4.4 Immunodeficiency Syndromes

Conditions such as Wiskott-Aldrich syndrome, severe combined immunodeficiency disease (SCID), Bruton's X-linked agammaglobulinemia, Duncan's X-linked lymphoproliferative syndrome, and, more recently, acquired immunodeficiency syndrome (AIDS) have all been associated with a markedly increased frequency of cancer, usually leukemias or lymphomas, and these cancers have been recognized to cause a number of deaths in these children (HOOVER 1977; MILLER 1989; MULVIHILL 1989; PURTILO et al. 1982; FRAUMENI and HOOVER 1977; KINLEN et al. 1979). Hopefully, the advent of bone marrow transplantation procedures will permit eradication of many of these underlying disorders and thus prevent many of these tumors.

2.4.5 Down's Syndrome (Trisomy 21)

Children with Down's syndrome have a number of neurologic, cardiac, and mesenchymal abnormalities as well as an increased risk of both acute lymphoblastic and acute nonlymphoblastic leukemia (MULVIHILL 1989; MULVIHILL and MADIGAN 1984; SANDBERG and TURC-CARE 1987).

2.4.6 Klinefelter's Syndrome (47,XXY) and Turner's Syndrome (45,SY or 45,XO)

Both Klinefelter's syndrome and Turner's syndrome are associated with gonadal and extragonadal germ cell tumors. An increased incidence of many other tumor types, including breast cancer and lymphoma/leukemias, has also been observed in the former condition (MULVIHILL 1989; SOGGE et al. 1979; MCCARTY et al. 1978).

2.4.7 Fanconi's Anemia, Bloom's Syndrome, and Ataxia Telangiectasia

Many children with these conditions will develop lymphoma or leukemias and, less frequently, other malignancies. Increased cellular radiation sensitivity is clinically relevant.

2.4.8 von Hippel-Lindau Disease

von Hippel-Lindau disease, an autosomal dominant condition, is associated with angiomas of the cerebellum or retina. Children and adults have developed renal, cerebellar (Hemangioblastoma), and adrenal malignancies.

2.4.9 Congenital Anomalies

Aniridia, hemihypertrophy, and a variety of genitourinary anomalies (hypospadias, fused ectopic kidneys, horseshoe kidney, etc.) have all been observed to be associated with an increased tumor risk in childhood. Aniridia with loss of a portion of the short arm of chromosome 11 is well known to predispose to Wilms' tumor. Children with hemihypertrophy have a significant excess risk of developing Wilms' tumor, adrenal tumors, and hepatoblastoma of the liver.

References

Abramson DH, Ellsworth RM, Kitchen FD, Tung G (1988) Second non-ocular tumors in retinoblastoma survivors. Are they radiation induced? Ophthalmology 91: 1351–1355

Bader JL, Miller RW (1978) Neurofibromatosis and childhood leukemia. J Pediatr 92: 925–929

Bader JL, Meadows AT, Zimmerman LE et al. (1982) Bilateral retinoblastoma with ectopic retinoblastoma: trilateral retinoblastoma. Cancer Genet Cytogenet 5: 203–213

Beebe GW (1979) Reflections on the work of the atomic bomb casualty commission in Japan. Epidemiol Rev 1: 184–210

Bithell JF, Stewart AM (1975) Pre–natal irradiation and childhood malignancy. A review of British data from the Ford survey. Br J Cancer 31: 271–287

Burkitt DP (1958) A sarcoma involving the jaws of African children. Br J Surg 46: 218–223

Darby SC, Nakashima E, Kato H (1985) A parallel analysis of cancer mortality among atomic bomb survivors and patients with ankylosing spondylitis given x-ray therapy. JNCI 75: 1–21

Draper, GJ, Sanders BM, Kingston JE (1986) Second primary neoplasms in patients with retinoblastoma. Br J Cancer 53: 661–671

Duffy BJ, Fitzgerald P (1950) Cancer of the thyroid in children: a report of 28 cases. J Clin Endocrinol Metab 10: 1296–1308

Fraumeni JF Jr, Hoover RN (1977) Immunosurveillance of cancer: epidemiologic observations. NCI Monogr 47: 121–126

Fraumeni JF Jr, Miller RW, Hill JA (1968) Primary carcinoma of the liver in childhood: an epidemiologic study. JNCI 40: 1087–1099

Hempelmann LH, Hall WJ, Phillips M et al. (1975) Neoplasms in persons treated with x-rays in infancy. Fourth survey in 20 years. JNCI 55: 519–530

Herbst AL, Ulfelder H, Poskanzer DC (1971) Adenocarcinoma of the vagina. N Engl J Med 284: 878–881

Hoover R (1977) Effects of drugs—immunosuppression. In: Hiatt HH, Watson JD, Weinstein JA (eds) Origins of human cancer. Cold Spring Harbor Laboratory, Cold Spring Harbor NY, pp 369–379

Ichimaru M, Ohkita T, Ishimaru T (1986) Leukemia, multiple myeloma and malignant lymphoma. Gann Monogr Cancer Res 32: 113–127

Innis MD (1972) Nephroblastoma. Possible index cancer of childhood. Med J Aust 1: 18–20

Jablon S, Kato H (1970) Childhood cancer in relation to prenatal exposure to atomic-bomb radiation. Lancet II: 1000–1003

Jakobiec FA, Ts'o MOM, Zimmerman LE, Davis P (1977) Retinoblastoma and intracranial malignancy. Cancer 39: 2048–2058

Jensen RD, Miller RW (1987) Retinoblastoma: epidemiologic characteristics. N Engl J Med 283: 307–311

Johnson FL, Feagler JR, Lerner KG et al. (1972) Association of androgenic–anabolic steroid therapy with development of hepatocellular carcinoma. Lancet II: 1273–1276

Kinlen U, Shiel AGR, Peto J, Doll R (1979) Collaborative United Kingdom–Australian study of cancer in patients treated with imunosuppressive drugs. Br Med J 2: 1461–1466

Kinney H, Faix R, Brazy J (1980) The fetal alcohol syndrome and neuroblastoma. Pediatrics 66: 130–132

Knudson AG Jr, Amromin GD (1966) Neuroblastoma and ganglioneuroma in a child with multiple neurofibromatosis—implications for the mutational origin of neuroblastoma. Cancer 19: 1032–1037

Koide O, Watanabe Y, Sato K (1980) A pathologic survey of intracranial germinoma and pinealoma in Japan. Cancer 45: 2119–2130

Li FP, Willard DR, Goodman R, Vawter G (1975) Malignant lymphoma after diphenyl hydantoin (Dilantin) therapy. Cancer 36: 1359–1362

Listernick R, Charrow J (1990) Neurofibromatosis type 1 in childhood. J Pediatr 116: 845–852

MacMahon B (1985) Prenatal x-ray exposure and twins. N Engl J Med 312: 576–577

Mauch P, Weinstein H, Botnick L, Belli J, Cassady JR (1983) An evaluation of long-term survival and complications in children with Hodgkin's disease. Cancer 51: 925–932

McCarty KS Jr, Barton TK, Peete CH Jr, Creasman WT (1978) Gonadal dysgenesis with adenocarcinoma of the endometrium. An electron microscopic and steroid receptor analysis with a review of the literature. Cancer 42: 512–520

McCaughan GW, Bilous MJ, Gallagher ND (1985) Long-term survival with tumor regression in androgen-induced liver tumors. Cancer 56: 2622–2626

McKeen EA, Bodurtha J, Meadows AT, Douglas EC, Mulvihill JJ (1978) Rhabdomyosarcoma complicating multiple neurofibromatosis. J Pediatr 93: 992–993

Meadows A, Baum E, Fossati-Bellani F et al. (1985) Second malignant neoplasms in children: an update from the late-effects study group. J Clin Oncol 3: 532–537

Melnich S, Cole P, Anderson D, et al. (1987) Rates and risks of diethylstilbestrol related clear-cell adenocarcinoma of the vagina and cervix. An update. N Engl J Med 316: 514–516

Miller RW (1977) Ethnic differences in cancer occurrence. Genetic and environmental influences with particular reference to neuroblastoma. In: Mulvihill JJ, Miller RW, Fraumeni JF Jr (eds) Genetics of human cancer. Raven, New York, pp 1–14

Miller RW (1979) Delayed radiation effects in atomic bomb survivors. Science 166: 569–574

Miller RW (1989) Frequency and environmental epidemiology of childhood cancer. In: Pizzo P, Poplack D (eds). Principles and practice of pediatric oncology. JB Lippincot, New York, pp 3–18

Miller RW, Myers MH (1983) Age distribution of epithelial cancers. Lancet II: 1250

Miller RW, Fraumeni JF Jr, Manning MD (1964) Association of Wilms' tumor with aniridia, hemihypertrophy and other congenital malformations. N Engl J Med 270: 922–927

Modan B, Ron E, Werner A (1977) Thyroid cancer following scalp irradiation. Radiology 123: 741–744

Mulvihill JJ (1980) Clinical observations of ecogenetics in human cancer. Ann Intern Med 92: 809–813

Mulvihill JJ (1982) Ecogenetic origins of cancer in the young. Environmental and genetic determinants. In: Levine As (ed) Cancer in the young. Masson, New York, pp 13–27

Mulvihill JJ (1989) Clinical genetics of pediatric cancer. In: Pizzo P, Poplack D (eds) Principles and practice of pediatric oncology. Lippincott, New York, pp 19–37

Mulvihill JJ, Madigan P (1984) Neoplasia of man (*Homo sapiens*). In: O'Brien SJ (ed) Genetics maps 1984. A compilation of linkage and restriction maps of genetically studied organisms, vol 3. Cold Spring Harbor Laboratory, Cold Spring Harbor, NY, pp 446–449

Mulvihill JJ, Parry DM, Sherman JL, Pikus A, Kaiser-Kupfer MI, Eldridge R (1990) Neurofibromatosis 1 (Reckling-hausen disease) and neurofibromatosis 2 (bilateral acoustic neurofibromatosis). Ann Intern Med 113: 40–52

Okoro AN (1975) Albinism in Nigeria. A clinical and social study. Br J Dermatol 92: 485–492

Otten J, Smets R, De Jager R, Gerard R, Maurus R (1977) Hepatoblastoma in an infant after contraceptive intake during pregnancy (letter). N Engl J Med 297: 222

Pendergrass TW, Hanson JW (1976) Fetal hydantoin syndrome and neuroblastoma (letter). Lancet II: 150

Purtilo DT, Sakamoto K, Barnabei V, et al. (1982) Epstein-Barr Virus-induced diseases in boys with the x-linked lymphoproliferative syndrome (XLP). Update on studies of the registry. Am J Med 73: 48–56

Riccardi VM, Sujansky E, Smith AC, Francke U (1978) Chromosomal imbalance in the aniridia–Wilms' tumor association. 11p interstitial deletion. Pediatrics 61: 604–610

Roartz JD, McLean I-W, Zimmerman LE (1988) Incidence of second neoplasms in patients with bilateral retinoblastoma. Ophthalmology 95: 1583–1587

Ron E, Modan B (1984) Thyroid and other neoplasms following childhood scalp irradiation. In: Boice JD Jr Fraumeni JF Jr (eds) Radiation carcinogenesis: epidemiology and biological significance. Raven, New York, pp 139–151

Sagerman RH, Cassady JR, Tretter P et al. (1969) Radiation induced neoplasia following external-beam therapy for children with retinoblastoma. AJR 105: 529–535

Sandberg AA, Turc-Carel C (1987) The cytogenetics of solid tumors. Relation to diagnosis, classification and pathology. Cancer 59: 387–395

Seeler RA, Israel JN, Royal JE, Kaye CL, Rao S, Abulaban M (1979) Ganglioneuroblastoma and fetal hydantoin-alcohol syndromes. Pediatrics 63: 524–527

Sherman S, Roizen N (1976) Fetal hydantoin syndrome and neuroblastoma (letter). Lancet II: 517

Shore RE, Woodward E, Hildreth N et al. (1985) Thyroid tumors following thymus irradiation. JNCI 74: 1177–1184

Sogge MR, McDonald SD, Cofold PB (1979) The malignant potential of the dysgenetic germ cell in Klinefelter's syndrome. Am J Med 66: 515–518

Sotelo-Avila C, Gooch WM III (1976) Neoplasms associated with the Beckwith-Wiedemann syndrome. Perspect Pediatr Pathol 3: 255–271

Stay EJ, Vawter G (1977) The relationship between nephroblastoma and neurofibromatosis (von Recklinghausen's disease). Cancer 39: 2550–2555

Trabonlsi EI, Zimmerman LE, Manz HJ (1988) Cutaneous malignant melanoma in survivors of heritable retinoblastoma. Arch Ophthalmol 106: 1057–1061

Witzleben CL, Lindy RA (1974) Disseminated neuroblastoma in a child with von Recklinghausen's disease. Cancer 34: 786–790

3 Acute and Chronic Normal Tissue Effects and Potential Modification in Pediatric Radiation Therapy

PATRICIA J. EIFEL

CONTENTS

3.1   Introduction   13
3.2   Skin.   14
3.3   Hematopoietic Tissues   15
3.3.1   Bone Marrow   15
3.3.2   Spleen   16
3.4   Musculoskeletal Tissues   16
3.4.1   Growing Bone.   16
3.4.2   Muscle and Soft Tissue.   22
3.5   Oral Cavity and Salivary Glands   22
3.6   Special Sensory Organs   23
3.6.1   The Eye   23
3.6.2   Olfactory Mucosa.   25
3.6.3   Taste Buds   26
3.6.4   The Ear   26
3.7   Cardiovascular System.   27
3.7.1   Heart.   27
3.7.2   Large Vessels   30
3.8   Lungs   31
3.8.1   Growth and Development   31
3.8.2   Radiation Pneumonitis.   31
3.8.3   Chronic Radiation Injury   31
3.8.4   Drug-Radiation Interactions   32
3.8.5   Pulmonary Toxicity After
        Bone Marrow Transplantation.   33
3.9   Gastrointestinal Tract   34
3.9.1   Esophagus   34
3.9.2   Liver   34
3.9.3   Small Bowel   35
3.10   Urinary Tract   36
3.10.1 Kidney.   36
3.10.2 Bladder   39
3.11   Reproductive Organs   39
3.11.1 Ovary.   39
3.11.2 Testis   40
3.12   Breast   42
3.13   Endocrine Effects   42
3.13.1 Thyroid   42
3.13.2 Parathyroid   44
3.13.3 Pituitary/Hypothalamus   44
        References   46

PATRICIA J. EIFEL, M.D., Associate Professor, Department of Clinical Radiotherapy, The University of Texas, MD Anderson Cancer Center, 1515 Holcombe Blvd., Houston, TX 77030, USA

3.1 Introduction

During the past three decades, changes in the overall approach to management of children with malignancy have had a dramatic impact on survival rates and, potentially, on the incidence and severity of major complications of treatment. In the early to mid 1960s, megavoltage radiotherapy equipment first became widely available. The more homogeneous dose distributions, sharper beam edges, and decreased bone absorption achieved with these machines promised a substantial improvement in the side-effects of radiotherapy. During the same period, the critical role of chemotherapy in the curative management of childhood malignancies was first appreciated. Over the years, chemotherapy regimens of increasing intensity have been used in an effort to control refractory malignancies. Today, almost all children with extracranial malignancy are treated with some form of chemotherapy. New drugs are being developed and employed every year. As the role of chemotherapy has evolved, the role of radiotherapy has changed as well. Radiotherapy has been eliminated from the treatment program of some children, and changes have occurred in the doses and volume of radiotherapy given to others. Because these dramatic changes in the quality of pediatric radiotherapy practice and in the use of chemotherapy have occurred simultaneously, it has been extremely difficult, sometimes impossible, to separate the effects of radiation and chemotherapy and to identify possible drug-radiation interactions.

Because treatment practices are continuing to evolve, we have incomplete information about the long-term complications of many of today's treatment approaches. We have, at most, 30–35 years of follow-up on children treated with any form of megavoltage radiotherapy and chemotherapy. This represents less than half the normal life expectancy of an American infant. Decades may be required to fully evaluate the toxic effects of new forms and combinations of treatment. Clearly, important questions about the long-term durability of organs that have been exposed to drugs, radiation, and serious illness during critical stages of development remain to be answered.

The damaging effects of radiation on developing musculoskeletal tissues are dominant clinical concerns and determine the most important differences between pediatric and adult radiotherapy. Infants and very young children are most vulnerable to these effects because of their greater capacity for growth. However, there is little empirical evidence to suggest that the visceral organs of children are inherently more susceptible to radiation damage than those of adults. Although our understanding of the relative radiosensitivity of rapidly dividing adult stem cell populations would suggest that rapidly developing, immature lung, kidney, and liver should be more vulnerable than mature tissues, the tolerance doses to radiation alone appear to be similar. It may be that developing tissues have a capacity for regeneration that compensates for any increased parenchymal response. However, the widespread use of radiosensitizing chemotherapeutic agents undoubtedly influences the radiation tolerance of normal tissues. Radiotherapy treatment plans must be designed with an understanding of the possible toxic interactions between drugs and radiation.

The following sections will summarize our current understanding of the acute and late effects of radiation in normal tissues with particular attention to the similarities and differences between pediatric and adult tolerances and to the important drug-radiation interactions that influence current pediatric radiotherapeutic practice.

3.2 Skin

Prior to the megavoltage era, skin was an important dose-limiting tissue in the radiotherapeutic management of malignancy. Kilovoltage radiotherapy units frequently delivered higher doses to the skin than to the target, and acute and late skin reactions were often severe. The poor skin quality of many children treated 25 or more years ago reflects the unfavorable therapeutic ratio achieved with these machines. The high-energy linear accelerators now used for most treatments produce photon beams that achieve maximum dose several millimeters or centimeters below the skin surface, providing considerable sparing of superficial tissues. Severe skin reactions are rarely observed with modern radiotherapy unless the skin is specifically being treated with a high dose

or, in some cases, when chemotherapy is being administered concurrently.

The severity of acute skin reactions depends upon the total dose and overall treatment time (TURESSON and NOTTER 1984a). The patient may not be aware of a subtle dryness of the skin that develops early in the course of treatment. This may be followed by progressive erythema in the distribution of the radiation field, which is accompanied by pruritis and a burning sensation. If the skin is treated with a high dose, moist desquamation of the skin may occur. The skin adnexa are also affected by a course of radiation. Epilation within the treatment field typically begins 2–3 weeks into a course of irradiation but also depends upon the beam energy and treatment technique. Sebaceous and sweat glands are affected by radiation, leaving the irradiated skin dry. Sometimes the irradiated skin has an increased tendency to develop furuncles. The hyperpigmentation that is often present in the radiation field gradually fades after treatment. Occasionally, dark-complected patients will develop areas of hypopigmentation. Telangiectasia may develop in the irradiated skin 1 or more years after treatment. TURESSON (1989) has documented the progressive nature of these changes. Skin ulceration is rarely seen as a late complication of radiation in patients treated with megavoltage equipment, but fibrosis of the subcutaneous tissues may occur in patients who have been treated with high total doses. The incidence and severity of late cutaneous reactions are also related to the fraction size and to the size of the irradiated area (TURESSON and NOTTER 1984b; SHYMKO et al. 1985). Increased skin reactions may be observed in skin folds where skin surfaces are located beneath the build-up region and in regions where the radiation beam strikes the skin surface tangentially. Failure to compensate adequately for sloping surfaces may also result in an increased dose to the skin in narrow portions of the neck and extremities, increasing the risk of acute and late radiation effects.

It is now well recognized that chemotherapeutic agents, particularly doxorubicin and actinomycin D, may augment the skin's reaction to radiation (CASSADY et al. 1975; D'ANGIO et al. 1959; DONALDSON et al. 1974; GRECO et al. 1976). Patients who are administered doxorubicin or actinomycin D during a course of radiation may develop sudden, severe skin reactions within the treatment field during the few days after chemotherapy administration. These reactions may be observed even when the drug is delivered early in the course of radiotherapy after relatively low doses of 20–30 Gy. When these drugs are delivered after a course of radiation, a "recall" of the radiation reaction may be observed within the previously treated field. These interactions probably contribute to late as well as acute skin reactions although the late effects of combined treatment are less well documented.

Skin damage can be minimized by careful attention to skin dose and possible drug-radiation interactions during treatment planning and by careful skin care following treatment. Patients should be discouraged from applying topical ointments immediately before treatment, as this may decrease skin sparing from a megavoltage beam by bolusing the skin surface. Ultraviolet light exacerbates skin damage and patients should be strongly encouraged to avoid sun exposure to the treated area during and after treatment. Young people may find this particularly difficult, and careful counseling may be required to achieve compliance.

3.3 Hematopoietic Tissues

3.3.1 Bone Marrow

Although proliferating bone marrow cells may be damaged by radiation doses of 0.5 Gy or less (FLIEDNER and NOTHDURFT 1986), mature granulocytes, platelets, and erythrocytes are relatively resistant, maintaining their functional integrity after doses of 50 Gy (BUTTON et al. 1981). Lymphocytes (with the exception of some subsets) are the most sensitive cells to irradiation. Unlike most cells, they may be killed immediately after small doses of irradiation, during nonmitotic phases of the cell cycle— so-called interphase death. For this reason, lymphocyte concentrations are the first to fall after a dose of ionizing irradiation; SCHREK (1961) reported a 75% decline in lymphocyte concentration 4 h after 1 Gy of total body irradiation. Because peripheral lymphocytes are so sensitive to radiation, measurable declines in the peripheral lymphocyte count may be observed after relatively small fields of irradiation. Changes in the peripheral blood concentrations of the other lineages depends primarily upon the volume of irradiated marrow, the life span of mature cells in the peripheral blood and tissues, and the transit time through compartments of proliferating and maturing hematopoietic cells (NOTHDURFT 1991). Granulocytes, which have a half-life of less than 24 h, begin to decline within 5–8 days. Platelets, which have a half-life of 9–10 days, usually begin to decline and reach their nadir shortly after the granulocytes.

The impact of radiation on erythrocyte concentrations may not be seen for several months because of their long half-life of about 120 days. Seeding of marrow by circulating progenitor cells is probably an important factor in bone marrow recovery after regional irradiation (FLIEDNER and NOTHDURFT 1986; NOTHDUREF 1991).

The distribution of active bone marrow changes as a function of age in humans (CRISTY, 1981). Compared with adults, young children have a larger proportion of their active bone marrow in the skull and extremities. These sites are relatively inactive in adults but may have increased marrow activity after extensive truncal irradiation.

Damage to bone marrow stroma also influences the rate of recovery. Most of the clinical data on bone marrow recovery after regional radiation therapy come from studies of patients treated for Hodgkin's disease and other lymphomas. The maximum depression of marrow activity after 40 Gy occurs about 6 months after irradiation (HILL et al. 1980), but hematopoietic activity may be depressed within the irradiated field for many years after regional irradiation. This is compensated by hyperactivity in unirradiated sites (PARMENTIER et al. 1983). Hematopoiesis may extend to extramedullary sites and to marrow that is usually dormant. Children may have prolonged hematopoiesis in the cranium and extremities after extensive truncal irradiation. Recovery of hematopoietic activity within the irradiated area is dependent upon volume of irradiated marrow—PARMENTIER et al. (1983) and SACKS et al. (1978) found more activity within the treated field of patients treated with total nodal irradiation than of patients treated with a mantle only. Regeneration within treatment fields is also influenced by the age of the patient and by the dose of irradiation (SACKS et al. 1978). The regenerative capacity of irradiated marrow may be particularly good in children. SACKS et al. (1978) reported full regeneration in 13 of 15 irradiated sites treated with doses as high as 40–50 Gy in five patients who were 17 years of age or less at the time of total nodal irradiation.

Although regional irradiation alone rarely causes clinically significant bone marrow toxicity, mild to moderate decreases in peripheral blood counts and in circulating granulocyte-monocyte precursor colony-forming units may occur, particularly when large volumes are irradiated (ABRAMS et al. 1985). The hematologic toxicity of concurrent regional irradiation and chemotherapy appears to be additive. The risk of significant radiation-induced hematologic toxicity is also increased in patients who have received previous chemotherapy (ABRAMS et al. 1985; PLOWMAN 1983).

Bone marrow toxicity is the dose-limiting acute effect of total body irradiation. Without bone marrow rescue, the $LD_{50/60}$ in humans has been estimated to be approximately 4.5 Gy, with the steep portion of the dose-effect curve between 3 and 6 Gy (NOTHDURFT 1991). Higher doses are required for complete bone marrow ablation, and even after single doses of 7.5–10 Gy combined with chemotherapy prior to allogeneic bone marrow transplantation, chimeric recovery has been observed in a minority of patients (PETZ et al. 1987). Bone marrow progenitor cells are relatively insensitive to fractionation. Fractionated and low-dose-rate schedules probably result in insignificant sparing of bone marrow toxicity (PETERS 1980; PETERS et al. 1979).

3.3.2 Spleen

In 1980, Dailey et al. reported a case of fulminant pneumococcal sepsis in a patient 12 years after she had received 40 Gy of splenic irradiation as part of the treatment for Hodgkin's disease. In a review of their autopsy experience, the authors found that the spleens of patients who had 40 Gy of splenic irradiation were atrophic compared with patients with the same disease who had not received splenic irradiation. They estimated the risk of significant splenic atrophy to be 30%–40% after 40 Gy. They also found clinical evidence of hyposplenism in three surviving patients who had received similar doses of splenic irradiation. Relatively high doses seem to be required for radiation-induced hyposplenism. In a review of 14 children treated with 17.5–35 Gy to the spleen for Wilms' tumor, Stevens et al. (1986) found no evidence of hyposplenism using a quantitative assessment of vacuolated ("pitted") red cells.

3.4 Musculoskeletal Tissues

3.4.1 Growing Bone

Growth arrest is undoubtedly the most important dose-limiting toxicity of radiation therapy in children. Rapidly proliferating populations of the epiphyseal plate are exquisitely sensitive to the effects of radiation. Fractionated doses as low as 10 Gy may have measurable effects on the growth of young children, and 30–40 Gy may cause dramatic growth-related sequelae.

The human skeleton develops initially as a preformed model of hyaline cartilage and, in the case of the skull and mandible, condensed mesenchyme. This framework is converted to osseous tissue from numerous ossification centers, which first appear in a predictable order and time during fetal and postnatal life. Some bones are ossified from a single ossification center (e.g., the bones of the wrist and ankle, nasal and zygomatic bones), while others are ossified from several separate foci. In these cases, a primary ossification center appears near the center of the future bone during the first half of fetal life. At varying times after birth, secondary ossification centers develop in the cartilagenous ends or *epiphyses* of the bone. As these secondary centers expands in the articular ends of the bone, a plate of growth cartilage is left between the epiphysis and diaphysis. This growth cartilage or epiphyseal plate is a complex, highly ordered structure composed of a number of specialized cell populations, several of which may be important targets for radiation damage. The cells of the growth plate are organized in columns surrounded by a complex matrix of collagen and proteoglycans.

The growth plate can be divided into zones extending from the secondary bony epiphysis to the metaphysis. The reserve or resting cell zone begins just below the secondary bony epiphysis and consists of scattered, roughly spherical cells that divide infrequently. Although they may serve a nutritional or storage function, the role of the reserve cells remains unclear. Below the reserve cell zone is the proliferative zone of rapidly dividing, flattened chondrocytes organized in columns that extend through the other zones of the growth plate to the metaphysis. In rodents, nearly 100% of the cells in the proliferative zone are dividing, with a cell cycle time that has been estimated at about 43 h (KEMBER 1971; WALKER and KEMBER 1972). Using serial radiographs from growing children and available histologic specimens, KEMBER and SISSONS (1976) have estimated the cell cycle time in the human distal femoral epiphysis to be longer—20–30 days at age 5–8 years (KEMBER and SISSONS 1976). Responding to an as yet undetermined signal, chondrocytes stop proliferating when they reach a certain distance from the top of the growth plate. As they progress down the cartilage columns, they expand progressively. As cells reach the base of the columns, calcium is released, and endothelial growth buds penetrate vascular orifices to occupy the space of the last hypertrophic cell. Growth rate is directly proportional to the rate of proliferation in the proliferative zone and the height of the last cell in the cartilage column (KEMBER 1978). Variations in all these parameters may contribute to differences in the growth rate of different bones, but the responsible control mechanisms are not well understood (KEMBER 1972). In humans, the growth rate is fastest during the first few years of life, then gradually slows, and accelerates again during the pubertal growth spurt, following which the growth plate fuses.

The rapidly dividing endothelial growth buds and the cells of the proliferative zone are both highly vulnerable to the effects of radiation. Although these populations may recover if the dose of irradiation is not excessive, the columns of the recovered growth plate tend to be less well defined (HINKEL 1943b). The epiphyseal vessels supply oxygen to the entire thickness (up to 1 mm) of the epiphyseal plate. Consequently, an oxygen gradient exists from epiphysis to metaphysis. TRUETA and AMATO (1960) demonstrated that disruption of the epiphyseal vessels caused necrosis of the growth plate, while disruption of the metaphyseal vasculature (supplying the endothelial growth buds) caused elongation of the chondrocyte columns and cessation of normal osteogenesis. In rodents, radiation has been shown to cause dose-related changes in the epiphyseal vessels (HINKEL 1943a), but the influence this may have on the epiphyseal growth rate is not understood.

The severity of treatment-related damage to growing bone is determined by a number of factors: the total radiation dose, fractionation, dose homogeneity, beam energy, and treatment volume, as well as the age of the patient, symmetry of the treatment volume, and nature of the irradiated growth centers.

It is difficult to estimate accurately the dose-effect relationship from the very heterogeneous retrospective clinical literature. However, taken together, the literature suggests that there is a fairly continuous dose-effect relationship between about 10 and 35–40 Gy which may be particularly steep between doses of approximately 15 and 25 Gy in standard fractions.

The fractionation sensitivity of growing bone in humans is not really known. Clinical impression suggests that the use of large fraction sizes is associated with particularly severe complications although other factors may have confounded these assessments. EIFEL et al. (1990) have determined the α/β ratio for growing bone in weanling rats to be approximately 4.5, suggesting an intermediate fractionation sensitivity. The rat is probably not an ideal model for estimating the fractionation sensitivity in humans because the acute response of the proliferative zone during the 1–2 weeks after radiation has

such a large impact on the short overall growth period of the animal. However, the rat data do suggest that the growth plate may be relatively sensitive to fractionation, and several multi- and single-institutional studies are currently investigating the use of hyperfractionated radiotherapy in children.

The clinical literature clearly indicates a strong inverse correlation between a child's age at the time of treatment and the severity of subsequent growth-related morbidity. However, animal studies have indicated that, if the growth remaining at the moment of irradiation is taken into account, there is no relationship between age and the radiation sensitivity of the growth plate (GONZALEZ and VAN DIJK 1983).

Before about 1965, many children who received radiation therapy were treated with kilovoltage units. For this reason, most of the studies that have reported long-term follow-up (past the age of puberty) of children who were treated in early childhood have included children who were treated with these low-energy units. Because much of the energy from these machines is absorbed through the photoelectric effect rather than Compton scatter, the dose absorbed in bone may be several times that in soft tissues. The degree to which this factor contributed to the incidence and character of morbidity is not well understood. The proliferative zone of the growth plate is not directly adjacent to calcified tissues and may not be seriously affected by the increased bone absorption. However, the intracellular calcium concentration of cells at the base of the cartilage column is high, and other critical populations such as the metaphyseal and epiphyseal vasculature that are adjacent to ossified or ossifying tissues may be affected. Of possibly greater importance are the dose inhomogeneities that may be present in treatment volumes irradiated with orthovoltage beams. Most studies have not carefully analyzed the dose distributions of such treatments to determine the maximum doses and fraction sizes that were actually delivered.

The influence of concurrent chemotherapy administration has rarely been addressed, but a recent observation by WALLACE and SHALET (1992) suggests that this may be an important contributory factor. They reported significantly less disproportion between sitting and standing heights in children treated for Wilms' tumor during the orthovoltage era (but without chemotherapy) than in those treated more recently with a combination of actinomycin D and megavoltage radiation (using similar doses and techniques). They hypothesized that this unexpected finding reflected sensitization of the growth plate to the damaging effects of radiation by actinomycin D. Further studies will be necessary to confirm this and to determine whether the dose and timing of drug administration could influence the severity of radiation-induced growth arrest.

3.4.1.1 Spine

Most of the clinical studies of radiation-induced growth arrest have focused on disorders of spinal growth after craniospinal irradiation, extended field irradiation for Hodgkin's disease and abdominal irradiation for Wilms' tumor. In their classic review of the effects of spinal irradiation in 45 children, NEUHAUSER et al. (1952) described radiologic changes in irradiated vertebral bodies that included growth arrest lines (sometimes producing an *os in os* or vertebra within a vertebra appearance), irregularity or scalloping of the epiphyseal cartilage plates, and gross abnormalities of the vertebral contour (flattening of the bodies and blunting and rounding off of the anterior margins of the vertebral surfaces). Vertebral abnormalities were not seen in any child who received less than 800 R (kilovoltage irradiation), even when the treatment was delivered in infancy. Growth arrest lines were seen in most children treated with 1000–2000 R and children who received more than 2000 R (most were treated at less than 2 years of age) had the most severe abnormalities. The authors observed only three cases of radiation-related scoliosis and stressed the importance of uniform irradiation of the vertebral body.

In 1975, PROBERT and PARKER reported the results of a longitudinal study of 44 children treated with megavoltage irradiation to the entire spine for medulloblastoma, lymphoblastic leukemia, or Hodgkin's disease. Twenty-nine children received more than 35 Gy to the spine (usually 44 Gy). Most of these children had a disproportion between sitting and standing height and eight had sitting heights more than 2 standard deviations below normal. Six of 15 children treated with less than 25 Gy also had a sitting height less than 2 standard deviations below normal. Children who were treated at less than 6 years of age or during the pubertal growth spurt appeared to have the greatest shortening. However, the follow-up period was short for some of these children, and those treated in the middle years may not have been followed long enough to register the dis-

proportionate growth that would be expected to occur during their pubertal growth spurt. Only four of these children had any scoliosis—all less than 10°. Again, this may have underestimated the risk because not all of the children were followed through puberty.

In a study of children treated with partial spinal irradiation for Wilms' tumor, WALLACE et al. (1990) emphasized the significant increase in disproportion that occurs during puberty. In a review of *adult* heights (24 years of age or more) of Hodgkin's disease patients treated with 35–40 Gy during childhood, WILIMAS et al. (1980) found that almost all those treated at less than 14 years of age had significant retardation of total height and crown-rump height. The boys appeared to be most severely affected; 50% had adult height of less than 5 1/2 feet tall. However, all of these children were treated with chemotherapy (cyclophosphamide, vincristine, and, in some cases, procarbazine and prednisone) as well as high-dose radiation. The influence of these drugs on the severity of radiation-induced growth arrest is unknown. In 1990, SILBER et al. presented a model that could be used to predict adult stature in children treated to portions of the spine and pelvis. Although such a model cannot correct for as yet unknown influences of chemotherapy and altered fractionation schemes, it may provide a rough guide for clinicians to predict the effect of truncal irradiation on adult stature.

The effects of flank irradiation in children with Wilms' tumor have been reviewed by a number of authors (EVANS et al. 1991; HEASTON et al. 1979; JAFFE et al. 1984; OLIVER et al. 1978; RATE et al. 1991; RISEBOROUGH et al. 1976; RUBIN et al. 1962; WALLACE et al. 1990; WHITEHOUSE and LAMPE 1953; WILLICH et al. 1990). Most of the children in these series were less than 6 years of age at treatment and most were treated prior to 1975, when high doses of radiation (30–45 Gy) were standardly used in treating Wilms' tumor. The use of orthovoltage irradiation has been blamed for the relatively severe deformities reported in the earlier series (RATE et al. 1991). Those treated after 1960 generally received actinomycin D-containing chemotherapy. Most were treated with eccentric flank fields, although the authors usually report an effort to include the entire width of the vertebral bodies. All of these series report radiologic changes similar to those described by NEUHAUSER et al. (1952). The reported incidence of scoliosis varies with the length of follow-up. In a series of 25 long-term survivors treated to the flank with 30 Gy or more of megavoltage radiation, HEASTON et al. (1979) found some degree of scoliosis in all of the 15 children followed past puberty although only five had a curvature of more than 5° and none more than 20°. Half of these children also had some degree of abnormal kyphosis. In their experience, scoliosis was usually not manifest until at least 5 years after treatment and was frequently accentuated during the pubertal growth spurt. In another series of children followed through puberty, RATE et al. (1991) did not observe any cases of severe scoliosis (> 20°) in children treated with megavoltage radiation. Inhomogeneous irradiation of the vertebral body undoubtedly increases the incidence and severity of scoliosis (RISEBOROUGH et al. 1976; WILLICH et al. 1990), and all authors stress the importance of using fields that include the vertebral body entirely within the high-dose region if any portion of the bone must be exposed. It has been speculated that soft tissue atrophy caused by asymmetric flank irradiation contributes to the incidence of scoliosis in Wilms' survivors. Of possibly greater significance is the frequent inclusion of the iliac crest apophysis in flank irradiation. Unilateral pelvic hypoplasia has been reported in many cases and probably contributes to asymmetric stresses on the spine. Most of the growth of the iliac wing is contributed from this growth center, which is particularly active during the pubertal period. An effort should always be made to exclude this growth plate if doing so will not compromise tumor control.

Children who have received spinal irradiation should be followed closely for evidence of secondary orthopedic problems, particularly during the pubertal period, when scoliosis is likely to make its first appearance. Tailored exercise programs may help to decrease symptoms. Surgical intervention may be necessary in rare cases of severe deformity (KING and STOWE 1982). Children with Wilms' tumor have been found to have a high incidence of spina bifida occulta, which may also contribute to back problems (HEASTON et al. 1979; WILLICH et al. 1990). During the past decade we have learned that high-dose flank irradiation is rarely required for control of Wilms' tumor. Fortunately, many children no longer require any irradiation. The doses of 10–20 Gy usually used for those who do should cause significantly less morbidity but will not obviate the need for close attention to dose homogeneity, field placement, and careful follow-up of irradiated children.

3.4.1.2 Thorax

Each of the ribs has a primary ossification center responsible for ossification of the shaft and one to three secondary centers for the head and tubercle. The primary center appears prior to birth and is located near the posterior angle of the rib anatomically and just lateral to the edge of the transverse process radiologically. Most of the reports of thoracic hypoplasia have been in children who have received whole lung irradiation (see Sect. 3.8.1). Some growth also occurs from the anterior pseudoepiphysis at the costochondral junction. Remodeling through appositional new bone formation also contributes to the shaping and possibly to the expansion of the rib cage with growth. The relative clinical importance of these factors is poorly described. Although the relationship between the width of spine and mantle fields and rib growth has not been studied in detail, presumably fields that include the primary ossification centers of the ribs will have a greater effect on subsequent rib growth.

Although early reports of mantle treatment with orthovoltage irradiation described severe sternal changes, including necrosis, this is not seen with the more homogeneous dose distributions delivered with megavoltage units (MORRIS et al. 1975). High-dose mantle irradiation in children causes a characteristic deformity of the chest, with shortened clavicles, decreased thoracic height, pectus excavatum, and a relative prominence of the lower ribs. Irradiation of primary ossification centers and pseudoepiphyseal centers in costal cartilages adjacent to the sternum may contribute to the latter. As with most forms of growth arrest, the degree of deformity is related to the total radiation dose and the child's age at the time of treatment.

3.4.1.3 Femoral Heads

The femoral heads are particularly vulnerable to the damaging effects of radiation and drugs. The reasons for this are not clear. However, the variable, relatively vulnerable blood supply of the femoral head and the high stresses to which it is exposed may contribute. In addition to growth arrest, which may cause coxa valga or coxa vara deformities (RUTHERFORD and DODD 1974), the femoral heads of irradiated children may undergo avascular necrosis or slippage of the femoral capital epiphysis.

Avascular necrosis of the femoral head is a well-documented complication of corticosteroid administration and has been reported by several authors to occur in patients treated with prednisone-containing chemotherapy for Hodgkin's disease or breast cancer (IHDE and DEVITA 1975; KOLIN and SHERRY 1987; ROSSLEIGH et al. 1986; SWEET et al. 1976). The nonsteroidal agents included in these regimens may play a contributory role, since the doses of corticosteroids are less than those usually reported to cause avascular necrosis in other settings. In adults, most of the patients reported to have radiation-related avascular necrosis have received either doses in excess of 50 Gy or concurrent corticosteroid-containing chemotherapy regimens. Consequently, the role of radiation in the etiology of this treatment complication remains unclear. There have been relatively few reports of radiation-related aseptic necrosis in children, and these have also been confounded by the concurrent use of chemotherapy (LIBSHITZ and EDEIKIN 1981; MASCARIN et al. 1991). However, LIBSHITZ and EDEIKEN (1981) reported two cases in children who received 30–40 Gy without chemotherapy.

Several authors have reported slipped femoral capital epiphyses in children irradiated to the hip (DICKERMAN et al. 1979; LIBSHITZ and EDEIKIN 1981; SILVERMAN et al. 1981; WOLF et al. 1977). SILVERMAN et al. (1981) reported eight abnormal epiphyseal plates in 5 of 50 children treated to 83 epiphyses. Of these cases, three involved severe abnormalities, four symptomatic slippage, and one asymptomatic slippage. Seven of 15 children (47%) treated with 25–55 Gy at less than 4 years of age had abnormalities compared with 1/21 (4.7%) treated at older ages. In Silverman's review of the literature, all of the reported cases occurred 1–9 years after radiation doses of 25 Gy or more, and most of the children were less than 4 years old at the time of treatment. Although epiphyseal slippage did not occur in any of the children who received less than 25 Gy, there was no apparent dose-effect relationship between 30 and 60 Gy. In unirradiated children, slipped femoral capital epiphysis is most common in overweight children and usually occurs during the rapid pubertal growth spurt, with a peak incidence at 12 years of age in girls and 13 years in boys (DICKERMAN et al. 1979). In contrast, the peak incidence in irradiated children occurs at age 9 to 10 years. Radiation damage to the vascular supply and to the rapidly proliferating cell populations of the growth plate probably causes structural weaknesses in the bone and matrix of the epiphysis that leave it particularly vulnerable to the increasing stresses of weightbearing as the child grows and as the femoral capital epiphysis assumes a more oblique position.

When children must be treated to this region, an effort should always be made to use techniques that minimize irradiation of the femoral head. If possible, doses of more than 25 Gy to the femoral head should be avoided in children less than 4 years of age. Children who have undergone femoral head irradiation should be followed with serial hip films through the age of puberty. Early correction of leg length discrepancies (with shoe lifts) in asymmetrically treated children will avoid unnecessary stresses on the treated epiphysis. The child's parents should be counseled to respond promptly to any symptom of pain. When a diagnosis of slipped femoral capital epiphysis is made, the child should be referred immediately to an experienced orthopedist for evaluation and possible intervention. COWELL (1966) demonstrated that children who were treated within 3 months of diagnosis had significantly better functional results than those treated after a longer delay.

3.4.1.4 Long Bones

High-dose irradiation of lower extremity growth plates prior to the completion of puberty will usually cause a discrepancy between the lengths of the treated and untreated legs. The amount of shortening is dictated by the amount of unexpressed growth in the treated epiphyses. In animals, the growth rate of the proximal and distal epiphyses differ, usually favoring the distal femoral and proximal tibial epiphyses. Whether this is also true in humans is unknown, but the largest leg length discrepancies reported in a series by GONZALEZ and BREUER (1983) were in children treated to both the distal femoral and proximal tibial epiphyses. In their review, four children treated with 22, 37, 43, and 64 Gy (kilovoltage radiation) to these two growth plates at 1 year of age or less had shortening of the leg by 9.0, 5.0, 11.5, and 12 cm, respectively, following 17, 13, 10, and 13 years of follow-up. Older children had much less discrepancy after similar treatment—a girl and boy aged 10 and 15 years at the time of treatment to these two epiphyses had 4.0- and 4.5-cm discrepancies. These discrepancies are probably close to the maximum that can occur after treatment at that age. Treatment-related morbidity should be substantially less if only one epiphysis is included. In a review of leg function in Ewing's sarcoma patients, JENTZSCH et al. (1981) reported minor functional limitations and a leg length discrepancy <1.5 cm in 11 of 22 children treated at less than 15 years of age. Moderate limitations with <2.5 cm discrepancy were noted in 7 of 22 children. Two patients who suffered posttreatment fractures had 2.5–3.8 cm discrepancies and a substantially decreased range of motion. One patient who had circumferential treatment above and below the knee required amputation.

As in most other sites, treatment plans that include only a portion of the epiphysis should be avoided, but care should always be taken to spare a strip of soft tissue for lymphatic drainage. Treatment fields should never divide the epiphysis as partial treatment can lead to severe curving deformities in addition to shortening (KATZMAN et al. 1969). Children should be followed closely for leg length discrepancies. When a significant discrepancy occurs, corrective shoe lifts will help to prevent secondary back problems. Early use of physical therapy may help to decrease limitations in range of motion. The irradiated bone should not be biopsied without strong indication, as this increases the risk of a fracture, which may heal poorly and increase morbidity.

3.4.1.5 Teeth

Children who are cured of cancer are at high risk of having chronic dental complications secondary to radiation or chemotherapy. In some cases, the influences of various treatments and of the illness itself have been difficult to differentiate.

Direct irradiation of the developing tooth buds causes abnormalities that are related to the site of irradiation, the age of the child (and therefore the stage of tooth development), and the dose of irradiation. Abnormalities may include tooth agenesis, delayed or arrested tooth development, premature closure of the apices, enamel dysplasias, and foreshortening, blunting, and abnormal curvature of the roots (JAFFE et al. 1984; SONIS et al. 1990; WEYMAN 1968). In addition, radiation effects on growth of the mandible and facial bones may contribute to malocclusion. Effects on salivary gland function may promote dental caries (see Sect. 3.5).

SONIS et al. (1990) have demonstrated a very steep dose-effect relationship between 18 Gy and 24 Gy (at 2 Gy/fraction). They studied late dental effects in 97 children with acute leukemia who received either chemotherapy alone or with 18 or 24 Gy to the brain for cranial prophylaxis. Their treatment fields routinely included the ramus of the mandible and posterior tooth buds. Children who received 24 Gy had much more severe dental sequelae within the treatment field than those treated with 18 Gy. Of those treated at less than 5 years of age with 24 Gy, 75% had microdontia, 25% had agenesis, and all had total root arrest. Of those treated with 18 Gy, 23% had microdontia, none had agenesis, and root development was present, though abnormal with V-shaped roots, blunted roots, and altered root numbers, in all children. In addition, 90% of the children treated with 24 Gy had cephalometric values indicating significant underdevelopment of the mandible. None of the children treated with 18 Gy and none of those treated after the age of 5 years had this finding.

High doses of radiation to the temporomandibular joint may cause trismus in addition to problems with malocclusion. As in adults, osteoradionecrosis of the mandible may be a late complication of high-dose radiation, particularly in patients with poor dental hygiene.

The effects of chemotherapy have not yet been fully defined, but many of the agents used to treat pediatric malignancies can cause abnormal tooth development (ROSENBERG 1990). Recent reports demonstrate that children who have received no radiation to the head and neck may develop chemotherapy-related abnormalities including tooth agenesis, microdontia, abnormal root development, and enamel dysplasias (MAGUIRE et al. 1987; ROSENBERG 1990; ROSENBERG et al. 1987; SONIS et al. 1990). The severity of chemotherapy-related damage is related to the age of the child and probably to the drugs and doses employed. MAGUIRE et al. (1987) found that treatment given during the first 3.5 years of life was most likely to affect crown development. Children treated after the age of 9 years were most likely to suffer altered root development. The premolar root structures are most commonly affected because of their later development. ROSENBERG et al. (1987) found evidence of abnormal premolar root length in 76% of leukemia patients treated at 4–10 years of age. These changes should not be erroneously attributed to scatter doses of irradiation from fields that did not include developing tooth buds.

All children should have a careful dental evaluation and treatment prior to the initiation of radiation therapy. Careful treatment planning and field-shaping should always be employed whenever such techniques can reduce the dose to developing teeth. However, doses of 24 Gy or more to the developing growth buds and mandible of small children can be expected to cause significant developmental disturbances. The dental development and hygiene of all children who have been treated with chemotherapy or radiation should be followed closely, preferably by a dentist who is experienced in the special problems of this population. Recommendations for the long-term evaluation of treated patients are evolving. A review of the extensive literature on this topic is beyond the scope of this work, but the subject has been summarized by ROSENBERG (1990).

3.4.2 Muscle and Soft Tissue

Children who have received radiation therapy, particularly at high doses, may have impaired development of muscle and soft tissue within the radiation field. Hypodevelopment of neck musculature has been noted following orthovoltage or megavoltage irradiation to the neck for Hodgkin's disease (DAWSON 1968; MAUCH et al. 1983); children treated to the face may have hypoplastic development of soft tissue as well as bone (GUYURON et al. 1983); young children treated for Wilms' tumor frequently have atrophy of the flank musculature, which may contribute to the development of scoliosis (EVANS et al. 1991; OLIVER et al. 1978; RUBIN et al. 1962); and children treated to the extremities may have muscle-atrophy with decreased extremity circumference (DAWSON 1968; JENTZSCH et al. 1981). There have as yet been no systematic studies relating dose, fractionation, and age at treatment with muscle atrophy and function. In an early review, DAWSON (1968) pointed out that patients with marked soft tissue atrophy in irradiated extremities often had surprisingly good strength and function. The histologic appearance of these underdeveloped muscles is not well described, and the mechanism of injury is poorly understood. However, in a recent study of magnetic resonance imaging studies in irradiated children, FLETCHER et al. (1990) found evidence of muscle atrophy as early as 6 weeks after completion of high-dose (60–65 Gy, 1.1–1.2 Gy per fraction) radiation and enhanced reticular densities in the subcutaneous fat as early as 15 weeks after radiation. In most cases, gadolinium-DTPA enhanced T_1-weighted and T_2-weight images revealed increased signal intensity of uninvolved tissues within the radiation field. These changes in signal intensity, which are also observed in irradiated adult tissue, should not be confused with tumor recurrence (FLETCHER et al. 1990).

3.5 Oral Cavity and Salivary Glands

The oral mucous membranes are covered by a nonkeratinizing, stratified squamous epithelium with a high rate of cell renewal. Sloughing senescent cells are replaced from rapidly proliferating stem cells in the basal layer of the epithelium. Radiation causes rapid depletion of this stem cell population, and radiation mucositis results when cells shed from the superficial epithelial layers are no longer being replaced at a sufficient rate—usually 2–3 weeks after the start of treatment. The severity of the mucosal reaction is related to the relative protraction or acceleration of treatment (FLETCHER et al. 1962; PERRACHIA and SALTI 1981). For this reason, radiation mucositis is usually the limiting factor in the rate of accelerated fractionation schedules in the treatment of head and neck tumors.

There is no evidence that the mucosal sensitivity of children is any different than that of adults. However, when chemotherapy is given concurrently or sequentially with radiation, mucosal reactions may be more severe. Bleomycin, hydroxyurea, and methotrexate may increase the severity of mucosal reactions during radiation (KNOWLTON et al. 1975; STEFANI et al. 1971; VERMUND et al. 1985). Actinomycin D and doxorubicin can increase mucosal reactions when given concurrently with radiation and can induce a radiation-recall phenomenon when given after a course of head and neck irradiation (D'ANGIO et al. 1959; DONALDSON et al. 1974).

The three major salivary glands, the parotid, submandibular, and sublingual, are connected to the oral cavity by ducts and are responsible for producing most of the saliva that lubricates the oral cavity. The parotid gland is composed of serous acini, while the others are mixed serous and mucin-producing glands. In addition, numerous small, primarily mucin-secreting minor salivary glands are scattered thoughout the upper aerodigestive tract. The serous acini of the salivary glands are exquisitely sensitive to the effects of radiation. Decreased salivation may occur within hours of the first radiation treatment. Occasionally, during the first few days of treatment, patients will develop acute symptoms of pain and swelling that subside after several days. Xerostomia may contribute to hypogeusia and decreased appetite. The severity of chronic xerostomia is related to the dose of radiation, the volume of irradiated salivary gland tissue, and the initial salivary flow rate of the individual. Young patients and males appear to have greater salivary flow rates and seem to have somewhat less severe xerostomia (ENEROTH et al. 1971; MIRA et al. 1981). Radiation has a proportionately greater effect on serous- than on mucous-producing acini, causing the remaining saliva to have a decreased water content, increased viscosity, and decreased pH (DREIZEN et al. 1976; SHANNON et al. 1978). Radiation of the parotid also causes a decrease in the secretory immunoglobulin content of saliva (MARKS et al. 1981). These changes in the amount and character of saliva encourage carious tooth decay, a problem that may be particularly severe in irradiated children whose tooth enamel may be defective because of direct effects of radiation on the developing teeth (see Sect. 3.4.1.5). These children require close dental follow-up and topical fluoride application for life to minimize the risk of severe tooth decay.

3.6 Special Sensory Organs

Decreased visual and auditory acuity can have a devastating effect upon the growth and development of children, particularly if the problem is not recognized immediately. Decreased taste and olfactory acuity can affect appetite and ultimately result in poor eating, suboptimal nutrition, and decreased tolerance to treatment. The radiation tolerance of these organs should be respected and children followed closely for any evidence of compromise following treatment.

3.6.1 The Eye

3.6.1.1 Lens

A radiation cataract may first be detected on ophthalmologic examination when a small opacified dot forms as cellular debris and abnormal lens fibers migrate from the germinal zone at the equator of the lens to the posterior pole. The opacity gradually increases in size and satellite granules or vacuoles appear around the central opacity; as the main opacity enlarges to 3–4 mm, a central lucency may appear. If this progresses, opacities may appear in the anterior subcapsular region and after relatively high doses, degeneration of lens fibers formed prior to irradiation may cause a diffuse cloudiness of the lens (FAJARDO 1982; RUBIN and CASARETT 1968).

The incidence, severity, and time to development of cataracts all depend upon both total radiation dose and fractionation. Children have more rapidly developing lenses and may be more susceptible to the effects of radiation than adults although this has not been clearly established. The latency period for cataract formation ranges from 6 months to many years, with an average of 2–3 years (RUBIN and CASARETT 1968). Estimates of the threshold dose for radiation cataract formation vary widely, probably because of varying methods of dose estimation and specification. In a classic paper published in 1957, MERRIAM and FOCHT estimated the lens doses of 173 patients using phantom reconstructions of the patients' clinical set-ups and described a minimum cataractogenic dose of 2 Gy in a single fraction and 4 Gy in fractionated doses over 3–12 weeks. All patients believed to have received more than 11.5 Gy developed cataracts. These measurements, based upon data collected using large ionization chambers, probably represent an underestimate of the threshold dose for cataractogenesis. In a series of patients treated with radon seed implants for eyelid tumors, BRITTEN et al. (1966) did not observe any cataracts in lenses that were thought to have received a dose less than 2000 R. In a more recent study of children treated with fractionated irradiation for retinoblastoma, the minimum cataractogenic dose was described as 8 Gy (SCHIPPER et al. 1985). In a review of 277 patients treated with total body irradiation as preparation for bone marrow transplantation, DEEG et al. (1984) clearly demonstrated the importance of fractionation in the development of cataracts. In their study the Kaplan-Meier product limit estimate of the probability of cataract formation was 80% after a single dose of 10 Gy (4–8 cGy/min) compared with 18% after fractionated total body irradiation for a total dose of 12–15.75 Gy at 2–2.25 Gy/fraction. Nineteen percent of patients treated with chemotherapy alone developed cataracts. Prolonged exogenous corticosteroid exposure (associated with the presence of chronic graft versus host disease) was also an important risk factor in cataract formation.

Small variations in treatment technique can dramatically influence the dose to the lens (HARNETT et al. 1987; KLINE et al. 1979). Whenever possible, lateral fields should be angled posteriorly to avoid unwanted dose to the contralateral eye from a divergent beam. Linear accelerators are preferred over cobalt-60 for treatment near the eyes because of their smaller penumbras. When cataracts do develop, vision can frequently be restored by surgical removal of the damaged lens. Removal of radiation cataracts is complicated somewhat by the need to remove the posterior capsule, which tends to opacify if left in situ. However, recent advances in microsurgical techniques have improved the results of lens extraction in children who have been irradiated to the eye for retinoblastoma and other malignancies (BROOKS et al. 1990).

3.6.1.2 Lacrimal Apparatus

The tear film consists of three layers: a superficial lipid layer produced by the meibomian glands located in the upper and lower lids, an aqueous layer produced by the major and accessory lacrimal glands, and a deep mucinous layer produced by conjunctival goblet cells (PARSONS et al. 1983). Basal tear secretions are thought to be produced primarily by the relatively small accessory lacrimal glands located in the conjunctival fornices and at the superior margin of the upper lid, whereas reflex tear secretion is thought to arise primarily from the main lacrimal gland located beneath the frontal bone superolateral to the outer canthus (JONES 1966). Deficiency of any of the components of the tear film may lead to a dry eye, with subsequent corneal and conjunctival damage. Although doses of 50–60 Gy are known to cause lacrimal gland atrophy (MERRIAM et al. 1972), very little is known about the radiosensitivity of the meibomian glands and the conjunctival goblet cells. Patients who develop severe dry eye syndrome complain of pain and photophobia during or shortly after treatment and then proceed over one or more years to lose vision because of progressive corneal ulceration, opacification, and vascularization. PARSONS et al. (1983) reported severe injury in all eyes that received ≥57 Gy and two slowly progressive injuries in nine eyes that received 32–45 Gy to the entire lacrimal tissue.

Doses of 50–60 Gy may cause obliteration of the puncta and canaliculi of the lacrimal ducts and, less frequently, obstruction of the nasolacrimal duct, causing increased tearing. In a review of 50 children treated for orbital rhabdomyosarcomas with tumor doses of 50–60 Gy in the Intergroup Rhabdomyosarcoma Study seven had stenosis of the nasolacrimal duct. Radiation doses to the duct were not estimated (HEYN et al. 1986). Although excess tearing may be annoying, treatment of lacrimal duct obstruction is usually not necessary. However, surgical correction is sometimes successful.

The risk of severe injury can be minimized by shielding at least a portion of the upper lateral lid and the major lacrimal gland. Lateral fields will exclude much of the major lacrimal gland and the accessory glands if the field border is at or behind the lateral bony canthus. Placement of the anterior field border at the fleshy canthus will usually result in inclusion of at least one-half of the major gland in the primary beam and will increase the contribution to the accessory glands from the lateral fields. Consequently, when the eye is to be treated with a high dose using a wedged-pair technique, care must be taken to ensure exclusion of the lacrimal gland from at least one field. Useful vision can rarely be preserved if the entire eye and lacrimal apparatus have received more than 50 Gy. Patients who have received a significant dose to the eye must be followed closely by an ophthalmologist and should be treated early and aggressively for any evidence of corneal injury. Use of sterile ophthalmic lubricating ointment at night and artificial tears may control mild to moderate symptoms and prevent secondary infection (PARSONS et al. 1983). A painful blind eye usually requires enucleation.

3.6.1.3 Cornea

Corneal complications probably reflect secondary effects of damage to the lacrimal apparatus more often than direct damage to the corneal epithelium. In their detailed review of eye complications from radiation, PARSONS et al. (1983) reported that no patients lost vision as a result of corneal injury if the major lacrimal gland was shielded from high-dose radiation. Whatever the etiology, keratitis must be treated aggressively as described above. Whenever possible, anterior megavoltage fields should be treated with the eyelids open to reduce the corneal dose.

3.6.1.4 Retina

Radiation retinopathy occurs as a relatively late ocular complications; initial symptoms rarely appear earlier than 1–3 years after treatment. Signs and symptoms are similar to those of diabetic retinopathy: capillary microaneurysms, cotton-wool spots, retinal hemorrhages, and hard exudates. Progressive microvascular occlusion leads to retinal ischemia and edema. Neovascularization may lead to vitreous hemorrhage, retinal detachment, rubeosis iridis, and angle closure glaucoma (ALBERTI 1991; PARSONS et al. 1983). The relatively avascular region of the macula may be particularly sensitive to the effects of radiation (SHUKOVSKY and FLETCHER 1972). In PARSONS et al.'s review, 10 of 13 patients with radiation retinopathy developed glaucoma which necessitated enucleation in most cases.

Radiation retinopathy appears to be rare after doses less than or equal to 50 Gy in 25 fractions (PARSONS et al. 1983), although WARA et al. (1979) reported four cases in adults treated with 45–50 Gy at 1.8–2.0 Gy/fraction. In PARSONS et al.'s review, all patients who received at least 60 Gy had severe damage. Their experience did not provide clear information about the dose-response relationship between 50 and 55 Gy because three of the four patients treated within this range (the three with retinal complications) either had received combined chemotherapy and radiation (one patient) or were treated with large doses per fraction (two patients). Fraction size appears to be an important factor in the development of radiation injury (ARISTIZABAL et al. 1977; HARRIS and LEVENE 1976; PARSONS et al. 1983). Most authors now recommend a daily fraction size of no more than 2 Gy. It has been suggested that chemotherapy may increase the risk and decrease the latency period of radiation retinopathy (BROWN et al. 1982; CHAN and SHUKOVSKY 1976). Concurrent medical conditions such as hypertension and diabetes mellitus may, when present, contribute to the development of retinal pathology.

There is no evidence that children are more susceptible to retinal damage than adults. In the review of the Intergroup Rhabdomyosarcoma Study experience, only 3 of 50 children followed for more than 3 years after treatment with 50–60 Gy (at 2 Gy/fraction) and concurrent chemotherapy developed retinal complications (HEYN et al. 1986). SCHIPPER et al. (1985) observed retinal vascular injury in 3 of 54 children treated with 45 Gy at 3 Gy/fraction for retinoblastoma. EGBERT et al. (1978) reported only one case of retinopathy in 28 children treated with 35–60 Gy (50–60 Gy in most cases) at 2 Gy/fraction for retinoblastoma. Retinal and optic nerve complications are extremely rare after low dose (18–24 Gy) whole brain irradiation for cranial prophylaxis (WEAVER et al. 1986). However, MARGILETH et al. (1977) reported two cases of apparently treatment-related blindness that developed approximately 8 months after 24 Gy of central nervous system irradiation combined with aggressive chemotherapy and intrathecal cytosine arabinoside.

Central retinal artery occlusion with sudden onset of blindness has been reported as a rare complication occurring very late (15–20 years) after radiation treatment of children for retinoblastoma (EGBERT et al. 1978; GAGNON et al. 1980). EGBERT et al. (1978) reported that one patient who had received more than 90 Gy in two courses of treatment for retinoblastoma had useful vision in both eyes for 19 years before developing sudden retinal artery occlusion.

3.6.1.5 Optic Nerve

Optic nerve injury usually presents as sudden painless loss of vision in one or both eyes. PARSONS et al. (1983) described two forms of optic nerve injury caused by irradiation. Anterior ischemic optic neuropathy was characterized by edema and pallor of the optic disc and splinter hemorrhages on or adjacent to the disc and generally occurred 2–4 years after treatment. In contrast, patients with retrobulbar optic neuropathy had no evidence of disc edema or hemorrhage but experienced sudden loss of vision 1–9 years after radiation. KLINE et al. (1985) restricted their definition of radiation-induced optic neuropathy to the second group of patients, who in their experience had a sudden loss of vision in one or both eyes within 3 years of treatment. The mechanism of injury is thought to be ischemia secondary to late vascular occlusion.

The incidence of optic nerve injury appears to be strongly correlated with radiation fraction size. In PARSONS et al.'s review, only 2 of 24 (8%) patients who had received 60–73 Gy at 1.65–1.9 Gy/fraction had evidence of optic nerve injury, compared with 7 of 17 (41%) patients treated with daily fractions of at least 1.95 Gy. RODEN et al. (1990) described 13 cases of optic neuropathy with sudden loss of vision 9–35 months after treatment with 45–72 Gy at 1.8–2.0 Gy/fraction. Despite aggressive management with steroids and hyperbaric oxygen, no patient experienced an improvement in vision. All of the patients who developed neuropathy after doses ≤ 50 Gy had been treated for pituitary adenomas. PARSONS et al. (1983) suggested that optic nerve compromise due to compression by tumor in such patients may have increased the risk of radiation injury.

When the optic nerve must be treated to doses above 45 Gy, the dose per fraction should not exceed 1.8–1.9 Gy. As much of the length of the nerve and optic chiasm as possible should be shielded from receiving more than 50 Gy. Although there are relatively few data about the affect of chemotherapy on radiation tolerance, it has been suggested that chemotherapeutic agents, particularly the nitrosoureas, may increase the risk of radiation optic neuropathy (WILSON et al. 1987). Special care should be taken in patients who are receiving aggressive combined modality regimens.

3.6.2 Olfactory Mucosa

The olfactory region of the nasal mucous membrane extends over the superior concha and the lateral walls above it and over the upper few millimeters of the nasal septum. The olfactory apparatus is fully functional before birth, but the thickness and surface area of the olfactory epithelium probably expand during the postnatal period through recruitment of blastemal cells located at the base of the olfactory epithelium. Although the olfactory receptor cells are primary sensory neurons, they are unique in their rapid rate of turnover with new receptor cells differentiating from the immature blastemal cells.

Radiation treatment of the olfactory mucosa results in a prompt decline in smell acuity. In a study of 12 patients treated either with 45 Gy for pituitary adenomas or to 65 Gy for nasopharyngeal carcinomas, OPHIR et al. (1988) found dramatically increased thresholds for detection of two odorants in all patients. Smell acuity improved continuously in all patients between 1 and 6 months after treatment but had not returned to normal in any patient by 6 months posttreatment (the last follow-up time in the study). Loss of smell acuity is rarely voiced as a specific complaint but it can contribute to loss of appetite and associated nutritional problems. The influence of patient age on the severity or duration of this effect of radiation has not been studied.

Some patients who receive radiation therapy to the olfactory mucosa experience a pungent, unpleasant odor during treatment that is thought to be caused by the radiochemical formation of ozone and free radicals in the mucus overlying the olfactory mucosa (SAGAR et al. 1991).

3.6.3 Taste Buds

Taste is mediated through taste buds consisting of a rapidly renewing cell population (with an average life span of 10–10.50 days) supplied from surrounding epithelial cells. Antimitotic agents, including radiation and drug therapy or poor nutrition, can influence taste by interrupting the renewal process. Taste buds are located throughout much of the upper aerodigestive tract but are most concentrated on the tongue. The concentration of buds on the lips and cheeks is greatest in the newborn (SCHIFFMAN 1983).

A profound decline in taste acuity occurs 3–6 weeks after the beginning of a course of radiation therapy to the oral cavity. Salt and bitter taste detection and thresholds are impaired earliest (at about 3 weeks) and most severely while the detection of sweets declines in the fifth or sixth week of irradiation (MOSSMAN and HENKIN 1978; MOSSMAN et al. 1982). Because the taste buds responsible for the detection of various taste qualities are clustered (sweet in the anterior tongue, sour in the mid tongue, and bitter in the posterior tongue), the character of dysgeusia may

vary according to the region irradiated (CONGER 1973). Reduced input from the taste buds tends to increase awareness of foods that stimulate free trigeminal nerve endings in the oral cavity, causing spicy foods and carbonated beverages to be irritating or even painful (SCHIFFMAN 1983). Xerostomia caused by concomitant irradiation to the salivary glands contributes to radiation-induced impairment. However, most patients experience a near complete recovery of taste acuity 2–4 months after completion of radiation despite continued, often profound impairment of salivary function (CONGER 1973; MOSSMAN and HENKIN 1978). Postradiation chemotherapy may prolong taste impairment. Uncontrolled studies suggest that zinc administration may reduce taste impairment in some patients (HENKIN 1972).

3.6.4 The Ear

The auditory apparatus itself appears to be relatively resistant to radiation (DIAS 1966). Osteonecrosis of the ossicles is extremely rare, even after very high therapeutic doses of radiotherapy to the normal ear. Examinations of the irradiated inner ear have not demonstrated any histologic changes after high doses of irradiation (NOVOTNY 1951). However, in a prospective study of 22 patients treated for nasopharyngeal carcinoma, GRAU et al. (1991) reported a significant relationship between radiation dose to the inner ear and subsequent evidence of high-frequency hearing loss. The latent period for this late sensorineural hearing loss was 12 months or more. The hearing disturbances that may occur in patients during and immediately after radiotherapy are chiefly related to a serous otitis media resulting from edema and blockage of the eustachian tube. Hearing tests usually reveal a mixed perceptive and conductive loss. In a study of adults with cancers of the head and neck, BRILL et al. (1974) reported only one case of serous otitis media in 27 patients (4%) treated with high-dose radiotherapy without surgery. In contrast, 13% of 101 patients who had had surgery in addition to radiotherapy developed symptoms. Presumably the surgery contributed to disruption of the normal lymphatic drainage of tissues surrounding the eustachian tube. Tumor infiltration in the region of the nasopharynx may also be a contributing factor in some cases. If the symptoms persist, decompression may be necessary with myringotomy tubes. The relatively low doses used for cranial prophylaxis in the treatment of leukemia are rarely associated with any auditory disturbance. THIBADOUX et al. (1980) found no evidence of hearing loss in 61 children tested 6–36 months after 24 Gy in 14–15 fractions.

Hearing loss is a well-described complication of cisplatin administration. The effect is related to the dose and schedule of administration and appears to be much more frequent in children than in adults. BROCK et al. (1991) and SCHELL et al. (1989) both found an inverse correlation between patient age and the severity of cisplatin ototoxicity. BROCK et al. reported moderate to severe high frequency hearing loss in 14 of 29 young children (median age 26 months) treated with standard doses of cisplatin. One-third of the children required hearing aids. Radiation does not appear to cause additional hearing loss in children who have received prior cisplatin (KRETSCHMAR et al. 1990), but several studies have suggested that cisplatin ototoxicity is enhanced in patients who are receiving concurrent radiation or who have received prior radiotherapy to a field encompassing the ears (KHAN et al. 1982; SCHELL et al. 1989; SEXAUER et al. 1985; WALKER et al. 1989). In patients who had received prior cranial irradiation, SCHELL et al. reported a high probability of significant hearing loss following cumulative doses of cisplatin as low as 270 mg/m^2—a dose that was associated with negligible risk in unirradiated patients. However, the authors also found an increased risk of cisplatin ototoxicity in *unirradiated* patients with central nervous system tumors. The apparent susceptibility of such patients may have influenced the results, since most of the patients who had been irradiated also had central nervous system neoplasms.

3.7 Cardiovascular System

3.7.1 Heart

Although therapeutic doses of radiation can damage the pericardium, myocardium, coronary arteries, cardiac valves, and conduction pathways, clinically evident injury to the heart is a relatively rare complication of modern radiation therapy.

3.7.1.1 Pericardium

During the 1970s and early 1980s, the literature tended to emphasize the pericardial effects of treatment, which, when present, cause specific symptoms readily attributable to radiation. Although, rarely, acute

pericarditis may present during treatment in patients with extensive pericardiac disease, most cases are somewhat delayed in onset (FAJARDO 1982). Pericardial effusion may be discovered incidentally and resolve spontaneously. In some cases, fluid may accumulate rapidly, causing tamponade. After large doses of radiation, pericardial fibrosis can cause constrictive heart disease necessitating pericardiectomy. Estimates of the latency period vary with the endpoint studied. Most effusions develop within the first year after treatment, but occasionally the onset of symptoms occurs several years after irradiation (BYHARDT et al. 1975; FAJARDO 1982; MILL et al. 1984).

Most of the published studies concern patients treated for Hodgkin's disease. Nearly all of the reported cases of symptomatic pericarditis have occurred in patients treated with techniques that delivered doses of more than 40 Gy to part or all of the pericardium, often with large daily fractions, one field treated per day and usually with large volumes of the heart treated at the full tumor dose. The experience at the National Cancer Institute (NCI) has been reported in numerous publications and is frequently cited in the literature (APPLEFIELD et al. 1981; BROSIUS III et al. 1981; BYHARDT et al. 1975; GOTTDIENER et al. 1983). These authors reported a high incidence of acute and chronic pericarditis with severe symptomatology experienced by some patients. However, the patients in these reviews were treated with fields that were heavily weighted to the anterior (in many cases with an anterior field only) without subcarinal shielding. Many of the patients were treated with cobalt-60, van der Graaf units, or 4 MV accelerators, which resulted in large dose gradients across the treated volume. In the NCI review reported in 1975 by BYHARDT et al., the mean anterior pericardial dose in treated patients was 53.3 Gy, with a prescribed dose to midplane of 40 Gy. With anteriorly weighted techniques, the high dose absorbed by the anterior pericardium is also delivered in relatively large doses per fraction (a mean of 2.67 Gy/fraction in the Byhardt series), further increasing the risk of late tissue injury. MILL et al. (1984) found a strong correlation between the dose to the anterior pericardium and the incidence of pericarditis. In 193 patients treated to mantle fields with various anterior-to-posterior weightings, there were no cases of pericarditis if the dose to the anterior pericardium (5 cm from the anterior skin surface) was less than 40 Gy, but the incidence was 3.4% if patients received 40–44.9 Gy, 8.6% if they received 45–49.9 Gy, and 31% if they received more than 50 Gy to the anterior pericardium. COSSET et al. (1991) also found an increased incidence of pericarditis in patients who received more than 41 Gy to the heart and in those who were treated with daily fractions of 3 Gy or more. In a review of clinical and laboratory experience, STEWART and FAJARDO (1971) concluded that pericardial toxicity was related to dose, fractionation, and volume treated. Rapid withdrawal of steroids in previously irradiated patients has been reported to precipitate symptoms of latent radiation injury to the pericardium (CASTELLINO et al. 1974).

With equally weighted treatment fields and modifications in the volume of pericardium treated and in the dose of radiation delivered to the heart, radiation pericarditis is now rarely seen after treatment for Hodgkin's disease. Reports of patients who received less than 40 Gy to the heart with evenly weighted fields have documented an incidence of acute pericarditis of less than 3% (CARMEL and KAPLAN 1976; TARBELL et al. 1990). All of the 13 patients who experienced acute pericarditis in TARBELL et al's series of 590 patients were successfully managed conservatively either with no treatment, with anti-inflammatory agents, or, in one case, with steroids. The frequency of pericardial disease in children who receive high-dose treatment for Hodgkin's disease seems to be similar to that observed in adults (DONALDSON and KAPLAN 1982).

3.7.1.2 Myocardium

While symptomatic myocardial damage is unusual following treatment with moderate doses of radiation alone, the increasing use of anthracyclines in cancer management has raised clinical awareness of relatively subtle radiation-induced abnormalities which, when combined with the effects of cardiotoxic drugs, can have an important effect on ventricular function. High doses of radiation may cause microvascular damage and interstitial myocardial fibrosis but do not appear to affect individual myocardial cells (BROSIUS III et al. 1981; FAJARDO 1982). In contrast, the anthracyclines doxorubicin and daunorubicin have little effect upon blood capillaries but have a direct effect upon myocytes which are eventually replaced by patches of fibrosis (FAJARDO and BERTHRONG 1976). Patients may suffer acute anthracycline cardiotoxicity or develop delayed (subacute) signs and symptoms of decreased contractility leading to cardiac failure 1–30 months after administration of the drug. Recent studies demonstrate that patients who have been asymp-

tomatic may have subclinical myocardial damage which is revealed only when they develop abnormalities of cardiac contractility and rhythm 10 or more years after completion of treatment (LIPSHULTZ et al. 1989, 1990; STEINHERZ et al. 1991). Endomyocardial biopsies of these patients reveal myocardial fibrosis with hypertrophy of surviving myocytes. The risk of late cardiac complications is strongly correlated with the cumulative dose of anthracycline, with the results of end-therapy echocardiogram, with a history of mediastinal radiotherapy, and with the total dose of mediastinal irradiation (STEINHERZ et al., 1991). Although many of the observations of late toxic effects have been in patients who were treated as children, STEINHERZ et al. (1991) found no correlation with age ($P = 0.50$). However, there was a strong correlation between the length of follow-up and the incidence of abnormal cardiac studies, with a steady increase in the percentage of abnormal studies with time (14% after 4–6 years, 24% after 7–9 years, and 38% after 10 years or more).

Even relatively low doses of radiation may increase the risk of anthracycline-related cardiac complications. MEFFERD et al. (1989) evaluated 14 children a mean of 15 months after treatment with 15–25 Gy and 150 mg/m^2 of doxorubicin in ABVD/MOPP. Despite relatively low doses of doxorubicin and radiation, 2 of 14 children had an abnormal resting or stress ejection fraction. One child in the second National Wilms' Tumor Study developed evidence of reduced left ventricular function after only 90 mg/m^2 and 27 Gy to the heart (THOMAS et al. 1988). Another child who had received 14.4 Gy to the heart in the first National Wilms' Tumor Study developed congestive heart failure following delivery of only 60 mg/m^2 of doxorubicin for recurrent pulmonary disease (TEFFT 1977). However, FRYER et al. (1990) have found no evidence of cardiac toxicity (by clinical examination, echocardiogram, or electrocardiogram) in 64 children 3–5 years after treatment for advanced Hodgkin's disease with 12 cycles of ABVD (total 400 mg/m^2) and 21 Gy.

Radiation can cause changes in resting electrocardiographic findings. STRENDER et al. (1986) noted an increase in T wave abnormalities 6 months after radiation treatment in 69 patients. These had generally returned to normal when the patients were reexamined 10 years after treatment. Although there was a somewhat increased incidence in ST abnormalities 10 years after treatment, this was felt to be consistent with the aging of the population. Conduction defects (primarily right bundle branch block and first degree

AV block) have been reported in a few patients following mantle radiation but the role of radiation in their etiology is unclear (POHJOLA-SINTONEN et al. 1987; WATCHIE et al. 1987). These findings appear to be somewhat more frequent in patients who were treated for extensive intrathoracic disease (WATCHIE et al. 1987).

3.7.1.3 Coronary Artery Disease

During the past decade, anecdotal reports of apparent premature narrowing of coronary vessels in irradiated patients have raised concern about this risk although most analyses of large populations failed to demonstrate conclusively that premature coronary artery disease was a serious risk in patients treated with modern radiotherapy techniques. In a detailed review of the subject, SCHULTZ-HECTOR (1991) found 32 case reports of myocardial infarctions that occurred in patients under 42 years of age who had been previously irradiated. The average time between radiation and the onset of ischemic heart disease was 5.5 years. The author noted that one-half of these patients had no other apparent risk factors for coronary artery disease. This contrasted with findings of studies of unirradiated young patients suffering myocardial infarction, in which very few lacked significant risk factors for heart disease. In addition, there have been a few anecdotal reports of premature coronary artery disease in irradiated children. DONALDSON and KAPLAN (1982) reported two cases, one of which was fatal (at age 15; COHN et al., 1967), in a series of 120 children treated with high-dose mantle irradiation and POHJOLA-SINTONEN et al. (1987) described one case of fatal myocardial infarction in a 12-year-old boy who was treated with mantle irradiation for a total dose of 33 Gy at age 6. Although such reports seem to provide compelling evidence of a damaging effect of radiation on the coronary arteries, they represent a very small proportion of the thousands of children and young adults who have been treated for Hodgkin's disease. The patients' histories provide no obvious clue to any common factor that would explain why a small subset of patients seem to suffer unusually severe radiation-induced vascular damage.

Of more general concern is the possibility that radiation may subtly accelerate the atherosclerotic process as treated patients age. In an autopsy study from the NCI, BROSIUS III, et al. (1981) evaluated the degree of narrowing in 482 serial sections of the coronary arteries from 11 irradiated patients (aged 15–33 at death) and compared them with those of 10 unirradiated control patients matched for age and sex who had not been irradiated to the heart. He found more than 75% narrowing in 6% of the sections from treated patients compared with 0.2% of those from controls ($p = 0.06$), 51–75% narrowing in 28% of sections from treated patients versus 13% of those from controls (p = NS) and 26–50% narrowing in 44% of those from treated patients versus 65% of controls (p<0.05). The total number of sections showing more than 25% narrowing was actually slightly greater in controls than in the treated patients. Although the authors concluded that this study demonstrated radiation-induced coronary artery disease, the evidence is of marginal significance, particularly in view of the small number of patients from whom the sections were taken. Of note was the substantial amount of coronary artery narrowing present in the unirradiated controls, illustrating the fallacy of assuming that all changes in young irradiated hearts are attributable to treatment. Histologically Brosius found somewhat more adventitial fibrosis and loss of smooth muscle cells from the media of irradiated patients, but no specific changes that could be used to differentiate radiation damage from the types of atherosclerotic vascular disease. FAJARDO (1982) concluded from clinical experience and laboratory studies that it was not possible to distinguish spontaneous atherosclerosis from that associated with radiation.

The nonspecific nature of radiation-induced vessel changes and the high incidence of coronary artery disease in the general population have made it very difficult to determine the relative importance of therapeutic radiation in the etiology of ischemic heart disease. Several authors have reported suggestive evidence of an increased incidence of heart disease in populations of patients who have received mediastinal irradiation for Hodgkin's disease or seminoma, but appropriate control populations have been difficult to define (COSSET et al., 1991; LEDERMAN et al., 1987; TARBELL et al., 1990). In a careful analysis from the Harvard School of Public Health, BOIVIN and HUTCHISON (1982) obtained follow-up information on 98% of the 957 patients diagnosed and treated for Hodgkin's disease at the hospitals of the Joint Center for Radiation Therapy and the Massachusetts General Hospital during the period 1942–1975 (BOIVIN and HUTCHISON, 1982). No information was available about treatment techniques. Death certificates were examined to determine the cause of death for 374 of 381 patients who had died. There were a total of 25 deaths from coronary heart disease, 14 in the 678 patients who had been irradiated to the heart and 10 in the 279 patients who had not. There was no significant difference in age, stage and interval-adjusted death rates from coronary heart disease between patients who did or did not receive heart irradiation. Adjusted comparison with death rates in the general population yielded a relative death rate from ischemic heart disease of 2.1 for the irradiated patients and 1.5 for the unirradiated patients, neither of which was significantly different from unity. Despite the large number of patients in the cohort, this study was not large enough to rule out a moderate increase in the risk of coronary heart disease, nor were there enough patients followed for more than 10 years to predict what the relative risk might be to children who would be expected to be at risk for more than 50 years after treatment.

The most convincing evidence for radiation-induced acceleration of coronary artery disease comes from two recent studies. In 1992, RUTQVIST et al. reported a significantly greater risk of death due to ischemic heart disease in women treated with post operative radiation for left-sided breast cancers compared with those treated for right-sided lesions (relative hazard: 3.2, p <0.05). In the same year, HANCOCK and HOPPE (1992) reported the results of a study of 2232 patients treated for Hodgkin's disease at Stanford between 1961 and 1990. The relative risk of death from heart disease was compared with an age, sex, and racially matched normal population. The relative risk of death from heart disease for treated patients was 3.1 times that of the control group. The risk was only increased in patients who received more than 30 Gy to the mediastinum. The relative risk increased significantly with increasing periods of observation and was highest in patients who were irradiated before the age of 20.

To minimize the risk of cardiac complications, treatment plans should be designed to avoid cardiac doses of more than 30–35 Gy and fraction sizes of more than 2 Gy. Careful shielding should be used to minimize the volume of heart in the treatment field. All fields should be treated daily. Treatment plans that include both anthracyclines and mediastinal irradiation should be considered very carefully. Combinations of high anthracycline doses and even moderate doses of cardiac irradiation attend a high risk of late complications and should be avoided if at all possible. Any previously irradiated patient (of any age) who displays symptoms that could suggest ischemic heart disease should be evaluated thoroughly. Patients who have received anthracyclines as well as mediastinal irradiation should be followed closely with periodic echocardiograms and, depending upon the level of risk, with radionuclide angiography, Holter monitoring, and Doppler examination (STEINHERZ and STEINHERZ, 1991). Although the published literature has contributed a great deal to our understanding of the cardiotoxic effects of drugs and radiation in both children and adults, many additional years of close observation and accurate documentation of cardiac function in patients treated with modern techniques will be necessary for clinicians to fully understand the influence of these agents on the long-term durability of the heart.

3.7.2 Large Vessels

The risk of accelerated atherosclerotic narrowing of critical arterial vessels in irradiated fields continues to be poorly defined. The clinical literature on this subject consists largely of case reports. Because the histopathologic changes associated with radiation-induced vascular narrowing are nonspecific, cases of apparent radiation vascular damage have been defined on the basis of the pattern of narrowing and the age of the patient. The large literature concerning the controversial subject of radiation-induced coronary artery disease is reviewed above and the subject of radiation-associated renal vascular narrowing is summarized in Sect. 3.10.1. In addition, the literature contains a number of case reports and small series of patients who have experienced symptoms of carotid or vertebral artery narrowing following neck irradiation. These were summarized by CALL et al. in 1990. Most of the reported cases were of patients who had received doses of more than 50 Gy although the authors reported two of their own patients who developed symptoms of carotid artery narrowing 2–3 years after mantle treatment for Hodgkin's disease to a prescribed dose of 38–39 Gy. The authors note that the actual carotid artery doses (and fraction size) in these patients and in others reported in the literature may have been significantly higher since compensators were not used. It is significant that fewer than 30 cases of purported radiation-induced carotid artery disease have been reported in view of the thousands of patients who have been treated successfully with radiation for lymphomas and cancers of the head and neck. However, such cases continue to raise appropriate concern about the vascular integrity of such patients. Any patient who develops neurologic signs or symptoms following neck irradiation should be evaluated for vascular disease.

Relatively little is known about the relative risk of serious vascular disease in irradiated children. As was mentioned in Sect. 3.10.1, hypoplasia of the renal arteries and adjacent aorta has been observed in several patients treated in infancy with abdominal irradiation. In 1966 COLQUHOUN reported two cases of aortic hypoplasia in children who were treated at age 1 month and 17 months with 2850 R and 6054 R, respectively. These cases appear to be rare, but they raise concern that the developing large vessels may not develop properly after large doses of irradiation. It is possible that such arterial narrowing is sometimes masked by collateral flow that develops during years of growth. Fortunately, magnetic resonance imaging provides a noninvasive method of evaluating such patients that may yield future information about the caliber of irradiated vessels in patients who received irradiation in infancy.

3.8 Lungs

Pulmonary morbidity is a critical dose-limiting factor in the treatment of tumors in or adjacent to the thoracic cavity. The clinical symptoms of radiation-induced lung disease can be divided into an acute pneumonitic phase that occurs 2–6 months after treatment and a chronic phase that is usually apparent radiographically 6 or more months after irradiation. In children, the effects of irradiation on growing bone may contribute to pulmonary dysfunction by decreasing the capacity of the thoracic cavity and the development of thoracic musculature. In young children, radiation may also affect the development of new alveoli.

3.8.1 Growth and Development

The effects of radiation on pulmonary growth and development are of particular concern in young children. The newborn lung, which weighs approximately 60 g, increases about ten fold in weight by adulthood (THURLBECK 1975). The total lung *volume* increases more than 20-fold as the ratio of volume to tissue mass more than doubles from birth to 6 years of age. The lung grows by cell multiplication and extensive remodeling of gas-exchanging units. At birth the human lung has few, if any, alveoli. The most rapid phase of cell division and alveolar multiplication occurs during the first year of life, reflecting the rapid growth rate of the organism as a whole. Relatively little alveolar multiplication appears to

occur after 4–8 years of age. Studies of children with congenital kyphoscoliosis suggest that children with secondarily diminished thoracic volumes develop fewer alveoli. The number of nonalveolated airways dose not increase after birth, but airways do increase in diameter, paralleling the increase in body size. Very little is known about the nature or extent of lung regeneration (in adults or children) following surgical or radiation-induced loss of lung volume or about the forces that might stimulate an increase in alveolar multiplication if it occurs. The influence of radiation, cytotoxic drugs, and steroids on alveolar multiplication and development is not known.

3.8.2 Radiation Pneumonitis

The symptoms of acute radiation pneumonitis include cough, fever, and shortness of breath. Histologic studies of the irradiated lung during the pneumonitic phase have demonstrated edema, fibrinous exudates in alveoli, hypertrophic and desquamating alveolar cells, and evidence of microvascular damage. Experimental studies suggest that damage to type I and II pneumocytes disrupts the pulmonary surfactant system (PENNEY and RUBIN 1977) and that pulmonary endothelial damage may cause changes in capillary permeability resulting in leakage of proteinaceous fluid into alveolar spaces (GROSS 1980). The incidence and severity of clinical symptoms depend on the radiation dose and fractionation schedule and the volume of lung irradiated (PHILLIPS and MARGOLIS 1972; RUBIN and CASARETT 1968). Radiographic findings of increased density corresponding to the radiation treatment field may be seen in patients who have little or no clinical symptomatology. Mild symptoms usually resolve spontaneously after 2–3 months. However, acute radiation pneumonitis can be life threatening, particularly in patients who have had a large volume of lung irradiated.

3.8.3 Chronic Radiation Injury

Histologically, chronic radiation damage is characterized by alveolar wall thickening, fibrosis, and microvascular changes. Radiographically, a region of increased density and volume loss corresponds to the treatment field. Patients who have been treated with relatively small volumes may be entirely asymptomatic despite radiographic evidence of localized fibrosis. Several studies have reported transient, mild restrictive ventilatory defects during the first year after treatment (ELLIS et al. 1992; SMITH et al. 1989; WATCHIE et al. 1987). Studies by MAH et al. (1987) and WARA et al. (1973) have described a strong relationship between radiation dose and the incidence of radiographically evident radiation injury. MAH et al. demonstrated a 50% incidence of radiation-induced radiographic changes in the lung that had received a fractionated dose equivalent of about 33 Gy in 15 fractions. The reported incidence of chronic or acute radiation injury varies with the endpoint studied. Studies that quote an incidence based on the results of radiographic studies or detailed pulmonary function tests tend to quote a higher incidence of radiation injury than studies that use clinical symptoms as an endpoint.

Because most children with malignant diseases that metastasize to the lung receive some form of chemotherapy, very little information is available about the effects of radiation alone, particularly in young children. BREUER et al. (1978) reported no clinical evidence of pulmonary toxicity in 30 children under 15 year of age treated with 20 Gy in 2 weeks to the bilateral lungs (cobalt-60 or megavoltage). ZAHARIA et al. (1986) reported no clinical evidence of pulmonary toxicity in 36 osteosarcoma patients (mean age 14.6 years) treated prophylactically to the lungs with 20 Gy (1.5 Gy/fraction) with or without doxorubicin. Several authors have reported on the pulmonary toxicity of partial lung irradiation for Hodgkin's disease. Pulmonary function following mantle treatment is influenced by the total dose, the volume irradiated, the use of low-dose whole lung irradiation, the initial size of mediastinal disease, and the use of adjuvant chemotherapy (MEFFERD et al. 1989; MORGAN et al. 1985; TARBELL et al. 1990), although detailed prospective studies of pulmonary function in adults have concluded that most Hodgkin's disease patients have minimal long-term pulmonary dysfunction from mantle irradiation (SMITH et al. 1989; WATCHIE et al. 1987). DONALDSON and KAPLAN (1982) reported a 3.6% incidence of pulmonary reactions in 55 children receiving mantle irradiation without chemotherapy, similar to the adult incidence. In a review of posttreatment pulmonary function testing in 20 children treated with low-dose mantle irradiation and alternating MOPP-ABVD chemotherapy, MEFFERD et al. (1989) found evidence of restrictive abnormalities in six (30%) and obstructive abnormalities in two (10%) children, although all were asymptomatic. Six of 11 children tested for carbon monoxide diffusion capacity had abnormal values.

Bleomycin was believed to have contributed to this toxicity.

3.8.4 Drug-Radiation Interactions

Experimental studies have demonstrated that several chemotherapeutic agents, including cyclophosphamide, vincristine, doxorubicin, actinomycin, bleomycin, and mitomycin C, enhance the pulmonary toxicity of radiation, particularly when given concurrently (STEEL et al. 1979; VAN DER MAASE et al. 1986).

Clinical studies suggest that chemotherapy increases both the acute and the chronic pulmonary effects of radiation. In particular, children who receive actinomycin D or doxorubicin during the first 3–4 months after pulmonary radiation seem to be at an increased risk of developing diffuse interstitial pneumonitis. In 1973, WARA et al. demonstrated a marked increase in the incidence of radiation pneumonitis in children and adults who received actinomycin D in addition to radiation and concluded that 25 Gy in 20 fractions without chemotherapy or 15 Gy in 10 fractions with actinomycin D could be delivered with no more than a 5% probability of inducing radiation pneumonitis. In a more recent analysis from the third National Wilms' Tumor Study, GREEN et al. (1989) reported a 13% incidence of diffuse interstitial pneumonitis in 153 children treated for stage IV favorable histology Wilms' tumor. Most children received 12 Gy to the lungs at 1.5 Gy/fraction and 66 weeks of chemotherapy, including doxorubicin and actinomycin D in alternating cycles with vincristine and, in some cases, cyclophosphamide. The first course of actinomycin D was given at the start of pulmonary irradiation. All cases of diffuse pneumonitis occurred during the first 16 weeks of treatment and between 4 and 14 weeks after the completion of pulmonary irradiation. Twelve of the 16 occurred 21–54 days after the first course of doxorubicin, which was planned in the sixth week of treatment. Three of 11 patients who underwent open lung biopsy had *Pneumocystis carinii* infections, and one had *Varicella zoster*. Eleven of the 18 patients with diffuse pneumonitis died despite treatment with trimethoprim/sulfamethoxazole and, in some cases, corticosteroids. The three patients with documented *Pneumocystis* recovered. Although the combination of pulmonary radiation and chemotherapy including actinomycin D and doxorubicin was undoubtedly the primary cause of the life-threatening pneumonitis in these children, superinfection with

Pneumocystis may have played a greater role than would be suggested by the three positive biopsies since many children were started on antibiotics prior to open lung biopsy. In 1991, COHEN et al. reported a case of fatal radiation pneumonitis in a child with Ewing's sarcoma who experienced the onset of pulmonary symptoms 1 day after a course of VACA and 3 months after 12 Gy in 8 fractions to both lungs. The authors suggested that dactinomycin and doxorubicin may have induced a radiation "recall" phenomenon and commented upon the patient's rapid deterioration following rapid withdrawal of a course of methylprednisolone. In 1974, CASTELLINO et al. reported six cases of apparent reactivation of latent pulmonary radiation injury following rapid withdrawal of a course of steroids (included in MOPP chemotherapy for Hodgkin's disease). The interval between pulmonary radiation and the onset of pulmonary symptoms following steroid withdrawal ranged between 3 months and 6 years.

Several retrospective studies have reported on the long-term follow-up of pulmonary function in children treated with radiation and chemotherapy for Wilms' tumor metastatic to the lung. BENOIST et al. (1982) performed sequential pulmonary function tests in 48 patients treated between 1960 and 1976 with actinomycin D and bilateral lung irradiation to a dose of 20 Gy in 21 days (fraction size and beam energy were not mentioned). The mean age of the children was 4 years (range 1–13 years) at the time of pulmonary irradiation, and they were followed for a mean of 7 years. The incidence of pulmonary function abnormalities increased with time, and nearly all the patients studied had a significant reduction in total lung capacity and dynamic lung compliance 5 years after the completion of treatment. Skeletal growth abnormalities probably contributed to the findings. Most children had reduced sagittal and frontal thoracic diameters 3–4 years after treatment, and about 20% had mild to moderate thoracolumbar scoliosis caused by flank irradiation. Despite this, the authors commented that these patients were not disabled, that most experienced no dyspnea on moderate exertion, and that there were no pulmonary radiographic findings after the first 2 years after radiation therapy. In an earlier study of Wilms' tumor patients, WOHL et al. (1975) reported similar impairment of total lung capacity and vital capacity in six children who received 8.5–12.5 Gy with 250-kV x-rays and unspecified fractionation. A second group of children who were reirradiated to a partial lung volume had particularly severe pulmonary function abnormalities. In another review from the Children's

Hospital of Philadelphia, LITTMAN et al. (1976) reported similar findings of decreased lung volume in children treated with orthovoltage irradiation for metastatic Wilms' tumor. Interestingly, a small group of children without lung metastases who were treated with similar doses of prophylactic pulmonary irradiation had normal vital capacities and total lung capacities. Although these studies suggest that low doses of pulmonary radiation in combination with actinomycin D cause significant late pulmonary function abnormalities, they are almost impossible to interpret in terms of current practice. The use of orthovoltage irradiation could have had a disproportionate effect on rib growth and, without lung density corrections, the specified doses of radiation from these low-energy beams will have significantly underestimated the real dose delivered to the lung.

3.8.5 Pulmonary Toxicity After Bone Marrow Transplantation

Pulmonary toxicity is an important cause of morbidity and mortality following bone marrow transplantation. Transient mild restrictive changes may be seen during the first year after treatment, and subsequent follow-up may reveal varying degrees of obstructive disease (SPRINGMEYER et al. 1983). However, interstitial pneumonitis represents the most serious threat to the transplant patient. Radiation therapy is only one of several factors, including chemotherapy, graft versus host disease, and opportunistic infections, that may contribute to interstitial pneumonitis following bone marrow transplantation. Patients who receive a syngeneic transplant have a significantly lower incidence of interstitial pneumonitis than those treated with the same total body irradiation prior to allogeneic transplant (NEIMAN et al. 1977). However, NEIMAN et al. also found that patients who have total body irradiation as part of the preparation for allogeneic transplant have twice the incidence of interstitial and idiopathic pneumonitis as those prepared with chemotherapy alone for aplastic anemia.

A number of radiation parameters, including total dose, dose rate, fractionation, and the method of dose specification (i.e., with or without lung density corrections), may influence radiation-related morbidity. In a detailed review of the literature, KEANE et al. (1981) demonstrated a clear dose-response relationship for patients treated with low-dose-rate whole lung irradiation. Patients who received an absolute dose to the lung (corrected for lung density) of 9 Gy or less (dose rate of 0.028–0.15 Gy/min) had a very low incidence of idiopathic pneumonitis (<50%). The incidence rises steeply, reaching approximately 50% after an absolute dose of 12 Gy. In the Seattle experience, the median time of onset of idiopathic pneumonitis was about 50 days after radiation, with 90% of cases occurring between 10 and 120 days. More than 50% of cases were fatal. Dose rate is also a critical factor. The incidence of radiation pneumonitis rises steeply from 5% to 50% with doses of 8–9 Gy (absolute) to the lung given at a high dose rate (VAN DYK et al. 1981). The use of low dose rates of 0.02–0.50 Gy/min appears to shift this threshold by approximately 2 Gy (BARRETT et al. 1987; VAN DYK et al. 1981; WEINER et al. 1986). A review of 932 patients entered in the International Bone Marrow Transplant Registry suggested an increasing frequency of interstitial pneumonitis (from 5% to 35% with an increasing dose rate from 0.02 to 0.1 Gy/min) (WEINER et al., 1986). This study found no evidence that fractionation reduced the risk of interstitial pneumonitis, although a number of investigators have reported decreased pulmonary morbidity with fractionated total body irradiation (DEEG et al. 1986; MEYERS et al. 1983; THOMAS et al. 1982).

3.9 Gastrointestinal Tract

3.9.1 Esophagus

Children whose radiation field encompasses the esophagus will experience symptoms of acute radiation esophagitis 2–4 weeks after the start of a course of standardly fractionated radiation. Symptoms may include substernal pain and dysphagia. These symptoms may cause transient nutritional problems but are usually self-limited in patients treated with less than 45 Gy of radiation alone. Higher doses may cause severe esophagitis with stricture or fistula formation. However, patients who receive relatively low doses may also experience severe symptoms when chemotherapy (particularly doxorubicin or, less frequently, actinomycin D) is delivered during or after radiation (BOAL et al. 1979; GRECO et al. 1976; NEWBURGER et al. 1978). Patients who receive doxorubicin concurrent with doses of radiation as low as 5–20 Gy may develop severe dysphagia, sometimes necessitating hospitalization and parenteral nutrition. Subsequent courses of chemotherapy may be associated with episodes of "recall" esophagitis,

which may also be severe. Chronic abnormalities in esophageal motility and even irreversible stricture may result.

3.9.2 Liver

The radiosensitivity of the liver was only recognized in the early 1960s, when the advent of megavoltage radiotherapy made it possible to treat the entire liver with relatively high doses. In 1963, INGOLD et al. published a detailed description of the clinical presentation and dose-dependence of radiation hepatitis in a series of patients treated to the abdomen. The first clinical signs of radiation toxicity included hepatomegaly, ascites, and portal hypertension and generally occurred 2–6 weeks after the completion of radiotherapy. An elevated alkaline phosphatase was the most reliable indicator of radiation hepatitis, but most liver function tests became abnormal as the process developed. Sudden, profound thrombocytopenia was occasionally observed but is more commonly seen in children who have also received actinomycin D (TEFFT et al. 1970).

Histologic changes associated with the acute phase of radiation hepatitis include sinusoidal congestion and atrophy of liver plates surrounding the central veins of liver lobules (FAJARDO 1982). The veno-occlusive lesions characteristic of radiation hepatitis appear 2.5–6 months after treatment. Progressive occlusion of small central (lobular) and sublobular veins is accompanied by increasing congestion and liver cell atrophy. In the chronic stages, congestion may decrease, and atrophied liver tissue is replaced by fibrosis with collagen deposition. Following partial volume irradiation, radioisotope scans demonstrate a sharply demarcated region of diminished uptake corresponding to the radiation portal (TEFFT et al. 1970).

In INGOLD et al.'s experience, which included primarily adults treated for metastatic disease, radiation hepatitis did not occur after doses less than 25 Gy but was observed in all patients who had received 45 Gy or more to the entire liver volume. Abnormalities were seen in 21% of patients who had received 30–36 Gy and in 42% of those who had received 38–42 Gy. For adults treated with radiation alone, toxicity is related to both the dose and the volume of liver irradiated (AUSTIN-SEYMOUR et al. 1986).

In 1970, TEFFT et al. reported their experience with partial or total liver irradiation in 115 children. They observed evidence of hepatotoxicity in children who had received radiation doses as low as 12–25 Gy—

well below the threshold described by INGOLD et al. Within their series no relationship between patient age and liver toxicity was observed. They were also unable to demonstrate any clear relationship between radiation dose or treatment volume and subsequent hepatotoxicity. In a more recent review of toxicity observed in the second National Wilms' Tumor Study, THOMAS et al. (1988) reported 16 cases of hepatic toxicity in 303 children. The incidence in patients treated to the right flank was significantly higher than that of patients treated to the left flank with fields encompassing relatively small liver volumes.

However, several other factors may have an important influence on liver tolerance in children. Because all of the children in TEFFT et al.'s series had been treated with actinomycin D as well as irradiation, the authors could not determine the influence of the drug upon observed hepatotoxicity. Subsequent experience has demonstrated that 1%–2% of children treated for Wilms' tumor with chemotherapy *alone* (actinomycin D and vincristine) develop veno-occlusive disease of the liver which may be severe and is usually associated with profound thrombocytopenia (GREEN et al. 1990; NYBONDE et al. 1988; RAINE et al. 1991). Actinomycin D is thought to be the responsible drug since hepatotoxicity has not been observed in children treated with vincristine alone (RAINE et al. 1991). In the fourth National Wilms' Tumor Study, the incidence of hepatic toxicity was significantly increased in children treated with a higher, single dose schedule of actinomycin D (GREEN et al. 1990). Infants appear to be particularly susceptible (MORGAN et al. 1988). Other drugs may contribute to liver toxicity in children treated for malignancy. Cytarabine (TEBBI et al. 1990) and ifosfamide (PRATT et al. 1989) can cause elevation of hepatic enzyme levels. Doxorubicin may potentiate radiation damage to the liver (KUN and CAMITTA 1978). Fatal veno-occlusive disease of the liver has also been reported following high-dose multiagent chemotherapy with or without total body irradiation for bone marrow transplantation (WOODS et al. 1980). RUCHELLI et al. (1990) have suggested that patients with α_1 antitrypsin deficiency may have an increased susceptibility to treatment-related hepatotoxicity.

FILLER et al. (1970) and TEFFT et al. (1970) demonstrated that children were particularly susceptible to treatment-related hepatotoxicity following partial hepatic resection. In their series, all five of the children who had had a partial hepatic resection had evidence of hepatic toxicity following radiation and chemotherapy, and two suffered severe hepatotoxic-

ity. The authors hypothesized that active liver regeneration following partial resection may have made the liver particularly susceptible to radiation damage. Toxicity seemed to have been greatest when treatment was initiated less than 1 month after partial hepatectomy. These patients also seemed to have unusually severe gastrointestinal and hematopoietic toxicity from their chemotherapy, and the authors suggested that prior resection may have impaired hepatic excretion, causing elevated drug levels that may also have contributed to treatment-related hepatic toxicity. GERACI et al. (1985) observed increased radiation-induced hepatotoxicity following partial hepatic resection in rats. However, animal studies of radiation hepatitis are difficult to relate to clinical radiotherapy because most animals do not develop the veno-occlusive hepatic lesions typically seen following radiation in humans (FAJARDO 1982).

Radiation hepatitis is rarely seen in patients treated with radiotherapy alone, since radiotherapists simply avoid treating large volumes of the liver with fractionated doses of more than 25–30 Gy. The developing livers of children may be somewhat more sensitive to the effects of radiation. More importantly, the frequent concurrent use of drugs that are known radiosensitizers and/or are themselves potential hepatotoxins makes the effect of liver radiation more unpredictable in children. Although radiation hepatitis is still uncommon in children who receive doses of less than 25 Gy to the liver, radiation to large volumes of liver should be given with caution and with a thorough knowledge of the current literature concerning drug-radiation interactions. Particular care should be taken when irradiating children who have experienced chemotherapy-related hepatopathy or who have undergone prior partial hepatic resection.

3.9.3 Small Bowel

The acute symptoms of radiation enteritis include nausea, diarrhea, and abdominal cramping. The severity is related to the volume of small bowel irradiated and the dose delivered per day. Occasionally symptoms may be severe, particularly when large volumes are treated with concurrent chemotherapy. Antispasmodic and anticholinergic drugs will often relieve mild symptoms but, in some cases, parenteral nutrition may be required to control diarrhea and maintain nutrition. Children who develop symptoms of enteritis must be followed closely for evidence of fluid and electrolyte disturbances. The frequent use of chemotherapy, particularly actinomycin D, may contribute to the apparently higher incidence of severe acute radiation enteritis in children than in adults. DONALDSON et al. (1975) reported severe vomiting and diarrhea in 29.5% and weight loss in 55% of children receiving whole abdominal irradiation. In some children, lactose malabsorption may contribute to the diarrhea associated with chemotherapy or radiation (HYAMS et al. 1982). Symptoms of acute radiation enteritis are usually self-limited, resolving completely 1–2 months after the completion of treatment.

A minority of patients develop late radiation enteropathy with gradual development of crampy abdominal pain and diarrhea 6–18 months after radiation. Most authors report little or no relationship between the severity of acute symptoms and the development of late radiation bowel disease although DONALDSON et al. (1975) found a strong correlation between severe acute effects and subsequent bowel obstructions in irradiated children. Previous abdominal surgery is probably the most important factor predisposing patients to late radiation injury (KINSELLA and BLOOMER 1980). The incidence of late radiation enteritis in irradiated children is poorly defined. DONALDSON et al. (1975) reported an 11% incidence of bowel obstruction in 44 children who had received whole abdominal irradiation and suggested that concurrent treatment with actinomycin D contributed to the development of late radiation complications. Ninety-eight percent of the children in their series had had major abdominal surgery prior to treatment. Small bowel damage has not been reported as a major complication by the National Wilms' Tumor Study Group, although many of the children entered on these studies were treated with relatively high radiation doses to large abdominal fields, often with actinomycin D or other chemotherapy (EVANS et al. 1991). This, combined with the young age of the these children and the frequent history of prior abdominal surgery, should have placed them at particularly high risk. A detailed study of bowel function in this population would be interesting.

3.10 Urinary Tract

3.10.1 Kidney

The clinical picture of radiation nephropathy can be divided into several periods or categories (LUXTON and KUNKLER 1964; RUBIN and CASARETT 1964).

During the first 6 months following radiation, an asymptomatic decrease in glomerular filtration rate may occur. Clinical symptoms of what has been variously termed acute or subacute radiation nephritis or nephropathy may appear after a latency period of 6–12 months. This latency period may be shorter in children (LUXTON and KUNKLER 1964). Presenting symptoms include dyspnea, edema, headache, and moderate hypertension. Patients may develop a severe normochromic, normocytic anemia and evidence of red blood cells and casts in the urine. Patients who survive the acute period usually progress to a chronic form of the disease with decreased renal function. Chronic radiation nephropathy may also develop in patients who have had no previous history of acute nephropathy. Patients may present with the first signs of radiation injury, including proteinuria, decreased renal function, and hypertension, many years after treatment.

Authors differ in their understanding of the pathogenesis of radiation injury. Most clinicopathologic studies are based on necropsy material or biopsies from patients already in renal failure and may reflect secondary changes of hypertension, terminal illness, or both. The applicability of various animal models has been questioned (FAJARDO 1982). However, the few biopsy specimens reported suggest that the earliest histologic changes in humans involve glomerular, endothelial, and mesangial cells (KEANE et al. 1976; LUXTON and KUNKLER 1964). Specimens from more advanced lesions show diffuse glomerular sclerosis and, with time, increasingly extensive tubular atrophy. Arterial lesions including myointimal proliferation and narrowing of arcuate and interlobular arteries are sometimes seen in association with glomerular and tubular changes (WHITE 1975). Although some authors argue that radiation injury is actually mediated through these arterial lesions, FAJARDO remarks that arteriolar lesions are proportionately less severe or even absent despite extensive glomerular and tubular changes in early biopsy specimens; he suggests that arterial narrowing is more often a secondary result of hypertension. Animal studies have been variously interpreted to support the glomerular (GLATSTEIN et al. 1977; LJUNGQVIST et al. 1971), tubular (JORDAN et al. 1978; PHILLIPS and ROSS 1973; WITHERS et al. 1986), or arterial (RUBIN and CASARETT 1964) theories of pathogenesis. It is, of course, possible that the constellation of symptoms and syndromes associated with radiation nephropathy reflect direct and indirect injury to multiple tissue compartments. These changes are generally not associated with any inflammatory exudate (FAJARDO 1982; GLATSTEIN et al. 1977). Consequently the term "radiation nephropathy" is currently considered a more appropriate term to describe radiation-induced renal damage than "radiation nephritis."

The kidneys are frequently a dose-limiting structure in the treatment of abdominal malignancies. In adults, radiation treatment with fractionated doses greater than 23–25 Gy to the entirety of both kidneys is associated with a high risk of radiation nephropathy, whereas fractionated doses less than 18 Gy are rarely associated with significant nephropathy (FAJARDO 1982; KEANE et al. 1976; KUNKLER et al. 1952; LUXTON and KUNKLER 1964). There is no clear evidence that renal tolerance in children differs from that in adults. However, comparisons are difficult because most children have received chemotherapy as well as radiation. With the maximum renal dose of 15 Gy recommended in the National Wilms' Tumor Studies, radiation nephropathy was not reported as a late complication in a recent review (EVANS et al. 1991). In an earlier report of complications experienced in children treated in the first National Wilms' Tumor Study, one child was reported as possibly having radiation nephritis, although the kidney appeared to have been outside the radiation field (TEFFT 1977). However, evidence of renal damage has been reported in children treated with relatively low doses of radiation in combination with chemotherapy. MITUS et al. (1969) studied subsequent renal function in 108 children treated with radiation and actinomycin D following unilateral nephrectomy for Wilms' tumor, neuroblastoma, or renal cell carcinoma. Seventy-six percent of children who had received more than 24 Gy to the remaining kidney had reduced creatinine clearance, as did 33% of children who had received 12–24 Gy and 18% of those who had received <12 Gy. Although renal toxicity has been an uncommon complication of most bone marrow transplantation regimens, TARBELL et al. (1988) have reported a disturbingly high incidence of renal dysfunction in children 4–7 months after very intensive multiagent chemotherapy and total body irradiation (12–14 Gy in 6–8 fractions at 9–11 cGy/min). Renal problems consistent with radiation nephropathy were diagnosed in 9 of 28 evaluable patients treated with autologous transplants for acute lymphoblastic leukemia and in 7 of 11 children who had received allogeneic transplants for neuroblastoma. VM-26, cytosine arabinoside, and cyclophosphamide were included in the preparatory regimen of the former group and cisplatin, VM–26, melphalan, and cyclophosphamide were included in the preparatory regimen for the latter. The authors warn that unexpected toxicity may result when relatively modest doses of irradiation are combined with very aggressive chemotherapeutic regimens.

Laboratory studies also indicate that drugs commonly used in the treatment of pediatric malignancies can influence radiation-induced renal damage. DONALDSON et al. (1980) reported enhancement of radiation toxicity by doxorubicin in the immature rat kidney. Cisplatin alone can produce dose-limiting renal toxicity characterized by tubular necrosis and atrophy. Several authors have described a modest increase in late renal damage when cisplatin is given before or during renal irradiation (JONGEJAN et al. 1987; MOULDER et al. 1986; STEWART et al. 1988). However, MOULDER et al. described a progressive increase in cisplatin toxicity as the interval between radiation therapy and drug administration was increased. Pathologic evaluation of the kidneys revealed changes consistent with radiation nephropathy which were greatest when the drug was given 3 or more months after irradiation. Decreased drug clearance following radiation may contribute to this toxicity. The same authors reported a decrease in clearance of methotrexate 9 or more months after renal irradiation. Ifosfamide has been associated with mild to severe nephrotoxicity in children, but very little is known about the combined effects of ifosfamide and radiation (SUAREZ et al. 1991).

The effect of fractionation on radiation-induced renal injury cannot be established from the clinical literature, but numerous investigators have addressed this issue in animal models. These experiments have suggested that the kidney is very sensitive to fractionation, with an α/β ratio of less than 4 in most studies (STEWART and WILLIAMS 1991). However, recent studies using very small doses per fraction suggest that the linear quadratic model may not accurately predict isoeffective doses with radiation fractions of less than 1–2 Gy (JOINER and JOHNS 1988; STEWART et al. 1988). The effect of age on fractionation sensitivity is unknown.

In children, low-dose irradiation partially suppresses the compensatory hypertrophy normally seen after unilateral nephrectomy but does not cause clinical impairment of renal function in most patients (CASSADY et al. 1981; DONALDSON et al. 1978). Chemotherapeutic agents may also blunt the hypertrophic response to unilateral nephrectomy (MOSKOWITZ et al. 1980; WIKSTAD et al. 1986).

Patients with two normal kidneys have substantial renal reserve and, in most cases, no clinically evident renal dysfunction results from partial treatment (as much as 70%–80% of one kidney) despite anatomic defects that can be demonstrated on radiologic studies (BIRKHEAD et al. 1979; LEBOURGEOIS et al. 1979). In adults, no compensatory hypertrophy of the unirradiated kidney is seen after partial renal irradiation (LEBOURGEOIS et al. 1979).

Hypertension secondary to renal artery stenosis and increased renin secretion from the juxtaglomerular apparatus has been reported as a rare complication of radiation therapy in children (GERLOCK et al. 1977; McGILL et al. 1979; SALVI et al. 1983; STAAB et al. 1976). Although this complication has been reported in older children and adults, it is interesting that most of the reported cases in children have occurred in patients who were treated in infancy (Table 3.1). It is important to differentiate this cause of hypertension from other forms of radiation-induced renal hypertension. Renal artery stenosis should cause increased renin levels and can be readily demonstrated by angiography. In some cases, medical management can maintain normal blood pressures. If successful, excision of the narrowed segment of renal artery usually reduces hypertension (STANLEY et al. 1978). However, damage to adjacent vessels may make vascular surgery difficult, and great caution must be taken particularly when there is bilateral involvement or when the affected kidney is the patient's only functioning renal unit. MILUTINOVIC et al. (1990) have reported the successful use, with a short follow-up, of transluminal angioplasty to improve radiation-induced renal artery stenosis in one patient.

Symptomatic radiation nephropathy can usually be avoided by careful treatment planning with accurate kidney localization by computed tomography, ultrasound, or intravenous pyelography. The position of the kidneys should always be known prior to external beam treatment of any site in the abdomen or pelvis. Anatomic anomalies such as a horseshoe kidney or a pelvic kidney may require major changes in treatment planning. Whenever possible, doses of more than 15 Gy to the entire renal volume should be avoided, particularly when the child will also be receiving chemotherapy. Small portions of one or both kidneys may be taken to significantly higher doses with relatively little risk. When multiple-field techniques are used, the dose per fraction to the kidneys can be minimized by treating all fields daily. Combined modality treatment regimens should be carefully planned. In patients who have had renal irradiation, particular care should be taken when giving drugs that are metabolized through renal excretion. Cisplatin should probably be avoided in patients who have received significant doses of irradiation to a large portion of the renal volume. Urinalysis and blood pressure determinations are part of the routine follow-up of patients who have received irradiation to the kidneys or renal arteries. Hypertension should be corrected immediately since prolonged blood pressure elevations can accelerate vascular damage from irradiation.

3.10.2 Bladder

The acute symptoms of high-dose bladder irradiation included dysuria, frequency, and urinary incon-

Table 3.1. Reported cases of hypertension resulting from renal artery stenosis following treatment with radiation in childhood

Reference	Age at RT	Latency (yrs)	Dose	Tumor diagnosis; comments
COLQUHOUN (1966)	1 mo	4	2850 R	Neuroblastoma, aortic hypoplasia
COLQUHOUN (1966)	17 mo	13	6054 R	Neuroblastoma, aortic hypoplasia
GERLOCK et al. (1977)	7 mo	12	30 Gy (abdomen) 22 Gy (kidney)	Wilms' tumor; ^{60}Co, 2 Gy/fraction, with actinomycin D; narrowing of proximal renal artery
McGILL et al. (1979)	9 mo	6	30 Gy	Wilms' tumor; with chemotherapy; compensatory renal hypertrophy noted; narrowing of proximal renal artery
McGILL et al. (1979)	14 mo	12	51 Gy	Neuroblastoma; bilateral renal artery stenosis, aortic, mesenteric artery hypoplasia
SALVI et al. (1983)	6 yrs	6	36 Gy	Hodgkin's lymphoma; inverted-Y field including spleen and >90% of left kidney, followed by chemotherapy; left renal artery stenosis
STAAB et al. (1976)	15 yrs	12	32.8 Gy	Lymphoma; 250 kV, 1 field/day, 1.7 Gy/fraction; As changes in proximal renal arteries and abdominal aorta but none outside RT volume

RT, radiotherapy; AS, atherosclorotic

tinence. The irradiated bladder may be more susceptible to infection, and it is important to rule out infection in any child who presents with these symptoms during radiotherapy. Cystoscopically, acute radiation cystitis is characterized by mucosal edema and hyperemia. Patients who have received high-dose irradiation may develop subsequent epithelial ulceration and occasionally hemorrhage or fistulization. Late effects may include fibrosis and reduced bladder capacity (STEWART and WILLIAMS 1991).

JAYALAKSHMAMMA and PINKEL (1976) have reported increased bladder toxicity in children receiving concurrent cyclophosphamide and pelvic radiotherapy. Cyclophosphamide alone is a specific bladder toxin that may cause urothelial ulceration and hemorrhage. Animal studies suggest that the drug may also increase the risk of late radiation cystitis, although the toxicities appear to be additive (ENDREES et al. 1988). Ifosfamide, another potent bladder toxin, is being used more frequently in the management of pediatric malignancies, but there is as yet little published information about possible combined toxicities.

3.11 Reproductive Organs

3.11.1 Ovary

With the increasing survival of children treated for malignancy, the effect of therapy on subsequent fertility and pregnancy outcome has become increasingly important. In general, the impact of cancer and its treatment upon fertility is less profound in female than in male survivors of malignancy. In a large retrospective cohort study of childhood cancer survivors and sibling controls, BYRNE et al. (1987) described a relative fertility rate of 94% for all females. Irradiation below the diaphragm was associated with a fertility rate of 78% compared with controls. Patients were not assessed in terms of ovarian dose or proximity of fields to the pelvis. Alkylating agents appeared to have little or no impact upon female fertility in this study. However, in women treated for Hodgkin's disease in childhood a strong correlation has been found between the number of cycles of MOPP chemotherapy and subsequent ovarian failure (ORTIN et al. 1990). In another study, three of three girls treated with adjuvant nitrosoureas for medulloblastoma had subsequent evidence of gonadal failure while all four girls treated with similar craniospinal fields without

chemotherapy had normal gonadal development (AHMED et al. 1983).

The effect of radiation on ovarian function is related to both radiation dose and the age at which treatment is given (FISHER and CHEUNG 1984). It has been estimated that as little as 6 Gy is sufficient to induce menopause in a 40-year-old woman whereas young women require a total fractionated exposure of 20 Gy to induce ovarian failure with 95% confidence (LUSHBAUGH and CASARETT 1976). This differential sensitivity may be related to the decline in the total population of oocytes that occurs with age (BAKER 1971). Several reports have demonstrated that some premenarchal girls treated to the whole abdomen with doses as high as 20–30 Gy may express subsequent ovarian function although most, if not all, will experience premature ovarian failure. WALLACE et al. (1989) found that 27 of 38 women treated in childhood to the whole abdomen with doses of 20–35 Gy developed pubertal ovarian failure and ten (treated with 22–30 Gy) experienced premature menopause. Only one of their patients demonstrated reversal of ovarian failure during a trial period off hormone replacement therapy. Few data are available about fertility rates of women who receive doses between 10 and 20 Gy to the uterus and ovaries. Studies of children treated to the pelvis with midline shielding of transposed ovaries suggest that radiation doses of 1–5 Gy to the ovaries do not have a significant impact on subsequent gonadal function (ORTIN et al. 1990). HORNING et al. (1981) reported that temporary amenorrhea lasting between several months and 4 years occurred in 68% of postmenarchal women treated with total lymphoid irradiation following oophoropexy and suggested that patients who experience a cessation of normal menses after receiving low doses of irradiation must be followed for a sufficient period to determine whether ovarian function has been preserved.

Factors other than ovarian dysfunction may contribute to infertility and reproductive problems in female survivors of childhood malignancy. LI et al. (1987) reviewed the pregnancy outcomes of 99 patients cured of childhood Wilms' tumor. Of 114 pregnancies in 60 females who had received abdominal irradiation (generally to the renal fossa or hemiabdomen, although details were not given), 34 (30%) had an adverse outcome. In particular, the rates of fetal mortality and perinatal mortality were significantly greater than those in the general United States' population or in the wives of male survivors. The authors suggested that radiation-induced somatic damage to abdominopelvic structures may have contributed to the high incidence of miscarriages and premature births. In WALLACE et al.'s 1989 series of patients treated to the abdomen and pelvis, four patients had six documented conceptions despite doses of 22–30 Gy to the pelvic structures. However, all of the pregnancies terminated in midtrimester spontaneous miscarriages. The authors speculate that radiation damage may have influenced uterine distensibility. Relatively little is known about the effects of modest doses of irradiation on the development and subsequent function of the uterine musculature. Some of the reproductive problems of female survivors of Wilms' tumors may be related to urogenital anomalies associated with various manifestations of the Wilms' tumor-malformation syndrome (BYRNE et al. 1988). To date, most of the studies of fecundity in Wilms' survivors have included small numbers of patients treated with relatively high doses of radiation. Few unirradiated Wilms' survivors have been available for comparison. Follow-up studies of the survivors of more recent Wilms' tumor studies in which many patients have been treated without radiotherapy or with more modest doses of 10–20 Gy to the abdomen or renal fossa should provide an opportunity to sort out the relative importance of these factors.

An effort should always be made to minimize ovarian dose when this can be done without compromising tumor control. Lateral or midline ovarian transposition should be performed when it will permit shielding of one or both ovaries from the primary radiation beam. Midline oophoropexy has been used successfully to place the ovaries in a protected position behind a midline block in patients treated to the pelvis for Hodgkin's or non-Hodgkin's lymphoma (HORNING et al. 1981; LEFLOCH et al. 1976). When midline structures will be included in the treatment field, the ovary must be transposed laterally or superiorly some distance from the uterus. This may be accomplished by dividing the ovarian ligament and transecting the fallopian tube. The ovary is then mobilized by incising the peritoneum along the infundibulopelvic ligament, taking care not to injure the fragile venous plexus that follows the ovarian artery. The ovaries can then be repositioned laterally or superiorly even above the renal vessels, although such a distant transposition is usually not necessary. Ovarian transposition should always be considered when abdominal exploration is performed and may warrant a special procedure in a girl who will require future pelvic radiation, as this simple procedure can

avoid a lifetime of exogenous estrogenic support. However, lateral ovarian transposition has been associated with ovarian cysts and may make diagnosis of subsequent ovarian abnormalities more difficult (GABRIEL et al. 1986).

In children who have been treated to the pelvis, elevated serum follicle-stimulating hormone (FSH) values may give evidence of ovarian dysfunction well before the usual age of menarche (PERRONE et al. 1988; SHALET et al. 1976), although few follow-up data have been published concerning the outcome of girls with elevated prepubertal FSH levels. Girls who experience pubertal ovarian failure will require hormonal support to develop appropriate secondary sex characteristics, and women who have experienced premature ovarian failure require long-term support to avoid the deleterious effects of hypoestrogenism. Women who maintain ovarian function and wish to become pregnant after having been irradiated to the pelvis in childhood should be counseled about the possibility of an increased risk of miscarriage and premature delivery, particularly if the pelvic structures have received more than 20 Gy. In women with irreversible ovarian failure, pregnancies have been established through artificial endometrial stimulation and surrogate embryo transfer (NAVOT et al. 1986). There is little evidence that gonadal irradiation leads to an increased incidence of birth defects, although hereditary deficits may be associated with some childhood neoplasms (BYRNE et al. 1988; HORNING et al. 1981; LI et al. 1987; MULVIHILL et al. 1987; ORTIN et al. 1990).

3.11.2 Testis

A number of detailed studies have demonstrated the extreme sensitivity of the adult male testis to radiation. ROWLEY et al. (1974) reported impairment of seminiferous tubule function after single fraction doses as low as 0.2 Gy and evidence of Leydig cell dysfunction [elevated leutinizing hormone (LH) levels] at doses ≥ 0.75 Gy. In a careful study of the effects of low-dose scatter irradiation on testicular function of adult males treated for Hodgkin's disease, KINSELLA et al. (1989) found that testicular doses of 0.2–0.7 Gy caused a dose-dependent increase in serum FSH values, with a maximum rise 6 months after irradiation and a return to normal in all patients within 12–24 months following irradiation. There was no evidence of Leydig cell injury (as measured by LH and testosterone levels) following these doses. Another study of the effects of somewhat higher doses of scatter radiation (0.5–25 Gy) in adult men treated for soft tissue sarcomas demonstrated dose-dependent elevations of both serum LH and FSH values. Serial determinations demonstrated a gradual decline in elevated values, although values had not yet returned to normal 30 months after doses greater than 2 Gy to the testis. The apparently subtle Leydig cell dysfunction caused by these doses of radiation was not associated with any alteration in testosterone levels (SHAPIRO et al. 1985). Other authors have reported transient oligospermia in men receiving scatter doses to the testis from pelvic radiation with recovery as late as 2–3 years after treatment (HAHN et al. 1982; PEDRICK and HOPPE 1986). The time from treatment to the first recovery of sperm in the semen is clearly dose related (PEDRICK and HOPPE 1986; ROWLEY et al. 1974).

Much less information is available about the effects of testicular irradiation in childhood. In prepubertal boys, basal gonadotropin levels may remain normal despite severe testicular damage (SHALET et al. 1978). Prior to puberty, radiation-induced Leydig cell dysfunction can be assessed by measuring the testosterone response to human chorionic gonadotropin (HCG) stimulation (LEIPER et al. 1983). There are no detailed prospective studies of the effects of scatter doses of testicular irradiation in children. SHALET et al. described oligo- or azoospermia in eight of ten men who had received doses of 2.68–9.83 Gy (estimated retrospectively) at age 1–11 years. Only one patient had an elevated LH with a low plasma testosterone level, but HCG-stimulated LH levels were not measured in this study (SHALET et al. 1978). DONALDSON and KAPLAN (1982) reported that three of five boys who were 15 years old or younger at the time of treatment with pelvic radiotherapy (without chemotherapy) for Hodgkin's disease fathered normal children. Two others were oligospermic or azoospermic, and all five boys who also received MOPP chemotherapy were azoospermic.

Several investigators have studied the effects of direct testicular irradiation in boys with acute lymphoblastic leukemia (BLATT et al. 1980; BRAUNER et al. 1983; SHALET et al. 1985; SHAPIRO et al. 1985; SKLAR et al. 1990). SKLAR et al. found evidence of primary germ cell dysfunction in 55% of boys treated prophylactically with 12 Gy to the testes on Children's Cancer Study Group protocols. The authors note that this incidence, which was judged on the basis of elevated FSH levels and reduced testicular volume, probably represents an under-

estimate (SKLAR et al. 1990). Studies of boys treated for testicular relapse demonstrate that testosterone deficiency is a frequent complication of doses of 20–25 Gy, although some patients will maintain a compensated Leydig cell deficiency with normal testosterone levels for some time after irradiation. In a study of 11 boys, SHALET et al. (1985) reported an absent testosterone response to HCG stimulation in six of seven boys treated before puberty and a subnormal response in three of four treated during puberty. Two of the boys treated during puberty maintained normal basal levels of testosterone, and the author suggested that the pubertal testis may be more resistant to radiation-induced Leydig cell damage than the prepubertal testis. BLATT et al. (1980) described delayed sexual maturation and increased LH levels in three of seven boys treated with 24 Gy in 12 fractions. All three were among the four boys in their series who had had documented bilateral testicular involvement, and the authors suggested that damage done by leukemic infiltration could contribute to testicular damage. In boys treated for testicular leukemic involvement, the influence of direct testicular irradiation may also be confused by possible concurrent influences of cranial irradiation, nutritional influences, and multiagent chemotherapy.

The deleterious effects of chemotherapy, particularly alkylating agents, on adult male seminiferous tubular function are well documented and appear to be dose related (CHAPMAN et al. 1981; QURESHI et al. 1972; RICHTER et al. 1970). In their review, BYRNE et al. (1987) reported a 34% relative fertility compared with controls for men who had received alkylating agents as part of treatment for childhood malignancy. In children, both tubular and stromal cell function may be affected. SHERINS et al. (1978) found that 9 of 13 adolescent boys (aged 10–17 years) treated for Hodgkin's disease with MOPP alone had evidence of Leydig cell dysfunction with elevated levels of LH, decreased testosterone levels, and symptoms of gynecomastia that developed 1–3 years after treatment. Testicular biopsies from six of these boys revealed normal-appearing Leydig cells and no evidence of seminiferous tubular sclerosis despite complete germinal aplasia. Of four boys followed with serial LH levels, two had gradual normalization of LH levels and two did not. None of the six boys treated at less than 10 years of age had evidence of stromal cell dysfunction after a minimum follow-up of 2 years. In a detailed study of 75 boys treated with chemotherapy for Hodgkin's disease, BRÄMSWIG et al. (1990) found elevated basal levels of LH in 24%

and elevated stimulated LH levels in 88% despite apparently normal pubertal development and testosterone levels in all patients. The authors described a clear relationship between the cumulative dose of chemotherapy and the frequency of elevated basal LH and FSH levels.

Since dose-related testicular damage is observed even with very low doses of scatter radiation, treatment fields should always be designed to keep testicular doses at an absolute minimum consistent with adequate tumor coverage. Whenever the pelvis is treated, the collimator should coincide with the lower margin of the field to avoid even small amounts of transmission through secondary blocks. Additional secondary blocking at the lower margin of the field will reduce the dose from external scatter. Testicular shielding at the level of the patient is difficult in small children but may be helpful in adolescents. In older adolescents who are being treated to the upper thigh or hemipelvis, the scrotal contents may be positioned laterally to maximize their distance from the field. As they approach puberty, boys who have received testicular irradiation or treatment with alkylating agents should be followed with biochemical asessments of testicular function. Androgen replacement therapy will be required if there is no evidence of pubertal development by 13–14 years of age. In some areas sperm banking is available for older boys who are at high risk of becoming infertile as a result of treatment.

3.12 Breast

Although inhibition of normal breast development is often overlooked as a complication of radiotherapy, this is an expected and potentially distressing late side-effect of radiation to the nipple region of prepubertal girls. KOLAR et al. (1987) reported mild breast hypoplasia after doses as low as 300 R to the infant breast bud, and several authors have reported disturbed breast development in girls who received doses as low as 10 Gy with standard fractionation (DAWSON 1968; KOLAR et al. 1967; MOSS et al. 1979; RUBIN and CASARETT 1968). In KOLAR et al.'s series, three patients who received 40–100 R had no subsequent breast deformity. Breasts that are hypoplastic usually do not lactate during pregnancy. Although the scant literature on this subject stresses the influence of radiation to the breast buds during infancy, doses of 15–20 Gy also impair breast development in perimenarchal girls (MOSS et al. 1979), suggesting that, prior to puberty, age is probably

not an important factor. Little is known about the influence of radiation fractionation or of concurrent chemotherapy administration. Radiation fields that bisect the nipple region may cause hypoplasia of the treated portions of the breast with relatively normal development of the untreated quadrants (DAWSON 1968). MOSS et al. suggest that treatment of the soft tissue adjacent to the areola may also affect breast development, but little is known about the size of the region of importance or whether this expands during the perimenarchal period. Males who receive radiation to the nipple region may have hypoplastic development of the nipple-areolar complex during puberty (DAWSON 1968). The doses used for whole lung irradiation of children with Wilms' tumor and other pediatric neoplasms (10–20 Gy) are high enough to cause hypoplastic breast development although this has not yet been mentioned as a late complication in the National Wilms' Tumor Studies. Such patients would be expected to have symmetrical hypoplasia, which may be less noticeable than that caused by partial or unilateral irradiation.

Hypoplastic breast (or nipple) development should be mentioned as a possible complication to the parents of any child who will receive radiation therapy to the region of the nipple-areolar complex. The child's pediatrician should also be informed when the breast rudiment has been treated so that he or she can help to counsel the child when she reaches puberty. In some cases, plastic surgery may be indicated to improve cosmesis or symmetry.

3.13 Endocrine Effects

3.13.1 Thyroid

Much of the available data about radiation-related thyroid dysfunction has been derived from studies of patients treated for Hodgkin's disease. Most cases are asymptomatic, with compensated hypothyroidism manifested as an elevated serum thyrotropin (TSH) level but with normal T4 and T3 resin uptake (Table 3.2). A smaller proportion develop an uncompensated primary hypothyroidism. Most authors have found no correlation between patient age (within the pediatric group) and the incidence of thyroid dysfunction (CONSTINE et al. 1984; DEVNEY et al. 1984; KAPLAN et al. 1983), although GREEN et al. (1980) reported a correlation in a small series of patients. TARBELL et al. (1990) reported that, in their experience, Hodgkin's disease patients who were less

Table 3.2. Thyroid dysfunction after neck irradiation in children

Reference	No. of patients	% with elevated TSH	% with decreased T4	Neck dose (Gy)
Low dose				
Constine et al. (1984)	24	17	0	≤26[a]
Kaplan et al. (1983)	41	15	2	≤30
High dose				
Constine et al. (1984)	95	78	1	>26[b]
Kaplan et al. (1983)	50	68	6	>30
Green et al. (1980)	27	37	0	34–40
Devney et al. (1984)	24	88	24	44
Mauch et al. (1983)	37	57	5	36–40

TSH, thyroid-stimulating hormone
[a] Mean dose 22 Gy
[b] Mean dose 44 Gy

than 16 years of age at the time of treatment had a significantly greater actuarial risk of developing thyroid complications than those who were more than 16 years of age, and in general the rates of thyroid dysfunction reported in children who have received high-dose radiotherapy tend to be higher than those quoted for the adult population.

Both Constine et al. (1984) and Kaplan et al. (1983) have demonstrated a strong correlation between radiation dose and the incidence of thyroid dysfunction in children (Table 3.2). With continued follow-up, at least 20%–30% of children appear to have a normalization of initially elevated TSH levels (Constine et al. 1984; Devney et al. 1984). This may be an underestimate, because children are generally placed on thyroid replacement as soon as elevated TSH levels are detected; normalization may be discovered only as a result of noncompliance. For this reason, very little information is available about the time course of these changes. Estimates of the latency of thyroid dysfunction vary with the frequency of testing in different series. Constine et al. reported that 46% of abnormal values in their high-dose treatment group were detected within 2 years, 73% within 3 years, and 89% within 5 years of radiation.

Little information is available about the effect of radiation fractionation on thyroid complications. However, Sklar et al. (1982) reported a relatively high rate of thyroid dysfunction (43%) in a population of children and young adults treated with 7.5 Gy in a single fraction (26 cGy/min) of total body irradiation as part of a bone marrow transplant regimen. The authors suggested that the large fraction size may have been responsible for this but could not rule out the possible role of high-dose chemotherapy which was administered concurrently. Neither Constine et al. nor Kaplan et al. reported any greater risk of hypothyroidism in children who had received chemotherapy in addition to radiation.

The role of lymphangiography in the etiology of radiation-induced thyroid dysfunction remains incompletely understood. Both Schimpff et al. (1980) and Smith et al. (1981) reported an inverse correlation between the length of the time interval between lymphangiography and radiation treatment and the incidence of thyroid dysfunction in Hodgkin's patients. Glatstein et al. (1971) reported a higher incidence of thyroid dysfunction in children who had had a lymphangiogram, Green et al. reported a *lower* incidence, and Kaplan et al. (1983) and Tamura et al. (1981) found no correlation. The mechanism by which the slow release of iodine from the fat-soluble lymphangiogram preparation might potentiate radiation-induced hypothyroidism is unclear.

Hyperthyroidism similar to Graves' disease has been reported as a rare complication of treatment for Hodgkin's disease. Loeffler et al. (1988) reported seven cases in a series of 437 adult patients treated for Hodgkin's disease, for an actuarial risk at 10 years of 3.3% in females and 1% in males. All seven patients had classic symptoms of Graves' ophthalmopathy. Constine and McDougall (1982) reported one child who initially developed hypothyroidism following treatment but subsequently became hyperthyroid with classic symptoms of Graves' ophthalmopathy.

The follow-up of any child who has received radiation therapy to the neck should include periodic determinations of serum TSH, T4, and T3 resin uptake, as well as physical examination of the thyroid. In animal studies, thyrotropin has been demonstrated to play an important role in the development of radiation-induced thyroid tumors (LINDSAY and CHAIKOFF 1964) and although this association has been less clearly demonstrated in humans, it is still recommended that any patient who develops an elevated TSH following irradiation should be given thyroid replacement. Thyroxine administration during radiation therapy does not prevent dysfunction (BANTLE et al. 1985).

3.13.2 Parathyroid

A number of studies have documented the increased incidence of autonomous hyperparathyroidism caused by functioning parathyroid adenomas following head and neck irradiation (CHRISTENSSON 1978; NETELENBOS and VAN DER MEER 1983; RAO et al. 1980; TISELL et al. 1976, 1985). Incidental parathyroid adenomas are sometimes discovered at the time of thyroid surgery in normocalcemic patients who have received prior radiotherapy. The latency period for development of this complication is long, an average of 34 years (range 15–52) in a series reported by NETELENBOS and VAN DER MEER (1983) and 44 years (range 28–62) in a series reported by TISELL et al. (1985). The incidence of hyperparathyroidism appears to be dose-related with a frequency as high as 20%–30% (with long follow-up) in patients who receive more than 14 Gy to the neck (TISELL et al. 1985). TISELL et al. also reported a greater frequency in females and a somewhat higher incidence in patients less than 20 years of age at the time of treatment. Surgical removal of the adenoma is curative.

3.13.3 Pituitary/Hypothalamus

Although radiation may damage the pituitary gland directly, the hypothalamus is probably the major site of radiation injury. Studies of pituitary response to hypothalamic releasing factors demonstrate that irradiated patients often develop profound hypothalamic dysfunction in the absence of primary hypopituitarism (LUSTIG et al. 1985; SAMAAN et al. 1975). In a detailed study of hypothalamic and pituitary function in 110 patients treated with radiotherapy for nasopharyngeal and paranasal sinus cancers, SAMAAN et al. (1982) found some evidence of hypothalamic dysfunction in 27% of patients studied 1–2 years after treatment and in 98% of patients studied 5 years or more after radiotherapy. The results suggested primary pituitary failure in only 40%–50% of patients 3–10 years after treatment, despite pituitary doses that were generally higher than those delivered to the hypothalamus.

3.13.3.1 Growth Hormone Deficiency

Although production of all the anterior pituitary hormones may be affected by radiation, growth hormone (GH) deficiency is the most common abnormality in children. SAMAAN et al. (1975) found clinical evidence of growth failure in 21 of 27 children (78%) treated at 12 years of age or less with doses of 17–70 Gy. Their data revealed no clear relationship between the dose to the hypothalamus or pituitary gland and subsequent growth failure, although there were few children treated at the lower dose levels. CLAYTON and SHALET (1991) also found no relationship between dose and the late incidence of GH deficiency but reported a strong relationship between radiation dose and the speed of onset of GH deficiency during the first few years after treatment (CLAYTON and SHALET 1991). In a prospective study of GH responses to arginine and insulin stimulation, DUFFNER et al. (1985) found evidence of a blunted response within 1 year of radiation in seven of eight children treated for brain tumors with doses of 24–60 Gy to the hypothalamus and pituitary. However, three of the seven had a normal linear growth rate despite an abnormal GH response to stimulation.

Studies of the possible growth effects of relatively low doses of cranial irradiation used to prevent central nervous system relapse of leukemia are more controversial. In 1985, ROBISON et al. reported that the heights of children with acute lymphoblastic leukemia tended to fall below their pretreatment percentile levels 6–9 years after treatment with chemotherapy and 24 Gy to the brain. A number of factors other than radiotherapy may contribute to this, including chemotherapy, chronic illness, poor nutrition, and infection. SCHROICK et al. (1991) found that the amount of growth retardation was inversely correlated with the age of the child at diagnosis. Investigators who attempted to define the role of cranial irradiation have drawn various conclusions. Several studies have demonstrated that children may have a blunted response to an insulin tolerance test after prophylactic cranial irradiation. However, both SHALET et al. (1979) and SWIFT et al. (1978) have reported normal growth rates in children who received 24–25 Gy despite blunted GH responses, suggesting that subtle abnormalities in the GH response may not always indicate a need for GH therapy.

The importance of radiation dose and fractionation are not well defined. SHALET et al. (1979) found an abnormal GH response in 14 of 17 children who received cranial irradiation at a dose of 25 Gy at 2.5 Gy per fraction compared with one of nine children treated with 24 Gy at 1.2 Gy per fraction in 4 weeks, suggesting that the effect may be sensitive to fractionation. Studies using similar doses and fractionation have quoted very different rates of growth retardation (CLAYTON et al. 1988; KIRK et al. 1987). LITTLEY et al. (1991) conclude that this reflects the effects of different chemotherapy regimens. Studies comparing the effects of 18 Gy with those of 24 Gy have also drawn different conclusions (CICOGNANI et al. 1988; CLAYTON et al. 1988; STARCESKI et al. 1987).

In a study of ten girls treated with chemotherapy and 20–24 Gy cranial or craniospinal irradiation, MOËLL et al. (1987) observed normal growth during the premenarchal period but found that the girls had significant blunting of the pubertal growth spurt resulting in a final standing height 1 standard deviation less than would have been expected from their heights 1 year after completion of therapy. The results of SCHRIOCK et al. (1991) demonstrate a similar blunting of the pubertal growth spurt in males and females treated at less than 8 years of age.

During the last decade, many children with leukemia have been treated without any cranial irradiation, but few studies have been published about the growth effects of such treatment. In one small study of 30 children treated for acute leukemia without cranial irradiation, KATZ et al. (1991) found a decline in standardized height percentile during the first year postdiagnosis followed by a subsequent period of accelerated growth, resulting in absolute growth and growth velocity similar to normal children 5 years after treatment (KATZ et al. 1991). However, MÁRKY et al. (1991) demonstrated a similar pattern of catch-up growth in children who received treatment that included prophylactic brain irradiation (24 Gy). Their data also suggest that aggressive maintenance chemotherapy may suppress the period of accelerated growth usually seen during the second and third posttreatment year. MOËLL et al. (1984) reported similar patterns of growth retardation and recovery in irradiated and unirradiated children with leukemia. Ultimately,

large studies with a variety of chemotherapy regimens and with extended follow-up through the pubertal growth period are needed to define the impact of various factors on the growth of these children.

3.13.3.2 Hypogonadism

Hypogonadism may also result from high-dose irradiation of the hypothalamic-pituitary axis. SAMAAN et al. (1982) reported evidence of primary amenorrhea in six of ten girls over the age of 16 who were treated with high-dose radiotherapy prior to the age of menarche. SHALET et al. reported details of several cases of amenorrhea resulting from primary pituitary failure, from hypothalamic failure with decreased production of leuteinizing hormone releasing factor, or from hyperprolactinemia due to hypothalamic damage affecting the prolactine inhibitory center. In his study, most of the boys who had reached the age of puberty were also hypogonadal.

3.13.3.3 Precocious Puberty

Precocious puberty has been reported following treatment for primary brain tumors (BRAUNER et al. 1984; WINTER and GREEN 1985) and in a small proportion of children treated with prophylactic brain irradiation for lymphoblastic leukemia (LEIPER et al. 1987; MOËLL et al. 1987). The nature of the lesion that causes disturbed timing of pubertal development is not well understood. In children who have this complication, the age of pubertal onset tends to correlate with the child's age at the time of treatment (LEIPER et al. 1987; LITTLEY et al. 1991). Precocious puberty may contribute to short stature by accelerating epiphyseal maturity and shortening the length of time available for growth hormone treatment.

3.13.3.4 Hypothyroidism/Hypoadrenalism

Thyroid and adrenal function are affected less frequently than growth hormone (POMAREDE et al. 1984; SAMAAN et al. 1982). In SAMAAN et al.'s study, adrenal insufficiency was detected in 8 of 35 (23%) of the children studied. This was similar to the incidence quoted for adults in the study. Hypothyroidism was detected in 16 of 35 (46%) of the children studied but was most commonly seen in children who had also received a significant dose of irradiation to the thyroid region (9 of 14, 64%). Hypothyroidism was detected in 33% of the 21 children who did not have neck irradiation. The posterior pituitary is rarely affected clinically.

Any child who has received radiotherapy to the hypothalamic-pituitary axis must be regularly followed by an endocrinologist experienced in the management of such children. Growth hormone deficiency should be anticipated in any child who has received more than 40–50 Gy to the region. Growth deficiency should be identified and treated promptly. Children with combined deficiencies pose particularly challenging management problems. Aggressive treatment of delayed puberty may contribute to short stature by accelerating epiphyseal maturation.

References

Abrams R, Lichter A, Bromer R, Minna J, Cohen M, Deisseroth A (1985) The hematopoietic toxicity of regional radiation therapy. Correlations for combined modality therapy with systemic chemotherapy. Cancer 55: 1429–1435

Ahmed S, Shalet S, Campbell R, Deakin D (1983) Primary gonadal damage following treatment of brain tumors in childhood. J Pediatr 103: 562–565

Alberti W (1991) Effects of radiation on the eye and ocular adnexa. In: Scherer E, Streffer C, Trott K (eds) Radiopathology of organs and tissues. Springer, Berlin Heidelberg New York, pp 269–282

Applefield M, Cole J, Pollock S, Sutton F, Slawson R, Singleton R, Wiernik P (1981) The late appearance of chronic pericardial disease in patients treated by radiotherapy for Hodgkin's disease. Ann Intern Med 94: 338–341

Aristizabal S, Caldwell W, Avita J (1977) The relationship of time-dose fractionation factors of complications in the treatment of pituitary tumors by irradiation. Int J Radiat Oncol Biol Phys 2: 667–673

Austin-Seymour M, Chen G, Castro J, Saunders W, Pitludk S, Woodruff K, Kessler M (1986) Dose volume histogram analysis of liver radiation tolerance. Int J Radiat Oncol Biol Phys 12: 31–35

Baker T (1971) Radiosensitivity of mammalian oocytes with particular reference to the human female. Obstet Gynecol 110: 746–761

Bantle J, Lee C, Levitt S (1985) Thyroxine administration during radiation therapy to the neck does not prevent subsequent thyroid dysfunction. Int J Radiat Oncol Biol Phys 11: 1999–2002

Barrett A, Depledge M, Powles R (1987) Interstitial pneumonitis following bone marrow transplantation after low dose rate total body irradiation. Int J Radiat Oncol Biol Phys 9: 1029–1033

Benoist M, Lemerle J, Jean R (1982) Effects on pulmonary function of whole lung irradiation for Wilms' tumor in children. Thorax 37: 175–180

Birkhead B, Dobbs C, Beard M, Tyson J, Fuller E (1979) Assessment of renal function following irradiation of the intact spleen for Hodgkin's disease. Radiology 130: 473–475

Blatt J, Sherins R, Niebrugge D, Bleyer W, Poplack D (1980) Leydig cell function in boys following treatment for testicular relapse of lymphoblastic leukemia. J Clin Oncol 3: 1227–1231

Boal D, Newburger P, Teele R (1979) Esophagitis induced by combined radiation Adriamycin. Am J Roentgenol 132: 567–570

Boivin J, Hutchison G (1982) Coronary heart disease mortality after irradiation for Hodgkin's disease. Cancer 49: 2470–2475

Brämswig J, Heimes U, Heiermann E, Schlegel W, Nieschlag E, Schellong G (1990) The effects of different cumulative doses of chemotherapy on testicular function. Results in 75 patients treated for Hodgkin's disease during childhood or adolescence. Cancer 65: 1298–1302

Brauner R, Czernichow P, Cramer PH, Schaison G, Rappaport R (1983) Leydig-cell function in children after direct testicular irradiation for acute lymphoblastic leukemia. N Engl J Med 309: 25–28

Brauner R, Czernichow P, Rappaport R (1984) Precocious puberty after hypothalamic and pituitary irradiation in young children. N Engl J Med 311: 920

Breuer K, Cohen P, Schweisguth O, Hart A (1978) Irradiation of the lungs as an adjuvant therapy in the treatment of osteosarcoma of the limbs. An E.O.R.T.C. randomized study. Eur J Cancer 14: 461–471

Brill A, Martin M, Fitz-Hugh G, Constable W (1974) Postoperative and postradiotherapeutic serous otitis media. Arch Otolaryngol 99: 406–408

Britten M, Halnan K, Meredith W (1966) Radiation cataract—new evidence on radiation dosage to the lens. Br J Radiol 39: 612–617

Brock P, Bellman S, Yeomans E, Pinkerton C, Pritchard J (1991) Cisplatin ototoxicity in children: a practical grading system. Med Pediatr Oncol 19: 295–300

Brooks H, Meyer D, Shields J, Balas A, Nelson L, Fontanesi J (1990) Removal of radiation-induced cataracts in patients treated for retinoblastoma. Arch Ophthamol 108: 1701–1708

Brosius F III, Waller B, Roberts W (1981) Radiation heart disease. Analysis of 16 young (aged 15–33 years) necropsy patients who received over 3,500 rads to the heart. Am J Med 70: 519–530

Brown G, Shields J, Sanborn G, Augsburger J, Savino P, Schatz N (1982) Radiation optic neuropathy. Ophthalmology 89: 1489–1493

Button L, DeWolf WC, Newburger P, Jacobsen M, Kevy S (1981) The effects of irradiation on blood components. Transfusion 21: 419–426

Byhardt R, Brace K, Ruckdeschel J, Chang P, Martin R, Wiernik P (1975) Dose and treatment factors in radiation-related pericardial effusion associated with the mantle technique for Hodgkin's disease. Cancer 35: 795

Byrne J, Mulvihill J, Myers M et al. (1987) Effects of treatment on fertility in long-term survivors of childhood or adolescent cancer. N Engl J Med 317: 1315–1321

Byrne J, Mulvihill J, Connelly R et al. (1988) Reproductive problems and birth defects in survivors of Wilms' tumor and their relatives. Med Pediatr Oncol 16: 233–240

Call G, Bray P, Smoker W, Buys S, Hays J (1990) Carotid thrombosis following neck irradiation. Int J Radiat Oncol Biol Phys 18: 635–640

Carmel R, Kaplan H (1976) Mantle irradiation in Hodgkin's disease. Cancer 37: 2813–2825

Cassady J, Richter M, Piro A, Jaffe N (1975) Radiation-Adriamycin interactions: preliminary clinical observations. Cancer 36: 946–949

Cassady J, Lebowitz R, Jaffe N, Hoffman A (1981) Effect of low dose irradiation on renal enlargement in children following nephrectomy for Wilms' tumor. Acta Radiol Oncol 20: 5–8

Castellino R, Glatstein E, Turbow M, Rosenberg S, Kaplan H (1974) Latent radiation injury of lungs or heart activated by steroid withdrawal. Ann Intern Med 80: 593–599

Chan R, Shukovsky L (1976) Effects of irradiation on the eye. Radiology 120: 673–675

Chapman R, Sutcliffe S, Malpas J (1981) Male gonadal dysfunction in Hodgkin's disease. JAMA 245: 1323–1328

Christensson T (1978) Hyperparathyroidism and radiation therapy. Ann Intern Med 89: 216–217

Cicognani A, Cacciar E, Vecchi V (1988) Differential effects of 18- and 24-Gy cranial irradiation on growth rate and growth hormone release in children with prolonged survival after acute lymphocytic leukemia. Am J Dis Child 142: 1199–1202

Clayton P, Shalet S (1991) Dose dependency of time of onset of radiation-induced growth-hormone deficiency. J Pediatr 118: 226–228

Clayton P, Shalet S, Morris-Jones PDA (1988) Growth in children treated for acute lymphoblastic leukemia. Lancet I: 460–462

Cohen I, Loven D, Schoenfeld T, Sandbank J, Kapilinsky C, Yaniv Y, Jaber L, Zaizov R (1991) Dactinomycin potentiation of radiation pneumonitis: a forgotten interaction. Pediatr Hematol Oncol 8: 187–192

Cohn D, Stewart J, Fajardo L, Hancock E (1967) Heart disease following radiation. Medicine 46: 281–298

Colquhoun J (1966) Hypoplasia of abdominal aorta following therapeutic irradiation in infancy. Radiology 86: 454–456

Conger A (1973) Loss and recovery of taste acuity in patients irradiated to the oral cavity. Radiat Res 53: 338–347

Constine L, McDougall I (1982) Radiation therapy for Hodgkin's disease followed by hypothyroidism and then Graves' hyperthyroidism. Clin Nucl Med 7: 69–70

Constine L, Donaldson S, McDougall R, Cox R, Link M, Kaplan H (1984) Thyroid dysfunction after radiotherapy in children with Hodgkin's disease. Cancer 53: 878–883

Cosset J, Henry-Amar M, Pelae-Cosset B, Carde P, Girinski T, Tubiana M, Hayat M (1991) Pericarditis and myocardial infarctions after Hodgkin's disease therapy. Int J Radiat Oncol Biol Phys 21: 447–449

Cowell B (19660 The value of early diagnosis and treatment in slipped femoral capital epiphysis. Clin Orthop 48: 89–92

Cristy M (1981) Active bone marrow distribution as a function of age in humans. Phys Med Biol 26: 389–400

Dailey M, Coleman C, Kaplan H (1980) Radiation-induced splenic atrophy in patients with Hodgkin's disease and non-Hodgkin's lymphoma. N Engl J Med 3002: 215–217

D'Angio G, Farber S, Maddock C (1959) Potentiation of x-ray effects by actinomycin-D. Radiology 73: 175–177

Dawson W (1968) Growth impairment following radiotherapy in childhood. Clin Radiol 19: 241–256

Deeg H, Flournoy N, Sullivan D (1984) Cataracts after total body irradiation and marrow transplantation: a sparing effect of dose fractionation. Int J Radiat Oncol Biol Phys 10: 957–964

Deeg H, Sullivan K, Buckner C et al. (1986) Marrow transplantation for acute non lymphoblastic leukemia in first remission: toxicity and long-term follow-up of patients

conditioned with single dose or fractionated total body irradiation. Bone Marrow Transplant 1: 151–157

Devney R, Sklar C, Nesbit M, Kim T, Williamson J, Robison L, Ramsay N (1984) Serial thyroid function measurements in children with Hodgkin's disease. J Pediatr 105: 223

Dias A (1966) Effects on the hearing of patients treated by irradiation in the head and neck area. J Laryngol 80: 276–287

Dickerman J, Newberg A, Moreland M (1979) Slipped capital femoral epiphysis (SCFE) following pelvic irradiation for rhabdomyosarcoma. Cancer 44: 480–482

Donaldson S, Kaplan H (1982) Complications of treatment of Hodgkin's disease in children. Cancer Treat Rep 66: 977–989

Donaldson S, Glick J, Wilbur J (1974) Adriamycin activating a recall phenomenon after radiation therapy. Ann Intern Med 81: 407–408

Donaldson S, Jundt S, Ricour C, Sarrazin D, Lemerle J, Schweisguth O (1975) Radiation enteritis in children. Cancer 35: 1167–1178

Donaldson S, Moskowitz P, Canty E, Efron B (1978) Radiation-induced inhibition of compensatory renal growth in the weanling mouse kidney. Radiology 128: 491–495

Donaldson S, Moskowitz P, Canty E, Fajardo L (1980) Combination radiation-adriamycin therapy: renoprival growth, functional and structural effects in the immature mouse. Int J Radiat Oncol Biol Phys 6: 851–859

Dreizen S, Brown L, Handler S, Levy B (1976) Radiation-induced xerostomia in cancer patients. Cancer 38: 273–278

Duffner P, Cohen M, Voorhess M, MacGillivray M, Brecher M, Panahon A, Gilani B (1985) Long-term effects of cranial irradiation on endocrine function in children with brain tumors: a prospective study. Cancer 56: 2189–2193

Egbert P, Donaldson S, Moazed K, Rosenthal A (1978) Visual results and ocular complications following radiotherapy for retinoblastoma. Arch Ophthalmol 96: 1826–1830

Eifel P, Sampson C, Tucker S (1990) Radiation fractionation sensitivity of epiphysial cartilage in a weanling rat model. Int J Radiat Oncol Biol Phys 19: 661–664

Ellis E, Marcus R, Cicale M et al. (1992) Pulmonary function tests after whole-lung irradiation and doxorubicin in patients with osteogenic sarcoma. J Clin Oncol 10: 459–463

Endrees G, Luts A, Stewart F (1988) Bladder damage in mice after combined treatment with cyclophosphamide and x-rays. The influence of timing and sequence. Radiother Oncol 11: 349–360

Eneroth C, Henrickson C, Jakobsson P (1971) Effect of fractionated radiotherapy on salivary gland function. Cancer 30: 1147–1153

Evans A, Norkool P, Evans I, Breslow N, D'Angio G (1991) Late effects of treatment for Wilms' tumor. A report from the National Wilms' Tumor Study Group. Cancer 67: 331–336

Fajardo L (1982) Pathology of radiation injury. Masson, New York Fajardo L, Berthrong M (1976) Combined cardiotoxicity of Adriamycin and X-irradiation. Lab Invest 34: 159–199

Filler R, Tefft M, Vawter G (1970) Hepatic lobectomy in childhood: effects of X-ray and chemotherapy. J Pediatr Surg 4: 31–41

Fisher B, Cheung A (1984) Delayed effect of radiation therapy with or without chemotherapy on ovarian function in women with Hodgkin's disease. Acta Radiol Oncol 23: 43–48

Fletcher B, Hanna S, Kun L (1990) Changes in MR signal intensity and contrast enhancement of therapeutically irradiated soft tissue. Magn Reson Imaging 8: 771–777

Fletcher G, Maccomb W, Ballantyne A (1962) Radiation therapy in the management of cancer of the oral cavity and oropharynx. Charles C. Thomas, Springfield, Ill.

Fliedner T, Nothdurft W (1986) Cytological indicators: haematopoietic effects. In: Kaul A, Dehos A, Bögl W et al. (eds) Biological indicators for radiation dose assessment. MMV Medizin, Munich, pp 123–156

Fryer C, Hutchinson R, Krailo M et al. (1990) Efficacy and toxicity of 12 courses of ABVD chemotherapy followed by low-dose regional radiation in advanced Hodgkin's disease in children: a report from the Childrens Cancer Study Group. J Clin Oncol 8: 1971–1980

Gabriel D, Bernard S, Lambert J, Croom R III (1986) Oophoropexy and the management of Hodgkin's disease. A reevaluation of the risks and benefits. Arch Surg 121: 1083–1085

Gagnon J, Ware C, Moss W, Stevens K (1980) Radiation management of bilateral retinoblastoma: the need to preserve vision. Int J Radiat Oncol Biol Phys 6: 669–673

Geraci J, Jackson K, Mariam M, Leitch J (1985) Hepatic injury after whole-liver irradiation in the rat. Radiat Res 101: 508–518

Gerlock AJ, Goncharenko V, Edelund L (1977) Radiation-induced stenosis of the renal artery causing hypertension: case report. J Urol 118: 1064–1065

Glatstein E, McHardy-Young S, Brast N, Eltringham J, Kriss J (1971) Alterations in serum thyrotropin (TSH) and thyroid function following radiotherapy in patients with malignant lymphoma. J Clin Endocrinol Metabol 32: 833–841

Glatstein E, Fajardo L, Brown J (1977) Radiation injury in the mouse kidney. I. Sequential light microscopic study. Int J Radiat Oncol Biol Phys 2: 933–943

Gonzalez D, Breuer K (1983) Clinical data from irradiated growing long bones in children. Int J Radiat Oncol Biol Phys 9: 841–846

Gonzalez D, van Dijk J (1983) Experimental studies on the response of growing bones to x ray and neutron irradiation. Int J Radiat Oncol Biol Phys 9; 671–677

Gottdiener J, Katin M, Borer J, Bacharach S, Green M (1983) Late cardiac effects of therapeutic mediastinal irradiation. Assessment by echocardiography and radionuclide angiography. N Engl J Med 308: 569–572

Grau C, Møller K, Overgaard M, Overgaard J, Elbrønd O (1991) Sensori-neural hearing loss in patients treated with irradiation for nasopharyngeal carcinoma. Int J Radiat Oncol Biol Phys 21: 723–728

Greco F, Brereton H, Dent H, Zimbler H, Merrill J, Johnson R (1976) Adriamycin and enhanced radiation reaction in normal esophagus and skin. Ann Intern Med 85: 294–298

Green D, Brecher M, Yakar D et al. (1980) Thyroid function in pediatric patients after neck irradiation for Hodgkin's disease. Med pediatr Oncol 8: 127–136

Green D, Finklestein J, Tefft M, Norkool P (1989) Diffuse interstitial pneumonitis after pulmonary irradiation for metastatic Wilms' tumor. A report from the National Wilms' Tumor Study. Cancer 63: 450–453

Green D, Norkool P, Breslow N, Finkelstein J, D'Angio G (1990) Severe hepatic toxicity after treatment with vincristine and dactinomycin using single-dose or divided-dose schedules: a report from the National Wilms' Tumor Study. J Clin Oncol 8: 1525–1530

Gross N (1980) Experimental radiation pneumonitis IV.

Leakage of circulatory proteins onto the alveolar surface. J Lab Clin Med 95: 19–31

Guyuron B, Dagys A, Munro I, Ross R (1983) Effect of irradiation on facial growth: a 7–25 year follow-up. Ann Plast Surg 11: 423–427

Hahn E, Feingold S, Simpson L, Batata M (1982) Recovery from aspermia induced by low-dose radiation in seminoma patients. Cancer 50: 337–340

Hancock S, Hoppe R (1992) Heart disease mortality after treatment of Hodgkin's disease. Int J Radiat Oncol Biol Phys 24:Suppl 1: 240

Harnett A, Hirst A, Plowman P (1987) The eye in acute leukaemia. 1. Dosimetric analysis in cranial radiation prophylaxis. Radiother Oncol 10: 195–202

Harris J, Levene M (1976) Visual complications following irradiation for pituitary adenomas and craniopharyngiomas. Radiology 104: 629–634

Heaston D, Libshitz H, Chan R (1979) Skeletal effects of megavoltage irradiation in survivors of Wilms' tumor. Am J Roentgenol 133: 389–395

Henkin R (1972) Prevention and treatment of hypogeusia due to head and neck irradiation. JAMA 220: 870–871

Heyn R, Ragab A, Raney R (1986) Late effects of therapy in orbital rhabdomyosarcoma in children: a report from the Intergroup Rhabdomyosarcoma Study. Cancer 57: 1738–1743

Hill D, Benak S, Phillips T, Price D (1980) Bone marrow regeneration following fractionated radiation therapy. Int J Radiat Oncol Biol Phys 6: 1149–1155

Hinkel C (1943a) The effect of irradiation upon the composition and vascularity of growing rat bones. Am J Roentgenol Radiat Therapy 50: 516–526

Hinkel C (1943b) The effect of roentgen rays upon the growing long bones of albino rats. II. Histopathological changes involving endochondral growth centers. Am J Roentgenol Radiat Therapy 49: 321–348

Horning S, Hoppe R, Kaplan H, Rosenberg S (1981) Female reproductive potential after treatment of Hodgkin's disease. N Engl J Med 304: 1377–1382

Hyams J, Batrus C, Grand R, Sallan S (1982) Cancer chemotherapy-induced lactose malabsorption in children. Cancer 49: 646–650

Ihde D, DeVita V (1975) Osteonecrosis of the femoral head in patients with lymphoma treated with intermittent combination chemotherapy. Cancer 36: 1585–1588

Ingld J, Reed G, Kaplan H, Bagashaw M (1963) Radiation hepatitis. Am J Roentgenol 93: 200–208

Jaffe N, Toth B, Hoar R (1984) Dental and maxillofacial abnormalities in long-term survivors of childhood cancer: effects of treatment with chemotherapy and radiation to the head and neck. Pediatrics 73: 816–823

Jayalakshmamma B, Pinkel D (1976) Urinary bladder toxicity following pelvic irradiation and simultaneous cyclophosphamide therapy. Cancer 38: 701–707

Jentzsch K, Binder H, Cramer H et al. (1981) Leg function after radiotherapy for Ewing's sarcoma. Cancer 47: 1267–1278

Joiner M, Johns H (1988) Renal damage in the mouse: the response to very small doses per fraction. Radiat Res 114: 385–398

Jones L (1966) The lacrimal system and its treatment. Am J Ophthalmol 62: 47–70

Jongejan H, van der Koegel A, Provoost A, Molenaar J (1987) Interaction of cis-diamminedichloroplatin and renal irradiation on renal function in the young and adult rat. Radiother Oncol 10: 49–57

Jordan S, Key C, Gomez L, Agnew J, Barton S (1978) Late effects of radiation on the mouse kidney. Exp Mol Pathol 29: 115–129

Kaplan M, Garnick M, Gelber R et al. (1983) Risk factors for thyroid abnormalities after neck irradiation for childhood cancer. Am J Med 74: 272

Katz J, Chambers B, Everhart C, Marks J, Buchanan G (1991) Linear growth in children with acute lymphoblastic leukemia treated without cranial irradiation. J Pediatr 118; 575–578

Katzman H, Waugh T, Berdon W (1969) Skeletal changes following irradiation of childhood tumors. J Bone Joint Surg 51: 825

Keane T, van Dyke J, Rider W (1981) Idiopathic interstitial pneumonia following bone marrow transplantation: the relationship with total body irradiation. Int J Radiat Oncol Biol Phys 7: 1365–1370

Keane W, Crosson J, Staley N, Anderson W, Shapiro F (1976) Radiation-induced renal disease: a clinico-pathologic study. Am J Med 60: 127–137

Kember N (1971) Cell population kinetics of bone growth: the first ten years of autoradiographic studies with tritiated thymidine. Cline Orthop 76: 213–230

Kember N (1972) Comparative patterns of cell division in epiphyseal cartilage plates in the rat. J Anat 111: 137–142

Kember N (1978) Cell kinetics and the control of growth in long bones. Cell Tissue Kinet 11: 477–485

Kember N, Sissons H (1976) Quantitative histology of the human growth plate. J Bone Joint Surg [Br] 58: 426–435

Khan A, D'Souza B, Wharam M (1982) Cisplatinum therapy in recurrent childhood brain tumors. Cancer Treat Rep 66: 2013–2020

King J, Stowe S (1982) Results of spinal fusion for radiation scoliosis. Spine 7: 574 585

Kinsella T, Bloomer W (1980) Tolerance of the intestine to radiation therapy. Surg Gynecol Obstet 151: 273–284

Kinsella T, Trivette G, Rowland J et al. (1989) Long-term follow-up of testicular function following radiation therapy for early-stage Hodgkin's disease. J Clin Oncol 7: 718–724

Kirk J, Raghupathy P, Stevens M et al. (1987) Growth failure and growth hormone deficiency after treatment for acute lymphoblastic leukemia. Lancet I: 190–193

Kline L, Kim J, Ceballos R (1985) Radiation optic neuropathy. Ophthalmology 92: 1118–1126

Kline R, Gerlin M, Kun L (1979) Cranial irradiation in acute leukemia: dose estimate in the lens. Int J Radiat Oncol Biol Phys 5: 117–121

Knowlton A, Percarpio B, Bobrow S, Fischer J (1975) Methotrexate and radiation therapy in the treatment of advanced head and neck tumors. Radiology 116: 709–712

Kolar J, Bed V, Vrabec R (1967) Hypoplasia of the infant breast. Arch Dermatol 96: 427–432

Kolin E, Sherry H (1987) Avascular necrosis of the femoral head in patients being treated for malignancy. Mount Sinai J Med 54: 516–521

Kretschmar C, Warren M, Lavally B, Dyer S, Tarbell N (1990) Ototoxicity of preradiation cisplatin for children with central nervous system tumors. J Clin Oncol 8: 1191–1198

Kun L, Camitta B (1978) Hepatopathy following irradiation and Adriamycin. Cancer 42: 81–84

Kunkler P, Farr R, Luxton R (1952) The unit of renal tolerance to x-rays. Br J Radiol 25: 190–201

Lagrange J, Darcourt J, Benoliel J, Bensadoun R, Migneco O (1992) Acute cardiac effects of mediastinal irradiation: assessment by radionuclide angiography. Int J Radiat Oncol Biol Phys 22: 897–903

LeBourgeois J, Meignan M, Parmentier C, Tubiana M (1979) Renal consequences of irradiation of the spleen in lymphoma patients. Br J Radiol 52: 56–60

Lederman G, Sheldon T, Chaffey J, Herman T, Gelman R, Coleman C (1987) Cardiac disease after mediastinal irradiation for seminoma. Cancer 60: 772–776

LeFloch O, Donaldson S, Kaplan H (1976) Pregnancy following oophoropexy and total nodal irradiation in women with Hodgkin's disease. Cancer 38: 2263–2268

Leiper A, Grant D, Chessells J (1983) The effect of testicular irradiation on Leydig cell function in prepubertal boys with acute lymphoblastic leukemia. Arch Dis Child 58: 906–910

Leiper A, Stanhope R, Kitching P, Chessells J (1987) Precocious and premature puberty associated with the treatment of acute lymphoblastic leukemia. Arch Dis Child 62: 1107–1112

Li F, Gimbrere K, Gelber R et al. (1987) Outcome of pregnancy in survivors of Wilms' tumor. JAMA 257: 216–219

Libshitz H, Edeikin B (1981) Radiotherapy changes of the pediatric hip. Am J Roentgenol 137: 585–588

Lindsay S, Chaikoff I (1964) The effects of irraidation on the thyroid gland with particular reference to the induction of thyroid neoplasms: a review. Cancer Res 24: 1099–1107

Lipshultz S, Colan S, Sanders S (1989) Late myocardial growth impairment in children treated with adriamycin. Am J Cardiol 64: 416

Lipshultz S, Colan S, Walsh E (1990) Ventricular tachycardia and sudden unexplained death in late survivors of childhood malignancy treated with doxorubicin. Pediatr Res 27: 145

Littley M, Shalet S, Beardwell C (1991) Radiation and the hypothalamic-pituitary axis. In: Gutin P, Leibel S, Sheline G (eds) Radiation injury to the nervous system. Raven, New York, pp 303–324

Littman P, Meadows A, Polgar G, Borns P, Rubin E (1976) Pulmonary function in survivors of Wilms' tumor. Patterns of impairment. Cancer 37: 2773–2776

Ljungqvist A, Unge G, Lagergren C, Notter G (1971) The intrarenal vascular alterations in radiation nephritis and their relationship to the development of hypertension. Acta Pathol Microbiol Scand 79: 629–638

Loeffler J, Tarbell N, Garber J, Mauch P (1988) The development of Graves' disease following radiation therapy in Hodgkin's disease. Int J Radiat Oncol Biol Phys 14: 175–178

Lushbaugh C, Casarett G (1976) The effects of gonadal irradiation in clinical radiation therapy. A review. Cancer 37: 1111–1120

Lustig R, Schriock E, Kaplan S, Grumbach M (1985) Effect of growth hormone releasing factor on growth hormone release in children with radiation-induced growth hormone deficiency. Pediatrics 76: 274–279

Luxton R, Kunkler P (1964) Radiation nephritis. Acta Radiol 2: 169–178

Maguire A, Craft A, Evans R (1987) The long-term effects of treatment on the dental condition of children surviving malignant disease. Cancer 60: 2570–2575

Mah K, Van Dyk J, Keane T, Poon P (1987) Acute radiation-induced pulmonary damage: a clinical study on the response to fractionated radiation therapy. Int J Radiat Oncol Biol Phys 13: 179–188

Margileth D, Poplack D, Pizzo P, Leventhal B (1977) Blindness during remission in two patients with acute lymphoblastic leukemia. Cancer 39: 58–61

Marks J, Davis C, Gottsman V, Purdy J, Lee F (1981) The

effects of radiation on parotid salivary function. Int J Radiat Oncol Biol Phys 7: 1013–1019

Marky I, Samuelsson B, Mellander L, Karlberg J (1991) Longitudinal growth in children with non-Hodgkin's lymphoma and children with acute lymphoblastic leukemia: comparison between unirradiated and irradiated patients. Med Pediatr Oncol 19: 96–99

Mascarin M, Giavitto M, Zanazzo G, Andolina M, Cova M, Accorsi E, Tamaro P (1991) Avascular necrosis of bone in children undergoing allogeneic bone marrow transplantation. Cancer 68: 655–659

Mauch P, Weinstein H, Botnick L, Belli J, Cassady J (1983) An evaluation of long-term survival and treatment complications in children with Hodgkin's disease. Cancer 51: 925–932

McGill C, Holder T, Smith T, Ashcraft K (1979) Postradiation renovascular hypertension. J Pediatr Surg 14: 831–833

Mefferd J, Donaldson S, Link M (1989) Pediatric Hodgkin's disease: pulmonary, cardiac, and thyroid function following combined modality therapy. Int J Radiat Oncol Biol Phys 16: 679–685

Merriam G, Focht E (1957) A clinical study of radiation cataracts and the relationship to dose. Am J Roentgenol Radiat Ther Nucl Med 77: 759–785

Merriam G, Szechter A, Focht E (1972) The effects of ionizing radiations on the eye. Front Radiat Ther Oncol 6: 346–385

Meyers J, Flournoy N, Wade J, Hackman R, McDougall J, Neiman P, Thomas E (1983) Biology of interstitial pneumonia after marrow transplantation. In: Gale R (ed) Recent advances in bone marrow transplantation. Alan R. Liss, New York, pp 405–423

Mill W, Baglan R, Kurichety P, Prasad S, Lee J, Moller R (1984) Symptomatic radiation-induced pericarditis in Hodgkin's disease. Int J Radiat Oncol Biol Phys 10: 2061–2065

Milutinovic J, Darcy M, Thompson K (1990) Radiation-induced renovascular hypertension successfully treated with transluminal angioplasty: case report. Cardiovasc Intervent Radiol 13: 29–31

Mira J, Westcott W, Starcke E, Shannon J (1981) Some factors influencing salivary function when treating with radiotherapy. Int J Radiat Oncol Biol Phys 7: 535–541

Mitus A, Tefft J, Fellers G (1969) Long-term followup of renal functions of 108 children who underwent nephrectomy for malignant disease. Pediatrics 44: 912–921

Moëll C, Garwicz S, Westgren U, Aronsson A, Wiebe T, Landberg T (1984) Height, weight and growth hormone secretion in children treated for acute leukemia. Eur Pediatr Haematol Oncol 1: 167–172

Moëll C, Garwicz S, Westgren U, Wiebe T (1987) Disturbed pubertal growth in girls treated for acute lymphoblastic leukemia. Pediatr Hematol Oncol 4: 1–5

Morgan E, Baum E, Breslow N, Takashima J, D'Angio G (1988) Chemotherapy-related toxicity in infants treated according to the second National Wilms' Tumor Study. J Clin Oncol 6: 51–55

Morgan G, Freeman A, McLean R, Jarvie B, Giles R (1985) Late cardiac, thyroid, and pulmonary sequelae of mantle radiotherapy for Hodgkin's disease. Int J Radiat Oncol Biol Phys 11: 1925–1931

Morris L, Cassady J, Jaffe N (1975) Sternal changes following mediastinal irradiation for childhood Hodgkin's disease. Radiology 115: 701

Moskowitz P, Donaldson S, Canty E (1980) Chemotherapy-induced inhibition of compensatory renal growth in the immature mouse. Am J Radiol 134: 491–496

Moss W, Brand W, Battifora H (1979) Radiation oncology. Rationale, technique, results. C.V. Mosby, St. Louis

Mossman K, Henkin R (1978) Radiation-induced changes in taste acuity in cancer patients. Int J Radiat Oncol Biol Phys 4: 663–670

Mossman K, Shatzman A, Chencharick J (1982) Long-term effects of radiotherapy on taste and salivary function in man. Int J Radiat Oncol Biol Phys 8: 991–997

Moulder J, Holcenberg J, Kamen B, Cheng M, Fish B (1986) Renal irradiation and the pharmacology and toxicity of methotrexate and cisplatinum. Int J Radiat Oncol Biol Phys 12: 1415–1418

Mulvihill J, McKeen E, Rosner F, Zarrabi M (1987) Pregnancy outcome in cancer patients. Cancer 60: 1143–1150

Navot D, Laufer N, Kopopovic J et al. (1986) Artificially induced endometrial cycles and establishment of pregnancies in the absence of ovaries. N Engl J Med 314: 806–811

Neiman P, Reeves W, Ray G, Flournoy N, Lorner K, Sale G, Thomas E (1977) A prospective analysis of interstitial pneumonia and opportunistic viral infection among recipients of allogenic bone marrow grafts. J Infect Dis 136: 754–767

Netelenbos C, van der Meer C (1983) Hyperparathyroidism following irradiation of benign diseases of the head and neck. Cancer 52: 458–461

Neuhauser E, Wittenborg M, Berman C, Cohen J (1952) Irradiation effects of roentgen therapy on the growing spine. Radiology 59: 637–650

Newburger P, Cassady J, Jaffe N (1978) Esophagitis due to adriamycin and radiation therapy for childhood malignancy. Cancer 42: 417–423

Nothdurft W (1991) Bone marrow. In: Scherer E, Steffer C, Trott K (eds) Radiopathology of organs and tissues. Springer Berlin Heidelberg New York, pp 113–169

Novotny O (1951) Sull'azione dei raggi X sulla chiocciola della cavia. Arch Ital Otol 62: 15–19

Nybonde T, Eklüf O, Bjürk O (1988) Wilms' tumor complicated by veno-occlusive disease of the liver (VOD): current concepts and a case report. Pediatr Hematol Oncol 5: 53–60

Oliver J, Gluck G, Gledhill R, Chevalier L (1978) Musculoskeletal deformities following treatment of Wilms' tumour. Can Med Assoc J 119: 459–464

Ophir D, Guuerman A, Gross-Isseroff R (1988) Changes in smell acuity induced by radiation exposure of the olfactory mucosa. Arch Otolaryngol 114: 853–855

Ortin T, Shostak C, Donaldson S (1990) Gonadal status and reproductive function following treatment for Hodgkin's disease in childhood: the Stanford experience. Int J Radiat Oncol Biol Phys 19: 873–880

Parmentier C, Morardet N, Tubiana M (1983) Late effects on human bone marrow after extended field radiotherapy. Int J Radiat Oncol Biol Phys 9: 1303–1311

Parsons J, Fitzgerald C, Hood C, Ellingwood K, Bova F, Million R (1983) The effects of irradiation of the eye and optic nerve. Int J Radiat Oncol Biol Phys 9: 609–622

Pedrick T, Hoppe R (1986) Recovery of spermatogenesis following pelvic irradiation for Hodgkin's disease. Int J Radiat Oncol Biol Phys 12: 117–121

Penney D, Rubin P (1977) Specific early fine structural changes in the lung following irradiation. Int J Radiat Oncol Biol Phys 2: 1123–1132

Perrachia G, Salti C (1981) Radiotherapy with twice-a-day fractionation in a short overall time. Int J Radiat Oncol Biol Phys 7: 99–104

Perrone L, Sinisi A, Sicuranza R et al. (1988) Prepubertal

endocrine follow-up in subjects with Wilms' tumor. Med Pediatr Oncol 16: 255–258

Peters L (1980) Discussion: the radiobiological bases of TBI. Int J Radiat Oncol Biol Phys 6: 785–787

Peters L, Withers H, Cundiff J, Dicke K (1979) Radiobiological considerations in the use of total-body irradiation for bone-marrow transplantation. Radiology 131: 243–247

Petz L, Yam P, Wallace R et al. (1987) Mixed hematopoietic chimerism following bone marrow transplantation for hematologic malignancies. Blood 70: 1331–1337

Phillips T, Margolis L (1972) Radiation pathology and the clinical response of lung and oesophagus. Front Radiat Ther Oncol 6: 254 273

Phillips T, Ross G (1973) A quantitative technique for measuring renal damage after irradiation. Radiology 109: 457–462

Plowman P (1983) The effects of conventionally fractionated, extended portal radiotherapy on the human peripheral blood count. Int J Radiat Oncol Biol Phys 9: 829–839

Pohjola-Sintonen S, Tötterman K-J, Salmo M, Siltanen P (1987) Late cardiac effects of mediastinal radiotherapy in patients with Hodgkin's disease. Cancer 60: 31–37

Pomerede R, Czernichow P, Zucker J et al. (1984) Incidence of anterior pituitary deficiency after radiotherapy at an early age; study in retinoblastoma. Acta Paediatr Scand 73: 115–119

Pratt C, Douglass E, Etcubanas E et al. (1989) Ifosfamide in pediatric malignant solid tumors. Cancer Chemother Pharmacol 24: S24–S27

Probert J, Parker B (1975) The effects of radiation therapy on bone growth. Radiology 114: 155–162

Qureshi M, Pennington J, Goldsmith H (1972) Cyclophosphamide therapy and sterility. Lancet II: 1290–1291

Raine J, Bowman A, Wallendszus K, Pritchard J (1991) Hepatopathy-thrombocytopenia syndrome—a complication of dactinomycin therapy for Wilms' tumor: a report from the United Kingdom Children's Cancer Study Group. J Clin Oncol 9: 268–273

Rao S, Frame D, Miller M, Kleerkoper M, Block M, Parfitt A (1980) Hyperparathyroidism following head and neck irradiation. Arch Intern Med 140: 205–207

Rate W, Butler M, Robertson W, D'Angio G (1991) Late orthopedic effects in children with Wilms' tumor treated with abdominal irradiation. Med Pediatr Oncol 19: 265–268

Richter P, Calamera J, Morgenfeld M (1970) Effect of chlorambucil on spermatogenesis in the human with malignant lymphoma. Cancer 25: 1026–1030

Riseborough E, Grabias S, Burton R, Jaffe N (1976) Skeletal alterations following irradiation for Wilms' tumor. J Bone Joint Surg [Am] 50: 526–536

Robison L, Nesbit M, Sather H, Meadows A, Ortega J, Hammond G (1985) Height of children successfully treated for acute lymphoblastic leukemia: a report from the late effects study committee of the Children's Cancer Study Group. Med Pediatr Oncol 13: 14–21

Roden D, Bosley T, Fowble B, Clark J, Savino P, Sergott R, Schatz N (1990) Delayed radiation injury to the retrobulbar optic nerves and chiasm. Clinical syndrome and treatment with hyperbaric oxygen and corticosteroids. Ophthalmology 97: 346–351

Rosenberg S (1990) Chronic dental complications. NCI Monogr 9: 173–178

Rosenberg S, Kolodney H, Wong G, Murphy M (1987) Altered dental root development in long-term survivors of pediatric acute lymphoblastic leukemia. Cancer 59: 1640–1648

Rossleigh M, Smith J, Straus D, Engel I (1986) Osteonecrosis in patients with malignant lymphoma. A review of 31 cases. Cancer 58: 1112–1116

Rowley M, Leach D, Warner G, Heller C (1974) Effect of graded doses of ionizing radiation on the human testis. Radiat Res 59: 665–678

Rubin P, Casarett G (1964) Clinical radiation pathology. W.B. Saunders, Philadelphia

Rubin P, Casarett G (1968) Clinical radiation pathology. W.B. Saunders, Philadelphia

Rubin P, Duthie R, Young L (1962) The significance of scoliosis in postirradiated Wilms' tumor and neuroblastoma. Radiology 79: 539–558

Ruchelli E, Horn M, Taylor S (1990) Severe chemotherapy-related hepatic toxicity associated with MZ protease inhibitor phenotype. Am J Pediatr Hematol Oncol 12: 351–354

Rutherford H, Dodd G (1974) Complications of radiation therapy; growing bone. Semin Roentgenol 9: 15

Sacks E, Goris M, Glatstein E, Kaplan H (1978) Bone marrow regeneration following large field irradiation. Influence of volume, age, dose and time. Cancer 42: 1057–1065

Sagar S, Thomas R, Loverock L, Spittle M (1991) Olfactory sensations produced by high-energy photon irradiation of the olfactory receptor mucosa in humans. Int J Radiat Oncol Biol Phys 20: 771–776

Salvi S, Green D, Grecher M et al. (1983) Renal artery stenosis and hypertension following abdominal irradiation for Hodgkin's disease: successful treatment with nephrectomy. Urology 21: 611–615

Samaan N, Bakdash M, Caderao J, Cangir A, Jesse R, Ballatyne A (1975) Hypopituitarism after external irradiation. Evidence for both hypothalamic and pituitary origin. Ann Intern Med 83: 771–777

Samaan N, Vieto R, Schultz P et al. (1982) Hypothalamic, pituitary and thyroid dysfunction after radiotherapy to the head and neck. Int J Radiat Oncol Biol Phys 8: 1857–1867

Schell M, McHaney V, Green A, Kun L, Hayes A, Horowitz M, Meyer W (1989) Hearing loss in children and young adults receiving cisplatin with or without prior cranial irradiation. Am J Clin Oncol 7: 754–760

Schiffman S (1983) Taste and smell in disease. N Engl J Med 308: 1275–1279

Schimpff S, Diggs C, Wiswell J, Salvatore P, Wiernik P (1980) Radiation-related thyroid dysfunction: implications for the treatment of Hodgkin's disease. JAMA 245: 46–49

Schipper J, Tan K, van Peperzeel H (1985) Treatment of retinoblastoma by precision megavoltage radiation therapy. Radiother Oncol 3: 117–132

Schrek R (1961) Qualitative and quantitative reactions of lymphocytes to x-rays. Ann NY Acad Sci 95: 839–848

Schroick E, Schell M, Carter M, Hustu O, Ochs J (1991) Abnormal growth patterns and adult short stature in 115 long-term survivors of childhood leukemia. J Clin Oncol 9: 400–405

Schultz-Hector S (1991) Heart. In: Scherer E, Streffer C, Trott K (eds) Radiopathology of organs and tissues. Springer Berlin Heidelberg New York, pp 347–368

Sexauer C, Khan A, Burger P, Krischer J, Van Eys J, Vats T, Ragab A (1985) Cisplatin in recurrent pediatric brain tumors: a POG phase II study. Cancer 56: 1497–1501

Shalet S, Beardwell C, Morris-Jones P, Pearson D, Orrell D (1976) Ovarian failure following abdominal irradiation in childhood. Br J Cancer 33: 655–658

Shalet S, Beardwell C, Jacobs H, Pearson D (1978) Testicular function following irradiation of the human prepubertal testis. Clin Endocrinol (Oxf) 9: 483–490

Shalet S, Price D, Beardwell C, Morris-Jones P, Pearson D (1979) Normal growth despite abnormalities of growth hormone secretion in children treated for acute leukemia. J Pediatr 94: 719

Shalet S, Horner A, Ahmed S, Morris-Jones P (1985) Leydig cell damage after testicular irradiation for lymphoblastic leukaemia. Med Pediatr Oncol 13: 65–68

Shannon I, Trodahl J, Starcke E (1978) Radiosensitivity of the human parotid gland. Proc Soc Exp Biol Med 157: 50–53

Shapiro E, Kinsella T, Makuch R, Fraass B, Glatstein E, Rosenberg S, Sherins R (1985) Effect of fractionated irradiation on endocrine aspects of testicular function. J Clin Oncol 3: 1232–1239

Sherins R, Olweny C, Ziegler J (1978) Gynecomastia and gonadal function in adolescent boys treated with combination therapy for Hodgkin's disease. N Engl J Med 299: 12–16

Shukovsky L, Fletcher G (1972) Retinal and optic nerve complications in a high dose irradiation technique of ethmoid sinus and nasal cavity. Radiology 104: 629–634

Shymko R, Hauser D, Archambeau J (1985) Field size dependence of radiation sensitivity and dose fractionation response in skin. Int J Radiat Oncol Biol Phys 11: 1143–1148

Silber J, Littman P, Meadows A (1990) Stature loss following skeletal irradiation for childhood cancer. J Clin Oncol 8: 304–312

Silverman C, Thomas P, McAlister W, Walder S, Whiteside L (1981) Slipped capital femoral epiphysis in irradiated children: dose volume and age relationships. Int J Radiat Oncol Biol Phys 7: 1357–1363

Sklar C, Kim T, Ramsay N (1982) Thyroid dysfunction among long-term survivors of bone marrow transplantation. Am J Med 73: 688–694

Sklar C, Robison L, Nesbit M et al. (1990) Effects of radiation on testicular function in long-term survivors of childhood acute lymphoblastic leukemia: a report from the Children's Cancer Study Group. J Clin Oncol 8: 1981–1987

Smith L, Mendenhall N, Cicale M, Block E, Carter R, Million R (1989) Results of a prospective study evaluating the effects of mantle irradiation on pulmonary function. Int J Radiat Oncol Biol Phys 16: 79–84

Smith R, Adler R, Clark P, Brinck-Johnsen T, Tulloh M, Colton T (1981) Thyroid function after mantle irradiation in Hodgkin's disease. JAMA 245: 46–49

Sonis A, Tarbell N, Valachovic R, Gelber R, Schwenn M, Sallan S (1990) Dentofacial development in long-term survivors of acute lymphoblastic leukemia. A comparison of three treatment modalities. Cancer 66: 2645–2652

Springmeyer S, Flournoy N, Sullivan K (1983) Pulmonary function changes in long-term survivors of allogeneic marrow transplantation. In: Gale R (ed) Recent advances in bone marrow transplantation. Alan R. Liss, New York, pp 343–353

Staab G, Tegtmeyer C, Constable W (1976) Radiation-induced renovascular hypertension. Am J Roentgenol 126: 634–637

Stanley P, Gyepes M, Olson D, Gates G (1978) Renovascular hypertension in children and adolescents. Radiology 129: 123–131

Starceski P, Lee P, Blatt J, Finegold D, Brown D (1987) Comparable effects of 1800 and 2400 rad (18 and 24 Gy) cranial irradiation on height and weight in children treated for acute lymphoblastic leukemia. Am J Dis Child 1987: 550–552

Steel G, Adams K, Peckham M (1979) Lung damage in C57B1 mice following thoracic irradiation: enhancement by chemotherapy. Br J Radiol 52: 741–747

Stefani S, Eells R, Abbate J (1971) Hydroxyurea and radiotherapy in advanced head and neck cancer. Radiology 101: 391–396

Steinherz L, Steinherz P (1991) Delayed anthracycline cardiac toxicity, vol 5, no. 4, J.B. Lippincott, New York

Steinherz L, Steinherz P, Tan C, Murphy L (1991) Cardiac toxicity 4–20 years after completing anthracycline therapy. JAMA 266: 1672–1677

Stevens M, Brown E, Zipursky A (1986) The effect of abdominal radiation on spleen function: a study in children with Wilms' tumor. Pediatr Hematol Oncol 3: 69–72

Stewart F, Williams M (1991) The urinary tract. In: Scherer E, Streffer C, Trott K (eds) Radiopathology of organs and tissues. Springer, Berlin Heidelberg New York, pp 405–431

Stewart F, Luts A, Oussoren Y, Begg A, Dewit L, Bartelink H (1988) Renal damage in mice after treatment with cisplatin and x-rays: comparison of fractionated and single dose studies. NCI Monogr 6: 23–27

Stewart J, Fajardo L (1971) Dose response in human and experimental radiation-induced heart disease. Radiology 99: 403–408

Strender L-E, Lindhal J, Larsson L-E (1986) Incidence of heart disease and functional significance of changes in the electrocardiogram 10 years after radiotherapy for breast cancer. Cancer 57: 929–934

Suarez A, McDowell P, Niaudet P, Comoy E, Flamant F (1991) Long-term follow-up of ifosfamide renal toxicity in children treated for malignant mesenchymal tumors: an International Society of Pediatric Oncology report. Am J Clin Oncol 9: 2177–2182

Sweet D, Roth D, Deseser R, Miller J, Ultmann J (1976) Avascular necrosis of the femoral head with combination chemotherapy. Ann Intern Med 85: 67–68

Swift P, Kearney P, Dalton R, Bullimore J, Mott M, Savage D (1978) Growth and hormonal status of children treated for acute lymphoblastic leukemia. Arch Dis Child 53: 890–894

Tamura K, Shimaoka K, Friedman M (1981) Thyroid abnormalities associated with treatment of malignant lymphoma. Cancer 47: 2704–2711

Tarbell N, Guinan E, Niemeyer C, Mauch P, Sallan S, Weinstein H (1988) Late onset of renal dysfunction in survivors of bone marrow transplantation. Int J Radiat Oncol Biol Phys 15: 99–104

Tarbell N, Thompson L, Mauch P (1990) Thoracic irradiation in Hodgkin's disease: disease control and long-term complications. Int J Radiat Oncol Biol Phys 18: 275–281

Tebbi C, Krischer J, Fernbach D, Mahoney D, Alvarado C, Camitta B (1990) Toxicity of high-dose cytosine arabinoside in the treatment of advanced childhood tumors resistant to conventional therapy. A Pediatric Oncology Group study. Cancer 66: 2064–2067

Tefft M (1977) Radiation related toxicities in National Wilms' Tumor Study Number 1. Int J Radiat Oncol Biol Phys 2: 455–463

Tefft M, Mitus A, Das L, Vawter G, Filler R (1970) Irradiation of the liver in children: review of experience in the acute and chronic phases, and in the intact normal and partially resected. Am J Roentgenol 108: 365–385

Thibdoux G, Pereira W, Hodges J, Aur R (1980) Effects of cranial radiation on hearing in children with acute lymphocytic leukemia. J Pediatr 96: 403–406

Thomas E, Clift R, Hersman J et al. (1982) Marrow transplantation for acute nonlymphoblastic leukemia in first remission using fractionated or single dose irradiation. Int J Radiat Oncol Biol Phys 8: 817–821

Thomas P, Tefft M, D'Angio G, Norkool P (1988) Acute toxicities associated with radiation in the second National Wilms' Tumor Study. J Clin Oncol 6: 1694–1698

Thurlbeck W (1975) Postnatal growth and development of the lung. Annu Rev Respir Dis 111: 803–843

Tisell L-E, Carlsson S, Lindberg S, Ragnhult I (1976) Autonomous hyperparathyroidism: a possible late complication of neck radiotherapy. Acta Chir Scand 142: 367–373

Tisell L, Carlsson C, Fjälling M, Hansson G, Lindberg S, Lundberg L, Odén A (1985) Hyperparathyroidism subsequent to neck irradiation. Risk factors. Cancer 56: 1529–1533

Trueta J, Amato V (1960) The vascular contribution to osteogenesis. III. Changes in the growth cartilage caused by experimentally induced ischaemia. J Bone Joint Surg [Br] 42: 571–587

Turesson I (1989) The progression rate of late radiation effects in normal tissue and its impact on dose-response relationships. Radiother Oncol 15: 217–226

Turesson I, Notter G (1984a) The influence of the overall treatment time in radiotherapy on the acute reaction: comparison of the effects of daily and twice-a-week fractionation on human skin. Int J Radiat Oncol Biol Phys 10: 607–618

Turesson I, Notter G (1984b) The influence of fraction size in radiotherapy on the late normal tissue reaction—I: Comparison of the effects of daily and once-a-week fractionation on human skin. Int J Radiat Oncol Biol Phys 10: 593–598

van der Maase H, Overgaard J, Valth M (1986) Effect of cancer chemotherapeutic drugs on radiation-induced lung damage in mice. Radiother Oncol 5: 245–259

Van Dyk J, Keane T, Kan S, Rider W, Fryer C (1981) Radiation pneumonitis following large single dose irradiation; a re-evaluation based on absolute dose to lung. Int J Radiat Oncol Biol Phys 7: 461–467

Vermund H, Kaalhus O, Winther F (1985) Bleomycin and radiation therapy in squamous cell carcinoma of the upper aerodigestive tract. A phase III clinical trial. Int J Radiat Oncol Biol Phys 11: 1877–1886

Walker D, Pilow J, Waters K (1989) Enhanced cis-platinum ototoxicity in children with brain tumours who have received simultaneous or prior cranial irradiation. Med Pediatr Oncol 17: 48–52

Walker K, Kember B (1972) Cell kinetics of growth cartilage in the rat tibia. I. Measurements in young rats. Cell Tissue Kinet 5: 401–408

Wallace W, Shalet S (1992) Letter to the editor: chemotherapy with actinomycin D influences the growth of the spine following abdominal irradiation. Med Pediatr Oncol 20: 177

Wallace W, Shalet S, Crowne E, Morris-Jones P, Gattamaneni H (1989) Ovarian failure following abdominal irradiation in childhood: natural history and prognosis. Clin Oncol 1: 75–79

Wallace W, Shalet S, Morris-Jones P, Swindell R, Gattamaneni H (1990) Effect of abdominal irradiation on growth in boys treated for a Wilms' tumor. Med Pediatr Oncol 18: 441–446

Wara W, Phillips T, Margolis L (1973) Radiation pneumonitis: a new approach to the derivation of time-dose factors. Cancer 32: 547–552

Wara W, Irvine A, Neger R, Howes E, Phillips T (1979) Radiation retinopathy. Int J Radiat Oncol Biol Phys 5: 81–83

Watchie J, Coleman C, Raffine T et al. (1987) Minimal long-term cardiopulmonary dysfunction following treatment for Hodgkin's disease. Int J Radiat Oncol Biol Phys 13: 517–524

Weaver G, Chauvenet A, Smith T, Schwartz A (1986) Ophthalmic evaluation of long-term survivors of childhood acute lymphoblastic leukemia. Cancer 58: 963–968

Weiner R, Bortin M, Gale R et al. (1986) Interstitial pneumonitis after bone marrow transplantation. Assessment of risk factors. Ann Intern Med 104: 168–175

Weyman J (1968) The effect of irradiation in developing teeth. Oral Surg 25: 623

While D (1975) An atlast of radiation histopathology. Technical Information Center, Office of Public Affairs, U.S. Energy Research and Development Administration, Washington, D.C

Whitehouse W, Lampe E (1953) Osseous damage in irradiation of renal tumors in infancy and childhood. Am J Roentgenol Radiat Ther Nucl Med 70: 721–729

Wikstad I, Pettersson B, Elinder G, Sökücü S, Aperia A (1986) A comparative study of size and function of the remnant kidney in patients nephrectomized in childhood for Wilms' tumor and hydronephrosis. Acta Pediatr Scand 75: 408–414

Wilimas J, Thompson E, Smith K (1980) Long-term results of treatment of children and adolescents with Hodgkin's disease. Cancer 46: 2123–2125

Willich E, Kuttig H, Pfeil G, Scheibel P (1990) Wirbelsäulenveränderungen nach Berstrahlung wegen Wilmstumor im Kleinkindesalter. Retrospektive interdisziplinäre Langzeit-studie an 82 Kindern. Strahlenther Onkol 166: 815–821

Wilson W, Perez G, Kleinschmidt-Demasters B (1987) Sudden onset of blindness in patients treated with oral CCNU and low-dose cranial irradiation. Cancer 59: 901–907

Winter R, Green O (1985) Irradiation-induced growth hormone deficiency: blunted growth hormone response and accelerated skeletal maturation to growth hormone therapy. J Pediatr 106: 609–612

Withers R, Mason K, Thames H (1986) Late radiation response of kidney assayed by tubule-cell survival. Br J Radiol 59: 587–595

Wohl M, Griscom N, Traggis D, Jaffe N (1975) Effects of therapeutic irradiation delivered in early childhood upon subsequent lung function. Pediatrics 55: 507–516

Wolf E, Berdon W, Cassady J, Baker D, Freiberger R, Pavlov H (1977) Slipped capital femoral epiphysis as a sequela to childhood irradiation for malignant tumors. Radiology 125: 781–784

Woods W, Dehner L, Nesbit M (1980) Fetal veno-occlusive disease of the liver following high dose chemotherapy, irradiation and bone marrow transplantation. Am J Med 60: 285–290

Zaharia M, Caceres E, Valdivia S, Moran M, Tejada F (1986) Postoperative whole lung irradiation with or without adriamycin in osteogenic sarcoma. Int J Radiat Oncol Biol Phys 12: 907–910

4 Molecular Biology and Genetic Advances in Childhood Malignancies

Paul S. Meltzer

CONTENTS

4.1 Introduction 55
4.2 Fundamentals of Cell and Molecular Genetics. . . 56
4.2.1 The Chromosomes 56
4.2.2 Recombinant DNA Techniques 57
4.3 Two Classes of Genes Are Altered in
Cancer Cells........................ 59
4.3.1 Oncogenes......................... 60
4.3.2 Functional Categories of Oncogenes......... 61
4.3.3 Tumor Suppressor Genes 61
4.4 Types of Genetic Alterations in
Human Tumors 62
4.4.1 Point Mutations: *ras* Genes.............. 62
4.4.2 Chromosomal Alterations 62
4.4.3 Gene Amplification................... 64
4.4.4 Gene Loss 64
4.5 Genetic Events in Specific Pediatric Cancers..... 65
4.5.1 Hematopoietic Neoplasms 65
4.5.2 Solid Tumors 66
4.6 Clinical Implications 69
4.6.1 Diagnosis.......................... 69
4.6.2 Therapeutic Applications 69
4.6.3 Cancer Prevention.................... 69
References........................ 70

4.1 Introduction

Pediatric oncology is replete with examples of therapeutic progress. Recently, these have been matched by dramatic breakthroughs elucidating the genetic mechanisms which underlie the development of childhood cancer. The powerful techniques of molecular biology have been brought to bear on the cancer problem with spectacular success. New information is being uncovered at a rapid pace. Of great importance, fundamental knowledge is being applied in the clinical setting, and there is ample reason to believe that applications will continue to increase. It is therefore essential that every clinician who cares for pediatric cancer patients has an understanding of molecular oncology which will serve as a

Paul S. Meltzer, M.D., Ph.D., Head, Section of Molecular Genetics, Laboratory of Cancer Genetics, National Center for Human Genome Research, 9000 Rockville Pike/Bldg 49 Rm 4A10, Bethesda, MD 20892, USA

foundation for the informed use of new DNA-based information in patient care.

The concept that cancer is a disease which originates due to acquired alterations in the genetic machinery of the cell dates back to the early cytologist Boveri (1929), who proposed that chromosome abnormalities in tumor cells were at the root of the disease process. This remarkably perceptive view could not be confirmed until the biologic sciences had evolved sufficiently to analyze the genetic make-up of the cancer cell. Boveri's concept can be restated in modern terms: tumor cells evolve from their normal progenitors by a series of genetic alterations which result in the malignant phenotype. Due to the multiple checks and balances on normal cell growth and development, several genetic alterations must occur before a cancer develops. The targets of these genetic events can be either growth-promoting genes or growth-suppressing genes. At the present time sufficient evidence has accumulated in support of this theory to place it in a central position in cancer biology (Bishop 1987; Weinberg 1989; Knudson 1986).

In order to confirm the genetic concept of cancer, it has been necessary to identify the specific genes postulated by the theory. For decades, this was the rate-limiting step affecting progress in this field. Certain specific developments led to rapid progress. With improvements in chromosome banding techniques, it became possible to identify specific human chromosomes in cytogenetic preparations. When this technique was applied to malignant cells, first in leukemias and more recently in solid tumors, disease-specific abnormalities were identified. The paradigm is the Philadelphia chromosome identified by Nowell (Nowell and Hungerford 1960) in chronic myelogenous leukemia, and numerous additional examples have followed (Solomon et al. 1991). The importance of these observations is twofold. First, they confirm that readily identifiable genetic alterations occur in cancer cells, and second, they identify specific chromosomes and chromosomal regions which are the targets of genetic alterations in neoplasia. The identification of specific genes at sites of chromosomal alteration has been a major route to the successful identification of cancer genes. Recombinant DNA technology has enabled the dissection of altered chromosomal regions at the molecular level, leading to the identification of specific target genes.

A second line of investigation transformed the field of tumor virology. Although many animal cancers can be caused by specific retroviruses, examples of human retrovirally induced cancer were difficult to find, casting doubt on any possible relevance of tumor virology to human cancer. However, genetic analysis of the acutely transforming retroviruses demonstrated that their oncogenic properties are the consequences of specific genes, termed oncogenes (BISHOP 1991). While this result is of intrinsic interest, it was startling when it was recognized that the viral oncogenes had been acquired by recombination events with the host genome. These oncogenic retroviruses have subverted the functions of normal cellular genes. The cellular precursor genes, referred to as proto-oncogenes, have turned out to be key genes which function to control the growth and proliferation of normal cells. In many instances the viral oncogene has been structurally altered relative to its cellular precursor in a fashion which promotes tumor growth. Several dozen oncogenes have been identified in various animal retroviruses. Although only a subset of the cellular oncogenes have been related to specific human cancers, all have proved to be of great interest in defining mechanisms of intracellular signal transduction (the mechanism by which a mitogenic signal leads to cell division).

Lines of investigation involving cytogenetic analysis of tumor cells and oncogenes have converged on several occasions with the demonstration that cellular oncogenes are the targets of tumor-specific chromosome rearrangements and may in some instances acquire transforming properties by point mutation. Additional lines of evidence implicating the same basic cellular mechanisms have emerged from the study of animal models of chemical carcinogenesis. Mice carrying oncogene constructs have become useful models for testing the effects of specific genes on tumorigenesis (HANAHAN 1989; CORY and ADAMS 1988).

Analysis of familial cancer has provided another important route to the identification of key genes in cancer cells. Certain pediatric cancers, most notably retinoblastoma, occur in a familial pattern suggesting the mendelian transmission of a cancer susceptibility gene. Investigation of familial cancer has led to major insights with broad general implications.

Progress in the identification of genetic alterations in cancer cells has continued at a rapid pace and is no longer the rate-limiting step affecting progress in cancer biology. At present, major efforts are focused at the difficult task of characterizing the functional networks of genes which control the cellular response to mitogenic signals at the levels of biochemistry and cell physiology. It has become clear that there is a significant redundancy in cellular control systems and that various mechanisms differ in their importance from one tissue to another. It is likely that in the final analysis, each individual cancer will have its own characteristic pattern of genetic alterations which is determined by the nature of the regulatory mechanisms which are operative in the normal progenitor cell.

4.2 Fundamentals of Cell and Molecular Genetics

To understand the molecular genetics of childhood cancer, it is necessary to have some familiarity with the language and techniques used in unraveling the cancer problem at the genetic level.

4.2.1 The Chromosomes

Normal human cells carry their genetic information in 23 pairs of chromosomes, 22 autosomes, and a pair of sex chromosomes. Chromosomes are visualized in mitotic cells by light microscopy of stained preparations. The key techniques which have led to cytogenetic progress are staining methods which produce a unique pattern of light and dark bands on each chromosome. This enables the identification of each normal chromosome as well as their abnormal derivatives seen in disease states. Cytogenetic analysis of cancer cells presents many unique problems. In particular, solid tumors present a major challenge because they frequently carry multiple complex chromosome abnormalities. It appears that genomic instability is part of the malignant phenotype of many cancers, and that numerous secondary changes become superimposed on the primary events which are associated with tumorigenesis. These secondary events may be associated with tumor progression in some instances. In others they may be random. Nonetheless, in spite of these difficulties, it has been possible to identify recurring patterns of chromosome alteration in numerous human cancers (HEIM and MITELMAN 1987). The goal of this analysis is to identify the recurring changes which characterize a given tumor in order to identify the target genes involved in tumorigenesis. Even short of achieving this ultimate objective, cytogenetic observations can reveal unexpected biologic information. One of the more intensively studied pediatric solid tumors is Ewing's sarcoma, which is characterized by the presence of a t(11;22) (AURIAS et al. 1984). Of considerable interest, the same translocation chromosome is observed in another small round blue cell tumor, peripheral neuroepithelioma (WHANG-PENG et al. 1984), suggesting that these apparently disparate tumors may share a common pathogenesis.

4.2.2 Recombinant DNA Techniques

The development of recombinant DNA technology is responsible more than any other factor for the rapid progress is molecular oncology. While it is beyond the scope of this chapter to present this technology in detail, a limited understanding of molecular biology has become essential for following the current literature in oncology. Most important are the techniques which are used to characterize genes and gene expression in tumor cells. These techniques all depend on the principle of base pair complementarity in the double-helical structure of DNA. Because of the stability of this structure, DNA which has been rendered single stranded (denatured) tend to return to the double-stranded configuration (Fig. 4.1).

The mapping of DNA segments largely depends on the utilization of restriction endonucleases, enyzmes which cleave DNA molecules at specific short sequences. Numerous restriction enzymes have been identified. Some enzymes cleave both strands of the substrate in a staggered fashion so that complementary overhanging ends remain (Fig. 4.2). These readily anneal to one another and can be spliced back together by DNA ligase. This is the basis

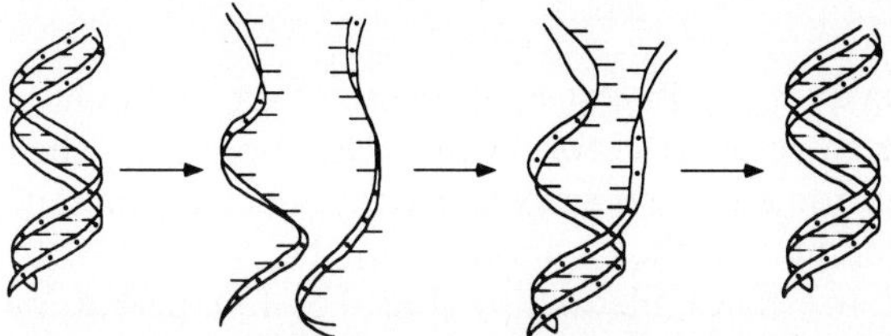

Fig. 4.1. Diagrammatic representation of the DNA double helix. The two strands can dissociate and reanneal in response to changes in conditions which affect the hydrogen bond stability

of many convenient recombinant DNA techniques. In addition, the sequence fidelity of the restriction endonucleases is sufficiently accurate that they can be used to map complex DNA such as the human genome.

The complementary strands of native double-stranded DNA can be separated by heat or alkali treatment. They then become accessible to annealing with a DNA probe of known constitution. If the probe has been labeled with a radioactive or chemical tag, it can be detected. These procedures are exquisitely sensitive and can easily detect target molecules in the picogram range. Frequently these experiments are conducted using target nucleic acids which have been immobilized to a solid support as a membrane and are often referred to as blot hybridization. Detection of DNA which has been digested by a restriction endonuclease and size fractionated by gel electrophoresis prior to transfer to a solid support is referred to as Southern blot hybridization (Fig. 4.3). RNA can be similarly detected following electrophoresis in a Northern blot procedure. These analytical techniques are made possible by preparative cloning techniques in which a small segment of human DNA is inserted into a microbial host using a cloning vector, usually a derivative of a bacterial plasmid or bacteriophage. The exogenous human DNA fragment can be either of genomic origin or prepared from mRNA by reverse transcriptase, in which case it is referred to as complementary DNA (cDNA). Although the human genome is large (over a billion base pairs), many important genes have been cloned, and sequenced at the nucleotide level. Progress in this field of genomic analysis is rapid, and in the context of the human genome initiative, plans are in place to sequence the entire human genome.

These procedures have been the major analytical tools of molecular oncology. Recently, the polymerase chain reaction technique (PCR) has become extremely important. PCR uses specific synthetic oligonucleotides to amplify a section of a given gene in vitro (SAIKI et al. 1988). By using automated equipment, it is possible to carry out this procedure in a few hours starting with minute quantities of DNA (Fig. 4.4). This makes it possible to analyze DNA from tumor biopsies for genetic changes. PCR products can be analyzed for the presence of mutations by a variety of electrophoretic or hybridization techniques as well as DNA sequence analysis. A new procedure, ligase-mediated PCR, promises to efficiently identify specific mutations (BARANY 1991).

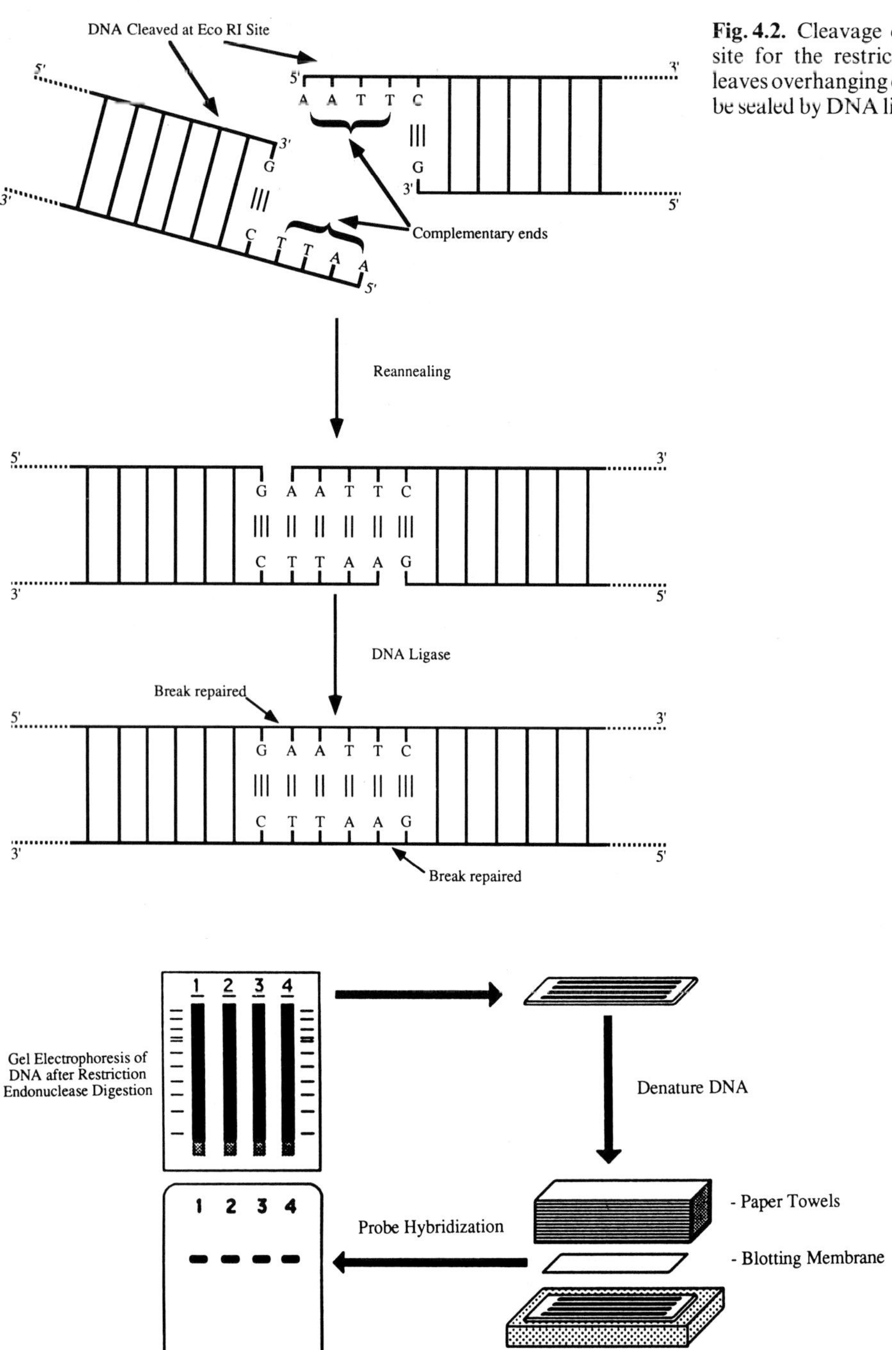

Fig. 4.2. Cleavage of DNA at the recognition site for the restriction endonuclease Eco RI leaves overhanging ends which can reanneal and be sealed by DNA ligase

Fig. 4.3. The Southern blot procedure (Southern 1975). DNA fragments generated by restriction endonuclease cleavage can be size fractionated by gel electrophoresis, transferred to membranes, and detected by DNA hybridization hybridization

Another new technique represents a fusion of molecular and cytogenetic methodologies. Fluorescence in situ hybridization (FISH) has dramatically improved the ability to analyze complex karyotypes (PINKEL et al. 1988). DNA probes have been prepared for whole chromosomes, their entromeres, and specific genes. Under appropriate conditions these probes can be visualized by fluorescence microscopy (Fig. 4.5, 4.6), permitting definitive mapping of chromosomes and genes in cancer cells at a higher level of resolution than is possible by banding techniques. In addition, FISH now enables a new type of analysis, interphase

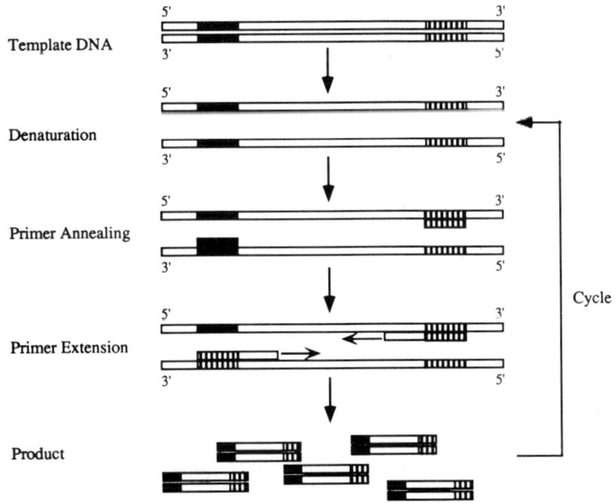

Fig. 4.4. The PCR can generate microgram quantities of DNA starting from a few template molecules by successive cycles of denaturation, primer annealing, and primer extension

cytogenetics. Using probes such as those specific for chromosome centromeres, it is possible to enumerate chromosomes in interphase nuclei. This type of analysis opens a new window on questions of tumor

Fig. 4.5. Fluorescence in situ hybridization (FISH). A chemically modified DNA probe is hybridized to chromosomal preparations in situ and visualized by fluorescence microscopy

heterogeneity and partially relieves the requirement of cytogenetic analysis for mitotic cells.

Unquestionably, techniques for characterizing genes in tumor cells will continue to be refined. For example, it has recently become possible to microdissect abnormal chromosomes in tumor cells in order to determine their genetic content (MELTZER et al. 1992). In addition to countless research applications, molecular diagnostic techniques can be expected to take an increasingly prominent role in clinical studies of pediatric cancers.

4.3 Two Classes of Genes Are Altered in Cancer Cells

It is now clear that genes which contribute to tumorigenesis fall into two broad categories. The first consists of genes with functions which drive cells toward proliferation. These genes, generally called oncogenes, become constitutively activated in cancer cells either by structural mutation or by events which lead to overexpression (BISHOP 1991). The second category consists of genes which in normal cells function to inhibit cell proliferation. These genes are referred to as tumor suppressor genes (MARSHALL 1991; SAGER 1989). Carcinogenic genetic damage to a normal cell can be envisioned as affecting either category of gene. Oncogenes, being dominant in function, are relatively easy to identify while tumor suppressor genes, being recessive, require much

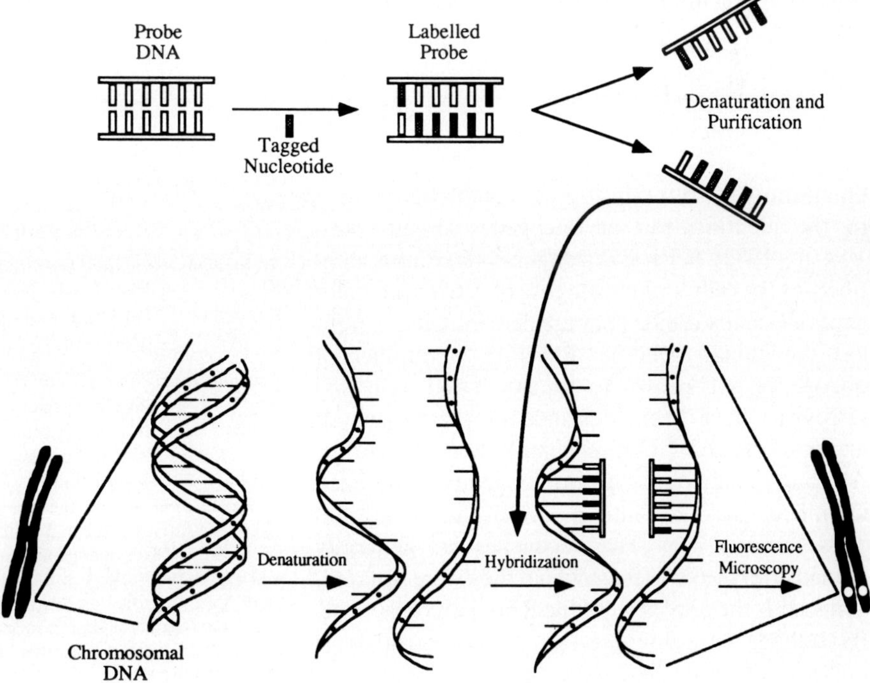

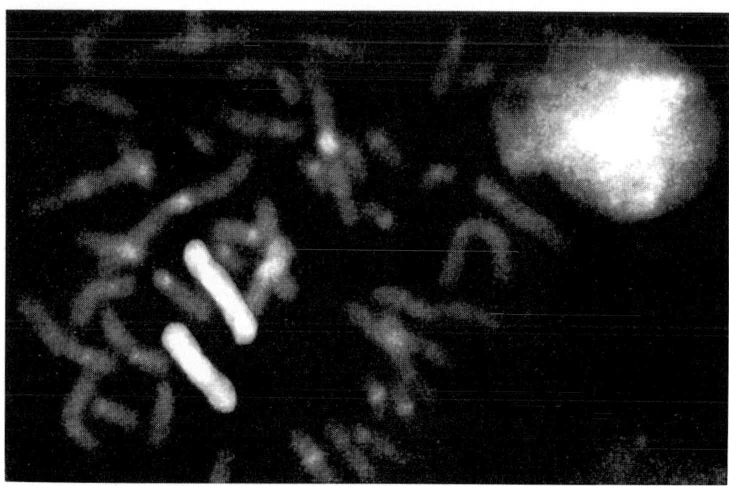

Fig. 4.6. "Chromosome painting" has been used to visualize both homologues of that chromosome in a normal cell. A complex probe derived from the X chromosome (Meltzer et al. 1992) was hybridized to a metaphase in situ on a microscope slide and visualized by fluorescence microscopy (FISH)

more elaborate strategies for their identification. Both are known to be important, but it now appears likely that the majority of steps which lead to the evolution of a fully malignant solid tumor, particularly one of epithelial origin, involves loss of tumor suppressor functions.

At the genetic level, the development of a malignant tumor involves multiple steps (often referred to as "hits"). The requirement for multiple hits explains the tendency for the vast majority of human cancers to occur in the elderly, who have accumulated decades of somatic mutations. The exact number and nature of the hits required varies from one type of cancer to another. It thus appears that cancer will prove to be as diverse and complex genetically as it is clinically. The molecular genetic analysis of human cancers has progressed rapidly, but remains incomplete.

4.3.1 Oncogenes

Quantitatively, retrovirology has contributed most to the identification of oncogenes (BISHOP and VARMUS 1982). Several dozen genes have been identified as the cellular homologues of retroviral oncogenes (VARMUS 1989). They are distributed throughout the human genome. Recently, a number of oncogenes not known to be associated with any retrovirus have been identified as the targets of leukemia-related chromosomal translocations. Although numerous proto-oncogenes have been identified, they fall into a few broad functional classes (Table 4.1). The oncogenes are generally named after the virus from which they were isolated. Thus *src* is the oncogene of the Rous sarcoma virus. Its cellular homologue is designated c-*src*. It is important to note that although all of these genes

clearly play a key role in the regulation of cellular proliferation in normal cells, only a few have been clearly implicated as targets of mutation or chromosomal alterations in human cancers. Further, not all of these genes are expressed in all tissues, and clearly different regulatory mechanisms function in cells of different lineages. It is likely that many additional genes remain to be identified, which may yet include critical targets of mutation in human cancer. Nonetheless, a general concept of oncogene function has emerged.

Table 4.1. Representative oncogenes in the major functional categories[a]

Growth factors:	
sis	PDGF B-chain growth factor
int-2	FGF-related growth factor

Receptor and nonreceptor protein-tyrosine kinases:	
src	Membrane-associated nonreceptor protein-tyrosine kinase
fps/fes	Nonreceptor protein-tyrosine kinase
abl/bcr-abl	Nonreceptor protein-tyrosine kinase
erbB	EGF receptor protein-tyrosine kinase
HER-2/neu	Receptor protein-tyrosine kinase

Membrane-associated G proteins:	
H-*ras*	Membrane-associated GTPase
K-*ras*	Membrane-associated GTPase
N-*ras*	Membrane-associated GTPase

Nuclear transcription factors:	
myc	Nuclear protein
N-*myc*	Nuclear protein
myb	Nuclear protein
erbA	Thyroxine (T_3) receptor

[a] Representatives of the major functional categories of oncogenes are listed. Certain oncogenes, such as *myc*, occur in retroviruses and are known targets in human cancer. Some, such as *fps/fes*, have been identified as retroviral oncogenes but have not been implicated to date as genetic targets in human tumors. Others such as N-*myc* are altered in human tumors but have not been isolated from retroviruses

4.3.2 Functional Categories of Oncogenes

Broadly oncogenes can be divided into several categories which correspond to steps in the transduction of extracellular mitogenic signals (Fig. 4.7). The c-*sis* gene is the homologue of the B-chain of the platelet-derived growth factor (JOHNSSON et al. 1984). This represents the most distal step, a soluble growth factor (CROSS and DEXTER 1991). A large group of genes constitute the membrane-bound proteins, which include receptors and other proteins that interact with receptors in the membrane (HUNTER 1991; ULLRICH and SCHLESSINGER 1990; YARDEN and ULLRICH 1988). An important example is the *erbB* gene, which is identical with the epidermal growth factor receptor (HAYMAN 1986). The effector mechanism of this and other related receptors occurs via a tyrosine kinase domain. There are nonreceptor tyrosine kinases also which can either be membrane bound (*src*) or cytoplasmic (*abl*) (VAN ETTEN et al. 1989; HUNTER 1989). Cytoplasmic serine/threonine kinases (*raf*) constitute another important link in the signal transduction pathway (HUNTER 1989; EDELMAN et al. 1987). The *ras* genes are important regulators of signal transduction with intrinsic GTPase activity similar to the G-proteins found associated with many cell surface receptors (BARBACID 1987; BOS 1988). *Ras* function is modulated by interaction with another protein designated GAP (PARSONS 1990). The most proximal category would include the nuclear oncogenes typified by c-*myc*, which are thought to function as transcription factors, proteins which are involved in the regulation

of gene expression (COLE 1986; EISENMAN 1989). As a group, the oncogenes can be considered positive regulators of cell proliferation. With more precise characterization of the biochemical interactions of these proteins it has become clear that they interact in a complex network rather than as part of a linear signaling pathway. The relative importance of each element of the network is dependent on cell lineage and the nature of the signal transduced (HUNTER 1991).

4.3.3 Tumor Suppressor Genes

If normal cells are induced to fuse with tumor cells, the hybrid cell frequently loses its ability to form tumors in experimental animals (STANBRIDGE 1990; HARRIS 1988). This effect can be demonstrated to depend on the introduction of specific normal chromosomes, suggesting that normal genes may suppress the ability of a cancer cell to form tumors. This is the operational definition of the term tumor suppressor gene.

Genetic analysis of tumors has identified several tumor suppressor genes. Most frequently altered is the *p53* gene. This gene has a fascinating history (LANE and BENCHIMOL 1990). It was originally identified as a tumor antigen associated with SV40 infection. Its increased expression in tumor cells led for a time to its misclassification as an oncogene. Careful studies of the loss of heterozygosity in colorectal cancer suggested the importance of a gene on chromosome 17p in the region where *p53* had been mapped. DNA sequence of *p53* in colorectal tumors identified inactivating mutations in *p53* (BAKER et al. 1989). It is now recognized that the normal *p53* gene functions to restrain cell growth and that mutations in this gene can act in a dominant negative fashion to promote cell growth. Hundreds of examples of *p53* mutations have been identified in a wide variety of human cancers including some pediatric tumors (e.g., rhabdomyosarcoma, osteosarcoma, and CNS tumors) (NIGRO et al. 1989; MULLIGAN et al. 1990; AHUJA et al. 1989). The mutations are not randomly distributed, but cluster at certain highly conserved locations in the *p53* gene. Gene transfer experiments which restore a normal *p53* gene to tumor cells carrying defective *p53* confirm that *p53* has tumor suppressor properties (BAKER et al. 1990; DILLER et al. 1990; ELIYAHU et al. 1989; FONG et al. 1989). The biochemistry of the *p53* gene is as yet incompletely understood. Current evidence suggests that it is involved in the regulation of gene expression and DNA synthesis in a fashion that regulates the cell cycle (FIELDS

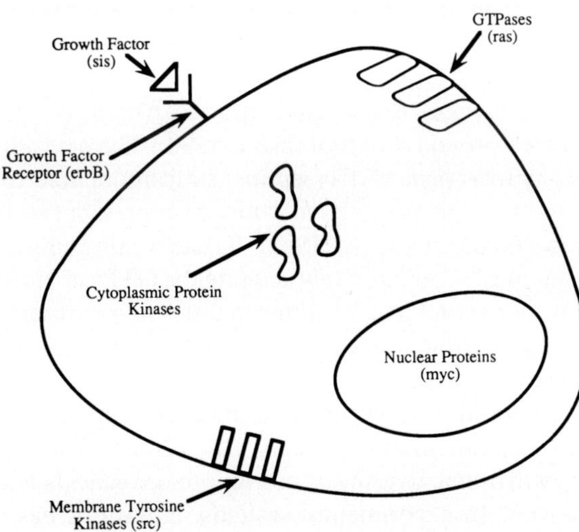

Fig. 4.7. Cellular oncogenes identify several levels of signal transduction from the extracellular mitogenic growth factors to nuclear DNA binding proteins

Table 4.2. Component tumors of Li-Fraumeni syndrome (MALKIN et al. 1990)

Definite component	Possible component
Soft tissue sarcoma	Lung carcinoma
Osteosarcoma	Prostate carcinoma
Brain tumors	Pancreas carcinoma
Breast carcinoma	Melanoma
Leukemia	
Adrenocortical carcinoma	

and JANG 1990; MILNER et al. 1990; STURZBECHER et al. 1990). In some human tumors, such as colorectal carcinoma, disturbance of this key regulatory mechanism by mutation appears to be one of the last steps in the evolution of the fully malignant phenotype (FEARON and VOGELSTEIN 1990). A tumor-prone phenotype has been observed in transgenic mice with a defect in *p53* (LAVIGUEUR et al. 1989; DONEHOWER et al. 1992). Remarkably, germ line *p53* mutations have been found in kindreds with the Li-Fraumeni syndrome, which predisposes to a variety of tumors including sarcomas, brain tumors, breast cancer, and leukemia (Table 4.2) (MALKIN et al. 1990). It remains to be demonstrated to what extent germline mutations in *p53* contribute to the occurrence of sporadic childhood cancers, but their presence should be suspected in patients with a family history suggestive of Li-Fraumeni syndrome or in those who develop two independent primary tumors.

Based on cytogenetic and molecular analyses of chromosome loss in human cancers, it is suspected that numerous additional tumor suppressor genes exist. Two childhood cancers, retinoblastoma and Wilms' tumor, which are regulated by tumor suppressor genes are discussed below.

4.4 Types of Genetic Alterations in Human Tumors

4.4.1 Point Mutations: ras Genes

Under appropriate conditions mammalian cells in culture can be induced to take up exogenous DNA. When this type of transfection experiment was carried out using DNA from a human bladder carcinoma cell line, and a mouse fibroblast cell line, NIH3T3, transformed foci of cells were identified (TABIN et al. 1982). These foci can be identified by their refractile appearance and consist of cells which have lost contact inhibition and pile up in an abnormal fashion. When injected into mice, the transformed cells are tumorigenic. Transformed foci can be plucked from the culture dish and clonally expanded. The DNA from these transformed cells retains transforming activity, suggesting that a gene from the tumor DNA has been transferred into the mouse cells, thereby conferring the transformed phenotype. By repeating the process of transfection, nontransforming "passenger" DNA is lost and the transforming gene itself can be readily isolated from the mouse genome. In this fashion, it was possible to isolate the responsible human gene. Nucleotide sequencing identified it as the H-*ras* gene, human homologue of the Harvey sarcoma virus oncogene. Remarkably, the gene isolated in this fashion differed from that found in normal cells by a mutation in codon 12 leading to a substitution of valine for glycine (TABIN et al. 1982; TAPAROWSKY et al. 1982). It is this mutant allele which carries transforming activity. Three members of the *ras* gene family, H-*ras*, K-*ras*, and N-*ras*, are now recognized in the human genome (BARBACID 1987; BOS 1988). All three have a generally similar structure, and transforming mutations are clustered in codons 12, 13, and 61. The introduction of PCR has made it possible to screen multiple tumor specimens for mutations in these genes, and it has become clear that *ras* mutations are frequent in certain human cancers such as colon cancer and occur sporadically in many other cancers. *Ras* gene mutations occur in a subset of pediatric leukemias and rhabdomyosarcomas, but do not seem to be frequent in neuroblastoma despite the fact that N-*ras* was isolated from a neuroblastoma cell line (BOS 1988; STRATTON et al. 1989; MOLEY et al. 1991).

Structural analysis of the *ras* gene family has demonstrated that the *ras* protein *p21* is a normal constituent of the inner surface of cell membranes (BARBACID 1987). *p21* has GTP-binding activity and GTPase activity (DOWNWARD et al. 1990) which is normally regulated by association with another regulatory protein, GAP (PARSONS 1990). The neurofibromatosis gene (NF1) is biochemically related to GAP and appears to have a tumor suppressor function (BALLESTER et al. 1990). Transforming mutations in *p21* constitutively activate the GTPase function of *ras* and lead to abnormalities in membrane signal transduction. The subsequent steps are not yet clearly defined.

In addition to point mutations activating oncogenes, point mutations may also promote cancer growth by inactivating tumor suppressor genes (such as *p53*). In experimental systems, mutations have been identified which are associated with drug resistance, but the importance of these phenomena in vivo has yet to be established.

4.4.2 Chromosomal Alterations

In general, cytogenetic analysis of human cancer cells reveals an abnormal karyotype. Human cancers frequently carry specific altered chromosomes which are characteristic of a given disease state. The classic example is the Philadelphia chromosome in chronic myelogenous leukemia (CML). Now dozens of alterations have been identified (HEIM and MITELMAN 1987). In several instances the genes which fall at the breakpoint of a translocation have been identified and have proved to be oncogenes. In CML the Philadelphia chromosome represents the fusion of the *abl* oncogene and the *bcr* (breakpoint cluster region) gene (HEISTERKAMP et al. 1983; HERMANS et al. 1987; LUGO et al. 1990). This gene fusion

event leads to the production of a fusion mRNA transcript leading to the production of an abnormal *bcr-abl* protein which does not occur in normal cells. Although the precise mechanism of action of this fusion protein has not been fully elucidated, extensive biochemical evidence suggests that its activity contributes to the proliferation of CML cell. *Abl* is a ubiquitous protein kinase gene and while the function of *bcr* has not been fully clarified, it also appears to possess protein kinase activity (LUGO et al. 1990). The *bcr-abl* fusion protein is highly characteristic of CML and even when the classic Philadelphia chromosome is not apparent on cytogenetic analysis, molecular evidence of *bcr-abl* joining can usually be identified by Southern blot or PCR analysis. Introduction of a *bcr/abl* gene into

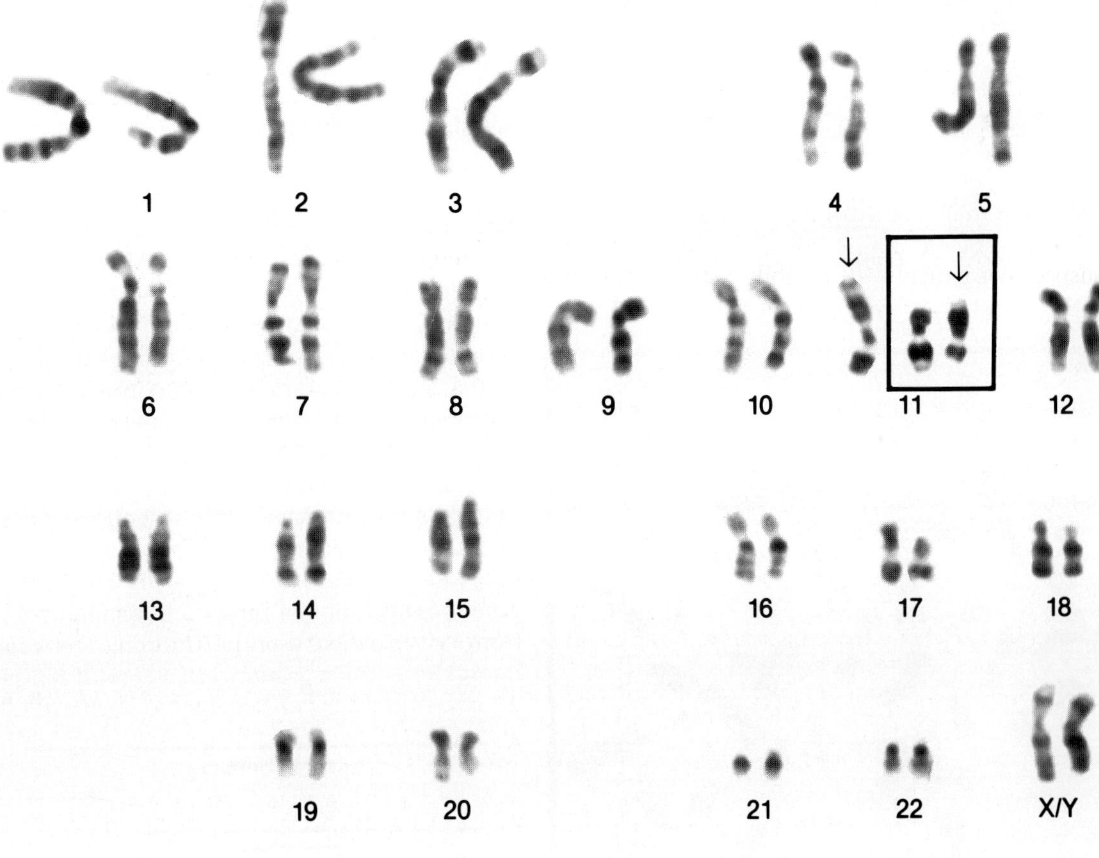

Fig. 4.8. G-banded karyotype from a Wilms' tumor isolated after short-term culture illustrates abnormalities in chromosome 11. *Arrows* indicate a chromosome 11 which has undergone a pericentric inversion with partial deletion of a portion of the short arm [der(11)inv(q22p14)del(p14)]. *Inset* shows a normal chromosome 11 and another example of the derivative 11 for comparison. An unidentifiable marker chromosome (*Umar*) is present (Courtesy of F. Thompson)

transgenic mice leads to a myeloproliferative disorder similar to CML (DALEY et al. 1990; KELLIHER et al. 1990).

Solid tumors also can be analyzed by cytogenetic techniques (Fig. 4.8), although these methods are not available in all centers. As a research tool, cytogenetic analysis of solid tumors has been an extremely important method for the identification of cancer genes.

4.4.3 Gene Amplification

A gene is amplified when its copy number is increased with respect to the cells' ploidy. Readily identifiable cytogenetic anomalies, double minutes, homogeneously staining regions are associated with gene amplification and have been demonstrated to be the cytologic manifestation of extra gene copies (ALITALO and SCHWAB 1986). Double minutes are small acentric paired chromatin bodies while homogeneously staining regions are expanded poorly banding intrachromosomal segments (Fig. 4.9A). Gene amplification is, as a rule, associated with increased gene expression. Amplification of a number of different oncogenes has been observed in human cancers. The best studied example in pediatric oncology is N-*myc* oncogene amplification in neuroblastoma (SCHWAB et al. 1983; KOHL et al. 1984). Numerous other examples exist in adult and pediatric tumors (ALITALO and SCHWAB 1986; SCHWAB and AMIER 1990). Gene amplification can be detected either by FISH or by Southern blot analysis of tumor preparations.

4.4.4 Gene Loss

Many cancers contain gains or losses of whole chromosomes or chromosome arms. The influence of chromosome gains is nuclear, although it is suspected that in some instances extra copies of chromosomes may be functionally analogous to low levels of gene amplification. Chromosome loss is now recognized as an important mechanism of inactivation of tumor suppressor genes. After attention is focused on a chromosomal region by cytogenetic analysis, gene loss is studied in tumor cells by comparing the genetic constitution of tumor cells and normal cells from a given patient using polymorphic DNA mark-

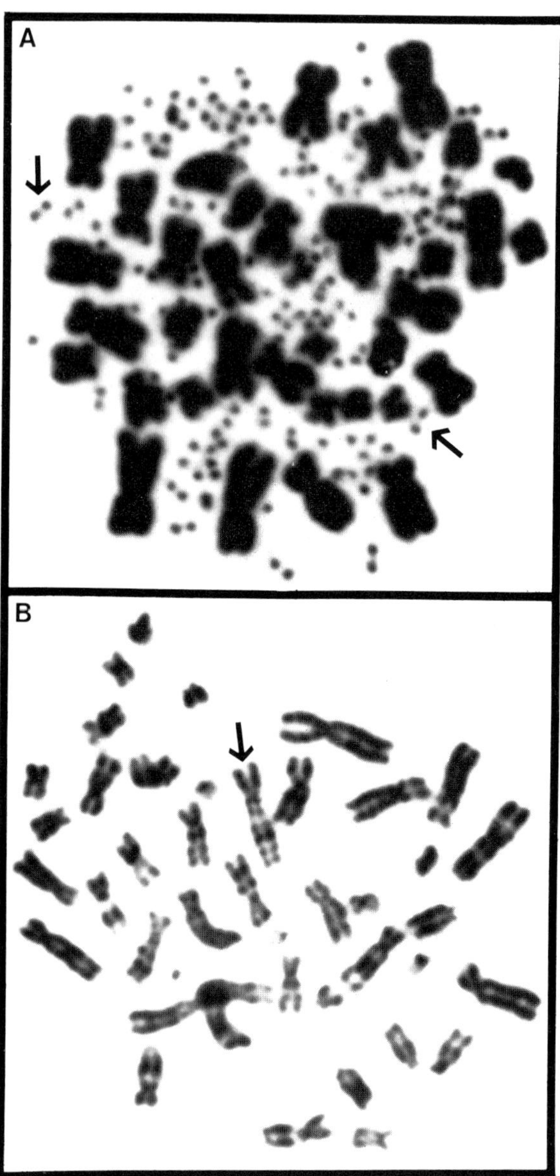

Fig. 4.9A,B. Cytogenetic analysis of a neuroblastoma cell line illustrates two abnormalities in this tumor. **A** Double minute chromosomes (dmins) which contain amplified N-*myc* sequences. **B** A partial deletion of the short arm of chromosome 1, del (1)(p31) (Courtesy of F. Thompson)

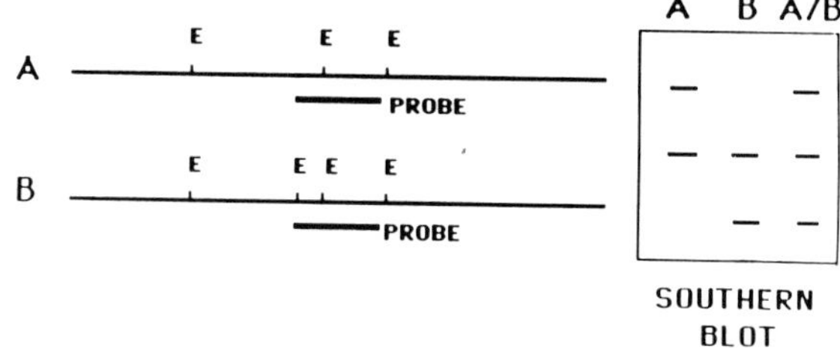

Fig. 4.10. Restriction fragment length polymorphism. Variants in the restriction map of different chromosomes can be used to track alleles during meiosis and to identify somatic loss of heterozygosity in tumor cells. The probe illustrated identifies a constant band and two variable bands. Two alleles would result in three bands on a Southern blot analysis

ers. Most studies have used restriction fragment length polymorphisms (Fig. 4.10). Loss of heterozygosity (LOH) for a given marker establishes loss at a particular point on the chromosome. By studying numerous cases with multiple markers, it is possible to define the minimal segment deleted in a given cancer and eventually identify the target gene of the deletion event. This strategy was used to identify the retinoblastoma susceptibility gene (discussed in detail below).

4.5 Genetic Events in Specific Pediatric Cancers

The analysis of genetic alterations in cancer cells is an ongoing process which is far from complete. As genes are identified, difficult biologic problems arise in their functional analysis. Key genetic events in many important pediatric tumors have yet to be defined. Current understanding resembles a jigsaw puzzle which is only partially assembled but nonetheless begins to suggest the emergence of a coherent picture.

4.5.1 Hematopoietic Neoplasms

The leukemias and lymphomas have been relatively amenable to molecular analysis (RABBITTS 1991). The malignant cells from these disorders often exhibit a single translocation chromosome which can be targeted for molecular analysis (PUI et al. 1990a). A significant series of these translocations have now been characterized (Table 4.3). They can be broadly divided into two groups. In the first group, which is characteristic of the lymphoid malignancies, an oncogene is translocated into a chromosomal region associated with the immunoglobulin genes or T-cell receptor genes (BISHOP 1989; HALUSKA et al. 1987; KAGAN et al. 1989; VON LINDERN et al. 1990; LE BEAU et al. 1986). Since these important gene clusters are well characterized, it is relatively straightforward to clone the breakpoint and identify the translocation target gene (CLEARY and SKLAR 1985; APLAN et al. 1990; BAKHSHI et al. 1985; BOEHM et al. 1988; CLEARY et al. 1986; CHEN et al. 1990; FINGER et al. 1989; ZUTTER et al. 1990). The majority of these have turned out to be nuclear proteins. Most contain structural features such as zinc finger domains or homeobox domains which suggest that they function to control the expression of other genes (McGUIRE et al. 1989). These gene products are referred to as transcription factors. In this type of translocation, a fusion protein is not formed. Positive regulatory elements derived from the lymphoid-specific genes presumably act on the translocated oncogene, leading to inappropriately high levels of oncogene expression (HALUSKA et al. 1987). Structural analysis of the translocations occurring in lymphoid malignancies has identified the presence of recognition sequences for the recombinase system which functions in the normal development of immunoglobulin and T-cell receptor diversity. It is likely that many of these translocations arise as a consequence of errors in the function of this system (HALUSKA et al. 1986).

The second type of translocation, exemplified by the t(9;22) of CML, results in the generation of a fusion protein which is never a constituent of normal cells. Several other examples such as the t(1:19) in acute lymphocytic leukemia (ALL) have been studied (KAMPS et al. 1990, 1991; MELLENTIN et al. 1989; NOURSE et al. 1990). Nonlymphoid leukemias are characterized by the presence of specific

Table 4.3. Representative translocations in leukemias[a]

Disease	Translocation	Target gene	Category
Burkitt Lymphoma	t(8;14)(q24;q32)	MYC	HLH nuclear protein
Pre-B ALL	t(1;19)(q23;p13)	E2A-PBX	Fusion protein (HLH/homeodomain)
T-ALL	t(1;14)(p32;q11)	TCL5 (TAL1, SCL)	HLH nuclear protein
T-ALL	t(10;14)(q24;q11)	HOX11 (TCL3)	Homeodomain protein
APL	t(15;17)(q22;q11.2-12)	PML-RARA	Fusion protein (Zn finger/Zn finger)
AML-M2, AML-M4	t(6;9)(p23;q34)	DEK-CAN	Fusion protein (nuclear/cytoplasmic)

ALL, acute lymphocytic leukemia; APL, acute promyelocytic leukemia; AML, acute myelocytic leukemia
[a] Selected examples of well-characterized translocations in hematopoietic malignancy. The first two examples involve immunoglobulin genes, the second two involve T-cell receptor genes, and the final two are fusion proteins

translocation chromosomes. These are so consistent that they can be associated with specific FAB classifications (KANEKO et al. 1982). Several of the translocation breakpoints in nonlymphoid leukemias have been characterized (BLAT et al. 1988). An important example is the t(15;17) translocation in acute promyelocytic leukemia (APL) (KANEKO and SAKURAI 1977; ROWLEY et al. 1977). This translocation has been shown to involve the retinoic acid receptor (RAR) α gene on chromosome 15 and the PML gene on chromosome 17 (DE THÉ et al. 1990). RAR-α belongs to the steroid receptor super family of ligand binding transcription factors, and PML is also likely to be a transcription factor on the basis of its structural analysis. Remarkably, patients with APL can be induced to enter remission by treatment with triretinoin alone (CHEN et al. 1991; LO COCO et al. 1991; WARRELL et al. 1991). Response to retinoids correlates strictly with the presence of the RAR/PML translocation. As the responses to retinoids, though dramatic, have been transient, the role of retinoid treatment in APL is not yet clear. The presence of a specific breakpoint junction region also provides a target for PCR analysis of minimal residual disease (BIONDI et al. 1992; MORGAN et al. 1989).

4.5.2 Solid Tumors

4.5.2.1 Retinoblastoma

Retinoblastoma is the paradigm of hereditary cancer. It is known to occur in two forms, sporadic cases, usually unilateral, and familial cases, often bilateral. Based on his analysis of the cumulative age of incidence of these two forms of retinoblastoma, KNUDSON (1971) proposed the "two hit" hypothesis. In this model, two genetic events are required to transform a retinoblast into a tumor cell. These two events correspond to the inactivation of both copies of the retinoblastoma susceptibility gene (*Rb*). This occurs at a low baseline rate in all cells and it is quite unlikely that two copies of Rb will be inactivated in more than one cell; hence the low incidence of bilateral disease in sporadic retinoblastoma patients. However, if the first "hit" is transmitted as a germline mutation, the age of onset is accelerated and it is substantially more likely that multiple sites will be affected, resulting in bilateral disease.

Since effective surgical treatment of retinoblastoma has been available for many years, the familial nature of bilateral disease has long been apparent. This meant that a number of multigeneration kindreds were available for genetic studies. Some of these kindreds carried deletions of the chromosome 13q, and 13q abnormalities were identifiable retinoblastoma tumors (BALABAN et al. 1982). With the development of techniques for gene mapping, the critical region of chromosome 13 was isolated, and the *Rb* gene was cloned (PARSONS 1990; LEE et al. 1987). Mutational analysis of the *Rb* gene has provided direct proof of the Knudson model at the DNA level (DRYJA et al. 1989; FUNG et al. 1987). The discovery of the *Rb* gene was associated with a number of surprises. Remarkably, the expression of the Rb protein is ubiquitous rather than limited to retinal tissue. Although the cell biology of *Rb* is not yet fully elucidated, *Rb* appears to be one of the key negative regulators of the cell cycle. The Rb protein has a binding site with high affinity for a number of proteins which function as positive regulators of cell division. Binding affinity of the *Rb* protein is regulated by cyclic phosphorylation and dephosphorylation during the cell cycle (MIHARA et al. 1989; LUDLOW et al. 1989; WEINBERG 1990; BUCHKOVICH et al. 1989; CHEN et al. 1989). Given the ubiquitous expression of *Rb*, the question arises of why germline *Rb* mutations predispose so dramatically to retinoblastoma and not to cancers of all tissues. In fact, patients with the hereditary form of retinoblastoma do have an increased susceptibility to cancer and may have a cumulative lifetime incidence of second malignancies approaching 100% (DRAPER et al. 1986). Most of these are sarcomas, often osteosarcomas, and importantly not all arise in previous radiation fields (ABRAMSON et al. 1989). Many of these second tumors represent a further manifestation of the cancer-prone phenotype. Nonetheless, second malignancies in retinoblastoma patients occur only in certain tissues, suggesting redundancy in control of the cell cycle in most tissues. Transgenic mice with two defective *Rb* alleles are nonviable, a result consistent with a central role for *Rb* in growth and differentiation. However, mice with a single inactive *Rb* allele develop pituitary tumors but not retinoblastoma, further emphasizing the tissue and species specificity of *Rb* function (LEE et al. 1992).

4.5.2.2 Wilms' Tumor

In Wilms' tumor as in retinoblastoma, certain affected individuals have clinical features which suggest the presence of a germline mutation in a tumor suppressor gene. These include multiple primary tumors and associated congenital anomalies (BRESLOW and BECKWITH 1982; MILLER et al. 1964). Several syndromes of congenital anomalies have been identified. The Wilms' tumor aniridia syndrome is particularly important because it is associated with cytogenetically detectable deletions of chromosome 11p13 (RICCARDI et al. 1980; FRANCKE et al. 1979; JUNIEN et al. 1980). Other patients have Beckwith-Wiedemann syndrome or urinary tract anomalies. The BWS gene is linked to chromosome 11p15, and appears to be distinct from the gene associated with Wilms' tumor aniridia syndrome (HENRY et al. 1989; NIIKAWA et al. 1986). Family studies strengthen the concept that the genetics of Wilms' tumor is considerably more complex than that of retinoblastoma since some kindreds with familial Wilms' tumor have not shown linkage to chromosome 11 (HUFF et al. 1988). Mapping studies of chromosome 11 have demonstrated that the BWS gene is distinct from the Wilms' tumor aniridia locus, confirming that additional genes contribute to Wilms' tumorigenesis in some patients (REEVE et al. 1989; KOUFOS et al. 1989; PETTENATI et al. 1986; PING et al. 1989). Acquired abnormalities of chromososme 11p are also apparent in Wilms' tumor tissue (Fig. 4.8). Using positional cloning methods, a gene designated *Wt-1* has been isolated from 11p13 (ROSE et al. 1990; CALL et al. 1990). *Wt-1* has structural features of a DNA binding protein. In vitro studies suggest that the *Wt-1* gene product is an inhibitor of gene expression which is probably involved in the normal process of renal morphogenesis. Acquired mutations in *Wt-1* have been identified in Wilms' tumor tissue, and germline mutations have been identified in patients with Wilms' tumor and urogenital anomalies (PRITCHARD-JONES et al. 1990). Clarification of this complex situation awaits the cloning of all the relevant genes from chromosome 11p. The well-known difference in clinical behavior between the favorable and unfavorable histologic variants of Wilms' tumor suggest that as yet unidentified genetic changes occur in addition to alterations of genes on chromosome 11. An additional genetic mechanism, germline imprinting, is illustrated by BWS patients who exhibit the phenomenon of uniparental disomy for chromosome 11 (BROWN et al. 1990; VILJOEN and RAMESAR 1992; MOUTOU et al. 1992). It has been proposed that, as part of the normal regulation of developmental gene expression, some tumor suppressor genes undergo selective inactivation by passage through either the male or the female germline (SCRABLE et al. 1989a).

The role of this process in oncogenesis is not yet fully defined.

4.5.2.3 Neuroblastoma

Although neuroblastoma rarely occurs in a familial form, most cases are sporadic, and so there has not been a straightforward approach to a "neuroblastoma gene." The current concept of the molecular genetics of neuroblastoma has arisen primarily from clues suggested by cytogenetic analysis. Neuroblastoma is well known to be characterized by abnormal structures called double minutes and homogeneously staining regions. Double minutes are small acentric paired extrachromosomal elements (Fig. 4.9A), and homogeneously staining regions are elongated poorly banding regions integrated within chromosomes. Studies in other systems had demonstrated that these structures are the cytologic hallmarks of gene amplification. Gene amplification can be defined as the presence of extra copies of a given gene in excess of a cell's ploidy. Analysis of DNA from neuroblastoma cell lines revealed that the double minutes and homogeneously staining region observed in neuroblastoma contained multiple copies of an oncogene designated N-*myc* (SCHWAB et al. 1983). N-*myc* copy number can vary from a few fold to several hundred fold but is remarkably consistent between sites and over time in an individual patient (BRODEUR et al. 1987). Surveys of neuroblastoma tumors have demonstrated N-*myc* amplification in approximately 40% of advanced stage patients, where it is clearly associated with early treatment failure (BRODEUR et al. 1984, 1992; SEEGER et al. 1985). N-*myc* amplification is rarely seen in early stage patients, but when present carries an adverse prognosis. In addition to N-*myc* amplification, chromosome 1p deletions are frequent in neuroblastomas, and it is suspected that a tumor suppressor gene important in this disorder is located there (FONG et al. 1989) (Fig. 4.9B). There is also evidence for an additional region of loss on chromosome 14 (FONG et al. 1992). A problem unique to neuroblastoma is the unusual behavior of stage IVS patients, who frequently exhibit spontaneous involution of their tumor. The genetic basis of this behavior is unclear. However, it has been recognized that stage IV patients with aggressive disease exhibit a near-diploid DNA index with many chromosome breaks, while stage IVS patients are near triploid with relatively few abnormal chromosomes (LOOK et al. 1984, 1991). As in stage IV neuroblastoma, N-*myc* amplification in stage IVS patients is associated with progressive disease.

4.5.2.4 Sarcomas

There has been considerable progress in understanding the molecular basis of sarcoma tumorigenesis. Evidence has accumulated implicating both oncogenes and tumor suppressor genes in sarcomas. Mutations in the *p53* gene are frequent in osteosarcomas, and soft tissue sarcomas are an important part of LFS. Inactivation of the retinoblastoma gene has been observed in sporadic osteosarcoma (Toguchida et al. 1989), and as noted above, osteosarcoma is a frequent second malignancy in survivors of hereditary retinoblastoma. Instances of N-*myc* amplification have been described in embryonal rhabdomyosarcoma (Dias et al. 1990; Hayashi et al. 1990). Recently, amplification of a gene, MDM2, has been described in sarcomas (Oliner et al.1992). MDM2 appears to interact with *p53*, and its overexpression may represent an alternative pathway to *p53* inactivation in tumors which lack *p53* mutations. This observation also emphasizes the likelihood that additional targets of gene amplification remain to be described in solid tumors. Additional tumor suppressor genes await discovery as suggested by well-defined examples of LOH in rhabdomyosarcoma (Scrable et al. 1989b; Loh et al. 1992; Koufos et al. 1985).

Some of the best-characterized chromosomal translocations of solid tumors occur in sarcomas (Table 4.4). Identification of the target genes has been possible in Ewing's sarcoma, alveolar rhabdomyosarcoma, and myxoid liposarcoma (Delattre et al. 1992; Barr et al. 1992; Gemmill et al. 1992; Åman et al. 1992). With a striking similarity to the leukemias, the genetic target of the translocation in each of these tumors includes a transcription factor.

Table 4.4. Chromosomal translocations in sarcomas

Tumor	Translocation
Ewing's sarcoma	t(11;22)(q24;q12)
Myxoid liposarcoma	t(12;16)(q13;p11)
Rhabdomyosarcoma	t(2;13)(q35–37;q14)
(alveolar) Synovial sarcoma	t(X;18)(p11;q11)
Myxoid chondrosarcoma	t(9;22)(q22;q11.2)

4.5.2.5 Brain Tumors

Despite their clinical importance, the molecular pathogenesis of CNS tumors has been incompletely elucidated. Gene amplification has been reported in a significant number of CNS tumors. Amplification of the epidermal growth factor receptor (EGFR), c-*myc*, N-*myc*, and GLI (Knizler et al. 1987; Wasson et al. 1990; Humphrey et al. 1988; Rasheed and Bigner 1991) genes has been reported particularly in high-grade glial tumors. Of these changes, EGFR amplification has been most frequently reported, and is likely to be an important step in the progression of glial tumors. Overexpression of EGFR is found in tumors carrying EGFR amplification, and the gene has frequently undergone rearrangement during the amplification process (Humphrey et al. 1988; Wong et al. 1987). Gene amplification also occurs in medulloblastoma (Wasson et al. 1990). Mutations in *p53* are relatively frequent in glial tumors (Nigro et al. 1989). Cytogenetic and LOH studies in CNS tumors have suggested the existence of as yet unidentified tumor suppressor genes at several sites, particularly chromosome 10 (Rasheed and Bigner 1991).

4.5.2.6 Genetic Alterations in Secondary Malignancies

It is apparent that certain subsets of cancer survivors have a substantially increased risk of developing a second malignancy. In some instances, such as Li-Fraumeni syndrome, the second tumor may be a manifestation of a hereditary predisposition to cancer. As the genes which predispose to childhood cancer are more completely defined, it is likely that genetic causes will be identified in an increasing proportion of patients with two independent cancers. However, in spite of these considerations, careful studies of patients who have developed second malignancies have shown that in some settings, second tumors result from the oncogenic effect of cancer therapy. Certain chemotherapeutic agents are clearly implicated in this process. In particular, secondary nonlymphoblastic leukemia has been associated with the use of nitrogen mustard in the treatment of Hodgkin's disease (Meadows et al. 1989; Blayney et al. 1987). The leukemic state typically develops after a latency of years following treatment and may initially present as a myelodysplastic syndrome. Cytogenetic studies frequently demonstrate complete or partial monosomy of chromosome 5 or

7 (HEIM and MITELMAN 1986; JOHANSSON et al. 1991; IURLO et al. 1988). Interestingly, similar cytogenetic abnormalities have been observed in patients whose leukemia has developed following exposure to genotoxic chemicals in the workplace (PASQUALETTI et al. 1991). Recently, secondary acute nonlymphoblastic leukemia has been observed in patients treated with epipodophyllotoxins. Abnormalities of chromosome 11 were frequent, and the carcinogenic properties of the drug appeared to be schedule dependent (PUI et al. 1989, 1990b; PRIETO et al. 1990). The development of oncogenic chromosomal abnormalities after exposure to epipodophyllotoxins is credible in view of their mechanism of action. These drugs are potent inhibitors of DNA topoisomerase II, a nuclear enzyme which can resolve knotted DNA structures. A consequence of topoisomerase II inhibition is the development of double-stranded breaks in the DNA backbone which could potentially lead to chromosome rearrangements. At the present time, the specific genetic targets associated with the development of secondary leukemia are the subject of intense investigation.

4.6 Clinical Implications

At the present time, the impact of molecular oncology is greatest in cancer cell biology, and the full clinical implications of this information may not be realized for some time. Nonetheless, a number of applications have reached the clinical arena; these are primarily in cancer diagnosis, but therapeutic and preventive applications are being intensively sought. Given the extraordinarily rapid rate of acquisition of new knowledge, molecular genetics is certain to have an increasing impact on clinical practice.

4.6.1 Diagnosis

The history of cancer diagnostics is in large part the history of establishing more precise classification of clinically similar but biologically distinct diseases. In this regard, genetic classification is just beginning to have a major impact. Perhaps the most straightforward application is the use of cancer cytogenetics. This technology is already well established in the hematopoietic malignancies. Solid tumor cytogenetics is currently limited by the fact that relatively few centers have the necessary resources to analyze this

material. It is likely that the development of FISH technology will facilitate the transition of solid tumor cytogenetics from a research to a clinical tool.

DNA studies are useful in the lymphoid malignancies, where clonality can be determined by southern blot analysis of the immunoglobulin and T-cell receptor genes (WALDMANN et al. 1985). Identification of specific translocations is currently routinely established by cytogenetic studies. FISH analysis of bone marrow aspirates can be used to identify the presence of leukemic cells in "remission." The powerful PCR technique also has the potential to detect translocations of specific genes. Bone marrow transplant patients can be followed for residual disease and chimerism after transplant by PCR analysis of leukemic translocation chromosomes and polymorphic loci (HANSON et al. 1990; ROTH et al. 1989; GRIBBEN et al. 1991, 1992; ROUX et al. 1992; THOMPSON et al. 1992; GABERT et al. 1989; MIYAMURA et al. 1992; LAWLER et al. 1989; GEHLY et al. 1991). In the pediatric solid tumors, the determination of N-*myc* copy number has become an important part of the diagnostic evaluation of neuroblastoma. As other molecular markers are identified, and appropriate clinical correlative studies are completed, molecular diagnostic studies may become routine in many more types of cancer.

4.6.2 Therapeutic Applications

At the present time only one promising investigational therapy, the use of triretinoin in APL, can be clearly related to the underlying genetic lesion. This example may serve as a model on which future therapies may be based. The recognition that cancer cells differ from their normal progenitors in definable ways opens the potential for the identification of multiple new therapeutic targets. Genes which are overexpressed in tumor cells may become attractive targets for toxin or radioisotope conjugated monoclonal antibody therapies. It is important that some of the cellular targets identified by molecular analysis, as exemplified by the RAR-PML fusion protein, are unique to cancer cells and never occur in normal cells. This observation suggests that it may be possible to develop novel therapies with unprecedented specificity for the tumor cell.

4.6.3 Cancer Prevention

Although concepts of cancer prevention may appear to apply mainly to adult oncology, there may well be

certain specific implications for pediatric cancer. The
ability to identify both germline and somatic oncogenic mutations at the DNA level creates novel possibilities for dissecting the influence of heredity and
environment. Specific types of mutations suggest the
signature of specific classes of mutagens. These may
potentially be traced to parental exposures or to
familial pharmacogenetic variants. The identification of germline mutations in Rb and Wt-1 enable
prenatal diagnosis of cancer susceptibility. The
recognition of *p53* mutations in the Li-Fraumeni
syndrome creates unique problems and opportunities. The phenotype and penetrance of germline
p53 mutations are highly variable. In contrast to
familial retinoblastoma, it is difficult to recommend
a reasonable screening program for affected individuals in LFS kindreds. In contrast, these families
may provide a unique opportunity to test chemopre-
ventive agents. Most likely multiple additional
genes will be identified which are associated with the
predisposition toward various cancers. The identification of cancer susceptibility genes is rapidly creat-
ing new challenges and opportunities for cancer
prevention.

References

Aaronson SA (1991) Growth factors and cancer. Science 254:
    1146–1153
Abramson DH, Ronner HJ, Ellsworth RM (1979) Second
    tumors in nonirradiated bilateral retinoblastoma. Am J
    Ophthalmol 87: 624–627
Adams JM, Harris AW, Pinkert CA et al. (1985) The c-*myc*
    oncogene driven by immunoglobulin enhancers induces
    lymphoid malignancy in transgenic mice. Nature 318:
    533–538
Ahuja H, Bar-Eli M, Advani SH, Benchimol S, Cline MJ
    (1989) Alterations in the p53 gene and the clonal evolution
    of the blast crisis of chronic myelocytic leukemia. Proc Natl
    Acad Sci USA 86: 6783–6787
Alitalo K, Schwab M (1986) Oncogene amplification in tumor
    cells. Adv Cancer Res 47: 235–282
Åman P, Ron D, Mandahl N, Fioretos T et al. (1992)
    Rearrangement of the transcription factor gene CHOP in
    myxoid liposarcomas with t(12;16) (q13;p11). Genes
    Chromosomes Cancer 5: 1–8
Aplan PD, Lombardi DP, Ginsberg AM, Cossman J, Bertness
    VL, Kirsch IR (1990) Disruption of the human SCL locus
    by "illegitimate" V-(D)-J recombinase activity. Science
    250: 1426–1429
Aurias A, Rimbaut C, Buffe D, Zucker JM, Mazabraud A
    (1984) Translocation of band q12 of chromosome 22 in
    Ewing's sarcoma. Cancer Genet Cytogenet 12: 21–25
Baker SJ, Fearon ER, Nigro JM et al. (1989) Chromosome 17
    deletions and p53 gene mutations in colorectal carcinomas.
    Science 244: 217–221
Baker SJ, Markowitz S, Fearon ER, Willson JKV,
    Vogelstein B (1990) Suppression of human colorectal
    carcinoma cell growth by wild-type p53. Science 249:
    912–914

Bakhshi A, Jensen JP, Goldman P, Wright JJ, McBride
    OW, Epstein AL, Korsmeyer SJ (1985) Cloning the
    chromosomal breakpoint of t(14;18) human lymphomas:
    clustering around J_H on chromosome 14 and near a tran-
    scriptional unit on 18. Cell 41: 899–906
Balaban G, Gilbert F, Nichols W, Meadows AT, Shields
    J (1982) Abnormalities of chromosome 13 in retino-
    blastomas from individuals with normal constitutional
    karyotypes. Cancer Genet Cytogenet 6: 213–221
Ballester R, Marchuk D, Boguski M, Saulino A, Letcher R,
    Wigler M, Collins F (1990) The *NF1* locus encodes a protein
    functionally related to mammalian GAP and yeast IRA
    proteins. Cell 63: 851–859
Barany F (1991) Genetic disease detection and DNA amplifi-
    cation using cloned thermostable ligase. Proc Nat Acad Sci
    USA 88: 189–193
Barbacid M (1987) *Ras* genes. Annu Rev Biochem 56: 779–827
Barr FG, Holick J, Nycum L, Biegel JA, Emanuel BS (1992)
    Localization of the t(2;13) breakpoint of alveolar rha-
    bodomyosarcoma on a physical map of chromosome 2.
    Genomics 13: 1150–1156
Biondi A, Rambaldi A, Pandolfi PP et al. (1992) Molecular
    monitoring of the myl/retinoic acid receptor-alpha fusion
    gene in acute promyelocytic leukemia by polymerase chain
    reaction. Blood 80: 492–497
Bishop JM (1987) The molecular genetics of cancer. Science
    235: 305–311
Bishop JM (1989) Oncogenes and clinical cancer. In:
    Weinberg RA (ed) Oncogenes and the molecular origins of
    cancer. Cold Spring Harbor Laboratory Press, New York,
    pp 327–358
Bishop JM (1991) Molecular themes in oncogenesis. Cell 64:
    235–248
Bishop JM, Varmus HE (1982) Functions and origins of retro-
    viral transforming genes. In: Weiss R, Telch N, Varmus H,
    Coffin J (eds) Molecular biology of tumor viruses. Part III,
    RNA tumor viruses. Cold Spring Harbor Laboratory
    Press, New York, pp 999–1108
Blat C, Aberdam D, Schwartz R, Sachs L (1988) DNA rear-
    rangement of a homeobox gene in myeloid leukaemic cells.
    EMBO J 7: 4283–4290
Blayney DW, Longo DL, Young RC et al. (1987) Decreasing
    risk of leukemia with prolonged follow-up after chemother-
    apy and radiotherapy for Hodgkin's disease. N Engl Med
    316: 710–714
Boehm T, Baer R, Lavenir I, Forster A, Waters JJ, Nacheva E,
    Rabbitts TH (1988) The mechanism of chromosomal
    translocation t(11;14) involving the T-cell receptor C delta
    locus on human chromosome 14q11 and a transcribed
    region of chromosome 11p15. EMBO J 7: 385–394
Bos JL (1988) The *ras* family and human carcinogenesis.
    Mutat Res 195: 255–271
Boveri T (1929) The origin of malignant tumors. Williams and
    Wilkins, Baltimore, pp 26–27
Breslow NE, Beckwith JB (1982) Epidemiological features of
    Wilms' tumor: results of the National Wilms' Tumor
    Study. J Natl Cancer Inst 68: 429–436
Brodeur GM, Seeger RC, Schwab M, Varmus HE, Bishop JM
    (1984) Amplification of N-*myc* in untreated human neu-
    roblastomas correlates with advanced disease stage.
    Science 224: 1121–1124
Brodeur GM, Hayes FA, Green AA, Casper JT, Wasson J,
    Wallach S, Seeger RC (1987) Consistent N-*myc* copy
    number in simultaneous or consecutive neuroblastoma
    samples from sixty individual patients. Cancer Res 47:
    4248–4253
Brodeur GM, Azar C, Brother M et al. (1992) Neuro-

blastoma, Effect of genetic factors on prognosis and treatment. Cancer 70: 1685–1694

Brown KW, Williams JC, Maitland NJ, Mott MG (1990) Genomic imprinting and the Beckwith-Wiedemann syndrome [letter]. Am J Hum Genet 46: 1000–1001

Buchkovich K, Duffy LA, Harlow E (1989) The retinoblastoma protein is phosphorylated during specific phases of the cell cycle. Cell 58: 1097–1105

Call KM, Glaser T, Ito CY et al. (1990) Isolation and characterization of a zinc finger polypeptide gene at the human chromosome 11 Wilms' tumor locus. Cell 60: 509–520

Chen PL, Scully P, Shew JY, Wang JYJ, Lee WH (1989) Phosphorylation of the retinoblastoma gene product is modulated during the cell cycle and cellular differentiation. Cell 58: 1193–1198

Chen Q, Cheng JT, Tsai LH et al. (1990) The *tal* gene undergoes chromosome translocation in T cell leukemia and potentia-lly encodes a helix-loop-helix protein. EMBO J 9: 415–424

Chen ZX, Xue YQ, Zhang R et al. (1991) A clinical and experimental study on all-*trans* retinoic acid-treated acute promyelocytic leukemia patients. Blood 78: 1413–1419

Cheng J, Haas M (1990) Frequent mutations in the p53 tumor suppressor gene in human leukemia T-cell lines. Mol Cell Biol 10: 5502–5509

Cleary ML, Sklar J (1985) Nucleotide sequence of a t(14;18) chromosomal breakpoint in follicular lymphoma and demonstration of a breakpoint cluster region near a transcriptionally active locus on chromosome 18. Proc Natl Acad Sci USA 82; 7439–7443

Cleary ML, Smith SD, Sklar J (1986) Cloning and structural analysis of cDNAs for *bcl*-2 and a hybrid *bcl*-2/immunoglobulin transcript resulting from the t(14;18) translocation. Cell 47:19–28

Cole MD (1986) The *myc* oncogene: its role in transformation and differentiation. Annu Rev Genet 20: 361–384

Cory SJ, Adams JM (1988) Transgenic mice and oncogenesis. Annu Rev Immunol 6: 25–48

Crist WC, Cleary ML, Grossi CE et al. (1985) Acute leukemias associated with the 4;11 chromosome translocation have rearranged immunoglobulin heavy chain genes. Blood 66: 33–38

Croce CM, Nowell PC (1985) Molecular basis of human B cell neoplasia. Blood 65: 1–7

Cross M, Dexter TM (1991) Growth factors in development, transformation, and tumorigenesis. Cell 64: 271–280

Daley GQ, Van Etten RA, Baltimore D (1990) Induction of chronic leukemia in mice by the p210*bcr/abl* gene of the Philadelphia chromosome. Science 247: 824–830

de Thé H, Chomienne C, Lanotte M, Degos L, Dejean A (1990) The t(15;17) translocation of acute promyelocytic leukaemia fuses the retinoic acid receptor α gene to a novel transcribed locus. Nature 347: 558–561

Delattre O, Zucman J, Plougastel B et al. (1992) Gene fusion with an *ETS* DNA-binding domain caused by chromosome translocation in human tumors. Nature 359: 162–165

Dias P, Kumar P, Marsden HB, Gattamaneni HR, Heighway J, Kumar S (1990) N-*myc* gene is amplified in alveolar rhabdomyosarcomas (RMS) but not in embryonal RMS. Int J Cancer 45: 593–596

Diller L, Kassel J, Nelson CE et al. (1990) p53 functions as a cell cycle control protein in osteosarcomas. Mol Cell Biol 10: 5772–5781

Donehower LA, Harvey M, Slagle BL, McArthur MJ, Montgomery CA Jr, Butel JS, Bradley A (1992) Mice deficient for p53 are developmentally normal but susceptible to spontaneous tumours. Nature 356: 215–221

Downward J, Riehl R, Wu L, Weinberg RA (1990) Identification of a nucleotide exchange promoting activity for p21*ras*. Proc Natl Acad Sci USA 87: 5998–6002

Draper GJ, Sanders BM, Kingston JE (1986) Second primary neoplasms in patients with retinoblastoma. Br J Cancer 53: 661

Dryja TP, Mukai S, Petersen R, Rapaport JM, Walton D, Yandell DW (1989) Parental origin of mutations of the retinoblastoma gene. Nature 339: 556–558

Edelman AM, Blumenthal DK, Krebs EG (1987) Protein serine/threonine kinase. Annu Rev Biochem 56: 567–613

Eisenman RN (1989) Nuclear oncogenes. In: Weinberg RA (ed) Oncogenes and the molecular origins of cancer, Cold Spring Harbor Laboratory Press, New York, pp 175–222

Eliyahu D, Michalovitz D, Eliyahu S, Pinhasikimhi O, Oren M (1989) Wild-type p53 can inhibit oncongene-mediated focus formation. Proc Natl Acad Sci USA 86: 8763–8767

Ellisen LW, Bird J, West DC, Soreng AL, Reynolds TC, Smith SD, Sklar J (1991) TAN-1, the human homolog of the *Drosophila* notch gene, is broken by chromosomal translocations in T lymphoblastic neoplasms. Cell 66: 649–661

Fearon ER, Vogelstein B (1990) A genetic model for colorectal tumorigenesis. Cell 61: 759–767

Fields S, Jang SK (1990) Presence of a potent transcription activating sequence in the p53 protein. Science 249: 1046–1048

Finger LR, Kagan J, Christopher G, Kurtzberg CG, Hershfield MS, Nowell PC, Croce CM (1989) Involvement of the *Tcl* 5 gene on human chromosome 1 in T-cell leukemia and melanoma. Proc Natl Acad Sci USA 86: 5039–5043

Fong CT, Dracopoli NC, White PS, Merrill PT, Griffith RC, Housman DE, Brodeur GM (1989) Loss of heterozygosity for the short arm of chromosome 1 in human neuroblastoma: correlation with N-*myc* amplification. Proc Natl Acad Sci USA 86: 3753–3758

Fong CT, White PS, Peterson K et al. (1992) Loss of heterozygosity for chromosomes 1 or 14 defines subsets of advanced neuroblastomas. Cancer Res 52: 1780–1785

Francke U, Holmes LB, Atkins L, Riccardi VM (1979) Aniridia-Wilms' tumor association: evidence for specific deletion of 11p13. Cytogenet Cell Genet 24: 185–192

Fung YK, Murphree AL, T Ang A, Quian J, Hinrichs SH, Benedict WF (1987) Structural evidence for the authenticity of the human retinoblastoma gene. Science 236: 1657–1661

Gabert J, Thuret I, Lafage M, Carcassonne Y, Maraninchi D, Mannoni P (1989) Detection of residual *bcr/abl* translocation by polymerase chain reaction in chronic myeloid leukaemia patients after bone-marrow transplantation. Lancet II: 1125–1128

Gehly GB, Bryant EM, Lee AM, Kidd PG, Thomas ED (1991) Chimeric BCR-abl messenger RNA as a marker for minimal residual disease in patients transplanted for Philadelphia chromosome-positive acute lymphoblastic leukemia. Blood 78: 458–465

Gemmill RM, Mendez MJ, Dougherty CM et al. (1992) Isolation of a yeast artificial chromosome clone that spans the (12;16) translocation breakpoint chracteristic of myxoid liposarcoma. Cancer Genet Cytogenet 62: 166–170

Gribben JG, Freedman AS, Woo SD et al. (1991) All advanced stage non-Hodgkin's lymphomas with a polymerase chain reaction amplifiable breakpoint of bcl-2 have residual cells containing the bcl-2 rearrangement at evaluation and after treatment. Blood 78: 3275–3280

Gribben JG, Saporito L, Barber M et al. (1992) Bone marrows of non-Hodgkin's lymphoma patients with a bcl-2 translocation can be purged of polymerase chain reaction-detectable lymphoma cells using monoclonal antibodies and immunomagnetic bead depletion. Blood 80: 1083–1089

Haluska FG, Finver S, Tsujimoto Y, Croce CM (1986) t(8;14) chromosomal translocation occurring in B-cell malignancies results from mistakes in V-D-J joining. Nature 324: 158–161

Haluska FG, Tsujimoto Y, Croce CM (1987) Oncogene activation by chromosome translocation in human malignancy. Annu Rev Genet 21: 321–347

Hanahan D (1989) Transgenic mice as probes into complex systems. Science 246: 1265–1275

Hanson CA, Holbrook EA, Sheldon S, Schnitzer B, Roth MS (1990) Detection of Philadelphia chromosome-positive cells from glass slide smears using the polymerase chain reaction. Am J Pathol 137: 1–6

Harris H (1988) The analysis of malignancy in cell fusion: the position in 1988. Cancer Res 48: 3302–3306

Hayashi Y, Sugimoto T, Horii et al. (1990) Characterization of an embryonal rhabdomyosarcoma cell line showing amplification and over-expression of the N-*myc* oncogene. Int J Cancer 45: 705–71

Hayman MJ (1986) *erb*-B, growth factor receptor turned oncogene. Trends Genet 2: 260–263

Heim S, Mitelman F (1986) Chromosome abnormalities in the myelodysplastic syndromes. Clin Haematol 15: 1003–1021

Heim S, Mitelman F (1987) Cancer cytogenetics. Alan R. Liss, New York

Heisterkamp N, Stephenson JR, Groffen J, Hansen PF, de Klein A, Bartram CR, Grosveld G (1983) Localization of the c-*abl* oncogene adjacent to a translocation breakpoint in chronic myelocytic leukaemia. Nature 306: 239–242

Henry I, Jeanpierre M, Couillin P et al. (1989) Molecular definition of the 11p15.5 region involved in Beckwith-Wiedemann syndrome and probably in predisposition to adrenocortical carcinoma. Hum Genet 81: 273–277

Hermans A, Heisterkamp N, von Lindern M et al. (1987) Unique fusion of *bcr* and c-*abl* genes in Philadelphia chromosome positive acute lymphoblastic leukemia. Cell 51: 33–40

Huff V, Compton DA, Chao LY, Strong LC, Geiser CF, Saunders GF (1988) Lack of linkage of familial Wilms' tumour to chromosomal band 11p13. Nature 336: 377–378

Humphrey PA, Wong AJ, Vogelstein B, Friedman HS, Werner MH, Bigner DD, Bigner SH (1988) Amplification and expression of the epidermal growth factor receptor gene in human glioma xenografts. Cancer Res 48: 2231–2238

Hunter T (1989) Oncogene products in the cytoplasm: the protein kinases. In: Weinberg RA (ed) Oncogenes and the molecular origins of cancer. Cold Spring Harbor Laboratory Press, New York, pp 147–173

Hunter T (1991) Cooperation between oncogenes. Cell 64: 249–270

Iurlo A, Mecucci C, Van Orshoven A, Michaux JL, Boogaerts M, Van den Berghe H (1988) The karyotype in secondary hematologic disorders after treatment for Hodgkin's disease. A study of 19 patients. Cancer Genet Cytogenet 36: 165–172

Johansson B, Mertens F, Heim S, Kristoffersson U, Mitelman F (1991) Cytogenetics of secondary myelodysplasia (sMDS) and acute nonlymphocytic leukemia (sANLL). Eur J Haematol 47: 17–27

Johnsson A, Heldin DH, Wasteson A et al. (1984) The c-*cis* gene encodes a precursor of the B chain of platelet-derived growth factor, EMBO J 3. 921–928

Junien C, Turleau C, de Grouchy J, Said R, Rethore MO, Tenconi R, Dufier JL (1980) Regional assignment of catalase (CAT) gene to band 11p13. Association with the aniridia-Wilms' tumor-gonadoblastoma (WAGR) complex. Ann Genet 23: 165–168

Kagan J, Finger LR, Letofsky J, Finan J, Nowell PC, Croce CM (1989) Clustering of breakpoints on chromosome 10 in acute T-cell leukemias with the t(10;14) chromosome translocation. Proc Natl Acad Sci USA 86: 4161–4165

Kamps MP, Murre C, Sun X, Baltimore D (1990) A new homeobox gene contributes the DNA binding domain of the t(1;19) translocation protein in pre-B ALL. Cell 60: 547–555

Kamps MP, Look T, Baltimore D (1991) The human t(1;19) translocation protein in pre-B ALL produces multiple E2A-Pbx1 fusion proteins with differing transforming potentials. Genes Dev 5: 358–368

Kaneko Y, Sakurai M (1977) 15/17 translocation in acute promyelocytic leukemia. Lancet I: 961

Kaneko Y, Rowley JD, Maurer HS, Variakojis D, Moohr JW (1982) Chromosome pattern in childhood acute non-lymphocytic leukemia. Blood 60: 389–399

Kelliher MA, McLaughlin J, Witte ON, Rosenberg N (1990) Induction of a chronic myelogenous leukemia-like syndrome in mice with v-*abl* and BCR/ABL. Proc Natl Acad Sci USA 87: 6649–6653

Kinzler KW, Bigner SH, Bigner DD et al. (1987) Identification of an amplified, highly expressed gene in a human glioma. Science 236: 70–73

Knudson AG (1971) Mutation and cancer: statistical study of retinoblastoma. Proc Natl Acad Sci USA 68: 820–823

Knudson AG Jr (1986) Genetics of human cancer. Annu Rev Genet 20: 231–51

Kohl NE, Gee CE, Alt FW (1984) Activated expression of the N-*myc* gene in human neuroblastomas and related tumors. Science 226: 1335–1337

Koufos A, Hansen MF, Copeland NG, Jenkins NA, Lampkin BC, Cavenee WK (1985) Loss of heterozygosity in three embryonal tumours suggests a common pathogenetic mechanism. Nature 316: 330–334

Koufos A, Grundy P, Morgan K et al. (1989) Familial Wiedemann-Beckwith syndrome and a second Wilms' tumor locus both map to 11p15.5. Am J Hum Genet 44: 711–719

Lane DP, Benchimol S (1990) p53: oncogene or anti-oncogene. Genes Dev 4: 1–8

Lavigueur A, Maltby V, Mock D, Rossant J, Pawson T, Bernstein A (1989) High incidence of lung, bone, and lymphoid tumors in transgenic mice overexpressing mutant alleles of the p53 oncogene. Mol Cell Biol 9: 3982–3991

Lawler M, McCann SR, Conneally E, Humphries P (1989) Chimaerism following allogeneic bone marrow transplantation: detection of residual host cells using the polymerase chain reaction. Br J Haematol 73: 205–210

Le Beau MM, McKeithan TW, Shima EA, Goldman-Leikin RA, Chan SJ, Bell GI, Rowley JD, Diaz MO (1986) T-cell receptor α-chain gene is split in a human T-cell leukemia cell line with a t(11;14)(p15;q11). Proc Natl Acad Sci USA 83: 9744–9748

Lee EYHP, Chang CY, Hu N et al. (1992) Mice deficient for Rb are nonviable and show defects in neurogenesis and haematopoiesis. Nature 359: 288–294

Lee WH, Bookstein R, Hong F, Young LJ, Shew JY, Lee

EYHP (1987) Human retinoblastoma susceptibility gene: cloning identification, and sequence. Science 235: 1394–1399

Lo Coco F, Avvisati G, Diverio D et al. (1991) Molecular evaluation of response to all-*trans*-retinoic acid therapy in patients with acute promyelocytic leukemia. Blood 77: 1657–1659

Loh WE Jr, Scrable HJ, Livanos E, Arboleda MJ, Cavence WK, Oshimura M, Weissman BE (1992) Human chromosome 11 contains two different growth suppressor genes for embryonal rhabdomyosarcoma. Proc Natl Acad Sci USA 89: 1755–1759

Look AT, Hayes FA, Nitschke R, McWilliams NB, Green AA (1984) Cellular DNA content as a predictor of response to chemotherapy in infants with unresectable neuroblastoma. N Engl J Med 311: 231–235

Look AT, Hayes FA, Shuster JJ et al. (1991) Clinical relevance of tumor cell ploidy and N-*myc* gene amplification in childhood neuroblastoma: a Pediatric Oncology Group study. J Clin Oncol 9: 581–591

Ludlow JW, DeCaprio JA, Huang CM, Lee WH, Paucha E, Livingston DM (1989) SV40 large T Antigen binds preferentially to an underphosphorylated member of the retinoblastoma susceptibility gene product family. Cell 56: 57–65

Lugo T, Pendergast AM, Muller AJ, Witte ON (1990) Tyrosine kinase activity and transformation potency of BCR-ABL oncogene products. Science 247: 1079–1082

Malkin D, Li FP, Strong LC et al. (1990) Germ line p53 mutations in a familial syndrome of breast cancer, sarcomas, and other neoplasms. Science 250: 1233–1238

Marshall CJ (1991) Tumor suppressor genes. Cell 64: 312–326

McGuire EA, Hockett RD, Pollock KM, Bartholdi MF, O'Brien SJ, Korsmeyer SJ (1989) The t(11;14)(p15;q11) in a T-cell acute lymphoblastic leukemia cell line activates multiple transcripts, including Ttg-1, a gene encoding a potential zinc finger protein. Mol Cell Biol 9: 2124–2132

Meadows AT, Obringer AC, Marrero O et al. (1989) Second malignant neoplasms following childhood Hodgkin's disease: treatment and splenectomy as risk factors. Med Pediatr Oncol 17: 477–487

Mellentin JD, Murre CM, Donlon TA et al. (1989) The gene for enhancer binding proteins E12/E47 lies at the t(1;19) breakpoint in acute leukemias. Science 246: 379–382

Meltzer PS, Guan XY, Burgess A, Trent JM (1992) Rapid generation of region specific probes by chromosome microdissection and their application. Nature Genet 1: 24–28

Mihara K, Cao XR, Yen A et al. (1989) Cell cycle dependent regulation of phosphorylation of the human retinoblastoma gene product. Science 246: 1300–1303

Miller RW, Fraumeni JF Jr. Manning MD (1964) Association of Wilms' tumor with aniridia, hemihypertrophy and other congential malformations. N Engl J Med 270: 922–927

Milner J, Cook A, Mason J (1990) p53 is associated with p34^{cdc2} in transformed cells. EMBO J 9: 2885–2889

Miyamura K, Tanimoto M, Morishima Y et al. (1992) Detection of Philadelphia chromosome-positive acute lymphoblastic leukemia by polymerase chain reaction: possible eradication of minimal residual disease by marrow transplantation. Blood 79: 1366–1370

Moley JF, Brother MB, Wells SA, Spengler BA, Biedler JL, Brodeur GM (1991) Low frequency of *ras* gene mutations in neuroblastomas, pheochromocytomas, and medulary thyroid cancers. Cancer Res 51: 1596–1599

Morgan GJ, Hughes T, Janssen JW et al. (1989) Polymerase chain reaction for detection of residual leukaemia. Lancet I: 928–929

Moutou C, Junien C, Henry I, Bonaiti-Pellie C (1992) Beckwith-Wiedemann syndrome: a demonstration of the mechanisms responsible for the excess of transmitting females. J Med Genet 29: 217–220

Mulligan LM, Matlashewski GJ, Scrable HJ, Cavenee WK (1990) Mechanisms of p53 loss in human sarcomas. Proc Natl Acad Sci USA 87: 5863–5867

Nigro JM, Baker SJ, Preisinger AC et al. (1989) Mutations in the p53 gene occur in diverse human tumour types. Nature 342: 705–708

Niikawa N, Ishikiriyama S, Takahashi S et al. (1986) The Wiedemann-Beckwith syndrome: pedigree studies on five families with evidence for autosomal dominant inheritance with variable expressivity. Am J Med Genet 24: 41–55

Nourse J, Mellentin JD, Galili N, Wilkinson J, Stanbridge E, Smith SD, Cleary ML (1990) Chromosomal translocation t(1;19) results in synthesis of a homeobox fusion mRNA that codes for a potential chimeric transcription factor. Cell 60: 535–545

Nowell PC, Hungerford DA (1960) A minute chromosome in human granulocytic leukemia. Science 132: 1497

Oliner JD, Kinzler KW, Meltzer PS, Geroge DL, Vogelstein B (1992) Amplification of a gene encoding a p53 associated protein in human sarcomas. Nature 358: 80–83

Parsons JT (1990) Closing the GAP in a signal transduction pathway. Trends Genet 6: 169–171

Pasqualetti P, Casale R, Colantonio D, Collacciani A (1991) Occupational risk for hematological malignancies. Am J Hematol 38: 147–149

Pettenati MJ, Haines JL, Higgins RR, Wappner RS, Palmer CG, Weaver DD (1986) Wiedemann-Beckwith syndrome: presentation of clinical and cytogenetic data on 22 new cases and review of the literature. Hum Genet 74: 143–154

Ping AJ, Reeve AE, Law DJ, Young MR, Boehnke M, Feinberg AP (1989) Genetic linkage of Beckwith-Wiedemann syndrome to 11p15. Am J Hum Genet 44: 720–723

Pinkel D, Landegent J, Collins C, Fuscoe J, Segraves R, Lucas J, Gray J (1988) Fluorescence in situ hybridization with human chromosome-specific libraries: detection of trisomy 21 and translocations of chromosome 4. Proc Natl Acad Sci USA 85: 9138–9142

Prieto F, Palau F, Badia L, Beneyto M, Perez-Sirvent ML, Orts A, Castle V (1990) 11q23 abnormalities in children with acute nonlymphocytic leukemia (M4-M5): association with previous chemotherapy. Cancer Genet cytogenet 45: 1–11

Pritchard-Jones K, Fleming S, Davidson D et al. (1990) The candidate Wilms' tumour gene is involved in genitourinary development. Nature 346: 194–197

Pui CH, Behm FG, Raimondi SC et al. (1989) Secondary acute myeloid leukemia in children treated for acute lymphoid leukemia. N Engl J Med 321: 136–142

Pui CH, Crist WM, Look AT (1990a) Biology and clinical significance of cytogenetic abnormalities in childhood acute lymphoblastic leukemia. Blood 76: 1449–1463

Pui CH, Hancock KL, Raimondi SC et al. (1990b) Myeloid neoplasia in children treated for solid tumors. Lancet 336: 417–421

Rabbitts TH (1991) Translocations, master genes, and differences between the origins of acute and chronic leukemias. Cell 67: 641–644

Rasheed BK, Bigner SH (1991) Genetic alterations in glioma and medulloblastoma. Cancer Metastasis Rev 10: 289–299

Reeve AE, Sih SA, Raizis AM, Feinberg AP (1989) Loss of

allelic heterozygosity at a second locus on chromosome 11 in sporadic Wilms' tumor cells. Mol Cell Biol 9: 1799–1803

Riccardi VM, Hittner HM, Francke U, Yunis JJ, Ledbetter D, Borges W (1980) The aniridia-Wilms' tumor association: the critical role of chromosome band 11p13. Cancer Genet Cytogenet 2: 131–137

Rose EA, Glaser T, Jones C et al. (1990) Complete physical map of the WAGR region of 11p13 localizes a candidate Wilms' tumor gene. Cell 60: 495–508

Roth MS, Antin JH, Bingham EL, Ginsburg D (1989) Detection of Philadelphia chromosome-positive cells by the polymerase chain reaction following bone marrow transplant for chronic myelogenous leukemia. Blood 74: 882–885

Roux E, Helg C, Chapuis B, Jeannet M, Roosnek E (1992) Evolution of mixed chimerism after allogeneic bone marrow transplantation as determined on granulocytes and mononuclear cells by the polymerase chain reaction. Blood 79: 2775–2783

Rowley JD, Golomb HM, Vardman JW, Fukuhara S, Dougherty C, Potter D (1977) Further evidence for nonrandom chromosomal abnormality in acute promyelocytic leukemia. Int J Cancer 20: 869–872

Sager R (1989) Tumor suppressor genes: the puzzle and the promise. Science 246: 1406–1412

Saiki RK, Gelfand DH, Stoffel S et al. (1988) Primer-directed enzymatic amplification of DNA with a thermostable DNA polymerase. Science 239: 487–491

Schwab M, Amier LC (1990) Amplification of cellular oncogenes: a predictor of clinical outcome in human cancer. Genes Cromosomes Cancer 1: 181–194

Schwab M, Alitalo K, Klempnauer KH et al. (1983) Amplified DNA with limited homology to *myc* cellular oncogene is shared by human neuroblastoma cell lines and a neuroblastoma tumour. Nature 305: 245–248

Scrable H, Cavenee W, Ghavimi F, Lovell M, Morgan K, Sapienza C (1989a) A model for embryonal rhabdomyosarcoma tumorigenesis that involves genome imprinting. Proc Natl Acad Sci USA 86: 7480–7484

Scrable H, Witte D, Shimada H et al. (1989b) Molecular differential pathology of rhabdomyosarcoma. Genes Chromosomes Cancer 1: 23–35

Seeger RC, Brodeur GM, Sather H, Dalton A, Siegel SE, Wong KY, Hammond D (1985) Association of multiple copies of the N-*myc* oncogene with rapid progression of neuroblastomas. N Engl J Med 313: 1111–1116

Solomon E, Borrow J, Goddard AD (1991) Chromosome aberrations and cancer. Science 254: 1153–1160

Southern EM (1975) Detection of specific sequences among DNA fragments separated by gel electrophoresis. J Mol Biol 98: 503–517

Stanbridge EJ (1990) Human tumor suppressor genes. Annu Rev Genet 24: 615–657

Stratton MR, Fisher C, Gusterson BA, Cooper CS (1989) Detection of point mutations in N-*ras* and K-*ras* genes of human embryonal rhabdomyosarcomas using oligonucleotide probes and the polymerase chain reaction. Cancer Res 49: 6324–6327

Sturzbecher HW, Maimets T, Chumakov P et al. (1990) p53 interacts with p34^{cdc2} in mammalian cells: implications for cell cycle control and oncogenesis. Oncogene 5: 795–801

Tabin C, Bradley S, Bargmann C et al. (1982) Mechanism of activation of a human oncogene. Nature 300: 143–148

Taparowsky E, Suard Y, Fassano O, Simizu K, Godlfarb M, Wigler M (1982) Activation of T24 bladder carcinoma transforming gene is linked to a single amino acid change. Nature 300: 762–765

Thompson JD, Brodsky I, Yunis JJ (1992) Molecular quantification of residual disease in chronic myelogenous leukemia after bone marrow transplantation. Blood 79: 1629–1635

Toguchida J, Ishizaki K, Sasaki MS et al. (1989) Preferential mutation of paternally derived RB gene as the initial event in sporadic osteosarcoma. Nature 338: 156–158

Ullrich A, Schlessinger J (1990) Signal transduction by receptors with tyrosine kinase activity. Cell 61: 203–212

Van Etten RA, Jackson P, Baltimore D (1989) The mouse type IVc-*abl* gene product is a nuclear protein and activation of transforming ability is associated with cytoplasmic localization. Cell 58: 669–678

Varmus H (1989) An historical overview of oncogenes. In: Weinberg RA (ed) Oncogenes and the molecular origins of cancer. Cold Spring Harbor Laboratory Press, New York, pp 3–44

Viljoen D, Ramesar R (1992) Evidence for paternal imprinting in familial Beckwith-Wiedemann syndrome. J Med Genet 29: 221–225

von Lindern M, Poustka A, Lerach H, Grosveld G (1990) The (6;9) chromosome translocation, associated with a specific subtype of acute nonlymphocytic leukemia, leads to aberrant transcription of a target gene on 9q34. Mol Cell Biol 10: 4016–4026

Waldmann TA, Davis MM, Bongiovanni KF, Korsmeyer SJ (1985) Rearrangements of genes for the antigen receptor on T cells as markers of lineage and clonality in human lymphoid neoplasms. N Engl J Med 313 (13): 776–83

Warrell RP Jr, Frankel SR, Miller WH Jr et al. (1991) Differentiation therapy of acute promylocytic leukemia with tretinoin (all-*trans*-retinoic acid). N Engl J Med 324: 324: 1385–1393

Wasson JC, Saylors RL, Zeltzer P et al. (1990) Oncogene amplification in pediatric brain tumors. Cancer Res 50: 2987–2990

Weinberg RA (1989) Oncogenes, anti-oncogenes, and the molecular bases of multistep carcinogenesis. Cancer Res 49: 3713–3721

Weinberg RA (1990) The retinoblastoma gene and cell growth control. Trends Biochem Sci 15: 199–202

Whang-Peng J, Triche TJ, Knutsen T, Miser J, Douglass EC, Israel MA (1984) Chromosome translocation in peripheral neuroepithelioma. N Engl J Med 311: 584–585

Wong AJ, Bigner SH, Bigner DD, Kinzler KW, Hamilton SR, Vogelstein B (1987) Increased expression of the epidermal growth factor receptor gene in malignant gliomas is invariably associated with gene amplification. Proc Natl Acad Sci USA 84: 6899–6903

Yarden Y, Ullrich A (1988) Growth factor receptor tyrosine kinases. Annu Rev Biochem 57: 443–478

Zutter M, Hockett RD, Roberts CWM et al. (1990) Th t(10;14)(q24;q11) of T-cell acute lymphoblastic leukemia juxtaposes the δ T-cell receptor with *tcl*-3, a conserved and activated locus at 10q24. Proc Natl Acad Sci USA 87: 3161–3165

5 Principles of Damage Interactions Between Radiation and Chemotherapeutic Agents

JAMES A. BELLI

CONTENTS

5.1   Introduction 75
5.2   Definitions........................... 75
5.2.1 Radiation Sensitivity 75
5.2.2 Sublethal Damage..................... 76
5.2.3 Cell Cycle Effects...................... 76
5.2.4 Repair of Sublethal Radiation Damage 77
5.2.5 Potentially Lethal Damage and Repair 77
5.3   Principles of Damage Interaction 78
5.4   Endpoints in the Study of Damage Interactions. . 79
5.4.1 Cells in Culture 79
5.4.2 Animal Tumor Studies.................. 79
5.5   Damage Interaction Models 80
5.5.1 Actinomycin D and Radiation............ 80
5.5.2 Repair of Sublethal Radiation Damage 81
5.6   Damage Interaction Between
       Doxorubicin and Radiation............... 82
5.7   Radiation Response of Multidrug Resistant
       Mammalian Cells 83
5.8   Damage Interaction Between Radiation and
       Other Chemotherapeutic Agents 84
5.9   Summary............................. 85
       References 85

5.1 Introduction

With the advent of effective chemotherapeutic agents in the treatment of childhood cancer, the use of radiation therapy in various therapeutic strategies is undergoing continual evaluation and evolution. Nonetheless, the pediatric radiation oncologist must have a detailed understanding of the possible interactions between radiation and chemotherapeutic agents for a number of reasons:

1. While concerns related to the late effects of radiation therapy have commanded substantial attention in recent years, the late effects of chemotherapy with or without the addition of radiation should not be neglected in the study of survivors of childhood cancer.

JAMES A. BELLI, M.D., Professor and John Sealy Centennial Chair, Department of Radiation Therapy, The University of Texas Medical Branch, Galveston, TX 77550-2780, USA

2. The acute reactions, when radiation is combined with chemotherapy, can be predicted by careful damage interaction studies in well-controlled cellular systems in vitro and in vivo.
3. Each of these therapeutic modalities, when used together or sequentially, may significantly alter the response of both tumors and normal tissues (therapeutic ratio).

This chapter will explore the damage interactions between radiation and those chemotherapeutic agents most commonly used in the treatment of childhood solid tumors. It is not intended to present a detailed review of the large number of studies devoted to the examination of these interactions in both cellular and animal systems. Rather, appropriate examples will be used to illustrate the major expressions of these interactions.

5.2 Definitions

5.2.1 Radiation Sensitivity

The definition of radiation sensitivity of cellular systems can be conceptualized in a number of ways. Figure 5.1 shows several single-dose radiation survival curves and illustrates these points. Curves A and B are drawn as having parallel final slopes. The major difference between these curves is in the width of the threshold region of the curve. Therefore, both of these cell populations exhibit the *same rate* of cell killing with increasing radiation dose; they are equally radiation sensitive. In contrast, curve C has a less steep final slope and represents a population which is radiation resistant compared to either population A or population B. It can be argued that the dose required to produce the same survival fraction (isoeffect) is higher for B than A, thus identifying population B as being more "radiation-resistant" than population A. Similarly, the same radiation dose results in a higher survival fraction for population B than for population A. However, the

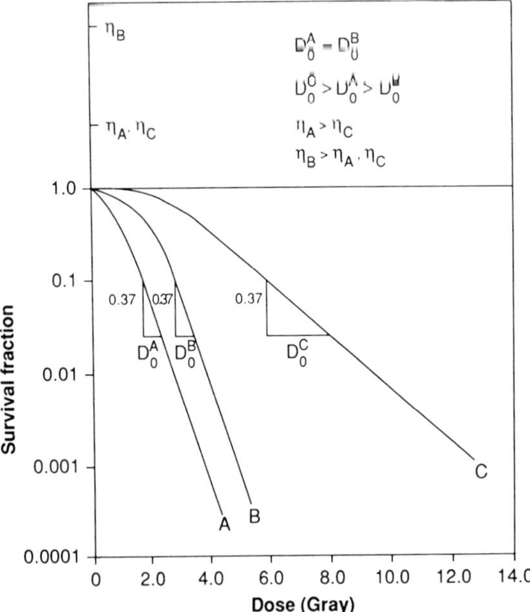

Fig. 5.1. Schematic representation of single-dose radiation survival curves. See text for details

important principle is that the use of single radiation doses and/or survival fractions are inappropriate determinants to compare cellular populations with regard to their relative radiation sensitivities. These comparisons are possible only if the entire single-dose radiation survival curve is known with confidence. This principle has important clinical implications. For example, it is inappropriate to speak of a particular childhood cancer as either "radiation sensitive" or "radiation resistant." Rather, extensive radiotherapeutic experience identifies childhood tumors which may or may not be radiation responsive.

Note that the single-dose radiation survival curves illustrated in Fig. 5.1 are probability statements that predict whether or not a proportion of the cellular population will survive a given level of radiation. This probability is best given by the reciprocal of the slope of the exponential portion of the curve. This reciprocal defines the D_0, which is that radiation dose required to reduce survival in the exponential portion of the curve by e^{-1} (0.368). Therefore, populations A and B in Fig. 5.1 have equal D_0's and, therefore, are equally radiation sensitive. On the other hand, the D_0 for population C is substantially larger and this population is more radiation resistant than population A and B.

5.2.2 Sublethal Damage

The concept of sublethal injury was first introduced, for mammalian cells, by ELKIND and SUTTON (1960). Sublethal damage is that level of radiation damage registered in mammalian cells which does not result in the suppression of a chosen endpoint. The registration of sublethal radiation damage is characterized by the presence of a threshold on the single-dose radiation survival curve (see Fig. 5.1). The capacity to tolerate sublethal radiation injury is given by the extrapolation number (n) which results when the exponential portion of the single-dose radiation survival curve is back-extrapolated to dose = 0. The larger this number, the larger the capacity for sublethal damage. Curves A and C in Fig. 5.1 have the same extrapolation number and therefore have the same capacity to accumulate sublethal radiation injury. The difference in these two curves, as pointed out above, is in the value of the D_0. On the other hand, curve B has a substantially higher extrapolation number than either curve A or curve C and, therefore, has a higher capacity for the registration of sublethal damage before exponential cell survival is observed.

5.2.3 Cell Cycle Effects

As exponentially growing cells progress from one division to the next, variation in survival response to radiation is observed. The four compartments of the cell cycle are G_1, S, G_2, and M. The most resistant cell cycle compartment for exponentially growing mammalian cells is the period of DNA synthesis, S. The sensitive compartments are G_2/M. G_1 also constitutes a sensitive compartment in those cell lines in which the length of G_1 is short. In those cell cycles in which G_1 is lengthy, there is a period of increased radiation resistance just prior to the onset of DNA synthesis. Therefore, radiation can be considered a true cell cycle-dependent modality with regard to cell killing. The damage interactions between radiation and certain chemotherapeutic agents are dependent upon the action of each of these modalities on cells as they progress through the cell cycle. For example, hydroxyurea preferentially kills cells in DNA synthesis, a radiation-resistant cell cycle compartment. Theoretically, these two modalities should interact when used in the treatment of solid tumors, resulting in a greater total cell killing than is produced by either agent alone. As is known from clinical experience, this expectation is very seldom realized. The chief reason is that cell growth kinetics of solid tumors are not comparable to those observed with exponentially growing cells in culture. Not all tumor cells may be in cycle: a substantial portion of cells may be deficient with regard to nutrients and oxygen, and a substantial proportion of the tumor cell population may be in a so-called quiescent phase, G_0.

5.2.4 Repair of Sublethal Radiation Damage

ELKIND and SUTTON (1960) investigated the consequences of delivering a total radiation dose in two fractions separated by time. Figure 5.2 illustrates the essential features of these investigations. Curve A is the single-dose radiation survival curve. Curve B is the fluctuations in survival as a total dose is divided into two portions separated by time. The initial survival increase is generally accepted to be indicative of the repair of sublethal radiation damage. The subsequent fall in survival represents the progression of the partially radiation-synchronized cell population into radiation-sensitive cell cycle compartments. This is followed by survival increase which can be attributed to cell division. Curve C results when cells are irradiated with a conditioning dose, allowed sufficient time for complete repair of sublethal damage, and irradiated with variable second doses. This level of repair is demonstrated by the capacity of surviving cells to accumulate the same level of sublethal injury as nonirradiated cells. If it is assumed that mammalian cells have the capacity for repeated cycles of damage and repair, it follows that the biologic effect on cells and tissues during a protracted course of radiation therapy will be substantially less compared to the same total radiation dose delivered in one fraction. Note, also, that the repair of sublethal radiation damage is defined in operational terms. Two-dose studies do not identify the molecular basis for the damage registered and/or its repair.

5.2.5 Potentially Lethal Damage and Repair

Operationally, three levels of radiation damage can be defined (BELLI and SHELTON 1969): (a) lethal damage, i.e., that level which completely suppresses a particular endpoint; (b) sublethal radiation damage which, if registered, does not suppress an endpoint; and (c) potentially lethal radiation damage which, when registered and the cell population placed in optimal postirradiation conditions, is expressed as lethal. PHILLIPS and TOLMACH (1966) first showed, in mammalian cells, that a nutritionally deficient postirradiation environment resulted in survival increases with time after a single radiation exposure. These observations, found with postirradiation inhibition of protein synthesis, were expanded to include incubation of irradiation cells in buffer (BELLI and SHELTON 1969), low temperature (WHITMORE and GULYAS 1967), postirradiation hypoxia (BELLI et al.1970), and cells in plateau phase maintained in depleted medium (LITTLE 1973; DRITSCHILO et al. 1979). Thus the repair of potentially lethal radiation injury is defined as the increase in survival following a single radiation dose under postirradiation conditions which are suboptimal, thus delaying or preventing progression of cells toward the first postirradiation division. Figure 5.3 illustrates the survival increase of irradiated cells as a function of time after exposure in a suboptimal environment. Survival increase is illustrated relative to survival for cells placed in an optimal environment immediately after irradiation (XR = 0, relative survival = 1.0). As shown, the survival increase reaches a plateau, the level of which is dependent upon the radiation dose; the maximum relative survival increases as the radiation exposure increases and as the survival level in optimal conditions decreases. The reason for this is that the repair of potentially lethal radiation damage

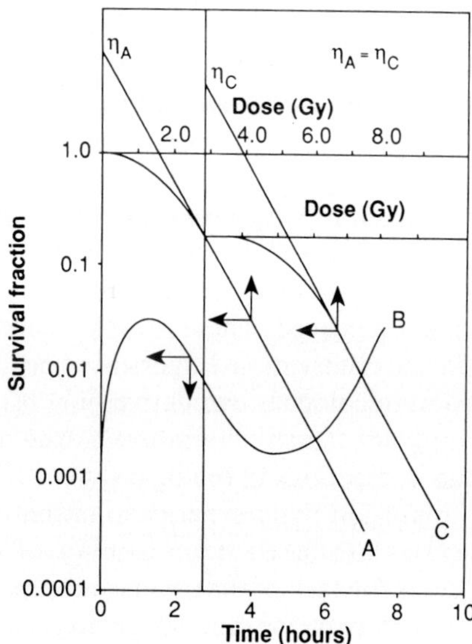

Fig. 5.2. Schematic representation of sublethal damage repair. *Curve A*, single-dose survival curve. *Curve B*, survival fluctuations when a total radiation dose is delivered in two fractions separated by time. *Curve C*, single-dose survival curve for the *survivors* of a conditioning dose irradiated with variable second doses after a time sufficiently long to allow for complete repair of sublethal damage. See text for further details

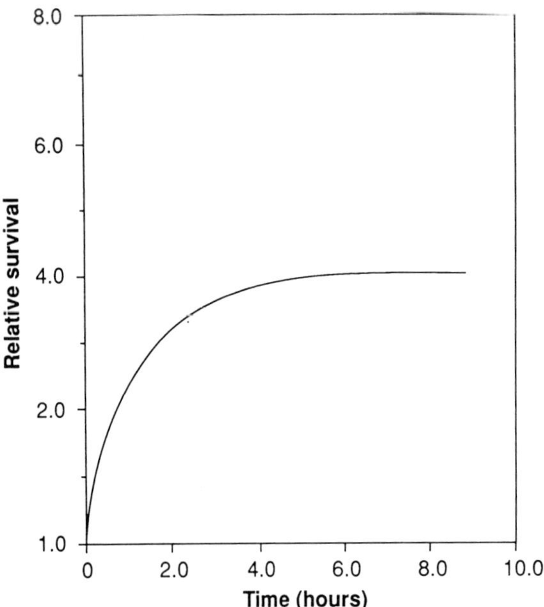

Fig. 5.3. Time course of the repair of potentially lethal radiation damage. See text for details

is expressed by an increase in D_0 (decreased slope) of the single-dose survival curve in suboptimal conditions.

5.3 Principles of Damage Interaction

Attempts to gain usable clinical insight into the consequences of combining radiation and chemotherapeutic agents have achieved only modest success. The reasons for this include:

1. A lack of sufficient information on the complete survival curves for radiation and the chemotherapeutic agent(s) of interest
2. Inappropriate experimental design to allow prediction of responses of normal tissues and tumors when multiple chemotherapeutic agents are used within the context of a fractionated course of radiation therapy, e.g., most in vitro and in vivo studies involve a single radiation exposure related in time to a single exposure to a single chemotherapeutic agent
3. Confusion surrounding the definition of the terms "synergy" and "additive"
4. Lack of detailed knowledge concerning the cellular and molecular mechanisms of cell killing by radiation and/or important chemotherapeutic agents.

A number of reviews have attempted to address some of these issues (HILL and BELLAMY 1984; BELLAMY and HILL 1984; BEGG 1987; STEEL and PECKHAM 1979).

Attempts to utilize experimental data to clarify and provide insight into clinical observations when chemotherapeutic agents are combined with radiation therapy suffer because these data are, in general, derived from biologic models which have little relevance to clinical experience. For example, STEEL and PECKHAM (1979) and STEEL (1979) suggested isobologram analysis to determine whether or not the interactions between chemotherapeutic agents and radiation are subadditive or superadditive. As these investigations pointed out, the validity of the isobologram analysis depends upon a detailed knowledge of the survival curves for each of the agents considered in the analysis. Often, such detailed information is not available. Reasons for this may include inappropriate experimental design, inappropriate endpoints, assumptions that the mode of action of cell killing by radiation and chemotherapeutic agents follow the same statistical models, or failure to recognize that the analysis is complicated if the curve shapes are different for drugs and radiation.

Clearly, the clinical objective in combined modality treatment is to increase the probability for local tumor control without an increase in normal tissue toxicity. It should be noted that clinical advantage for the child is achieved if the same tumor control probability occurs with lower radiation doses when combined with single or multiple chemotherapeutic agents. This is true even if the normal tissue toxicity remains the same. Rather, if a reduced radiation dose achieves higher local tumor control when used in conjunction with appropriate chemotherapeutic agents and normal tissue toxicity remains the same, a distinct and even more important clinical advantage is achieved. These principles are derived from clinical observation. Experienced pediatric and radiation oncologists can derive only broad guidelines from the extensive literature on drug/radiation damage interactions in biologic systems. Thus, the concepts of additivity, synergism, and antagonistic interactions are based upon analysis of dose-response curves for each of the agents and depend upon these curves having the same shape. In general, most dose-response curves available for radiation and some chemotherapeutic agents are the results of single exposures. The use of isobologram analysis to predict efficacy for various radiotherapeutic and chemotherapeutic combinations must be approached with caution. The success or failure of such expectations will depend upon whether or not the effect on a particular tumor cell population is greater than that on important normal tissues, e.g., whether or not the therapeutic index is increased. Strictly speaking, isobologram analysis, by itself, of single dose-response curves will not satisfy this requirement.

5.4 Endpoints in the Study of Damage Interactions

5.4.1 Cells in Culture

The success of any therapeutic strategy in the treatment of neoplastic disease is directly related to the probability that all tumor cells in the treated population do not retain the capacity for unlimited division. This endpoint has a precise counterpart in cell culture studies in which the endpoint is the capacity for a treated cell to divide without limit and form a visible colony on a suitable growth surface. This endpoint has been used to advantage in the identification of dose-response curves for radiation and/or chemotherapeutic agents, the characteristics of cellular repair, the influence of time between therapeutic agents, identification of the influence of cell cycle effects, and the relationship between response and various physiologic conditions (hypoxia, phase of growth, etc.). The disadvantage of this experimental approach, however, is that damage interaction studies usually involve a single exposure to each of the agents studied.

5.4.2 Animal Tumor Studies

There are three major endpoints in use when studying the effects of various therapeutic agents on animal tumors in vivo.

5.4.2.1 Tumor Control Dose50 (TCD 50)

In this assay system, transplantable tumors, generally in murine systems, are exposed to radiation and/or single chemotherapeutic agents and a dose-response curve constructed. The dose required to control tumors in 50% of the animals is used to compare various therapeutic approaches.

5.4.2.2 Growth Delay

Similar to the TCD50 endpoint, this assay system is used to measure the time required for a tumor of given size to reach that size after treatment. It is generally assumed that the longer this time, the more effective the treatment schedule. It should be remembered that this endpoint is most valid when the posttreatment tumor growth curves are parallel.

5.4.2.3 In Vivo/In Vitro Clonogenic Assays for Animal Tumors

In this assay system, transplantable animal tumors are irradiated and/or treated with chemotherapeutic agents in situ, tumors removed, and cells dispersed and plated for colony formation. Not all animal tumors are suitable for this assay. One of the important requirements is that untreated tumor cells have a high plating efficiency. If untreated tumor cells have a plating efficiency which is less than 50%, one cannot be confident that the responses noted under experimental conditions reflect the response of the entire tumor cell population in the host. This is true even though the plating efficiency from experiment to experiment remains the same, but low. One cannot be certain that these low plating efficiencies reflect the response of the *same* subpopulation of the isolate. However, this particular assay system allows for some therapeutic manipulation including the use of multiple radiation fractions and/or drug exposures.

5.4.2.4 Normal Tissue Assays

A number of assay techniques have been developed to study the effects of radiation and/or chemotherapeutic agents on important normal tissues. Among these are the bone marrow, small intestine, and skin. TILL and McCULLOCH (1961) developed an assay for the proliferative survival of mouse bone marrow stem cells. Recipient animals were lethally irradiated and subsequently injected with normal or irradiated bone marrow cells from donors. After a suitable period, recipient animals were sacrificed and the number of colonies in the spleen counted. These colonies were found to represent the proliferation of surviving "stem" cells from the donor animals. Relating the number of colonies to the number of cells injected allowed for the determination of a survival fraction to a given radiation dose. This assay system has been used to advantage in many studies, some of which will be reviewed below.

An equally imaginative assay system was refined by WITHERS and ELKIND (1970). In this assay system, groups of animals are irradiated with total body irradiation of varying doses and 3.5 days later sections of the jejunum are removed and fixed for histologic section. The endpoint is the number of regenerating crypts within a given circumference. Because the number of crypt cells irradiated cannot be determined, and since the regenerating crypt is due to the proliferation of more than one cell, a complete single-dose radiation survival curve (from dose = 0) cannot be plotted. Utilizing split-dose type experiments, these investigators were able to estimate that the extrapolation number for the crypt cells of the mouse small intestine was between 10 and 15. The D_0 value was similar to that found with other mammalian cells in vivo and in culture (1.3–1.7 Gy). WITHERS (1967) developed an assay system for the determination of radiation survival curves for mouse skin. This assay system depends upon irradiating areas of plucked skin in the shape of a doughnut to high dose. The purpose of this is to inactivate all cells in the basal layer to ensure that these will be reproductively suppressed. The center, which has been protected, is then exposed to varying doses of radiation and observed for skin regrowth. Thus, three important normal tissues bone marrow, crypt cells of the small intestine, and the basal cells of the skin have been characterized for their single-radiation-dose survival properties. This body of information, originally developed by radiation biologists, constitutes an important base upon which to study, in detail, damage interactions between radiation and chemotherapeutic agents in normal tissues.

5.5 Damage Interaction Models

Table 5.1 lists the commonly used chemotherapeutic agents in the treatment of many solid tumors in children, the tumors for which activity is found, and the normal tissues which are known to demonstrate increased toxicity when used in conjunction with radiation therapy. Of these, actinomycin D and doxorubicin represent two of the more important agents used in this age group. The damage interactions between radiation and these antibiotics will be used as a paradigm to illustrate important principles in the analysis of damage interactions in general and to identify putative models for other chemotherapeutic agents.

5.5.1 Actinomycin D and Radiation

Actinomycin D is an antibiotic which has activity against many solid tumors in children. Its principal

Table 5.1. Chemotherapeutic agents and radiation: toxicity in normal tissues

Agent	Normal Tissue
Actinomycin D	Gastrointestinal
	Skin
	Liver
	Esophagus
	Lung
	Bone marrow
Doxorubicin	Heart
	Skin
	Lung
	Gastrointestinal
	Esophagus
	Kidney
	Bone marrow
Cytoxan	Bladder
	Mucous membranes
	Bone marrow
Vincristine	Bone marrow
	Peripheral nerves
	Mucous membranes
Plantinum agents	Kidney
	Skin
	Mucous membranes
	Auditory apparatus
5-Fluorouracil	Skin
	Mucous membranes
	Bone marrow
	Gastrointestinal
Methotrexate	Central nervous system
	Bone marrow
	Mucous Membranes
Bleomycin	Lung
Nitrosoureas	Central nervous system
	Bone marrow

mode of action is suppression of RNA transcription following intercalation of the antibiotic into G-C-rich regions of DNA. Its principal action with regard to modification of radiation response is dependent upon the level of toxicity produced by actinomycin D alone. With cells in culture, antinomycin D at nontoxic levels modifies the single-dose radiation survival curve by reducing the extent of the threshold. The most appropriate interpretation of this finding is that actinomycin D at nontoxic levels reduces the capacity of mammalian cells in culture to accumulate sublethal radiation damage. When actinomycin D is given preirradiation, at levels which produce cell killing alone, the extrapolation number of the single-dose survival curve approaches 1.0 and the D_0 of the curve is reduced. The latter indicates that at toxic levels, actinomycin D sensitizes cells to radiation.

It is generally agreed that exponentially growing mammalian cells in culture do not constitute the most appropriate cell model for clarifying important damage interactions between chemotherapeutic agents and radiation as these pertain to a clinical situation. An important growth characteristic of mammalian cells in culture is that cell growth continues until density-inhibition occurs and cells enter a plateau phase. Such a population is characterized by a reduction in the number of cells in cycle and, therefore, may constitute a more appropriate model for those normal tissue populations which do not depend upon the cell division of a stem cell population for their structural and functional integrity. The liver, kidney, and lung are three examples of these normal tissue populations.

PIRO et al.(1975) have shown that the actinomycin D response of Chinese hamster cells in plateau phase growth 3 days following fractionated irradiation (2.1 Gy per day for 5 days) are significantly more sensitive to actinomycin D than nonirradiated cells. This observation may partially explain the clinical experience in children receiving actinomycin D at times after a course of radiation therapy. In such children, so-called recall phenomena are observed. For example, the skin which was included in the irradiated volume, which may appear normal before the administration of actinomycin D, may become erythematous after receiving the drug. Such recall phenomena have also been observed in the lung, esophagus, and heart. At the cellular level, these clinical observations have been seen in those tissues which have slowly proliferating or nonproliferating cells such as the skin, vascular endothelium, lung, and kidney.

Thus, in summary, the damage interaction between actinomycin D and radiation in exponentially growing mammalian cells is predominantly on the capacity for drug-treated cells to tolerate radiation damage. This effect may be important for both bone marrow stem cells, which have a small threshold on the single-dose radiation survival curve, and for the stem cells in the crypt of the small intestine, which have a large threshold on the single-dose radiation survival curve. Pretreatment with actinomycin D may lead to increased radiation toxicity when the abdomen is irradiated because the reduction in the threshold of the crypt cells of the small intestine may be reflected in the level of sublethal damage repair, thus interfering with the advantage of fractionated radiation therapy.

5.5.2 Repair of Sublethal Radiation Damage

Actinomycin D interferes with the repair of sublethal radiation injury as measured by the delivery of two radiation exposures separated by time and depends upon the level of actinomycin D between fractions (ELKIND et al. 1964). As the level of actinomycin D is increased between two fractions of radiation, the survival fluctuations reflecting repair of sublethal injury as modified by progression of the cells through the first postirradiation cell cycle are less prominent than those seen in untreated cells.

PIRO et al. (1976) studied the effects of actinomycin D between two radiation fractions delivered to Chinese hamster cells in plateau phase. Untreated cells demonstrated a survival increase with time, reflecting the repair of both sublethal and potentially lethal radiation damage. However, when actinomycin D was present between fractions, the survival increases observed were absent. To distinguish between the repair of potentially lethal and sublethal radiation damage in plateau phase cells, these investigators harvested cells immediately after the first dose and plated them into fresh medium. As a function of time, a second radiation dose was delivered. Under these conditions, the effect of actinomycin D, present during the time in fresh medium, was found to significantly inhibit the increases observed when nontreated cells were tested. It was also found that actinomycin D(0.04 µg/ml) present after plating irradiated plateau phase cells into fresh medium resulted in a significant amount of additional cell killing following a second radiation exposure. These observations were interpreted to mean that irradiated plateau phase cells demonstrate increased radiation sensitivity to a second radiation dose if actinomycin D has been present during the interval between the radiation fractions. Therefore, normal or malignant cells which are out of cycle and exposed to radiation (through some therapeutic manipulation), recruited into cycle, and subsequently exposed to actinomycin D may be at risk for cell killing out of proportion to the level of radiation and/or actinomycin D used.

FILLER et al. (1969) reported their clinical observations in children with Wilms' tumor with liver metastasis. These children were treated by partial hepatectomy followed immediately with actinomycin D and fractionated radiation therapy. It was found that these patients experienced severe and acute toxicity and eventually demonstrated chronic hepatic changes. These clinical observations prompted these investigators to delay treatment with actinomycin D and radiation therapy for at least 1 month following partial hepatectomy. These children did not demonstrate the severe toxicity shown by the children described above. This clinical observation can be interpreted in the following way. It is known that the liver represents a cell population which can be recruited into the cell cycle when a partial hepatectomy is performed. This recruitment is necessary to accomplish sufficient liver regeneration. When partial hepatectomy is followed by actinomycin D and fractionated radiation therapy, the severe toxicity observed may have been due to the increased sensitivity of "plateau" cells recruited into the cell cycle, representing a clinical counterpart to the work of Piro et al. (1976), described above. This increased cellular response to actinomycin D and radiation therapy was avoided if chemoradiation therapy was delayed following hepatectomy.

5.6 Damage Interaction Between Doxorubicin and Radiation

Doxorubicin is an aglycone sugar which has a side chain chromophore giving it its red color. This agent is active against a variety of solid tumors in both children and adults. In combination with other chemotherapeutic agents, it represents one of the more effective agents. The chemotherapeutic action of doxorubicin is similar to that of actinomycin D in that it also intercalates into DNA. However, this intercalation appears to be random rather than preferential at certain base pairs.

The single-dose survival curve for mammalian cells in culture that are exposed to doxorubicin is characterized by an initial steep slope followed by a resistant response. Figure 5.4 is a schematic representation of this biphasic response.

When mammalian cells in culture are exposed to doxorubicin prior to determination of a single-dose radiation survival curve, the major effect is to reduce the degree of threshold to radiation. This reduction eventually reaches exponential response from dose = 0. The decrease in the threshold of the single-dose radiation survival curve persists through at least 24 h. A reasonable interpretation of these result is that the damage induced by doxorubicin persists in progeny, at least through 1.5–2.0 divisions, and that this residual damage is reflected in the loss of ability of irradiated cells to accumulate sublethal radiation damage (Belli and Piro 1977).

When irradiated mammalian cells express a survival response which is exponential (extrapolation number = 1.0), the expectation is that such cells will not be capable of expressing the survival fluctuations observed in a two-dose radiation study. However, Belli and Piro (1977) showed that doxorubicin-treated cells which expressed exponential survival from zero-dose fully demonstrated the survival fluctuations seen in untreated cells. Therefore, doxorubicin and radiation interact in mammalian cells to reduce the capacity to accumulate sublethal damage, but doxorubicin does not interfere with the repair of such damage. These results imply that the damage interaction between doxorubicin and radiation occurs in a target which may determine whether or not a threshold is present, but not with a target which is important in the survival fluctuation seen in two-dose radiation studies.

Thus, the damage interactions, at the cellular level, between actinomycin D or doxorubicin and radiation differ with regard to their effects on the repair of sublethal radiation injury. Actinomycin D appears to interfere with this process, while doxorubicin does not though the latter influences the single-dose radiation survival curve by reducing the extrapolation number close to 1.0.

Lastly, Dritschilo et al. (1979) showed that doxorubicin does not interfere with the repair of potentially lethal damage in plateau-phase V79 cells. In these studies, the drug was present throughout the postirradiation interval. Thus, the major effect of doxorubicin on the radiation response of mam-

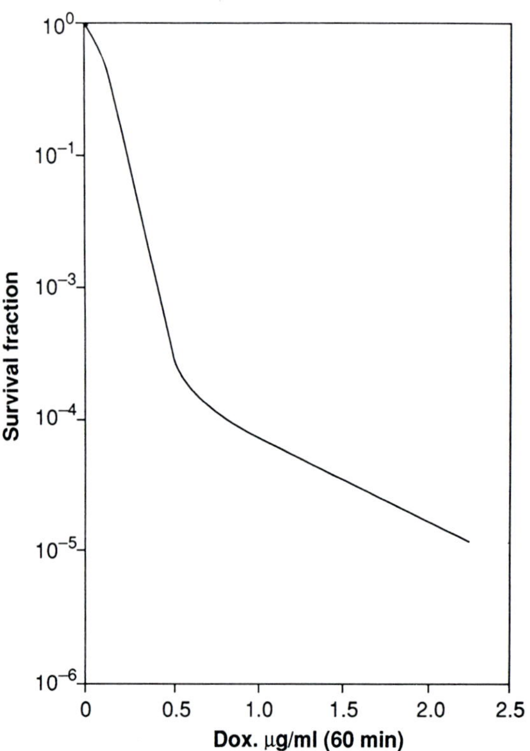

Fig. 5.4. Schematic survival curve for doxorubicin exposure illustrating the biphasic response typical for most mammalian cells studied

malian cells in culture is to reduce the single-dose radiation survival curve extrapolation number, but not to interfere with the repair of sublethal or potentially lethal radiation damage. The persistence of this effect of doxorubicin is measured in several doublings. Therefore, caution must be exercised when patients are treated with fractionated radiation who have received doxorubicin in the past as part of a general therapeutic strategy.

These cellular studies may serve to provide insight into several clinical observations. First, CASSADY et al. (1975) observed that children previously treated with doxorubicin experienced increased radiation toxicity primarily in the skin and lung. Two of these patients demonstrated delayed skin reactions similar to that seen with actinomycin D and represented an additional example of a recall phenomenon. In a large study, BILLINGHAM et al. (1977) explored the cardiotoxicity of doxorubicin. These investigators found that the histologic manifestation of cardiotoxicity was more extensive if doxorubicin was used in patients who had had previous irradiation to the mediastinum. Finally, STEIN (1978) and RANSOM et al. (1979) showed clinically important increased gastrointestinal toxicity when doxorubicin was part of a chemotherapeutic regimen following abdominal irradiation. Therefore, there is sufficient and extensive clinical experience with regard to the damage interactions between doxorubicin and radiation to alert oncologists to expect increased normal tissue reactions when these two modalities are used sequentially or together in the management of neoplastic disease. This is particularly true in children.

5.7 Radiation Response of Multidrug Resistant Mammalian Cells

The failure of chemotherapeutic agents to ultimately control solid tumors is generally ascribed to the emergence of tumors cells resistant to further treatment. A variety of mammalian cell lines have now been described which express the multidrug resistant (MDR) phenotype. These include cells resistant to actinomycin D (BIEDLER and RIEHM 1970), colchicine (BECH-HANSEN et al. 1976), and doxorubicin (HOWELL et al. 1984). The MDR phenotype is characterized by (a) collateral resistance to other agents; (b) the presence of a protein of 170 k Da in the cell membrane (p-glycoprotein); and (c) an ability to rapidly efflux toxic agents. This last characteristic is ascribed to the putative function of p-glycoprotein as an energy-dependent pump.

BELLI and co-workers (BELLI and HARRIS 1979; BELLI 1989; SOGNIER et al. 1991; ZHANG et al. 1992a) have characterized the phenotypic expression of multidrug resistance, including radiation response, in V79 Chinese hamster lung fibroblasts selected for resistance to doxorubicin. The single-dose radiation survival curve for resistant cells is characterized by a decrease in D_0 (increased radiation sensitivity) and a reduced extrapolation number (a reduced capacity for sublethal radiation damage). It was found that when V79 cells were selected for increased doxorubicin resistance, cells remained radiation sensitive, but the extrapolation number increased, suggesting a restoration of the capacity to tolerate sublethal radiation damage. Studies on the molecular mechanisms responsible for the increase in radiation sensitivity observed in doxorubicin-resistant cell lines indicate that there is no difference between these cells and wild-type cells with regard to rapair of single- or double stranded DNA breaks, or a lack of repair capacity for either sublethal or potentially lethal radiation injury. The lack of correlation between the increase in radiation sensitivity and the findings described above suggestes that other cellular structures may be important in the expression of increased radiation sensitivity in MDR cells. Possible candidates include the cell membrane, the nuclear membrane, signal transduction mechanisms, histones, or changes in DNA conformation which are not expressed as single- or double-stranded DNA breaks.

The damage interactions between doxorubicin and radiation in MDR cell lines are similar to those observed in non-MDR cells. These interactions take the form of a reduction in the extrapolation number, but little or no change in the sensitivity of such cells to radiation (no change in the D_0).

The common interpretation of a biphasic survival curve (see Fig. 5.4) is that at least two cell subpopulations are present, one of which has a sensitive and the other a resistant response state. Attempts to isolate V79 cells inherently resistant to doxorubicin have been unsuccessful, suggesting that this cell line does not contain a subpopulation which is inherently resistant to doxorubicin (BELLI 1979; BELLI and HARRIS 1979). An alternative explanation, therefore, is that mammalian cells may have at least two *targets* susceptible to doxorubicin, one of which results in a sensitive response state while the other is responsible for the resistant portion of the survival curve. It has been suggested that the cell membrane is an important target for doxorubicin cytotoxicity. This was first suggested by TRITTON and

YEE (1982) and is supported by more recent demonstrations that the cell membrane may constitute an important target for doxorubicin cytotoxicity (see BELLI et al. 1990). The presence of *p*-glycoprotein in the cell membrane of MDR cells may have a function in the expression of drug resistance, but may also render the cell membrane more susceptible to radiation damage, thus increasing the radiation sensitivity of MDR cells. For example, as the amount of *p*-glycoprotein increases in the cell membrane of MDR cells, radiation damage registered in the cell membrane, the level of which would ordinarily not result in an increase in radiation-induced cell killing, would be proprotionately higher in important normal constituents of the cell membrane because of the physical presence of high levels of *p*-glycoprotein.

As V79 cells are selected for increasing resistance to doxorubicin, at least two other phenotypic expressions for resistance are found. These are, in addition to efflux rates, (a) the ability to detoxify doxorubicin (ZHANG et al. 1992b) and (b) the capacity for cells to utilize *p*-glycoprotein to form intracellular vesicles which contain and sequester doxorubicin (SOGNIER et al. 1992). These findings have important clinical implications. Clinical studies designed to reverse multidrug resistance by the use of calcium channel blockers such as verapamil may enjoy only modest success if resistant tumor cells have other mechanisms of resistance such as drug detoxification and/or vesicle formation. This is especially true in pediatric oncology because doxorubicin occupies an important place in the chemotherapeutic management of childhood cancers and tumor recurrence and subsequent drug resistance may be due to a phenotype consisting of more than one mechanism.

Prior irradiation interferes with the participation of *p*-glycoprotein in vesicle formation. In cells highly resistant to doxorubicin, preirradiation reduces the number of vesicles formed and increases the sensitivity of cells to the drug (BELLI et al., unpublished). This observation strongly suggests that radiation exerts a major effect on the cell membrane and on the function of *p*-glycoprotein in particular.

The demonstration that *p*-glycoprotein assumes at least three functions in the expression of the MDR phenotype – as a pump, as a detoxification site for chemotherapeutic agents, and in vesicle formation – raises certain issues:

1. Are the three functions of *p*-glycoprotein present in MDR cells from the initiation of this phenotype or do these functions evolve as increasing resistance is achieved? In the former case, it is not necessary to assign a change in gene action as resistance increases. On the other hand, the latter possibility requires that sequences in the *mdr* gene become functional as cells acquire more resistance.

2. If the failure of chemotherapeutic agents in the treatment of both pediatric and adult tumors is ascribed to the MDR phenotype, the use of agents which are designed to address only one of the possible mechanisms of resistance is not likely to achieve significant clinical success.

5.8 Damage Interaction Between Radiation and Other Chemotherapeutic Agents

Important clinical observations have been made with regard to the response of important normal tissues to radiation in children receiving a variety of chemotherapeutic agents. The latter include bleomycin (lung tolerance), cisplatin (kidney tolerance), and cyclophosphamid (bladder tolerance). Relatively few in vitro data are available to identify the cellular factors important in these damage interactions. However, the extensive experimental data derived from studies on the damage interactions between radiation and actinomycin D and doxorubicin provide an important principle for the interpretation of clinical observation. It should be remembered that studies on the damage interaction between certain chemotherapeutic agents and radiation are generally performed in exponentially growing cells or in cells that have entered plateau-phase growth. When the latter are studied, release from plateau-phase growth is easily accomplished by simply subculturing the population. Decreases in extrapolation number, changes in the slope, or changes in the repair of sublethal or potentially lethal radiation damage as a consequence of the inclusion of a chemotherapeutic agent may have little relevance to the damage interaction between these agents and radiation in tissues such as the lung, central nervous system, kidney, liver or other tissues which have a very small or nonexistent proportion of cells in cycle. Table 5.1 summarizes the important normal tissues at risk for increased toxicity when chemotherapeutic agents used in most pediatric *solid* tumors are combined with radiation therapy. The table is not meant to be all-inclusive.

5.9 Summary

The principles of damage interaction between chemotherapeutic agents and radiation can be briefly stated. These damage interactions may be expressed by.

1. Change in the ability to accumulate sublethal radiation injury (a change in the extrapolation number).
2. Change in the slope of the exponential portion of the survival curve, indicating a change in radiation sensitivity
3. Suppression of the repair of sublethal radiation injury as demonstrated by two-dose radiation survival studies
4. Change in the ability of cells to repair potentially lethal radiation injury
5. Increase in the number of single- or double-stranded breaks observed
6. Suppression of the ability to repair single- or double-stranded breaks following drug and radiation exposure.

It is difficult for the clinician to relate observations in children treated with radiation and chemotherapeutic agents to any of the above cellular consequences observed with well-controlled cell culture models.

However, the clinician is well advised to keep these possibilites in mind when the therapeutic strategy in the treatment of pediatric solid tumors includes the use of multiple chemotherapeutic agents and radiation therapy.

References

Bech-Hansen NT, Till JE, Ling V (1976) Plieotropic phenotype of colchicine-resistant CHO cells: cross-resistance and collateral sensitivity. J Cell Physiol 88: 23–31

Begg AC (1987) Additivity versus repair inhibition in fractionated treatments combining drugs and x-rays: a theoretical analysis. Int J Radiat Oncol Biol Phys 13: 921–927

Bellamy AS, Hill BT (1984) Interactions between clinically effective antitumor drugs and radiation in expermental systems. Biophys Acts 738: 125–166

Belli JA (1979) Radiation response and Adriamycin resistance in mammalian cells in culture. Front Radiat Therap Oncol 13: 9–20

Belli JA (1989) Interaction between radiation and drug damage in mammalian cells. IV. Radiation response of Adriamycin-resistant V79 cells. Radiat Res 119: 88–100

Belli JA, Dicus EJ, Nagle W (1970) Repair of radiation damage as a factor in preoperative radiation therapy. Front Radiat Therap Oncol 5: 40–57

Belli JA, Harris JR (1979) Adriamycin resistance and radiation response. Int J Radiat Oncol Biol Phys 5: 1231–1234

Belli JA, Piro AJ (1977) The interaction between radiation and Adriamycin damage in mammalian cells. Cancer Res 37: 1624–1630

Belli JA, Shelton M (1969) Potentially lethal radiation damage: repair by mammalian cells in culture. Science 165: 490–492

Belli JA, Zhang Y, Fritz P (1990) Transfer of Adriamycin resistance by fusion of M_r 170,000 p-glycoprotein to the plasma membrane of sensitive cells. Cancer Res 50: 2191–2197

Bieldler JL, Riehm H (1970) Cellular resistance to actinomycin D in Chinese hamster cells in vitro: cross-resistance, radioautographic, and cytogenetic studies. Cancer Res 30: 1174–1184

Billingham ME, Bristow MR, Elabsten E, Mason JW, Masek MA, Daniels JR (1977) Adriamycin cardiotoxity: endomyocardial biopsy evidence of enhancement by irradiation. Am J Surg Pathol 1: 17–23

Cassady JR, Richter MP, Piro AJ, Jaffe N (1975) Radiation-Adriamycin interactions: preliminary clinical observations. Cancer 36: 946–949

Dritschilo A, Piro AJ, Belli JA (1979) Interaction between radiation and drug damage in mammalian cells. III. The effect of Adriamycin and actinomycin-D on the repair of potentially lethal radiation damage. Int J Radiat Biol 35: 549–560

Elkind MM, Sutton H (1960) Radiation response of mammalian cells grown in culture. I. Repair of x-ray damage in surviving Chinese hamster cells. Radiat Res 25: 359–376

Elkind MM, Whitmore GF, Alescio T (1964) Actinomycin D: suppression of recovery in x-irradiated mammalian cells. Science 143: 1454–1456

Filler RM, Tefft M, Varoter, GF-Maddock C, Mitus A (1969) Hepatic lobectomy in childhood: effects of x-ray and chemotherapy. J Pediatr Surg 4: 31

Hill BT, Bellamy AS (1984) An overview of experimental investigations of interactions between certain antitumor drugs and x-irradiations in vitro. Adv Radiat Biol 2: 211–267

Howell N, Belli TA, Zaczkiewicz LT, Belli JA (1984) High-level, unstable Adriamycin resistance in a Chinese hamster mutant cell line with double minute chromosomes. Cancer Res 44: 4023–4029

Little JB (1973) Factors influencing the repair of potentially lethal radiation damage in growth-inhibited human cells. Radiat Res 56: 320–333

Philips RA, Tolmach LJ (1966) Repair of potentially lethal damage in x-irradiated Hela cells. Radiat Res 29: 413–432

Piro AJ, Taylor CC, Belli JA (1975) Interaction between radiation and drug damage in mammalian cells. I. Delayed expression of actinomycin D/x-ray effects in exponential and plateau phase cells. Radiat Res 63: 346–362

Piro AJ, Taylor CC, Belli JA (1976) Interaction between radiation and drug damage in mammalian cells. II The effect of actinomycin-D on the repair of sublethal radiation damage in plateau phase cells. Cancer 37: 2697–2702

Ransom JL, Novak RW, Kumar APM, Hustu HO, Pratt CB (1979) Delayed gastrointestinal complications after combined modality therapy of childhood rhabdomyosarcoma. Int J Radiat Oncol Biol 5: 1275–1279

Sognier MA, Eberle RL, Zhang Y, Belli JA (1991) Interaction between radiation and drug damage in mammalian cells. V. DNA damage and repair induced in LZ cells by Adriamycin and/or radiation. Radiat Res 126: 80–87

Sognier MA, Zhang Y, Eberle RL, Belli JA (1992) Characterization of Adriamycin-resistant and radiation-sensitive Chinese hamster cell lines. Biochem Pharmacol 44: 1859–1868

Steel GG, Peckham M (1979) Exploitable mechanisms in combined radiotherapy-chemotherapy: the concept of additivity. Int J Radiat Oncol Biol Phys 5: 85–91

Stein RS (1978) Radiation-recall enteritis after actinomycin-D and Adriamycin therapy. South Med J 71: 960–961

Till JE, McCulloch EA (1961) A direct measurement of the radiation sensitivity of normal mouse bone marrow cells. Radiat Res 14: 213–222

Tritton TR, Yee G (1982) The anticancer agent Adriamycin can be actively cytotoxic without entering cells. Science 217: 248–250

Whitmore GF, Gulyas S (1967) Studies on recovery processes in mouse L cells. Natl Cancer Inst Monogr 24: 141–156

Withers HR (1967) Recovery and repopulation in vivo by mouse skin epithelium cells during fractionated irradiation. Radiat Res 32: 227–239

Withers HR, Elkind MM (1970) Microcolony survival assay for cells of mouse intestinal mucosa exposed to radiation. Int J Radiat Biol 17: 261–267

Zhang Y, Sweet K, Sognier M, Belli JA (1992a) Interaction between radiation and drug damage in mammalian cells. VI. Radiation and doxorubicin age-response function of doxorubicin-sensitive and resistant Chinese hamster cells. Radiat Res 132:105–111

Zhang Y, Sweet KM, Sognier MA, Belli JA (1992b) An enhanced ability for transforming Adriamycin into a non-cytotoxic form in a multidrug-resistant cell line (LZ8). Biochem Pharmacol 44: 1869–1877

6 Acute Lymphoblastic Leukemia

AMY LOUISE BILLET and STEPHEN E. SALLAN

CONTENTS

6.1 Introduction 87
6.2 Presentation 87
6.3 Diagnosis 87
6.4 Therapy 88
6.4.1 General Principles of Therapy 88
6.4.2 Treatment Factors 88
6.4.3 Remission Induction 88
6.4.4 CNS Treatment 88
6.4.5 Intensification and Continuation Therapy 88
6.5 Prevention of CNS Disease 89
6.5.1 Historical Background 89
6.5.2 Interpretation of Results 89
6.5.3 Use of Radiation 89
6.5.4 Use of Intrathecal and Systemic Chemotherapy . . 91
6.5.5 Comparison of Radiation and Chemotherapy . . . 92
6.5.6 CNS Preventive Therapy After Relapse 93
6.6 Treatment of Established CNS Disease 94
6.6.1 Early Randomized Trials 94
6.6.2 Efficacy of Craniospinal Radiation 94
6.6.3 Efficacy of Radiation, Induction and Maintenance
     Intrathecal Therapy, and Systemic Therapy 94
6.6.4 Effect of Prior Therapy 94
6.6.5 Other Pharmacologic Approaches 95
6.6.6 Role of Bone Marrow Transplantation 95
     References 95

6.1 Introduction

Acute lymphoblastic leukemia (ALL), the most common childhood malignancy, accounts for 75% of the 2000–2500 new cases of acute leukemia diagnosed each year in United States children under the age of 15 years. In the 1950s almost all children diagnosed with ALL died of their disease within months. In the 1990s we expect that 65%–70% of patients will be cured.

AMY LOUISE BILLET, M.D., Pediatric Oncology, Dana Farber Cancer Institute, Harvard Medical School, 44 Binney Street, Boston, MA 02115, USA.
STEPHEN F. SALLAN, M.D., Clinical Director, Pediatric Oncology, Dana Farber Cancer Institute, Harvard Medical School, 44 Binney Street, Boston, MA 02115, USA.

6.2 Presentation

Children with ALL usually present with the signs and symptoms of bone marrow replacement with or without extramedullary invasion: pallor, fatigue, bleeding, fever, and bone pain. Central nervous system (CNS) disease at presentation occurs in only 3% of children (BLEYER 1988). The most common manifestations of CNS involvement include the signs and symptoms of increased intracranial pressure such as headache, vomiting, papilledema, lethargy, and irritability; visual disturbances such as diplopia, blurred vision, blindness, or photophobia; meningismus; and cranial nerve palsies (especially sixth and seventh nerve palsies) (BLEYER and POPLACK 1985). Less common manifestations of CNS disease include hypothalamic syndrome with hyperphagia, sleep-wake disturbances, or pathologic weight gain, vertigo, auditory disturbances, cerebellar dysfunction, hallucinations, hyperpnea, or proptosis. Non-CNS extramedullary disease findings include adenopathy, arthralgias, hepatosplenomegaly, and testicular enlargement.

6.3 Diagnosis

The diagnosis of ALL is established by examination of the bone marrow including morphology, cytochemical stains, immunologic cell surface markers, and cytogenetics. The latter two studies are critical to identify treatment factors at the time of diagnosis, although initial treatment plans can often be developed on the basis of morphology and cytochemical stains alone. Once the diagnosis of leukemia is suspected or established, all patients should be referred to a center staffed by pediatric onclogists familar with the many aspects of the disease and its treatment. Specific therapy should not be instituted until the diagnosis has been established except in the rare instance when a patient is in imminent danger. Since ALL is a rare disease and each patient can contribute to the development of more effective, less morbid future treatments, we always recommend therapy on a research protocol.

6.4 Therapy

6.4.1 General Principles of Therapy

The treatment of ALL includes, multiple drug systemic and intrathecal chemotherapy for all patients and cranial irradiation for some. Treatment is usually divided into four phases, beginning with intensive *remission induction*, designed to eradicate all measurable disease. With modern era chemotherapy, 95% of children will achieve complete remission with restoration of normal bone marrow function and no detectable leukemia on bone marrow examination. There is, however, still unmeasurable residual disease at this time.

The next two phases of therapy, *central nervous system* (CNS) therapy and systemic *intensification*, are often administered concurrently. All children have leukemic invasion of the meninges at diagnosis, although only 3% have measurable CNS disease by examination of the cerebrospinal fluid. Since most systemic chemotherapy does not penetrate into the CNS, specific CNS therapy must be given. The role of radiation therapy to the cranium and intrathecal and/or systemic chemotherapy in the prophylaxis and treatment of CNS disease will be addressed in detail below. Concurrent with specific CNS therapy, it is important to treat intensively the residual systemic disease. *Intensification* therapy with multiple, non-cross-resistant drugs to prevent the emergence of drug-resistant leukemia is given for several months.

The final phase of treatment, *continuation* (or *maintenance*) chemotherapy, consists of less intensive therapy administered to eliminate any residual leukemia cells. Although mercaptopurine and methotrexate have been the mainstay of this phase of therapy, many successful programs also add prednisone and vincristine. Parenteral therapy is used when possible to obviate problems with poor compliance and drug absorption. The minimum duration of treatment is 2 years of continuous complete remission. Some programs continue for longer.

6.4.2 Treatment Factors

It is important to identify factors at the time of diagnosis than can guide treatment decisions. Once called prognostic factors, we believe that it is more appropriate to call them treatment factors, since intensive therapy can change outcome. The most important adverse factors that indicate the need for more intensive therapy include: high initial white blood cell count (greater than $20\,000/mm^3$), age less than 2 years or greater than 9 years, T-cell immunophenotype, CNS disease at diagnosis, and DNA index less than 1.16. Still more intensive therapy may be indicated for patients with initial WBC greater than $100000/mm^3$, age less than 1 year, or certain chromosomal translocations such as t(9;22) in all patients and t(4;11) in infants. Identification of treatment factors allows the use of the most intensive therapy for the patients at highest risk of relapse.

6.4.3 Remission Induction

Remission-induction chemotherapy includes the use of daily prednisone or dexamethasone, weekly vincristine, and one or more other systemic agents such as an anthracycline, high-dose methotrexate, and asparaginase, in addition to intrathecal drug over the course of the first month. Although some programs use less intensive remission-induction regimens for patients with lower risk treatment factors, previous studies have shown improved survival in the setting of more intensive induction and consolidation regimens (CLAVELL et al. 1986; HENZE et al. 1981). Improvements in supportive care have reduced the occurrence of toxic deaths during induction to approximately 3%. Most patients require hospitalization throughout remission induction.

6.4.4 CNS Treatment

Specific CNS therapy must be initiated during remission induction with intrathecal drug. Once complete remission has been obtained, definitive therapy is instituted. The approach to definitive preventive therapy is discussed below. After specific therapy is given, intrathecal drug is administered on a regular basis throughout all subsequent treatment.

6.4.5 Intensification and Continuation Therapy

Once complete remission has been obtained, intensive chemotherapy is instituted concurrent with specific CNS therapy. Treatment is stratified by risk factors. The antimetabolites, methotrexate and mercaptopurine, are the mainstay of therapy.

Intravenous high doses of these two drugs have been used by the Pediatric Oncology Group (POG) to intensify therapy (CAMITTA et al. 1989, 1992). Additional drugs such as asparaginase, vincristine, and prednisone in the Dana-Farber Cancer Institute (DFCI) consortium programs; cytosine arabinoside, cyclophosphamide, and asparaginase in the Berlin Frankfurt Muenster (BFM) programs; and the use of alternating non-cross-resistant drug pairs in the St. Jude Children's Research Hospital (SJCRH) program have contributed to improved survival (Clavell et al. 1986; HENZE et al. 1981; RIVERA et al. 1991).

Because modern chemotherapy results in cure for approximately two-thirds of children with ALL, bone marrow transplantation in first remission is reserved for very high risk patients such as those with the Philadelphia chromosome, t (9; 22).

6.5 Prevention of CNS Disease

6.5.1 Historical Background

In the era preceding effective systemic control of leukemia, CNS disease was a rare and usually preterminal event. As systemic therapy improved in the 1960s, however, the incidence of CNS relapse rose to approximately 4% per month of hematologic remission (EVANS et al. 1970). It was thus recognized that the CNS represented a sanctuary site, protected from systemic drugs, that required specific therapy (FREI et al. 1965). In addition, it became apparent that CNS relapse was a harbinger of bone marrow relapse, suggesting that the bone marrow was reseeded from leukemic cells in the CNS (HUSTU and AUR 1978). Thus, the concept of prophylactic CNS treatment was developed. Although the original term developed for this treatment was "CNS prophylaxis," the term "CNS preventive therapy" more accurately describes this concept. The institution of routine CNS preventive therapy has reduced the incidence of CNS relapse from more than 50% (AUR et al. 1972) to 5%–10% (HAGHBIN et al. 1980; MOE et al. 1981; POPLACK et al. 1984, INATI et al. 1983; SULLIVAN et al, 1982; GELBER et al. 1993). Routine CNS preventive therapy has thus contributed significantly to the increased numbers of long-term disease-free survivors in childhood ALL.

6.5.2 Interpretation of Results

In the following discussion of approaches to CNS preventive therapy, several issues must be considered in interpreting the results of any study, single-arm or comparative. *First*, it should be emphasized that the efficacy of CNS therapy must be interpreted in the context of overall treatment results. If the competing risk of bone marrow relapse is high, the observed occurrence of CNS relapse may be low no matter what CNS preventive therapy is used (GELBER et al. 1993). *Second*, the results must be interpreted in the context of the population under study. Since an increased risk of CNS leukemia is associated with high initial leukocyte count, T-cell disease, and very young ages (BLEYER and POPLACK 1985), exclusion of such patients may identify a regimen that is effective only for lower risk patients. *Third*, since risk criteria differ between different studies, the efficacy of a regimen for "standard risk" patients in one study is not necessarily applicable to " standard risk" patients in a different study. *Fourth*, the efficacy of a particular CNS preventive therapy can only be measured in the context of a particular systematic regimen. Since the drugs used in the systemic regimen will have varying effects in the CNS, a CNS preventive regimen that appears successful in the context of one systemic regimen may be less successful in the context of a different systemic regimen (BILLETT et al. 1993a).

Although the first attempts to control CNS disease began with intrathecal aminopterin or methotrexate (FREI et al. 1965), subsequent approaches involved irradiation, intrathecal drug, and/or systemic chemotherapy with CNS efficacy. Of note, one major advance in the use of intrathecal therapy was the recognition by Bleyer that the predictable cerebrospinal fluid levels of methotrexate were best achieved with dosing by age, not body surface area, and that dosing by age led to better control of CNS disease with less acute toxicity (BLEYER 1977; BLEYER et al. 1983). All subsequent and current trials have used this method.

6.5.3 Use of Radiation

Once the risk of leukemia in the CNS was recognized, approaches to specific CNS therapy were developed. The use of CNS irradiation was based on a mouse model of leukemia with L1210 leukemia cells where the combination of cyclophosphamide and cranial irradiation led to cures of leukemia (JOHNSON 1964). This led to the first clinical use of radiation therapy at SJCRH (HUSTU et al. 1973). As shown in Table 6.1, these studies demonstrated that 24 Gy of craniospinal radiation or 24 Gy of cranial radiation with five concurrent doses of intrathecal methotrexate

Table 6.1. Role of Radiation in the Prevention of CNS Disease

Study (Years)	CNS therapy	No.	Initial CNS relapse No. (%)		No. in CCR	EFS
SJCRH I–III[a] (1962–65)	5–12 Gy CSI	37	15	(40)	7	
SJCRH IV[a] (1965–67)	None	42	25	(60)	2	
SJCRH V[a] (1967–68)	24 Gy cranial + early IT MTX	31	3	(10)	18	
SJCRH VI[a] (1968–70)	24 Gy CSI	45	2	(4)	27	
	None	49	32	(67)	11	
SJCRH VII[a] (1970–71)	24 Gy C + early IT MTX	45	3	(7)	27	
	24 Gy CSI	49	3	(6)	28	
MRC[b] 1970–72	25 Gy C + 10 Gy spine + IT MTX × 1 yr	75	1		57	~75%
	None	80	26		48	< 50%
DFCI[c] (1971–74)	24 Gy C + IT MTX early and extended	65	0		41	
CCG 101[d] (1972–74)	24 Gy CSI	152	(9)			61%
	24 Gy C + early IT MTX	86	(17)			57%
CCG 143[d] (1974–75)	18 Gy CSI	159	(7)			62%
	18 Gy C + early IT MTX	81	(16)			64%
BFM[e] SR-High (1983–86)	18 Gy C + IT/ID MTX	71			51	70%
	12 Gy C + IT/ID MTX	72			54	74%

CSI, craniospinal irradiation; IT, intrathecal; MTX, methotrexate; C, cranial irradiation; ID, intermediate dose; CCR, continuous complete remission; EFS, event-free survival
[a] Hustu et al. (1973)
[b] Leukemia Committee and Working Party on Leukemia in Childhood (1973)
[c] Dritschilo et al. (1976)
[d] Nesbit et al. (1981)
[e] Henze et al. (1983)

reduced the occurrence of CNS relapse to approximately 10% and improved overall survival to approximately 50%. Of note, these early studies did not give maintenance intrathecal drug.

A number of other studies then examined different doses of cranial or craniospinal radiation, with or without the use of concurrently and/or subsequently administered intrathecal drug. These studies are summarized in Table 6.1 and discussed below.

Trials conducted in the United Kingdom showed that craniospinal radiation followed by intrathecal methotrexate for 1 year reduced the risk of CNS relapse from 30% to less than 1% and increased overall survival from less than 50% to 75% (Leukemia Committee and Working Party on Leukemia in Childhood 1973). Other studies then assessed differ-

ent doses of radiation in an attempt to identify an effective dose that might have less long-term toxicity than 24 Gy. Early studies at DFCI demonstrated good control of CNS disease with 24 Gy of cranial radiation and intrathecal methotrexate, the latter given concurrently with radiation and continued throughout treatment (Dritschilo et al. 1976). That study emphasized the importance of radiation therapy technique, especially the need to treat *all meningeal surfaces*, including the retro-orbital space, with the use of anesthesia if necessary. The C2-whole brain field for a meningeal seeding tumor differs from the whole brain field for a nonseeding brain tumor. Others have shown that one-third of treatment ports provide marginal or inadequate coverage for the base of the skull and that inadequately treated patients were more likely to relapse (KUN et al. 1984).

The Children's Cancer Group (CCG) compared patients who received 18 Gy radiation to historical controls who received 24 Gy and found no difference in the incidence of CNS relapse or overall survival (NESBIT et al. 1981). Of note, infants were excluded from the randomization and analysis of outcome. The CCG did observe a lower incidence of CNS relapse in patients who received craniospinal radiation versus cranial radiation with intrathecal drug. Although these were not randomized comparisons of radiation dose, they did provide the basis for subsequent studies with lower doses of radiation.

The German BFM group compared two doses of radiation, 18 Gy and 12 Gy, in the context of intensive systemic therapy including intermediate-dose methotrexate for "standard risk-high" patients (RIEHM et al. 1990; HENZE et al. 1983). There were no differences in the incidence of CNS relapse or in event-free survival in this population.

In summary, radiation provides an extremely effective approach to CNS disease prevention. A dose of 18 Gy is the minimum effective dose that has been studied for most patients, although a dose of 12 Gy may be effective for certain relatively low-risk patients in the context of highly effective systemic therapy.

6.5.4 Use of Intrathecal and Systemic Chemotherapy

Despite early studies showing the efficacy of prophylactic radiation in preventing subsequent CNS relapse, concerns about long-term toxicity related to radiation led to continued study of drug alone for specific CNS therapy. Several early studies had demonstrated that prophylactic administration of intrathecal drug could delay the onset of CNS leukemia (FREI et al. 1965; BERNARD et al. 1972). In 1969, the L-2 protocol was begun at Memorial Sloan Kettering Cancer Institute (MSKCI) to assess the efficacy of intrathecal drug alone in controlling CNS disease (HAGHBIN et al. 1975; GEE et al. 1976; CLARKSON et al. 1979). In this trial, methotrexate was administered intrathecally three times during induction and then twice every 2 months for the 3 years of therapy. In addition, the investigators hypothesized that some of the drugs that were administered systemically would have a therapeutic effect in the CNS. Only eight of 74 children who attained remission developed subsequent CNS disease. This study was one of the first to demonstrate that induction and maintenance intrathecal drug without irradiation could prevent CNS disease.

Subsequent trials looked at the duration of intrathecal therapy, different combinations of intrathecal drug, and use of systemic drugs with CNS effect in addition to intrathecal therapy. Low event-free survival in early studies of different intrathecal drug regimens obviated adequate assessment of CNS disease prevention (SULLIVAN et al. 1982; KOMP et al. 1982; SACKMANN et al. 1983; GREEN et al. 1980). As improvements in both systemic and CNS therapy led to increased event-free survival, subsequent studies showed that for lower risk patients, extended intrathecal therapy without radiation could adequately control CNS disease (PULLEN et al. 1993; TUBERGEN et al. 1993).

Systemic drugs with CNS effect have been added to intrathecal drug alone in order to better control CNS disease without irradiation. The addition of intermediate-dose methotrexate to intrathecal therapy has improved event-free survival and adequately controlled CNS disease without the use of irradiation in lower risk patients (RIEHM et al. 1990; GREEN et al. 1980; FREEMAN et al. 1983; ABROMOWITCH et al. 1988); however, good control of CNS disease was not demonstrated in higher risk patients (GREEN et al. 1980; FREEMAN et al. 1983; ABROMOWITCH et al. 1988; BUHRER et al. 1990). Intermediate-dose methotrexate alone, without extended intrathecal therapy, was inadequate to control CNS disease in lower risk patients (PULLEN et al. 1993). Very high-dose methotrexate without intrathecal drug has been shown to control CNS disease in average risk patients in a CCG study (POPLACK et al. 1984). The Pediatric Oncology Group and the DFCI consortium are studying the role of high-dose infusion mercaptopurine in CNS preventive therapy.

Thus, a number of studies have demonstrated that for lower risk patients, control of CNS can be achieved without the use of irradiation. Of note, a recent DFCI trial that omitted radiation for lower risk patients led to a significantly increased risk of CNS relapse and lower event-free survival for those patients compared to historical controls who received radiation and similar systemic therapy (BILLETT et al. 1993a). This result emphasizes the interaction between the CNS preventive regimen and systemic therapy. That drug alone can adequately control CNS disease in higher risk patients has yet to be shown, but is under investigation by a number of groups.

6.5.5 Comparison of Radiation and Chemotherapy

A retrospective analysis of trials conducted by three different groups compared three approaches to CNS disease prevention: intrathecal methotrexate alone, intermediate-dose intravenous and intrathecal, methotrexate, and 24 Gy cranial irradiation and intrathecal methotrexate (GREEN et al. 1980). Among standard risk patients, those who received intermediate-dose methotrexate had a significantly better event-free survival, although primary meningeal relapse was significantly less frequent in the irradiated group. Among high-risk patients, there were no significant differences in event-free survival. Again, there were significantly fewer meningeal relapses in the irradiated group. Because each of the CNS treatments was administered in the context of different systemic therapies and because

Table 6.2. Comparative Studies of Radiation Versus Drug for CNS Prevention

Study (Years)	CNS therapy	No.	1st relapse in CNS No. (%)		No. in CCR		EFS	
SWOG ALinC 9[a] (1971–73)	18–24 Gy C + TIT upfront + extended	92	4				~20%	
	TIT upfront + extended	102	7				~20%	
POG ALinC 11[b] (1974–76)	24 Gy C XRT + concurrent IT MTX	105	7				<40%	
	TIT upfront and extended	243	10				~50%	
GATLA 10-ALL-72[c] (1972–75)	24 Gy C + Concurrent IT MTX/DEX + extended IT MTX/DEX	172	(22%)		74		21%	
	24 Gy C + concurrent IT MTX/DEX	181						
GATLA 1-ALL-76[c] (1976–78)	IT MTX/DEX upfront and extended	349	(37%)		123		31%	
RPMI ID-MTX[d] (1973–76)	ID + IT MTX upfront	54	SR HR				~68% ~35%	
DFCI 73–01 (1973–77)	24 Gy C XRT + IT MTX upfront	137	SR HR				~55% ~55%	
CCG 101 (1972–74)	IT MTX upfront	143	SR HR				~35% ~28%	
CALGB 7611[e] (1976–79)	24 Gy C XRT + IT MTX	247	SR HR	7 7	SR 36 HR 35		SR HR	~50% <50%
	ID and IT MTX × 3	259	SR HR	18 20	SR 56 HR 66		SR HR	~60% < 50%
CCG[f]: average and high risk	24 Gy C XRT + IT MTX upfront	AR 131	AR	(4.6%)			AR	84%
	VHD MTX		AR	(4.6%)			AR	84%
BFM: low risk[g] (1981–83)	18 Gy C XRT + IT MTX	141	3	(2)	108		78%	
	IT + ID MTX	136	19	(15)	92		68%	
CCG 105[h]: intermediate risk[g] (1983–87)	18 Gy C XRT + IT MTX × 6 mos.	697	(7)				68%	
	IT MTX × 30–36 mos.	691	(9)				64%	

C, cranial irradiation; TIT, triple intrathecal; XRT, radiotherapy; IT, intrathecal; MTX, methotrexate; DEX, dexamethasone; ID, intermediate dose; VHD, very high dose; AR, average risk; SR, standard risk; HR, high risk; CCR, continuous complete remission; EFS, event-free survival;

[a] KOMP et al. (1982)
[b] SULLIVAN et al. (1982)
[c] SACKMANN et al. (1983)
[d] GREEN et al. (1980)
[e] FREEMAN et al. (1983)
[f] POPLACK et al. (1984)
[g] RIEHM et al. (1990)

this was not a prospective, randomized trial, clear conclusions regarding the relative efficacy of each approach cannot be made.

A number of prospective controlled trials have compared CNS treatments with and without irradiation. These trials are summarized in Table 6.2 and discussed below.

Three studies from two different groups compared cranial radiation with different intrathecal drug regimens and found no significant differences in CNS outcome. Poor overall survival in all three studies, however, prevented the conclusion that the intrathecal therapy alone was as effective as cranial radiation (SULLIVAN et al. 1982; KOMP et al. 1982; SACKMANN et al. 1983). A prospective study by the Cancer and Leukemia Group B (CALGB) compared treatment with three doses of intermediate-dose methotrexate to treatment with cranial irradiation, with no maintenance intrathecal therapy in either regimen (FREEMAN et al. 1983). For standard-risk patients, there were significantly more CNS relapses and significantly fewer bone marrow relapses in the unirradiated patients. Since the competing risk of bone marrow relapse was much higher in the irradiated group, it was difficult to ascertain the efficacy of the CNS treatment. For high-risk patients, there were significantly more CNS relapses in the non-irradiated group, but the event-free survival was less than 50%. A follow-up investigation of these patients, treated at a single institution, reported CNS relapses in 11/29 who received intermediate-dose methotrexate and 0/11 who were irradiated (SCHWENN et al. 1989).

A CCG study compared very high-dose methotrexate (33 g/m^2) to cranial radiation with concurrent intrathecal methotrexate in patients with intermediate- and high-risk disease (POPLACK et al. 1984). For the entire group, the incidence of isolated CNS relapse was 9% and event-free survival was 79% at 2 years. For intermediate-risk patients, there was no difference in CNS or overall outcome by treatment arm but the outcome of high-risk patients is not described. Long term results of this trial remain to be determined.

In 1983, the CCG undertook a prospective, randomized study to address the efficacy of cranial radiation versus intrathecal drug alone in patients who meet intermediate-risk criteria (TUBERGEN et al. 1993). Both groups received six doses of intrathecal drug in the first 8 weeks, and all intrathecal drug was dosed by age. This study also randomized patients to one of four systemic therapies of different intensities. A number of important observations can be made from this study.

1. There were no significant differences in CNS relapse-free survival, disease-free survival, or event-free survival by CNS treatment when all four systemic regimens were considered together.
2. The intensity of systemic therapy affected CNS outcome in that there was a significantly higher rate of isolated CNS relapses and lower event-free survival among patients who received less intensive systemic treatment and intrathecal drug compared to those who received the same systemic treatment and irradiation.
3. In older patients who received more intensive systemic therapy, cranial irradiation led to an improved event-free survival by reducing bone marrow relapses.

The study emphasized the need to evaluate the efficacy of CNS therapy in the context of effective systemic therapy.

In summary, more recent trials with prospective, randomized comparisons have shown that adequate control of CNS disease and good overall outcome for lower risk patients can be achieved without irradiation. For higher risk patients, however, radiation provides the most effective control of CNS disease.

6.5.6 CNS Preventive Therapy After Relapse

Survival after bone marrow relapse in ALL is extremely poor in most studies, and few have studied the role of CNS preventive therapy in this setting. One study from SJCRH compared (a) patients who received CNS preventive therapy with four doses of intrathecal cytosine arabinoside and methotrexate during reinduction and every 6 weeks subsequently and (b) historical controls who received similar systemic therapy but no specific CNS therapy (RIVERA et al. 1983). All patients had been irradiated during initial therapy. No CNS relapses were seen in the treated group, compared to seven relapses among the 16 historical controls. This study demonstrated the need for retreatment of the CNS after relapse. Since chemotherapy rarely leads to cure after bone marrow relapse, bone marrow transplantation is often the treatment of choice. For patients with documented CNS disease prior to transplantation who have not had cranial irradiation, options include a radiotherapy boost to the cranium immediately prior to total body irradiation or regular intrathecal therapy after transplanation (BILLETT et al. 1993b; BROCHSTEIN et al. 1987). The former approach is effective and reliable. For patients without prior CNS disease, we do not give additional radiation other than total body irradiation and have not seen isolated CNS relapse after autologous transplantation. For patients who do not undergo transplantation, intrathecal therapy is given throughout treatment, but specific CNS therapy is often delayed 6–12 months to allow intensive systemic chemotherapy. In current POG trials, this has not led to a high incidence of CNS relapse prior to preventive therapy.

6.6 Treatment of Established CNS Disease

Since the incidence of CNS disease at diagnosis is only 3%, the focus of this section will be on the treatment of isolated CNS relapse. The following discussion of the various studies that have been done for treatment of established CNS disease is generally limited to patients with their first isolated CNS relapse. Interpretation of trials for the treatment of isolated CNS relapse require consideration of several issues. *First*, prognosis after relapse may be affected by prior therapy, not only by initial CNS preventive therapy but also by the intensity of the initial systemic regimen. *Second*, the efficacy of the CNS regimen may be affected by the nature of the concurrent systemic therapy used. *Third*, if initial CNS preventive therapy included radiation, use of radiation at relapse may be limited by concerns about subsequent toxicity.

Although the efficacy of CNS preventive therapy has improved greatly, CNS relapse still occurs in 5%–10% of patients (HAGHBIN et al. 1980; MOE et al. 1981; POPLACK et al. 1984; INATI et al. 1983; SULLIVAN et al. 1982; GELBER et al. 1993). Second CNS remission can usually be achieved, but the eventual outcome is poor for most patients because of subsequent relapse (BLEYER and POPLACK 1983; GELBER et al. 1993; OCHS et al. 1985; GEORGE et al. 1985). As the incidence of CNS relapse has decreased, the number of patients eligible for randomized trials has also decreased. Thus, most randomized trials for the treatment of established CNS disease were done in the 1960s and 1970s. More recent reports are single-arm studies with smaller number of patients.

6.6.1 Early Randomized Trails

A series of randomized studies from 1962 to 1973 demonstrated that low-dose radiation alone was ineffective, that multiple doses of intrathecal drug or craniospinal radiation could achieve CNS remission, and that the addition of maintenance intrathecal drug with or without radiation could prolong the duration of remission (SULLIVAN et al. 1969, 1975, 1977). Most of those patients had been treated with little or no CNS preventive therapy prior to relapse. In addition, none of these early studies utilized additional systemic therapy at the time of relapse. The importance of maintenance intrathecal drug was demonstrated in a more recent study POG (LAND et al. 1985).

6.6.2 Efficacy of Craniospinal Radiation

KUN and co-workers demonstrated that craniospinal radiation could effectively control established CNS disease in 14 patients who had isolated CNS relapses after initial CNS preventive therapy with cranial radiation (KUN et al. 1984). Another small study showed that very intensive systemic and intrathecal chemotherapy followed by delayed craniospinal radiation was effective (MANDELL et al. 1990). Prior therapy was not described for the latter patients, and only some of them were treated at the time of their first CNS relapse.

6.6.3 Efficacy of Radiation, Induction and Maintenance Intrathecal Therapy, and Systemic Therapy

Several small studies have demonstrated the efficacy of induction intrathecal therapy followed by radiation and maintenance intrathecal therapy as well as systemic chemotherapy (WELLS et al. 1980, STEINHERZ et al. 1985, 1990). A POG study looked at the efficacy of induction and maintenance triple intrathecal therapy with 24 Gy cranial radiation as well as systemic reinduction and continuation therapy for 120 children with first isolated CNS relapse (WINICK et al. 1993). All patients attained second remission and the 4 year event-free survival was 46%. In a multivariate analysis, short first remission and prior therapy with an anthracycline were the only factors that predicted worse outcome. The incidence of leukoencephalopathy was somewhat higher in previously irradiated patients.

6.6.4 Effect of Prior Therapy

It is difficult to examine the effect of prior therapy because of its heterogeneity, for most patients entering relapse studies. ORTEGA and colleagues (1987) examined the effect of prior CNS preventive therapy on the outcome after relapse in patients who had received uniform systemic treatment on a CCG protocol, but who were randomized to one of four CNS preventive regimens. Event-free survival after relapse was significantly better for patients who received prior radiation compared to those who did not. The most significant predictor of poor outcome after relapse was short duration of initial remission.

6.6.5 Other Pharmacologic Approaches

Although intrathecal therapy remains the mainstay of the management of CNS relapse, systemically adminstered drugs that achieve therapeutic cerebrospinal fluid concentrations may play a role in clearing CNS disease. Both high-dose cytosine arabinoside with or without asparaginase and high-dose methotrexate have been shown to clear CNS disease. (FRICK et al. 1984; AMADORI et al. 1984; BALIS et al. 1985).

6.6.6 Role of Bone Marrow Transplantation

Since the outcome after relapse is poor in most studies, bone marrow transplantation may be a reasonable alternative treatment after a CNS relapse. We have performed purged autologous bone marrow transplantation in nine patients who had isolated CNS relapses. Seven patients were in second and two in third remission. All but two had a first remission of at least 2 years. All patients received systemic reinduction, consolidation, and intrathecal therapy prior to transplantation. With one exception, patients who had not had prior preventive CNS radiation were given additional cranial radiation immediately prior to total body irradiation. Three patients relapsed, and six were in continuous complete remisson at a median of 3 years from transplantation. The three patients who relapsed included the only patient who did not receive a cranial "boost" with total body irradiation, one patient who had a short first remission, and one patient transplanted in third remission.

In summary, CNS treatment remains an important aspect of ALL therapy. Multiple therapeutic approaches are available. The choice of an ideal modality for a given child remains unsettled and the subject of clinical investigation. Clearly, prevention of CNS leukemia is desirable because of the high risk of subsequent relapse. It is important that the CNS treatment efficacy be measured not only in the prevention of CNS leukemia but also by the event-free survival. The morbidity of the various treatment modalities must be clearly delineated.

References

Abromowitch M, Ochs J, Pui, C-H Fairclough D, Murphy SB, Rivera GK (1988) Efficacy of high-dose, methotrexate in childhood acute lymphocytic leukemia; Analysis by contemporary risk classifications. Blood 71: 866–869

Amadori S, Papa G, Avvisati G et al. (1984) Sequential combination of systemic high-dose ara-C and asparaginase for the treatment of central nervous system leukemia and lymphoma. J Clin Oncol 2: 98–101

Aur RJA, Simone JV, Hustu HO (1972) A comparative study of central nervous system irradiation and intensive chemotherapy early in remission of childhood acute lymphocytic leukemia. Cancer 29: 331–341.

Balis FM, Savith JL, Bleyer WA, Reaman GH, Poplack DG (1985) Remission induction of meningeal leukemia with high-dose intravenous methotrexate. J Clin Oncol 3: 485–489

Bernard J, Jackquillat C, Weil M (1972) Treatment of the acute leukemias. Semin Hematol 9: 181–191

Billet AL, Gelber RD, Tarbell NJ et al. (1993a) Sex differences in the risk of central nervous system relapse in childhood acute lymphoblastic leukemia. Proc Am Soc Clin Oncol 12: 316

Billet AL, Kornmehl E, Tarbell NJ, Weinstein HJ, Gelber RD, Ritz J, Sallan SE (1993b) Autologous bone marrow transplantation after a long first remission for children with recurrent acute lymphoblastic leukemia. Blood 81: 1651–1657

Bleyer WA (1977) Clinical pharmacology of intrathecal methotrexate. II. An improved dosage regimen derived from age-related pharmacokinetics. Cancer Treat Rep 61: 1419–1425

Bleyer WA (1988) Central nervous system leukemia. Pediatr Clin North Am 35: 789–814

Bleyer WA, Poplack DG (1985) Prophylaxis and treatment of leukemia in the central nervous system and other sanctuaries. Semin Oncol 12: 131–148

Bleyer WA, Coccia PF, Sather HN et al. (1983) Reduction in central nervous system leukemia with a pharmacokinetically derived intrathecal methotrexate dosage, J Clin Oncol 1: 317–325

Brochstein JA, Kernan NA, Groshen S et al. (1987) Allogeneic bone marrow transplantation after hyperfractionated total-body irradiation and cyclophosphamide in children with acute leukemia. N Engl J Med 317: 1618–1624

Buhrer C, Henze G, Hofmann J, Reiter A, Schellong G, Riehm H (1990) Central nervous system relapse prevention in 1165 standard-risk children with acute lymphoblastic leukemia in five BFM trials. In: Büchner T, Schellong G, Hiddemann W, Ritter J (eds) Haematology and blood transfusion 33: acute leukemia II. Springer, Berlin Heidelberg New York, pp 500–502

Camitta B, Leventhal B, Lauer S et al. (1989) Intermediate-dose intravenous methotrexate and mercaptopurine therapy for non-T, non-B acute lymphocytic leukemia of childhood: a Pediatric Oncology Group study. J Clin Oncol 7: 1539–1544

Camitta B, Lauer S, Leventhal B, Mahoney D, Shuster J (1992) Early intensive methotrexate/6-mercaptopurine for higher risk childhood acute lymphocytic leukemia: A Pediatric Oncology Group pilot study. Proc Am Soc Clin Oncol 11: 280

Clarkson BD, Haghbin M, Murphy ML et al. (1979) Prevention of central nervous system leukaemia in acute lymphoblastic leukemic with prophylactic chemotherapy alone. In: Whitehouse JMA, Kag HEM (eds) CNS complication of malignant disease. University Park Press, Baltimore, pp 36–58

Clavell LA, Gelber RD, Cohen HJ et al. (1986) Four-agent induction and intensive asparaginase therapy for treatment of childhood acute lymphoblastic leukemia. N Engl J Med 315: 657–663

Dritschilo A, Cassady JR, Camitta B, Jaffe N, Paed D, Furman L, Traggis D (1976) The role of irradiation in central nervous system treatment and prophylaxis for acute lymphoblastic leukemia. Cancer 37: 2729–2735

Evans AE, Gilbert ES, Zandstra R (1970) The increasing incidence of central nervous system leukemia in children. Cancer 26: 404–409

Freeman AI, Weinberg V, Brecher ML et al. (1983) Comparison of intermediate-dose methotrexate with cranial irradiation for the post-induction treatment of acute lymphocytic leukemia in children. N Engl J Med 308: 477–484

Frei E, Karon M, Levin RH et al. (1965) The effectiveness of combinations of antileukemia agents in inducing and maintaining remission in children with acute leukemia. Blood 26: 642–656.

Frick J, Ritch PS, Hansen RM, Anderson ZT (1984). Successful treatment of meningeal leukemia using systemic high-dose cytosine arabinoside. J Clin Oncol 2: 365–368

Gee TS, Haghbin M, Dowling MD, Cunningham I, Middleman MP, Clarkson B (1976) Acute lymphocytic leukemia in adults and children. Differences in response with similar therapeutic regimens. Cancer 37: 1256–1264

Gelber RD, Sallan SE, Cohen HJ et al. (1993) Central nervous system treatment in childhood acute lymphoblastic leukemia: long-term follow-up of patients diagnosed between 1973–1985. Cancer 72: 261–270

George SL, Ochs JJ, Mauer AM, Simone JV (1985) The importance of an isolated central nervous system relapse in children with acute lymphoblastic leukemia. J Clin Oncol 3: 776–781

Green DM, Freeman AI, Sallan SE, et al. (1980) Comparison of three methods of central nervous-systemic prophylaxis in childhood acute lymphoblastic leukemia. Lancet I: 1398–1401

Haghbin M, Tan CT, Clarkson B, Mike B, Burchenal JH, Murphy ML (1975) Treatment of acute lymphoblastic leukemia in children with "prophylactic" intrathecal methotrexate and intensive systemic chemotherapy. Cancer Res 35: 807–811

Haghbin M, Murphy ML, Tan CT, Clarkson BC, Thaler HT, Passe S, Burchenal J (1980) A long-term clinical follow-up of children with acute lymphoblastic leukemia treated with intensive chemotherapy regimens. Cancer 46: 241–252

Henze G, Lan German HJ, Ritter J, Schellong G, Riehm H (1981) Treatment strategy for different risk groups in childhood acute lymphoblastic leukemia: a report from the BFM group. In: Neth R, Gallo RC, Graf T, Mannweiler K, Winkler K (eds) Modern trends in human leukemia IV. Springer, Berlin Heidelberg New York, pp 87–98

Henze G, Langermann H-J, Bramswig J, Schellong G, Ludwin R, Riehm H (1983) Ergebnisse der präventiven Behandlung des Zentralnervensystems bei 275 Kindern mit acuter lymphoblastischer Leukämie. Klin Pädiatr 195: 168–175

Hustu HO Aur RJA (1978) Extramedullary leukemia. Clin Haematol 7: 313–317

Hustu HO, Aur RJA, Verzoa MS, Simone JV, Pinkel D (1973) Prevention of central nervous system leukemia by irradiation. Cancer 32: 585–597

Inati A, Sallan SE, Cassady JR, Hitchcock-Bryan S, Clavell LA, Belli JA, Solle N (1983) Efficacy and morbidity of central nervous system "prophylaxis" in childhood acute lymphoblastic leukemia: eight years' experience with cranial irradiation and intrathecal methotrexate. Blod 61: 297–303

Johnson RE (1964) An experimental therapeutic approach to L1210 leukemia in mice: combined chemotherapy and central nervous system irradiation. J Natl Cancer Inst 32: 1333–1340

Komp DM, Fernandez CH, Falletta JM et al. (1982) CNS prophylaxis in acute lymphoblastic leukemia comparison of two methods. Southwest Oncology Group Study. Cancer 50: 1031–1036

Kun LE, Camitta BM, Mulhern RK et al. (1984) Treatment of meningeal relapse in childhood acute lymphoblastic leukemia. I. Results of craniospinal irradiation. J Clin Oncol 2: 359–364

Land VJ, Thomas PRM, Boyett JM et al. (1985) Comparison of maintenance treatment regimens for first central nervous system relapse in children with acute lymphoblastic leukemia. A Pediatric Oncology Group study. Cancer 56: 81–87

Leukemia Committee and Working Party on Leukemia in childhood (1973) Treatment of acute lymphoblastic leukemia: effect of "prophylactic" therapy against central nervous system leukemia. Br Med J II: 381–384

Mandell LR, Stenherz P, Fuks Z (1990) Delayed central nervous system radiation in childhood CNS acute lymphoblastic leukemia. Cancer 66: 447–450

Moe PJ, Seip M, Finne PH (1981) Intermediate dose methotrexate in childhood acute lymphocyte leukemia. Acta Paediatr Scand 70: 73–79.

Nesbit ME, Robison LL, Littman PS, Sather HN, Ortega J, D'Angio GJ, Hammond GD (1981) Presymtomatic central nervous system therapy in previous untreated childhood acute lymphoblastic leukaemia: comparison of 1800 rad and 2400 rad. Lancet I: 461–466

Ochs JJ, River G, Aur RJ, Hustu HO, Berg R, Simone JV (1985) Central nervous system morbidity following an initial isolated central nervous system relapse and its subsequent therapy in childhood acute lymphoblastic leukemia. J Clin Oncol 3: 622–626

Ortega JA, Nesbit ME, Sather HN et al. (1987) Long-term evaluation of a CNS prophylaxis trial–treatment comparisons and outcome after CNS relapse in childhood ALL: A report from the Children's Cancer Study Group. J Clin Oncol 5: 1646–1654

Poplack DG, Reaman GH, Bleyer WA, Miser J, Feusner J, Wesley R, Hammond D (1984) Central nervous system (CNS) preventive therapy with high dose methotrexate (HDMTX) in acute lymphoblastic leukemia (ALL): a preliminary report (abstract) Proc Am Soc Clin Oncol 3: 204

Pullen J, Boyett J, Shuster J et al. (1993) Extended triple intrathecal chemotherapy trial for prevention of CNS relapse in good-risk and poor-risk patients with B-progenitor acute lymphoblastic leukemia: Pediatric Oncology Group study. J Clin Oncol 11: 839–849

Riehm H, Gadner H, Genze G et al. (1990) Results and significance of six randomized trials in four consecutive ALL-

BFM studies In: Buchner, Schellong G, Hiddeman, Ritter (eds) Haematology and blood transfusion 33: acute leukemias II. Springer, Berlin Heidelberg, New York, pp 439–450

Rivera GK, George SL, Bowman WP et al. (1983) Second central nervous system prophylaxis in children with acute lymphoblastic leukemia who relapse after effective cessation of therapy. J Clin Oncol 8: 471–476

Rivera GK, Raimondi SC, Hancock ML et al. (1991) Improved outcome in childhood acute lymohoblastic leukaemia with reinforced early treatment and rotational combination chemotherapy. Lancet 1: 61–66

Sackmann F, Svarch E, Pavlosky S et al. (1983) Comparison of central nervous system prophylaxis with cranial radiation and intrathecal methotrexate versus intrathecal methotrexate alone in acute lymphoblastic leukemia. Blood 62: 241–250

Schwenn M, Chun M, Wolfe L (1989) Long-term follow-up of childhood acute lymphoblastic leukemia: role of cranial irradiation. Proc Am Soc Clin Oncol 8: 216

Steinherz P, Jereb B, Galicich J (1985). Therapy of CNS leukemia with intraventricular chemotherapy and low-dose neuraxis radiotherapy. J Clin Oncol 3: 1217–1225

Steinherz P, Mandell L, Meyers P, Tan C, Fuks Z (1990) Periodic central nervous system reinduction and delayed craniospinal radiation in the treatment of CNS relapse in acute lymphoblastic leukemia. Proc Am Soc Clin Oncol 9: 221

Sullivan MP, Vietti TJ, Fernback JD, Griffith K, Haddy TB, Watkins WL (1969) Clinical investigations in the treatment of meningeal leukemia: radiation therapy regimens versus conventional intrathecal methotrexate. Blood 34: 301 319

Sullivan MP, Humphrey GH, Vietti TJ, Haggard ME, Lee E (1975) Superiority of conventional intrathecal methotrexate therapy with maintenance over intensive intrathecal methotrexate therapy, unmaintained, or radiotherapy (2000–2500 rads tumor dose) in treatment for meningeal leukemia. Cancer 35: 1066–1073

Sullivan MP, Moon TE, Trueworthy R, Vietti RJ, Humphrey GB, Komp D (1977) Combination intrathecal therapy for meningeal leukemia: Two versus three drugs. Blood 50: 471 479

Sullivan MP, Chen T, Dyment PG, Hvizdala E, Steuber CP (1982) Equivalence of intrathecal chemotherapy and radiotherapy as central nervous system prophylaxis in children with acute lymphatic leukemia: a Pediatric Oncology Group study. Blood 60: 948–958.

Tubergen DG, Gilchrist GS, O'Brian RT, Coccia PF, Sather HN, Waskerwotz MJ, Hammond GD (1993) Prevention of CNS disease in intermediate acute lymphoblastic leukemia: comparison of cranial radiation and intrathecal methotrexate and the importance of systemic therapy: a Children's Cancer Group report. J Clin Oncol 11: 520–526

Wells RJ, Weetman RM, Baehner FL (1980) The impact of central nervous system relapse following intitial complete remission in childhood acute lymphocytic leukemia. J Pediatr 97: 429–432

Winick NJ, Smith SD, Shuster J et al. (1993) Tratment of CNS relapse in children with acute lymphoblastic leukemia: a Pediatric Oncology Group study. J Clin Oncol 11: 271–278

7 Acute Nonlymphocytic Leukemia

BALDASSARRE STEA

CONTENTS

7.1   Introduction   99
7.2   Pathogenesis   99
7.3   Etiology   99
7.4   Biology and Cytogenetics 100
7.5   Classification 100
7.6   Clinical Presentation and Diagnosis 101
7.7   Treatment 102
7.7.1 Chemotherapy 102
7.7.2 Bone Marrow Transplantation 102
7.7.3 Radiation Therapy 105
7.7.4 Treatment of Leukostasis 107
7.7.5 Treatment of Extramedullary Lesions 107
7.8   Complications of Treatment 108
7.8.1 Complications Due to CNS Irradiation 108
7.8.2 Toxicities Due to Total Body Irradiation 109
7.9   Conclusion 110
       References 111

7.1 Introduction

Acute nonlymphocytic leukemias (ANLL) represent approximately 20%–25% of all the leukemias seen in childhood; therefore they account for approximately 400–500 newly diagnosed cases of childhood leukemia in the United States each year. Unlike acute lymphocytic leukemia (ALL), which has a peak occurrence at approximately age 4 years, the incidence of ANLL is constant from birth through age 10 years. However, most congenital leukemias are due to ANLL. Furthermore, there appears to be no sex-related or racial difference in the incidence of ANLL.

7.2 Pathogenesis

Several lines of evidence exist to support a clonal origin for the majority of the cases of ANLL. These lines are based on cytogenetic studies of bone marrow blast cells as well as studies involving female patients

BALDASSARRE STEA, Ph.D., M.D., Associate Professor, Department of Radiation Oncology, The University of Arizona Health Science Center, 1501 N. Campbell Avenue, Tucson, AZ 85724, USA

with heterozygosity in the X-linked enzyme glucose-6-phosphate dehydrogenase (G6PD). Blast cells from these patients with ANLL express only a single isozyme form of G6PD whereas their normal cells express both forms of this enzyme (FIALKOW et al. 1979, 1981). Additional evidence for the clonal origin of ANLL comes from molecular biology studies involving DNA polymorphism based on the DNA methylation that occurs with the X-chromosome inactivation (FEARON et al. 1986). The transforming event giving rise to the clonal expansion can occur at any level between the progenitor cells and the committed precursors such as the myeloblast or monoblast. After successful treatment and achievement of a complete remission (defined as less than 5% blasts in the bone marrow), polyclonal hematopoiesis resumes in the majority of the patients. However, recent studies have shown that some patients, apparently in a morphologic remission, continue to have clonal hematopoiesis (JACOBSON et al. 1984). This finding obviously raises some questions about the validity of a morphologically defined complete remission.

7.3 Etiology

A variety of possible etiologic factors for ANLL have been examined, including genetic and environmental factors. From a genetic point of view, it is known that the incidence of leukemia is increased in children with certain chromosomal abnormalities such as trisomy 21 (Down's syndrome) (ROSNER and LEE 1972). It is believed that predisposition of these children to develop leukemia is due to an inherent chromosomal instability that renders the DNA susceptible to other leukemogenic factors. Other conditions known to predispose children to ANLL are Fanconi's anemia and Bloom's syndrome (LI and BADER 1987), two recessively transmitted disorders associated with several congenital abnormalities and characterized by a defect in DNA repair mechanisms. From an environmental point of view, irradiation and exposure to toxic chemicals have been shown to predispose to ANLL. People exposed to the nuclear bombs exploded at Hiroshima and Nagasaki at the end of World War II showed an increased incidence of leukemia (SCHULL and WEISS 1992). Chronic exposure to benzene has been associated with a increased risk of ANLL (RINSKY et al. 1987), and the incidence of leukemia has been shown to be increased in patients treated with alkylating agents used to treat a variety of malignancies (BLAYNEY et al. 1987; PEDERSEN-BJERGAARD et al. 1981). Usually these patients will develop a myelodysplastic syndrome before ANLL becomes manifest. The incidence of this type of secondary leukemia appears to peak at 6 years following exposure to the alkylating agents and appears to be time limited (BLAYNEY et al. 1987).

7.4 Biology and Cytogenetics

It is believed that ANLL originates from a single precursor cell that undergoes transformation and gives rise to a poorly differentiated cell population (blast cells). With continued proliferation, these blast cells replace the bone marrow and it is estimated that at the time of diagnosis, the leukemic burden is approximately 10^{12} cells. A number of clonal cytogenetic abnormalities are present in more than 80% of patients with ANLL (YUNIS et al. 1981; KANEKO et al. 1982; BERNSTEIN et al. 1984). These chromosomal abnormalities are present in the malignant cells but not in the normal cells of the individual. The most frequent abnormalities observed are: trisomy of chromosome 8, loss of a sex chromosome, and several translocations, primarily t(8;21) and t(15;17) (LARSON et al. 1984; WOODS et al. 1985). Some chromosomal abnormalities have been identified as having prognostic significance; SCHIFFER et al. (1989) reported on a study with 198 patients diagnosed in one center, and identified t(8;21) and t(15;17) and a number of abnormalities in 16q22 as being associated with a favorable outcome whereas – 5/5q – and – 7/7q – and + 8 were found to be associated with a poor outcome in terms of remission rates and disease-free survival.

The molecular biologic events associated with the malignant transformation of leukemic cells are unknown. However, it is believed that a chromosomal translocation may be responsible for the transposition of a proto-oncogene from one chromosome to another, thus altering its expression, as in Burkitt's lymphoma and chronic myelogenous leukemia. A high frequency of *ras* oncogene activation has been found in both acute myeloid and lymphoid leukemias as well as in myelodysplastic syndrome (BOS 1990). Activation of this oncogene occurs by point mutation leading to a single amino acid substitution. The *ras* gene products are plasma membrane guanine nucleotide-binding proteins involved in the signal transduction pathways. The consequence of *ras* activation is the conversion of a normally regulated protein into one that is constantly activated. However, the exact mechanism of leukemogenesis by activated *ras* proteins is unknown.

7.5 Classification

Acute nonlymphocytic leukemia includes several subtypes which are defined most commonly according to the French-American-British (FAB) morphology. Initially developed in 1976 (BENNETT et al. 1976), the FAB classification divided ANLL into six

Table 7.1. French-American-British (FAB) classification of ANLL and relative frequency (adapted from GRIER and WEINSTEIN 1989)

FAB class	Common Name	Histochemistry[a]	Frequency in children ≥ 2 years old
M1	Acute myeloblastic leukemia without differentiation	MP +	25%
M2	Acute myeloblastic leukemia with differentiation	MP +	27%
M3	Acute promyelocytic leukemia	MP +	5%
M4	Acute myelomonocytic leukemia	MP + NSE +	26%
M5	Acute monocytic leukemia	NSE +	16%
M6	Erythroleukemia (D:G)	MP + (myeloblasts) PAS + (erythroid precursors)	2%
M7	Acute megakaryoblastic leukemia	PPO +	

[a]MP, myeloperoxidase; NSE, nonspecific esterase; PAS, perodic acid-Schiff; PPO, platelet peroxidase (by electron microscopy)

subtypes. This classification was updated in 1987 with the addition of megakaryocytic leukemia (BENNETT et al. 1985b) (Table 7.1). This type of classification has been found to have prognostic significance. In addition, certain FAB subtypes present unique clinical problems such as in the case of promyelocytic leukemia (M3) and its microgranular variant (M3v), which are frequently associated with a disseminated intravascular coagulation syndrome (ROVELLI et al. 1992). Acute monocytic leukemia is particularly frequent in children less than 3 years of age. In older children, the majority of the leukemias are of the myeloblastic (M1, M2) and the myelomonocytic type (M4) (Table 7.1). Furthermore, several cell surface and biochemical markers have been identified and found to be associated with specific subtypes of ANLL (BALL and FANGER 1983; VAN DER REIJDEN et al. 1993; GRIFFIN et al. 1981). A wide variety of both lineage- and differentiation-specific monoclonal antibodies have been developed and are being used to differentiate among myeloid surface markers (FOON and TODD 1986). These markers can be helpful in identifying unusual cases of undifferentiated leukemias, and can be used to predict outcome (CHAN et al. 1985; GRIFFIN et al. 1986).

7.6 Clinical Presentation and Diagnosis

The presenting signs and symptoms of children with ANLL are directly related to the depletion of normal bone marrow elements – a consequence of the abnormal proliferation of leukemic cells in the bone marrow. This abnormal proliferation leads to a hypercellular bone marrow with up to 80%–100% blast cells. Depletion of normal progenitor cells results in anemia, neutropenia, and thrombocytopenia. A child with ANLL may present with fatigue, dyspnea on exertion, and pallor, which would indicate the presence of profound anemia. The median presenting hemoglobin concentration in one large study was 7 g/dl (CHOI and SIMONE 1976). Additionally, thrombocytopenia leads to easy bruising, bleeding from gingivae, petchiae on the skin, and epistaxis. The platelet count in approximately 50% of newly diagnosed children with ANLL was below 50 000/mm^3 (CHOI and SIMONE 1976). Neutropenia often results in an absolute neutrophil count of less than 1000/mm^3 and this leads to prolonged bacterial infection usually originating from teeth, gingivae, sinuses, lungs, and perirectal areas.

Extramedullary leukemia spread can result in hepatomegaly and splenomegaly, conditions present in about 50% of the children with ANLL (CHOI and SIMONE 1976). In addition, lymphadenopathy is present at diagnosis in less than 25% of the patients, but is more common in the M4 and M5 subtypes. Leukemic infiltration of the periosteum leads to bone pain and may be associated with a limp or refusal to walk in very young children. Some patients develop localized extramedullary accumulation of leukemic cells that can occur in bones or soft tissues around the orbits and on epidural surfaces. These collections of leukemic cells have been called chloromas because they can appear green on the cut surface due to the high level of the enzyme myeloperoxidase (WIERNIK and SERPICK 1970). These tumors are usually associated with the M4 and M5 subtypes.

Leukemia cutis is an uncommon mode of presentation and consists of accumulation of leukemic infiltrates in the skin with the appearance of colorless or slightly purplish ("blueberry muffin") lesions often occurring in neonates with acute monocytic leukemia.

Involvement of the central nervous system (CNS) can occur in the form of chloromas, as indicated earlier, or in the more common form of meningeal involvement. CNS involvement has been reported in 5%–17% of children at diagnosis, a proportion that is higher than that noted in ALL (GRIER et al. 1987; PUI et al. 1985). Symptoms associated with CNS leukemia are nausea and vomiting, headaches, photophobia, and cranial nerve palsies. CNS involvement was found to be more common in patients with an initial WBC greater than 25 000/mm^3 and in children younger than 3 years of age at diagnosis (PUI et al. 1985). The monoblastic or myelomonoblastic subtype of leukemia has also been associated with the presence of CNS disease at diagnosis (GRIER et al. 1987; CREUTZIG et al. 1985).

The WBC at diagnosis can be quite variable despite profound infiltration of the bone marrow, and approximately one-third to one-fourth of children with ANLL will present with a leukocyte count greater than 100 000/mm^3 (GRIER et al. 1987). A definite diagnosis of leukemia is made by examination of a bone marrow aspirate. A minimum of greater than 30% blasts is necessary in order to make the diagnosis of leukemia (BENNETT et al. 1985). Careful morphologic examination of bone marrow aspirates which have been stained with Romanovsky's stain is mandatory. In addition, a number of histochemical studies using myeloperoxidase, Sudan black, periodic acid-Schiff, and various esterase-based stains are often necessary to distinguish ANLL from ALL.

Immunologic cell surface markers and biochemical markers may also help in the differentiation of the various subtypes of ANLL.

The diagnosis of acute megakaryoblastic leukemia (M7) requires demonstration of platelet peroxidase by electron microscopy or the presence of platelet-specific surface markers (Bennett et al. 1985b). Unlike ALL, no consistent prognostic factors have been identified in children with ANLL. The most commonly reported negative factors are an age of less than 2 years at presentation, the M4 and M5 FAB subtypes, a high leukocyte count greater than 100 000/mm³, the presence of splenomegaly greater than 5 cm, and a high labeling index (greater than 10% at diagnosis). These factors have been associated with an increased risk of relapse and decreased survival (Grier et al. 1987; Lampkin et al. 1983; Chessels et al. 1985; Dahl et al. 1982). Several specific cytogenetic abnormalities are now being used as prognostic indicators (Schiffer et al. 1989; Woods et al. 1985).

7.7 Treatment

7.7.1 Chemotherapy

Following diagnosis, the initial therapy is directed toward the prevention and the treatment of potentially life-threatening complications such as bleeding, overwhelming infections, and leukostasis.

The most effective regimens for remission induction incorporate cytosine arabinoside (Ara-C) plus an anthracycline (doxorubicin or daunorubicin). Most induction regimens involve the continuous infusion of Ara-C for 7 days plus a 3-day course of an anthracycline with or without additional drugs such as 6-thioguanine, prednisone, and vincristine. The objective of remission induction is to reduce the leukemic cell burden to undetectable levels (<5% of myeloblasts in the bone marrow). Drugs used to achieve this goal will induce profound marrow aplasia; consequently they have great potential for contributing to morbidity and mortality from infection and bleeding. With such regimens, remission rates of 70% and 80% have been achieved (Grier et al. 1992; Ritter et al. 1992; Hurwitz et al. 1992). Although these results represent a substantial improvement over previous trials, the median duration of remission infrequently exceeds 24 months. Following remission induction, continuation of therapy is usually instituted.

Although post remission chemotherapy is generally believed to be beneficial, the intensity and duration of therapy remain controversial. Three different types of strategy have been used to maintain the state of remission. The first involves an "intensification" phase in which the same drugs are used as during the induction phase, but at much higher doses, and often in conjunction with other non-cross-resistant drugs. Another strategy is that of "consolidation" chemotherapy, which involves the administration of the same drugs in the same doses as used in the induction phase. The third strategy used in the post remission period is that of "maintenance" chemotherapy consisting of the same drugs used for induction, but at less myelosuppressive doses than in the induction period, these drugs are given monthly for 2–3 years. Several studies utilizing induction chemotherapy followed by intensive postremission chemotherapy have reported a continuous complete remission rate of 30%–50% at 5 years (Grier et al. 1992; Ritter et al. 1992; Hurwitz et al. 1992). The value of "maintenance" chemotherapy remains controversial since long-term follow-up of children treated with this approach shows a disease-free survival rate of about 20% (Dahl et al. 1982; Baehner et al. 1981).

7.7.2 Bone Marrow Transplantation

Bone marrow transplantation (BMT) is increasingly being used as a form of intensification or consolidation therapy for children with ANLL. With this approach, supralethal doses of chemotherapy (usually cyclophosphamide at 120 mg/kg) plus total body irradiation (TBI) (7.5–14 Gy) are used as conditioning regimens. Recent trials from cooperative groups as well as single institutions indicate a 5-year actuarial leukemia-free survival of 45%–66% for children with ANLL in first remission (Santos et al. 1983; Zwaan et al. 1984; Bostrom et al. 1985; Sanders et al. 1985; Brochstein et al. 1987; Herve et al. 1991). Although these results are encouraging, controversy exists as to the relative value of BMT versus conventional chemotherapy for children with ANLL in first remission. The Children's Cancer Study Group (CCSG) has performed a prospective controlled study of BMT versus conventional chemotherapy and has thereby demonstrated a significantly better disease-free survival rate for BMT than for chemotherapy (49% versus 36%, p=0.03) (Nesbit et al. 1987; Buckley et al. 1989). The improved survival noted with BMT in this study, however is not greatly different from that achieved with traditional induction and intensification chemotherapy regimens (Grier et al. 1987; Creutzig et al. 1985).

The rationale for the use of BMT is that it allows the administration of supralethal doses of TBI and hematologically suppressive chemotherapy. Thus in theory BMT should achieve a greater dose-related tumor cell kill than conventional chemotherapy. In addition, the graft versus host reaction generated by the infused lymphocytes from the donor bone marrow may have a beneficial immunotherapeutic effect. BMT can be performed with either allogeneic marrow, in which case the bone marrow is obtained from an HLA-compatible sibling, or syngeneic marrow from an identical twin donor. Furthermore, several groups have performed BMT with autologous bone marrow (LINCH and BURNETT 1986; HERVE et al. 1991). In autotransplantation the bone marrow is removed from the patient usually during the first remission and reinfused following the preparative regimen of either chemotherapy or TBI or both. In autologous BMT, the bone marrow is transplanted either untreated or after exvivo purging. With the former technique, a differential effect of freezing on leukemic versus normal bone marrow cells, reinfusion of a sublethal dose of leukemic cells, or an autologous graft versus leukemia effect is presupposed to be operational. Alternatively, ex vivo drug or antibody treatments have been used to purge autologous bone marrow of leukemic cells (YEAGER et al. 1986). Although autologous BMT overcomes the problem of lack of HLA-compatible donors, it must be recognized that the relapse-free survival is usually better in patients who show some degree of graft versus host disease (GVHD) in comparison to those who have no GVHD following allogeneic transplantation or in

comparison to syngeneic transplantation (THOMAS 1983; CHAMPLIN and GALE 1987).

7.7.3 Radiation Therapy

7.7.3.1 Prophylactic CNS Irradiation

The CNS is a common site of occult leukemic cell infiltration. Without any specific CNS prophylaxis up to 36% of all relapses will occur in the CNS (GRIER et al. 1987). CNS prophylaxis with either irradiation or intrathecal chemotherapy or both has been shown to decrease the development of subsequent CNS relapses (Table 7.2). In a study performed at St. Jude Children's Research Hospital, craniospinal irradiation was used to prophylactically treat subclinical meningeal leukemia in 24 children with ANLL, and no prophylactic treatment was given to 20 children. This study showed that CNS relapses occurred in 6 of the 20 children without preventative therapy, but in none of the 24 children who received craniospinal irradiation to a dose of 24 Gy in 15 fractions (Table 7.2) (DAHL et al. 1978). More recently, CNS prophylaxis has been accomplished with intrathecal Ara-C, or intrathecal methotrexate with or without cranial irradiation (12–24 Gy). With these forms of prophylaxis, the rate of isolated CNS relapses has been reduced to 2%–15% (GRIER et al. 1987; CREUTZIG et al. 1985; DAHL et al. 1982). Although the use of CNS prophylaxis has lowered the number of CNS relapses, this practice has not led to improved disease-free survival (Table 7.2). This apparent lack of benefit

Table 7.2. CNS Prophylaxis

Study	CNS leukemia at diagnosis	CNS prophylaxis	Isolated CNS relapses/total relapses	Proportion of patients in CCR or DFS (duration of F/U)	References
St. Jude AML-72	12/83 (14%)	CSI (24 Gy)	0/24 (0%)	0.08 (2.9–3.3 yr)	DAHL et al. 1978
		None	6/20 (30%)	0.15 (1.9–2.8 yr)	DAHL et al. 1978
St. Jude AML-76	14/81 (17%)	IT MTX (monthly × 6)	3/50 (6%)	0.29 (3 yr)	DAHL et al. 1982
AML-BFM-78	14/151 (9%)	CRT (12–18 Gy) + IT MTX (weekly × 4)	1/47 (2%)	0.41 (4.75 yr)	CREUTZIG et al. 1985
VAPA	NA	None	8/22 (36%)	0.33 (5 yr)	GRIER et al. 1987
80–035	11/64 (17%)	IT AraC	3/20 (15%)	0.29 (3 yr)	GRIER et al. 1987
CCSG-241	NA	CRT (24 Gy) + IT MTX (weekly × 6)	14/118 (12%)	0.13 (4 yr)	BUCKLEY et al. 1989
CCSG-241A	NA	CRT (24 Gy) + IT MTX (monthly × 6)	7/126 (5%)	0.21 (4 yr)	BUCKLEY et al. 1989

CSI, craniospinal irradiation; IT MTX, intrathecal methotrexate; CRT, cranial irradiation; IT Ara-C, intrathecal cytosine arabinoside; CCR, continuous complete remission; DFS, disease-free survival; F/U, follow-up; NA, not available

from CNS prophylaxis in ANLL is believed to be due to the short duration of median disease-free survival; therefore, the full value and benefit of CNS prophylaxis will probably not become apparent until more durable bone marrow remissions are achieved. Although it is now clear that some form of CNS prophylaxis is needed for children with ANLL, it is not known whether intrathecal chemotherapy alone can provide adequate protection against CNS relapses.

7.7.3.2 Treatment of Overt CNS Disease

The incidence of overt CNS leukemia in ANLL is believed to be similar and probably greater than in ALL (KAY 1976). Pathophysiologically leukemic cells progressively infiltrate the walls of small subpial vessel, they invade the subarachnoid space and eventually extend into the brain parenchyma, thus giving rise to meningeal leukemia or to localized infiltration of the brain in the form of chloromas. CNS involvement at diagnosis has been reported in up to 17% of patients with ANLL, a proportion that indeed appears to be greater than in ALL (DAHL et al. 1982; LAMPKIN et al. 1983). Factors that have been found to be associated with an increased incidence of CNS leukemia have been an initial WBC greater than 25 000 mm^3, diagnosis of myelomonocytic or monocytic leukemia (M4 and M5), and an age less than 2 years (PUI et al. 1985; WEINSTEIN et al. 1983; MAYER et al. 1982).

Overt CNS leukemia is generally diagnosed by the presence of leukemic blasts in Wright-stained cytocentrifuged samples of cerebrospinal fluid. Clinical signs of CNS involvement include cranial nerve palsies and the presence of intracranial masses on computed tomographic scans. In one study, the presence of CNS leukemia at diagnosis did not adversely affect the rate of remission induction or for that matter the duration of complete remissions (PUI et al. 1985). Treatment of overt CNS leukemia present at the time of diagnosis or developing at the time of relapse consists of intrathecal chemotherapy (methotrexate with or without Ara-C) given weekly for 4 weeks and then monthly throughout the remainder of the course of therapy. Patients who achieve CNS remission then receive 24 Gy of cranial irradiation in combination with five doses of intrathecal methotrexate before cessation of chemotherapy. In one study, the probability of continuous complete remission in 32 patients who presented with CNS leukemia at diagnosis was 37%, a rate that is similar to the probablity of continuous

complete remission for patients without CNS leukemia (PUI et al. 1985).

7.7.3.3 Technique of CNS Irradiation

Although craniospinal irradiation was initially shown to be highly effective in the prevention of CNS relapses, it was later abandoned because of its profound myelosuppressive effect, which interfered with (delayed) the administration of systemic chemotherapy. This technique, however, is reviewed here because, as in ALL it could be applied in the treatment of overt or recurrent CNS disease.

Craniospinal irradiation involves the simultaneous treatment of the entire craniospinal axis, which is accomplished by irradiating the cranial content with opposed lateral beams, and the spinal content with one (or more) posterior-anterior field(s). The target volume for the cranial field includes the posterior half of the orbit (including the posterior half of the retina) and the region of the cribriform plate. The temporal fossa is also included in its entirety with enough margin to achieve an adequate dose profile. The caudal margin of the cranial field is usually placed at the bottom of the second cervical vertebra (C2) (Fig. 7.1). In order to treat the posterior half of the globe while sparing the contralateral eye, a 4°–5°

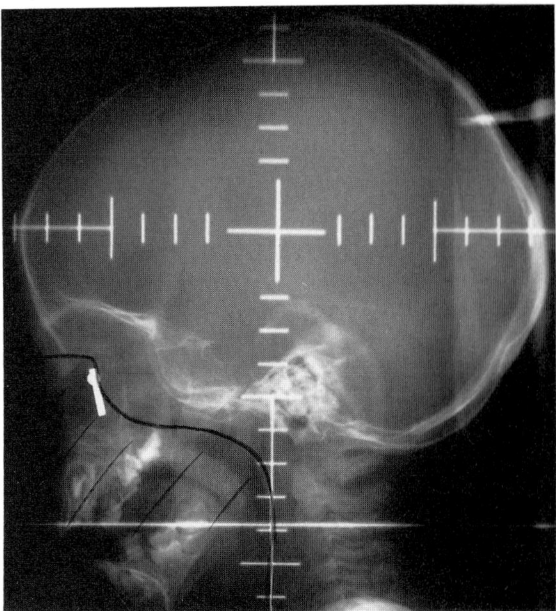

Fig 7.1. Simulation radiograph for whole brain irradiation. The *etched areas* indicate regions that were protected with custom-made blocks. Radiopaque markers have been placed on the lateral canthi and the gantry has been rotated 5° (see text for details)

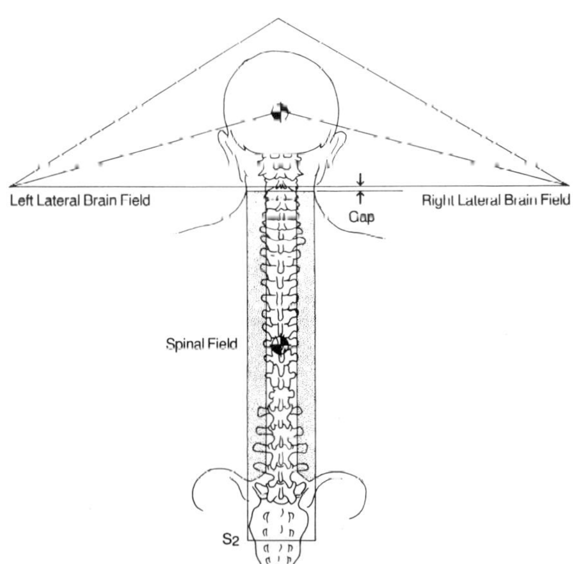

Fig 7.2. Schematic representation of fields used for craniospinal irradiation (view from top). The inferior edges of the lateral brain fields have been made coincident by adjusting the pedestal angle. The *etched area* in the spinal field represents shielding blocks used to protect underlying lungs and bowel. (Adapted from Buck et al. 1984)

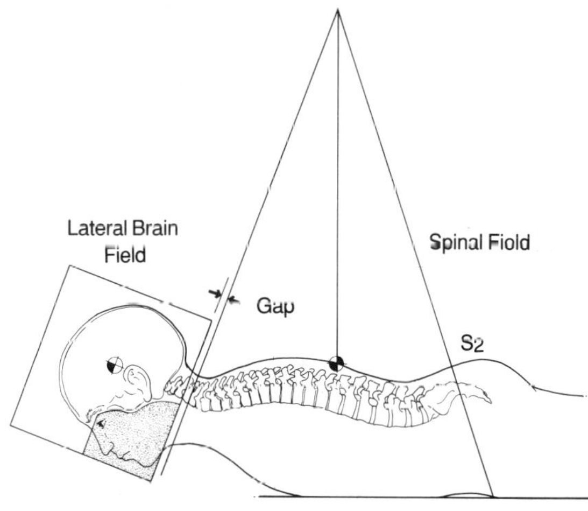

Fig 7.3. Schematic representation of fields used for craniospinal irradiation. The collimator angle of the lateral brain fields has been adjusted to match the divergence of the superior border of the spinal field. (Adapted from Buck et al. 1984)

gantry angle is necessary to correct for beam divergence. Alternatively, the isocenter of the field can be placed at the level of the bony canthi and a split-beam field then constructed. The target volume for the spinal field must include the lower limit for the sacral sac, which extends approximately to the level of S2–S3. This field is wider in the sacral area than in the remaining part of the spine in order to encompass the sacral foramina (Fig. 7.2). In order to achieve dose homogeneity and at the same time avoid overlap or overdosage at the junction sites between the cranial and the spinal radiation fields, extreme precautions must be taken to correct for divergence in three dimensions (Fig. 7.2). Since the lateral cranial fields diverge into the spinal field, the angle of divergence is calculated based on the length of the cranial field, and an appropriate adjustment is made in the pedestal angle to compensate for such divergence (Fig. 7.2). This maneuver makes the inferior edges of the brain field coincident. In addition, the collimator angle of the brain field is adjusted to match the divergent edge of the superior border of the spinal field (Fig. 7.3). Finally, three 1-cm gaps are used between the lateral cranial fields and the posterior spinal field. Moving the gap by 1 cm daily in a repetitive pattern every third day allows "feathering" or homogenization of the dose at the junction sites. Using this technique, the dose across the gap areas has been determined to be no less than 70% of the prescribed dose delivered to the craniospinal axis (Buck et al. 1984).

7.7.3.4. Total Body Irradiation

Total body irradiation (TBI) in conjunction with high-dose chemotherapy (usually cyclophosphamide) has been widely used as a preparative regimen for bone marrow transplantation (BMT). The objective of TBI is twofold: (1) to induce enough immunosuppression to allow allogeneic bone marrow engraftment and (2) to achieve a greater leukemic cell kill than would be possible with conventional chemotherapy.

In the early studies performed by Thomas (1983), TBI for both ALL and ANLL was given in one single fraction of 9.2–10 Gy at a dose rate of 5–6 cGy/min by means of a dual cobalt-60 source. Subsequently, patients with ANLL in first remission were randomized to receive 10 Gy in a single fraction vs 12 Gy in 6 fractions/6 days. Survival analysis of these two groups of patients showed a marginally better survival for the patients treated with the fractionated regimen ($P = 0.05$) (Thomas 1983).

Because of the relatively high rate of relapse after TBI with 12 Gy, attempts have been made to increase the total dose of radiation used in TBI for patients with acute myeloid leukemia (AML). A randomized study of 12 Gy in 6 fractions vs 15.75 Gy in 7 fractions (2.25 Gy/fraction) was performed in patients with AML undergoing BMT while in first complete remission. While the 3-year probability of disease-free survival was virtually identical (0.58 vs 0.59), the

3-year probability of relapse was 0.35 for the 12-Gy group vs 0.12 for the 15.75-Gy group ($P = 0.06$). However, the probabilities of transplant-related mortality were 0.12 and 0.32 for the low- and high-dose groups, respectively ($P = 0.04$) (CLIFT et al. 1990). Thus, high-dose TBI was associated with a significant increase in treatment-related deaths, which were almost all due to acute GVHD.

Studies of BMT conditioning regimens in ANLL have recently been reviewed and the transplant outcomes with such regimens have been compared with the data reported to the International Bone Marrow Transplant Registry (AURER and GALE 1991). Today, several TBI regimens are in use at different institutions: from single-dose (5 Gy), high-dose-rate (58 cGy/min) TBI (FYLES et al. 1991) to the hyperfractionated TBI (13.2 Gy at 1.2 Gy t.i.d. for 11 fractions) used at Memorial Sloan Kettering Cancer Center (BROCHSTEIN et al. 1987). Children with ANLL in first remission treated with the latter approach had an estimated 5-year disease-free survival rate of 65% ± 10% (BROCHSTEIN et al. 1987).

Technically, TBI is performed by positioning the patient in such a way as to ensure that the entire body is irradiated. Because of differences in the thickness of various body regions, tissue compensation is often necessary to achieve dose homogeneity. At the University of Arizona, this goal is achieved by placing bolus bags filled with rice around the thinnest parts of the patient (Fig. 7.4). Rice was selected as the tissue compensator because of its density, its tissue equivalency, and its ability to conform and fit around various body parts. The patient lies supine on a specially built treatment couch, mounted with a Plexiglass beam spoiler which itself is positioned at a distance of 555 cm from the radiation source (Fig. 7.4). At our institution, TBI consists of 12 Gy in 6 fractions of 2 Gy delivered in two fractions/day over 3 days at a dose rate of approximately 10 cGy/min.

One of the major causes of morbidity and mortality following TBI and BMT is the development of idiopathic interstitial pneumonitis, a complication which occurs in more than 10% of the patients undergoing BMT and is thought to be due in part to TBI. When TBI is delivered by opposed lateral beams, the lung dose is higher than the midplane prescription dose by about 15%–20%. Several measures can be taken to decrease the dose of radiation delivered to the lungs to a level approximately equal to the prescription dose. At our institution, a lung compen-

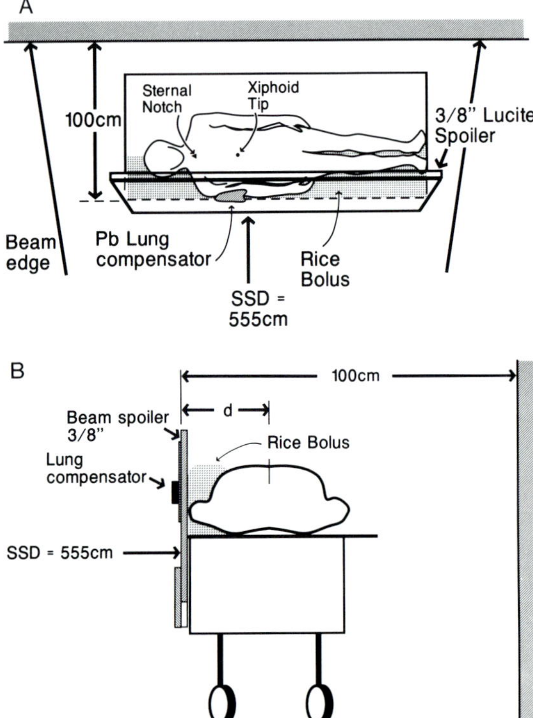

Fig 7.4 a,b. Schematic representation of patient setup for TBI. The patient lies on a special treatment couch positioned at 555 cm from the source. A 3/8″ beam spoiler (Lucite) is used to reduce Dmax with a high-energy beam. Rice bolus is placed around the head, neck, and lower extremities to achieve dose homogeneity. **a** Top view. **b** Side views. (Courtesy of Wendell Lutz, Ph.D., Department of Radiation Oncology, University of Arizona)

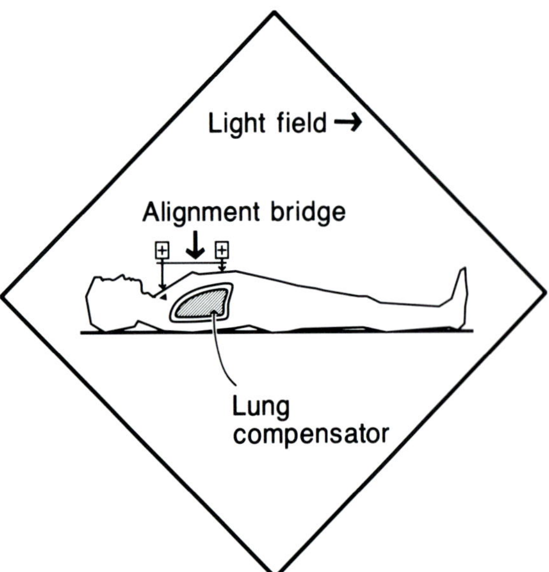

Fig 7.5. Schematic representation of the placement of the lung compensator. An alignment bridge is used to facilitate accurate positioning of the compensator by utilizing anatomic landmarks (sternal notch and xiphoid tip). (courtesy of Wendell Lutz, Ph.D., Department of Radiation Oncology, University of Arizona)

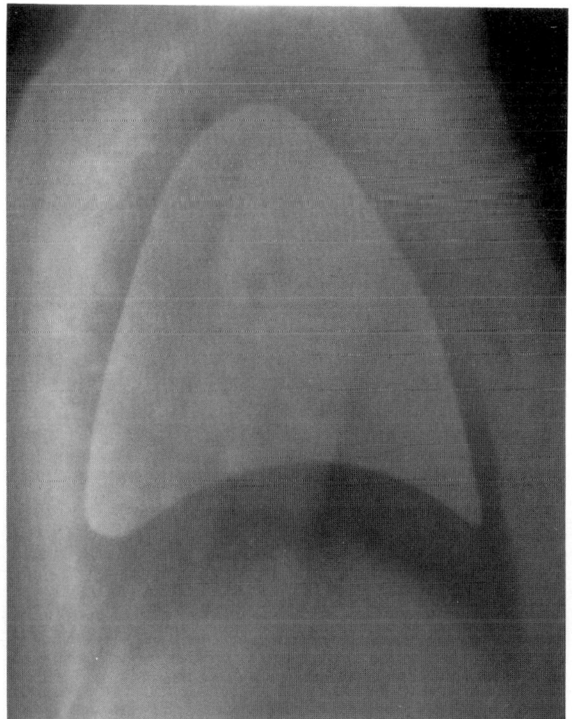

Fig. 7.6. Port film of lung compensator in place during TBI. The compensator conforms to the thoracic cavity and diaphragm and is slightly smaller than the lungs to avoid attenuating the beam over sternum and spine

sator is fabricated for each patient and mounted on the Plexiglass beam spoiler on the side of the patient (Fig 7.5). This compensator decreases the lung dose by approximately 15%. A port film is taken to verify the position of the attenuator before commencing each course of radiation (Fig. 7.6).

7.7.4 Treatment of Leukostasis

Leukostasis refers to the intravascular clumping of large blast cells within capillaries of the brain and lung. This situation is likely to occur with WBC counts $> 200\,000/mm^3$ and can lead to hypoxia, hemorrhage, and subsequent infarction. In the brain, this condition inevitably leads to stroke and coma (DEARTH et al. 1978; LICHTMAN and ROWE 1982; BUNIN and PUI 1985). Therefore when a patient presents with WBC $> 200\,000/mm^3$, it is imperative to commence therapy as soon as possible after confirmation of diagnosis. Hydroxyurea, in combination with allopurinol and hydration, is usually effective (GRUND et al. 1977). Leukapheresis can also be attempted, but it only works transiently and can be used in the initial management if the patient is symp-

tomatic (CUTTNER et al. 1983). Low dose cranial irradiation can be and is sometimes used (6 Gy in 3–4 fractions) although its benefit has not been proven in the setting of clinical trials.

7.7.5 Treatment of Extramedullary Lesions

With the advent of more effective chemotherapeutic regimens and the resultant prolongation of median survival of patients with ANLL, extramedullary leukemic deposits are being observed more frequently. Although the exact magnitude of this problem is not accurately known, in one large study of 171 children with ANLL 8% of the boys had testicular involvement and 12% of the children had involvement of bone and other extramedullary sites (CHOI and SIMONE 1976). Furthermore, 14% of the patients were found to have leukemic cells in the CSF at diagnosis and an additional 36% developed positive CSF cytology during the course of their disease.

The most frequent signs and symptoms of extramedullary leukemia masses (chloromas) or infiltrates are pain, soft tissue swelling, proptosis (GOLDBERG et al. 1982), gum hypertrophy, cranial nerve palsies. upper airway obstruction and superior vena cava syndrome. The most common sites of involvement are bones, soft tissues (eyes), and CNS. Less frequent sites are testicles, lymph nodes (including the mediastinum), pelvis, pleura, spleen, liver, and skin.

Radiation therapy has been widely used for the treatment of symptomatic leukemic lesions or chloromas (FOON and GALE 1982; WIERNIK and SERPICK 1970; TAKAUE et al. 1986). In a retrospective review of the Stanford experience with irradiation of extramedullary ANLL lesions (including 23 cases of granulocytic sarcoma), CHAK and co-authors (1983) showed that the complete response rate increased with the total dose of radiation (Table 7.3). Based on these results, the authors suggested tumor doses of 30 Gy in 15 fractions over 3 weeks in the treatment of sympomatic infiltrates secondary to leukemic lesions. Furthermore, since their highest response rate (with doses of $\geq$ 30 Gy) was 89% ±10%, they argued that for sites in which "a complete clinical response is desired, even higher doses of irradiation should be used." These doses are generally higher than those recommended for extramedullary sites of ALL involvement (SULLIVAN 1980) and suggest that nonlymphocytic leukemic cells may be less radioresponsive than their lymphocytic counterparts. Finally, superficial electron beam radiotherapy has been used in the treatment of diffuse skin

Table 7.3. Correlation between radiation dose and response in extramedullary leukemia (adapted from CHAK et al. 1983)

Total dose (Gy)	Total no. of courses	Response		
		CR[a](%)	PR[a]	NR
<10	17	3 (18%)	11	3
10–19.99	21	9 (43%)	11	1
20–29.99	7	6 (86%)	1	0
≥ 30	9	8 (89%)	1	0

CR, complete response; PR, partial response; NR, no response
[a] The difference in response rates to these dose ranges was statistically significant ($P = 0.003$)

involvement (leukemia cutis); total skin doses of 13–16.5 Gy have been used with partial success (MORRIS 1982).

7.8 Complications of Treatment

7.8.1 Complications Due to CNS Irradiation

Since information about late toxicities from CNS irradiation is generally more readily available from children with ALL and since the treatment philosophy for overt CNS leukemia or CNS prophylaxis is essentially the same for both types of leukemia, the information presented in this chapter about toxicities of CNS treatment has been extrapolated from the ALL literature.

At least three types of histologic changes have been reported in the brains of children with leukemia after CNS therapy: subacute leukoencephalopathy, mineralizing microangiopathy, and cortical atrophy. Radiographically, calcifications in the basal ganglia and at the gray-white matter junctions can be seen on CT scans. Furthermore, neuroendocrine and long-term cognitive dysfunction is induced by prophylactic CNS treatment (OCHS 1988).

Although differences in neuropsychological performance tests between children who received and those who did not receive prophylactic cranial irradiation (CRT) have not always been apparent among the general population of ALL survivors (OCHS et al. 1991; MULHERN et al. 1991), an increase in the incidence of neuropsychological deficits has been reported in very young children who received ≥ 18 Gy CRT (MULHERN et al. 1992). A recent study from St. Jude Children's Research Hospital compared the neuropsychological status of 26 long-term survivors of ALL who were diagnosed within the first 24 months of life (and received CRT) with the functional status of a matched group of Wilms' tumor patients who did not receive CRT. As a group, children with ALL treated with CRT [and intrathecal methotrexate (IT MTX) with or without hydrocortisone and Ara-C] did not differ significantly from the Wilms' tumor patients on measures of global functional status. However, on neuropsychological testing, children treated for ALL scored significantly lower than children with Wilms' tumor. More specifically, children with ALL had lower mean intelligent quotient (IQ) scores, performed less adequately on four of six measures of visual and auditory memory, and had lower scores in computational mathematics. Furthermore, a significant inverse correlation was found between total CRT dose and IQ, and significantly lower IQ scores were reported in children with calcification of the basal ganglia or of gray/white matter junctions on CT scans.

This CRT dose-adverse effect relationship has also been evaluated in a retrospective study from the University of California San Francisco (MOORE et al. 1991). Children receiving 24 Gy on the average scored 10 points lower than children who received 18 Gy in full-scale IQ and reading, spelling, or arithmetic achievement tests. All these children had received at least two cycles of IT MTX during remission induction and two to four cycles during the CNS prophylaxis. These findings suggest that the CNS of very young children is more vulnerable to adverse physiologic effects from CRT (in combination with IT MTX) than is the CNS of older children. However, the relative contribution of IT MTX vs CRT to the development of cognitive dysfunctions remains an area of controversy. For example, a study conducted on two groups of children with ALL who had received either CRT (24 Gy) with IT MTX (six doses) or IT Ara-C and IT MTX (ten doses) showed no difference in IQ, memory, learning, attention, and frontal tasks between the two groups (GIRALT et al. 1992). Both groups, however, scored approximately 10 points lower in mean IQ when compared to siblings or children with solid tumors. Similarly, a study from St. Jude (MULHERN et al. 1988) comparing children who had received CNS prophylaxis with either 18 Gy plus IT MTX or IT MTX plus high-dose intravenous (IV) MTX showed no treatment- or age-related differences on 16 standardized memory tests. However, as a group, patients who had received CNS therapy scored lower than age-corrected norms in verbal and visual-spatial memory abilities. These authors concluded that the long-term neuropsychological sequelae in ALL survivors treated with CNS therapy may be attributable to a common factor such as the presence of leukemic cells in the CNS or treatment with IV and IT MTX. Therefore, in evaluating neurotoxicity following successful leukemic treatment, it is important to consider systemic therapy in addition to CNS specific treatment.

A recent study from the Dana Farber Cancer Institute has disclosed a sex-dependent association between high-dose IV MTX and lower IQ scores in 51 long-term leukemia survivors who also received prophylactic CNS treatment with 18 or 28 Gy and IT MTX (WABER et al. 1992). In addition to CNS-specific treatment, these patients were randomized to receive IV MTX either as a low dose of 40 mg/m^2 or as a high dose of 4–33 g/m^2. Fifty percent of the girls versus 14% of the boys exhibited a low IQ score (IQ < 90, $P = 0.01$); furthermore, 80% of the girls who received high-dose IV MTX had low IQ scores compared to 25% in the low-dose IV MTX group ($P = 0.03$). This study documents that a single high dose of IV MTX during remission induction was associated with significant neurotoxicity and reinforces the view that systemic therapy, in addition to intrathecal chemotherapy and CRT, needs to be considered when evaluating the cognitive sequelae of CNS treatment.

A more ominous late sequela is the induction of brain tumors. A recent study describes three patients who developed supratentorial malignant brain tumors with histologic and immunohistochemical features of primitive neuroectodermal tumors. These tumors developed 7–9 years after prophylactic CNS treatment with CRT (18–24 Gy) and IT MTX (BRÜSTLE et al. 1992). Other secondary primary malignant tumors occurring in patients after CNS therapy are gliomas, meningiomas, and sarcomas (SHAPIRO et al. 1989). Whether children with lymphoid malignancies have a genetic predisposition to develop brain tumors and the exact etiologic roles of CRT and IT MTX in inducing these rare complications are a matter of speculation.

7.8.2 Toxicities Due to Total Body Irradiation

As in the case of CNS toxicities, much of the information regarding TBI-associated complications has been derived from childhood ALL and/or from the adult leukemia experience. Since the techniques and parameters of TBI used for the treatment of ANLL are similar to those used for ALL, we feel that the information derived from the latter clinical experience is applicable to children with the former condition.

The use of TBI in conjunction with high-dose chemotherapy as a conditioning regimen for BMT can be associated with acute, short-lived side-effects as well as with late, severe complications. Among the acute toxicities the most common are nausea and vomiting, mucositis, diarrhea, parotiditis, abdominal pain, and skin rashes. These side-effects resolve within hours to days with conservative medical management. In general, fractionated TBI appears to cause fewer acute side-effects than single-dose TBI (LATINI et al. 1992), though no statistically significant differences have been reported between the two regimens at institutions where both approaches have been used (OZSAHIN et al. 1992).

The late toxicities associated with the use of TBI have a more indolent course but can lead to significant morbidity and mortality. Interstitial pneumonitis (IP) is the most common of the late toxicities observed among BMT recipients. Approximately 10%–50% of transplanted patients will develop IP and the mortality of patients with this complication ranges from 20% to 80%. Infectious etiologies (especially cytomegalovirus) account for about 50%–60% of the cases of IP. In the other 40%–50% no cause can be found; these cases are classified as idiopathic IP (IIP) and are thought to be related to the use of TBI. The exact role of radiation in the pathogenesis of IIP is not well understood. Nevertheless, IIP occurring in the setting of BMT has clinical and pathophysiologic features similar to those encountered in localized radiation-induced pneumonitis occurring in routine clinical practice (KEANE et al. 1981; PINO-Y-TORRES et al. 1981). The total dose of radiation, the dose rate, and the fractionation are thought to contribute, in a multifactorial way with chemo-therapy and GVDH, to the development of IIP. Data from hemibody and total body irradiation have shown that even a 5% change in the lung dose can result in a 20% increase in IIP (VAN DYK et al. 1981). Therefore, much effort has been devoted to the accurate measurement of the radiation dose delivered to the lungs through the use of high-energy photon beams. Lower lung doses (relative to unit density tissues) can be achieved with high energy beams (EL-KHATIB et al. 1992). Dose rate is another factor thought to play a role in the development of IIP. Although several uncontrolled studies have indicated a greater lung tolerance at low dose rates (BARRETT et al. 1983; KIM et al. 1985; RINDGEN et al. 1983; TRAVIS et al. 1985; WEINER et al. 1986), a recent randomized study of low- vs high-dose-rate TBI failed to show any difference in the incidence of IIP (OZSAHIN et al. 1992). In a subgroup of allogeneic BMT, however, patients with GVHD had a significantly higher incidence of IP (54%) compared to those patients who did not develop a graft reaction (21%) (Ozsahin et al. 1992), suggesting that immunologic processes are also involved in the development of this severe complication. With regard to fractionation, some retrospective studies have shown that fractionated or hyperfractionated TBI is associated with a lower incidence of IP than single-dose TBI (Cosset et al. 1989; Shank et al. 1983). In the study from the Institute Gustave Roussy, an IP incidence of 13% was noted in the fractionated TBI group vs 45% for the single-dose group (Cosset et al. 1989). However, several other studies have failed to show a statistically significant difference in the incidence of IP between single-dose and fractionated TBI (Ozsahin et al. 1992; Deeg et al. 1986; Thomas et al. 1982).

Veno-occlusive disease (VOD) of the liver is another major complication of BMT, accounting for 5%–10% of deaths following transplantation. The role of radiation in the pathogenesis of this complication is not clearly established since the same clinico-pathologic syndrome can be seen in the absence of TBI. Pathophysiologically the development of VOD is manifested by marked enlargement and congestion of the liver. Microscopically, there is marked congestion of the central portion of the lobule and narrowing of the central vein with the appearance of entrapped erythrocytes and the formation of fibrin deposits. The diagnosis, however, is made on clinical grounds based on the presence of right upper quadrant pain, jaundice, and weight gain. Signs of VOD include hepatomegaly, ascites, and encephalopathy. Laboratory studies show elevated levels of bilirubin, alkaline phosphatase, and SGOT (McDonald et al. 1984). VOD carries a mortality of 30%–50%. Some authors have reported a lower incidence of VOD at a low dose rate (< 67cGy/min) both in experimental animals (Travis et al. 1985) and in retrospective clinical studies (Barrett 1982). These findings, however, were not reproduced in a randomized trial (Ozsahin et al. 1992). The effect of single-dose versus fractionated TBI on the incidence of VOD is also a matter of controversy, with some authors suggesting an increased incidence with single-dose regimens (Cosset et al. 1989; Deeg et al. 1986) and others showing no difference (McDonald et al. 1984; Ozsahin et al. 1992).

Renal toxicity has also been reported in 16 of 39 children with ALL or neuroblastoma who had undergone BMT. Nine of 28 children with ALL developed this complication (Guinan et al. 1988). They had received 12–14 Gy of TBI (in 6–8 fractions at 9–11 cGy/min) with chemotherapy consisting of VM-26, Ara-C, and cyclophosphamide. In addition, 7 of 11 children with neuroblastoma were affected by this complication as well. Their conditioning regimen had included the same TBI and intensive chemotherapy with cisplatin, VM-26, melphalan, and cyclophosphamide. Biopsies performed on two patients were consistent with radiation nephropathy. The median time for development of this complication was 5 months. The relative contribution of irradiation and chemotherapy for the development of renal toxicity is a subject for speculation (Tarbell et al. 1988). Nevertheless, tubular degeneration and depletion were noted in experimental animals that received only TBI. These histologic changes were late effects and demonstrated a dose-rate dependence (Travis et al. 1985).

Finally, cataract formation in the crystalline lens of the eye is also a known sequela of TBI, occurring months to years following exposure to ionizing radiation. The estimated incidence of this late event has been reported to be a function of fractionation of TBI (80% for the single-dose group vs 19% for the fractionated group; $P < 0.00005$) (Deeg et al. 1984). The incidence of cataract formation was also estimated to be higher (77% vs 33%) in patients who received high-dose-rate TBI than in those who received low-dose-rate TBI (Ozsahin et al. 1992).

7.9 Conclusion

Major advances have been made over the last two decades in the treatment of children with ANLL. Complete remissions can be achieved in 70%–80% of these patients, and long-term disease-free survival of 40%–50% has been reported. Recently published data indicate improved survival rates with BMT, though selection biases may account for some of these improvements. For children with ANLL in first or second remission, the 5-year disease-free estimates were 66% and 75%, respectively, with BMT after preparation with 13.2 Gy of hyperfractionated TBI and high-dose cyclophosphamide (Brochstein et al. 1987). Radiation therapy may play an important role in achieving sustained remission rates; a primary role may be in the delivery of CNS therapy for occult or overt CNS leukemia either alone or in conjunction with intrathecal chemotherapy. Another important contribution of radiation therapy is in preparation for BMT. Finally, radiation therapy is highly effective in the palliation of symptoms or dysfunction due to diffuse leukemic infiltration or to the presence of chloromas. CNS irradiation may assume an even greater role in the prevention of CNS relapses as remissions become more durable and as the rate of remission induction increases with new therapies.

Reference

Aurer I, Gale RP (1991) Are new conditioning regimens for transplants in acute myelogenous leukemia better? Bone Marrow Transplant 7: 255–261

Baehner RL, Kennedy A, Sather H et al. (1981) Characteristics of children with acute non-lymphocytic leukemia in long-term continuous remission: a report from Children's Cancer Study Group. Med Pediatr Oncol 9: 393–403

Ball ED, Fanger MW (1983) The expression of myeloid-specific antigens on myeloid leukemia cells: correlations with leukemia subclasses and implications for normal myeloid differentiation. Blood 61: 456–463

Barrett A (1982) Total body irradiation (TBI) before bone marrow transplantation in leukemia: a co-operative study from the European Group for Bone Marrow Transplantation. Br J Radiol 55: 562–567

Barrett A, Depledge MH, Powles RL (1983) Interstitial pneumonitis following bone marrow transplantation after low dose rate total body irradiation. Int J Radiat Oncol Biol Phys 9: 1029–1033

Bennett JM, Catovsky D, Daniel MT et al. (1976) Proposals for the classification of the acute leukemias. Br J Haematol 33: 451–458

Bennett JM, Catovsky D, Daniel MT et al. (1985a) Proposed revised criteria for the classification of acute myeloid leukemia. Ann Intern Med 103: 620–625

Bennett JM, Catovsky D, Daniel MT et al. (1985b) Criteria for the diagnosis of acute leukemia of megakaryocyte lineage (M7). A report of the French-American-British cooperative group. Ann Intern Med 103: 460–462

Bernstein R, Macdougall LG, Pinto MR (1984) Chromosome patterns in 26 South African children with acute nonlymphocytic leukemia. Cancer Genet Cytogenet 11: 199–214

Blayney DW, Longo DL, Young RC et al. (1987) Decreasing risk of leukemia with prolonged follow-up after chemotherapy and radiotherapy for Hodgkin's disease. N Engl J Med 316: 710–714

Bos LJ (1990) ras gene mutations and human cancer. In: Cossman J (ed) Molecular genetics in cancer diagnosis. Elsevier, New York, pp 272–287

Bostrom B, Brunning RD, McGlave P et al. (1985) Bone marrow transplantation for acute nonlymphocytic leukemia in first remission. Analysis of prognostic factors. Blood 65: 1191–1196

Brochstein J, Kernan N, Groshen S et al. (1987) Allogeneic bone marrow transplantation after hyperfractionated total-body irradiation and cyclophosphamide in children with acute leukemia. N Engl J Med 317: 1618–1624

Brüstle O, Ohgaki H, Schmitt H, Walter G, Ostertag H, Kleihues P (1992) Primitive neuroectodermal tumors after prophylactic central nervous system irradiation in children. Cancer 69: 2385–2392

Buck B, Diddon R, Svensson G (1984) A beam alignment device for matching fields. Int J Radiat Oncol Biol Phys 11: 1039–1043

Buckley J, Chard R, Baehner R, Nesbit M, Lampkin B, Woods W, Hammond GD (1989) Improvement in outcome of children with acute nonlymphocytic leukemia. Cancer 63: 1457–1464

Bunin NJ, Pui C-H (1985) Differing complications of hyperleukocytosis in children with acute lymphoblastic or acute nonlymphoblastic leukemia. J Clin Oncol 3: 1590–1595

Chak L, Sapozink M, Cox R (1983) Extramedullary lesions in non-lymphocytic leukemia: results of radiation therapy. J Radiat Oncol Biol Phys 9: 1173–1176

Champlin R, Gale RP (1987) Acute myelogenous leukemia: recent advances in therapy. Blood 69: 1551–1562

Chan LC, Pegram SM, Greaves MF (1985) Contribution of immunophenotype to the classification and differential diagnosis of acute leukaemia. Lancet I: 475–479

Chessels JM, Callaghan UO, Hardisty RM (1986) Acute myeloid leukaemia in childhood: clinical features and prognosis. Br J Haematol 63: 555–564

Choi S-I, Simone JV (1976) Acute nonlymphocytic leukemia in 171 children. Med Pediatr Oncol 2: 119–146

Clift R, Buckner CD, Appelbaum F (1990) Allogeneic marrow transplantation in patients with acute myeloid leukemia in first remission: a randomized trial of two irradiation regimens. Blood 76: 1867–1871

Cosset JM, Baume D, Pico JL et al. (1989) Single dose versus hyperfractionated total body irradiation before allogeneic bone marrow transplantation: a non-randomized comparative study of 54 patients at the Institut Gustave Roussy. Radiother Oncol 15: 151–160

Creutzig U, Ritter J, Riehm H et al. (1985) Improved treatment results in childhood acute myelogenous leukemia: a report of the German cooperative study AML-BFM-78. Blood 65: 298–304

Cuttner J, Holland JF, Norton L et al. (1983) Therapeutic leukapheresis for hyperleukocytosis in acute myelocytic leukemia. Med Pediatr Oncol 11: 76

Dahl GV, Simone J, Hustu O, Mason C (1978) Preventive central nervous system irradiation in children with acute nonlymphocytic leukemia. Cancer 42: 2187–2192

Dahl GV, Kalwinsky DS, Murphy S et al. (1982) Cytokinetically based induction chemotherapy and splenectomy for childhood acute nonlymphocytic leukemia. Blood 60: 856–863

Dearth JC, Fountain KS, Smithson WA et al. (1978) Extreme leukemic leukocytosis (blast crisis) in childhood. Mayo Clin Proc 53: 207–211

Deeg HJ, Flournoy N, Sullivan KM et al. (1984) Cataracts after total body irradiation and marrow transplantation: a sparing effect of dose fractionation. Int J Radiat Oncol Biol Phys 10: 957–964

Deeg HJ, Sullivan KM, Buckner CD et al. (1986) Marrow transplantation for acute nonlymphoblastic leukemia in first remission: toxicity and long-term follow-up of patients conditioned with single dose or fractionated total body irradiation. Bone Marrow Transplant 1: 151–157

El-Khatib E, Connors S, Logus W (1992) The influence of lung and bone dosimetry on the choice of radiation energy for total body irradiation. Int J Radiat Oncol Biol Phys 23: 1051–1057

Fearon ER, Burke PJ, Schiffer CA et al. (1986) Differentiation of leukemia cells in polymorphonuclear leukocytes in patients with acute nonlymphocytic leukemia. N Engl J Med 315: 15–24

Fialkow PJ, Singer JW, Adamson JW et al. (1979) Acute nonlymphocytic leukemia: expression in cells restricted to granulocytic and monocytic differentiation. N Engl J Med 301: 1–5

Fialkow PJ, Singer JW, Adamson JW et al. (1981) Acute nonlymphocytic leukemia: heterogencity of stem cell origin. Blood 57: 1068–1073

Foon KA, Gale RP (1982) Controversies in the therapy of acute myelogenous leukemia Am J Med 72: 963–978

Foon KA, Todd RF III (1986) Immunologic classification of leukemia and lymphoma. Blood 68: 1–31

Fyles G, Messner H, Lockwood et al. (1991) Long-term results of bone marrow transplantation for patients with AML, ALL and CML prepared with single dose total body irradiation of 500 cGy delivered with a high dose rate. Bone Marrow Transplant 8: 453–463

Giralt J, Ortega J, Olive T et al. (1992) Long-term neuropsychologic sequelae of childhood leukemia: comparison of two CNS prophylactic regimens. Int J Radiat Oncol Biol Phys 24: 49–53

Goldberg L, Tao A, Romano P (1982) Severe exophthalmos secondary to orbital myopathy not due to Graves's disease. Br J Ophthamol 66: 392–395

Grier H, Weinstein H (1989) Nonlymphocytic Leukemia. In: Pizzo P, Poplack D (ed) Principles and practice of pediatric oncology. J. B. Lippincott, Philadelphia, pp 367–382

Grier H, Gelber R, Camitta et al. (1987) Prognostic factors in childhood acute myelogenous leukemia. J Clin Oncol 5: 1026–1032

Grier H, Gelber R, Link M et al. (1992) Intensive sequential chemotherapy for children with acute myelogenous leukemia: VAPA, 80–035, and HI-C-Daze. Leukemia 6: 48–51

Griffin JD, Ritz J, Nadler LM et al. (1981) Expression of myeloid differentiation antigens on normal and malignant myeloid cells. J Clin Invest 68: 932–941

Griffin JD, Davis R, Nelson DA et al. (1986) Use of surface marker analysis to predict outcome of adult acute myeloblastic leukemia. Blood 68: 1232–1241

Grund FM, Armitage JO, Burns CP (1977) Hydroxyurea in the prevention of the effects of leukostasis in acute leukemia. Arch Intern Med 137: 1246–1249

Guinan E, Tarbell N, Niemeyer C et al. (1988) Intravascular hemolysis and renal insufficiency after bone marrow transplantation. Blood 72: 451–455

Herve P, Labopin M, Plouvier E et al. (1991) Autologous bone marrow transplantation for childhood acute myeloid leukemia-A European survey. Bone Marrow Transplant 8: 76–79

Hurwitz C, Krance R, Schell M et al. (1992) Current strategies for treatment of acute myeloid leukemia at St. Jude Children's Research Hospital, Leukemia 6: 39–43

Jacobson RJ, Temple MJ, Singer JW et al. (1984) A clonal complete remission in a patient with acute nonlymphocytic leukemia originating in a multipotent stem cell. N Engl J Med 310: 1513–1517

Kaneko Y, Rowley JD, Maurer HS et al. (1982) Chromosome pattern in childhood acute nonlymphocytic leukemia. Blood 60: 389–399

Kay H (1976) Development of CNS leukaemia in acute myeloid leukaemia in childhood. Arch Dis Child 51: 73–74

Keane TJ, Van Dyk J, Rider WD (1981) Idiopathic interstitial pneumonia following bone marrow transplantation: the relationship with total body irradiation. Int J Radiat Oncol Bio Phys 7: 1365–1370

Kim TH, Rybka WB, Lehnert S et al. (1985) Interstitial pneumonitis following total body irradiation for bone marrow transplantation using two different dose rates. Int J Radiat Oncol Biol Phys 11: 1285–1291

Lampkin BC, Woods W, Strauss R et al. (1983) Current status of the biology and treatment of acute non-lymphocytic leukemia in children (Report from the ANLL Strategy Group of the Children's Cancer Study Group). Blood 61: 215–218

Larson RA, Kondo K, Vardiman JW et al. (1984) Evidence for a 15; 17 translocation in every patient with acute promyelocytic leukemia. Am J Med 76: 827–841

Latini P, Aristei C, Aversa F et al. (1992) Interstitial pneumonitis after hyperfractionated total body irradiation in HLA-matched T-depleted bone marrow transplantation. Int J Radiat Oncol Biol Phys 23: 401–405

Li FP, Bader JL (1987) Epidemiology of cancer in childhood In:Nathan DG, Oski FA (eds) Hematology of infancy and childhood, vol 2. W.B. Saunders, Philadelphia, pp 908–937

Lichtman MA, Rowe JM (1982) Hyperleukocytic leukemias: rheological, clinical and therapeutic considerations. Blood 60: 279–293

Linch DC, Burnett AK (1986) Clonal studies of ABMT in acute myeloid leukemia. Clin Haematol 15: 167–186

Mayer RJ, Weinstein HJ, Carol FS et al. (1982) The role of intensive postinduction chemotherapy in the management of patients with acute myelogenous leukemia. Cancer Treat Rep 6: 1455–1462

McDonald GB, Sharma P, Matthews DE et al. (1984) Venoocclusive disease of the liver after bone marrow transplantation: diagnosis, incidence and predisposing factors. Hepatology 4: 116–122.

Moore I, Kramer J, Wara W et al. (1991) Cognitive function in children with leukemia. Cancer 68: 1913–1917

Morris TCM, Vincent P, Foster K, Johnson N, Thompson I (1982) Treatment of widespread skin infiltration in acute myeloblastic leukaemia with superficial penetrating whole body electron beam therapy. Eur J Cancer Clin Oncol 18: 321–324

Mulhern R, Wasserman A, Fairclough D, Ochs J (1988) Memory function in disease-free survivors of childhood acute lymphocytic leukemia given CNS prophylaxis with or without 1,800 cGy cranial irradiation. J Clin Oncol 6: 315–320

Mulhern R, Fairclough D, Ochs J (1991) A prospective comparison of neuropsychologic performance of children surviving leukemia who received 18-Gy, 24-Gy, or no cranial irradiation. J Clin Oncol 9: 1348–1356

Mulhern R, Kovnar E, Langston J et al. (1992) Long-term survivors of leukemia treated in infancy: factors associated with neuropsychologic status. J Clin Oncol 10: 1095–1102

Nesbit M, Buckley J, Lampkin B et al. (1987) Comparison of allogeneic bone marrow transplantation (BMT) with maintenance chemotherapy in previously untreated childhood acute nonlymphocytic leukemia (ANLL) (Abstract) Proc Am Soc Clin Oncol 6: 163–164

Ochs J (1988) Neurotoxicity due to central nervous system therapy for childhood leukemia. Am J Pediatr Hematol Oncol 11: 93–105

Ochs J, Mulhern R, Fairclough D et al. (1991) Comparison of neuropsychologic functioning and clinical indicators of neurotoxicity in long-term survivors of childhood leukemia given cranial radiation or parenteral methotrexate: a prospective study. J Clin Oncol 9: 145–151

Ozsahin M, Pene F, Touboul E et al. (1992) Total-body irradiation before bone marrow transplantation. Cancer 69: 2853–2865

Pedersen-Bjergaard J, Philip P, Mortensen BT et al. (1981) Acute nonlymphocytic leukemia, preleukemia, and acute myeloproliferative syndrome secondary to treatment of other malignant disease. Clinical and cytogenetic characteristics and results of in vitro culture of bone marrow and HLA typing. Blood 57: 712–723

Pino-y-Torres JL, Bross DS, Lam WL et al. (1981) Risk factors in interstitial pneumonitis following allogeneic bone marrow transplantation. Int J Radiat Oncol Biol Phys 8: 1301–1307

Pui CH, Dahl G, Kalwinsky D et al. (1985) Central nervous system leukemia in children with acute nonlymphoblastic leukemia. Blood 66: 1062–1067

Rindgen O, Baryd I, Johansson B et al. (1983) Increased mortality by septicemia, interstitial pneumonitis and pulmonary fibrosis among bone marrow transplant recipients receiving an increased mean dose rate of total irradiation. Acta Radiol Oncol 22: 423–428

Rinsky RA, Smith AB, Hornung R et al. (1987) Benzene and leukemia: an epidemiologic risk assessment. N Engl J Med 316: 1044–1050

Ritter J, Creutzig U, Schellong G (1992) Treatment results of three consecutive German childhood AML trials: BFM-78, -83, and -87. Leukemia 6: 59–62

Rosner F, Lee SL (1972) Down's syndrome and acute leukemia: myeloblastic or lymphoblastic? Am J Med 53: 203–218

Rovelli A, Biondi A, Rajnoldi A et al. (1992) Microgranular variant of acute promyelocytic leukemia in children. J Clin Oncol 9: 1413–1419

Sanders J, Thomas ED, Buckner CD et al. (1985) Marrow transplantation for children in first remission of acute nonlymphoblastic leukemia: an update. Blood 66: 460–462

Santos GW, Tutschka PJ, Brookmeyer R et al. (1983) Marrow transplantation for acute nonlymphocytic leukemia after treatment with busulfan and cyclophosphamide. N Engl J Med 309: 1347–1352

Schiffer CA, Lee EJ, Toniyasu T et al. (1989) Prognostic impact of cytogenetic abnormalities in patients with de novo acute nonlymphocytic leukemia. Blood 73: 263–270

Schull W, Weiss K (1992) Radiation carcinogenesis in humans. In: Nygaard OF, Sinclair WK, Lett JT (eds) Effects of low dose and low dose rate radiation, vol 16. Academic, San Diego, pp 215–258

Shank B, Chu FCH, Dinsmore R et al. (1983) Hyperfractionated total body irradiation for bone marrow transplanation: results in seventy leukemia patients with allogeneic transplants. Int J Radiat Oncol Biol Phys 9: 1607–1611

Shapiro S, Mealy J, Sartorius C (1989) Radiation-induced intracranial malignant gliomas. J Neurosurg 71: 77–82

Sullivan MP, Perez CA, Herson J et al. (1980) Radiotherapy (2500 rad) for testicular leukemia: local control and subsequent clinical events: a Southwest Oncology Group Study. Cancer 46: 508–515

Takaue Y, Culbert S, Van Eys J et al. (1986) Spontaneous cure of end-stage acute nonlymphocytic leukemia complicated with chloroma (granulocytic sarcoma). Cancer 58: 1101–1105

Tarbell N, Guinan E, Niemeyer C et al. (1988) Late onset of renal dysfunction in survivors of bone marrow transplantation. Int J Radiat Oncol Biol Phys 15: 99–104

Thomas E (1983) Marrow transplantation for malignant diseases. J Clin Oncol 9: 517–531

Thomas ED, Clift RA, Hersman J et al. (1982) Marrow transplantation for acute nonlymphoblastic leukemia in first remission using fractionated or single-dose irradiation. Int J Radiat Oncol Biol Phys 8: 817–821

Travis EL, Peters LJ, McNeill J et al. (1965) Effect of dose-rate on total body irradiation: lethality and pathologic findings. Radiother Oncol 4: 341–351.

van der Reijden HJ, van Rhenen DJ, Lansdorp PM et al. (1983) A comparison of the surface marker analysis and FAB classification in acute myeloid leukemia. Blood 61: 443–448

Van Dyk J, Keane T, Kan S, Rider WD, Fryer CJH (1981) Radiation pneumonitis following large single dose irradiation: a reevaluation based on absolute dose to lung. Int J Radiat Oncol Biol Phys 7: 461–467

Waber D, Tarbell N, Kahn C, Gelber R, Sallan S (1992) The relationship of sex and treatment modality to neuropsychologic outcome in childhood acute lymphoblastic leukemia. J Clin Oncol 10: 810–817

Weiner RS, Bortin MM, Gale RP et al. (1986) Interstitial pneumonitis after bone marrow transplantation. Assessment of risk factors. Ann Intern Med 104: 168–175

Weinstein HJ, Mayer RJ, Rosenthal DS et al. (1983) Chemotherapy for acute myelogenous leukemia in children and adults: VAPA update. Blood 62: 315–319

Wiernik P, Serpick AA (1970) Granulocytic sarcoma (chloroma). Blood 35: 361–369

Woods WG, Nesbit ME, Buckley J et al. (1985) Correlation of chromosome abnormalities with patient characteristics, histologic subtype and induction success in children with acute nonlymphocytic leukemia. J Clin Oncol 3: 3–11

Yeager AM, Kaiser H, Santos G et al. (1986) Autologous bone marrow transplantation in patients with acute nonlymphocytic leukemia, using ex vivo marrow treated with 4-hydroperoxycyclophosphamide. N Engl J Med 315: 141–147

Yunis JJ, Bloomfield CD, Ensrud K (1981) All patients with acute nonlymphocytic leukemia may have a chromosomal defect. N Engl J Med 305: 135–139

Zwaan FE, Hermans J, Barrett AJ et al. (1984) Bone marrow transplantation for acute nonlymphoblastic leukemia: a survey of the European Group for bone marrow transplantation (E.G.B.M.T.). Br J Haematol 56: 645–653

8 Biologic and Physical Principles of Total Body Irradiation for Allogeneic and Autologous Bone Marrow Transplantation in Children with Leukemia and Lymphoma

RICHARD G. EVANS

CONTENTS

8.1 Introduction 115
8.2 Linear Quadratic Model and Biologically
    Effective Dose 116
8.3 Caveats in the Clinical Application of the
    Linear Quadratic Model to TBI 116
8.4 Comparison of TBI Regimens. 117
8.5 Dose Effect Factor and Therapeutic Gain Factor . . 117
8.6 Influence of Dose Fractionation. 118
8.7 Influence of Dose Rate. 119
8.8 Chemotherapeutic Agents and TBI 120
    References. 121

8.1 Introduction

Following Roentgen's discovery of x-rays in the twilight of the nineteenth century, only a decade or so elapsed before the birth of total body irradiation (TBI), described by Dessauer in 1907 as the "x-ray bath." In 1927, Teschendorf first described the favorable results he had achieved using TBI in the treatment of the lymphomas. Five years later, Heublein reported on a group of patients with lymphoma, Hodgkin's disease, and leukemia treated with TBI at Memorial Hospital in New York. In the 1990s, we are still struggling with the nuances of TBI and, in particular, how it is best used in conditioning regimens for bone marrow trasplantation (BMT). The relatively new art of BMT remains fraught with complex issues, and the increasing use of BMT in the leukemias and lymphomas and its emerging role in the treatment of solid tumors have led to a re-examination of the effects of various conditioning regimens, not only in terms of tumor cell kill and prevention of rejection, but also in relation to long-term organ toxicity. Prior to receiving TBI as part of their conditioning regimens for BMT, children have often been exposed to various agents such as cyclophos-

phamide and cisplatin, causing subclinical damage to such organs as kidney and lung which must be factored into considerations of long-term organ toxicity.

Several different schools of thought exist on the impact of various conditioning regimens on long-term outcome and, in particular, whether fractionated TBI has been shown unequivocally to be beneficial compared to single-dose treatment. The effectiveness of any conditioning regimen that includes TBI must be balanced against the potential side-effects, especially irreparable damage to organs such as lung and kidney. There is a paucity of information in the literature on the radiation tolerance of different organs to TBI, but it is highly likely that the tolerances are lower than when the doses are delivered to a more restricted field. When considering conditioning regimens for the lymphomas and the leukemias, it is unclear from the literature what is the proper timing for use of cyclophosphamide with TBI for optimum leukemic cell kill with the least damage to lung tissue. Although the majority of centers in the United States utilize fractionated TBI regimens (with or without partial lung shielding), many centers in Europe remain committed to single-dose TBI (at various dose rates) and employ some type of lung shielding.

Despite the addition of cyclophosphamide to single-fraction TBI in the pioneering studies in BMT to obtain a greater leukemic cell kill, it became clear that larger doses of irradiation were necessary, which led in turn to the use of fractionated regimens and/or lung shielding to avoid lung toxicity. The development of conditioning regimens has progressed to the extent that BMT (a) is now the treatment of choice for children in first remission for acute nonlymphocytic leukemia (allogeneic) or those in second remission (autologous), and leads to long-term cure in over half the patients, and (b) is a viable treatment option for children with acute lymphoblastic leukemia (ALL) in second or third remission (allogeneic or autologous), curing a third of the patients. However, the role of BMT in the treatment of

RICHARD G. EVANS, Ph.D., M.D., Professor and Chairman, Department of Radiation Oncology, University of Kansas Medical Center, 3901 Rainbow Blvd., Kansas City, KS 66103, USA

recurrent or refractory lymphomas of childhood is still under investigation.

The literature is divided regarding the extent to which clinical outcomes are dependent upon the conditioning regimens used, leading one to conclude that the issues involved in the success and toxicity of BMT are multifactorial and that the conditioning regimen per se may not necessarily play a major role in the final outcome. Despite this caveat based on the conflicting conclusions in the literature, it remains desirable, from a clinical standpoint, to have a method of comparing the effectiveness of different conditioning regimens. However, the efficacy of any regimen is a complicated issue, and factors to be considered must include (a) its value as an immunosuppressive agent, with the sentinel effect being the engraftment rate, (b) tumor cell eradication, with the sentinel effect being relapse as a function of time following the transplant, and (c) the amount of damage caused to dose-limiting tissues such as the lung and kidney, where the sentinel effects would be pneumonitis/fibrosis and nephritis, respectively. Although the literature is replete with erudite discussions regarding the importance of dose rate and fractionation of the TBI in different conditioning regimens, it is perhaps more productive to consider the differential response of the acute-reacting cells of the bone marrow (including leukemic cells) and the late-reacting tissues, particularly of the lung and the kidney, when judging and comparing different regimens. The linear quadratic model (LQM), when appropriately applied, provides a clinically useful predictor of cell kill and tissue damage following TBI, in that it is sensitive to such factors as radiation dose, fractionation, dose rate, and tissue radiosensitivity, and some of the factors in the model could be modified to account for the impact of drugs, either given in combination with TBI or to which the patient has been previously exposed.

8.2 Linear Quadratic Model and Biologically Effective Dose

The LQM is based on the assumption that there are two components of cell killing. The α component, in which killing is proportional to dose (linear), represents cell damage by a "single-hit" phenomenon and is thought to be irreparable, at least between fractions or during prolonged exposures (type A damage). The β component, on the other hand, in which killing is proportional to the square of the dose (quadratic), represents cell damage by more than one event, and some of this damage is thought to be reparable (type B damage). At a dose equal to α/β, the linear component (αD) of cell killing is equal to the quadratic component (βD^2). Survival curves of late reacting tissues, such as the kidney and lung, are "curvier" than those for acute-reacting tissues, such as bone marrow, skin, and probably tumor cells. The consequence of the difference in curviness of the survival curves for the two tissue types is that the α/β for late-reacting tissue has a low value and is more influenced by the β (quadratic) component, whereas the α/β for acute-reacting tissue has a higher value and is more influenced by the α (linear) component. The late-reacting tissues, in view of curvier survival curves and low α/β, are more susceptible to the effects of fractionation and dose rate.

The mathematical expression $SF = e^{-n(\alpha D + \beta D^2)}$ where SF is equal to surviving fraction, n = number of fractions, and D = dose – describing cell survival in terms of the LQM, can, for a single dose, be replaced by:

$$\text{Effect } (E) = \alpha D + \beta D^2 = D(\alpha + \beta D)$$

and for n fractions of d each:

$$E = n(\alpha d + \beta d^2) = nd(\alpha + \beta d)$$

where E is the number of logs to base e of cells killed and represents the effect of a total dose $D = nd$ (Gy) on a tissue having a given α/β (Gy), where d is the size of the dose fraction also in Gy. In order to introduce the ratio α/β, we could divide through by β as recommended by THAMES and HENDRY (1987), but the result is in units of dose squared. An alternate, and possibly more convenient, method is to divide through by α, when the result is the *biologically effective dose* (BED) (BARENDSEN 1982; FOWLER 1989):

$$\text{BED} = \frac{E}{\alpha} = nd\left(1 + \frac{d}{\alpha/\beta}\right)$$

The factor in parentheses [$1 + d/(\alpha/\beta)$] has been referred to as the *relative effectiveness* (RE) (BARENDSEN 1982).

Late-reacting tissues such as lung and kidney tend to have low α/β values, of the order of 2–3 Gy, whereas acute-reacting tissues such as bone marrow and tumor cells tent to have α/β values of the order of 10 Gy.

8.3 Caveats in the Clinical Application of the Linear Quadratic Model to TBI

We have chosen for simplicity to use one α/β for each late-reacting tissue, although it is entirely possible in the case of lung, for example, that pneumonitis and fibrosis may involve different target cells and have somewhat different α/β values (VAN DYK et al. 1989). We did not consider dose inhomogeneity in the lung in the model, although we are aware that children are different from adults. For the kidney, where damage in children may be described as nephritis, we have chosen one α/β value. Finally, we chose one value to calculate bone marrow damage, i.e., we assumed the same radiosensitivity for normal and leukemic cells, although we know this not to be strictly true (KIMLER et al. 1985). Due to the lack of human data on repair half-times ($T_{1/2}$), we have chosen to use values based mainly on animal data, fully appreciating that values may be significantly longer in humans. For lung, we chosen a $T_{1/2}$ of 1.5 h and for kidney, a $T_{1/2}$ of 2 h. Finally, we would like to enumerate eight factors that impact on organ and tumor cell sensitivity to TBI and chemotherapy. The first three factors are notable in that clinicians have little or no control over them, namely, age of the patients, repair half-times of different tissues, and exposure to agents such as cyclophosphamide concurrent with TBI (lung damage) or any prior exposure to other nephrotoxic agents. The factors over which clinicians *do* have some control are total dose, radiation fraction size, number of fractions, time between fractions, and dose rate.

Bearing all these caveats and factors in mind, we feel it is still clinically useful to compare various TBI regimens using the LQM, and in the next several paragraphs it will be illustrated how the model can be used to develop a therapeutic gain factor.

8.4 Comparison of TBI Regimens

To demonstrate the application of the LQM, we have chosen to contrast two different TBI regimens employed at a large institution in Italy where, from 1981 to 1983, patients with ALL were treated with a TBI regimen of 3.3 Gy per day for 3 days to a total dose of 9.9 Gy and, from 1983 to 1988, with a hyperfractionated regimen using six fractions of 2 Gy 6 h apart over 3 days for a total dose of 12 Gy (cyclophosphamide was given for 2 days prior to each TBI regimen). Of interest is that the overall survival in these children with ALL was 60% for the hyperfractionated TBI versus 23% for the daily fraction treatment (CORVO et al. 1989). Assuming an α/β value of 10 Gy for normal or leukemic cells in the bone marrow (BM) and a value of 3 Gy for the critical cells of the lung (leading to pneumonitis or fibrosis), let *regimen I* be the hyperfractionated TBI of 12

Gy (D) in 2-Gy fractions, 6 h apart each day over 3 days, and let *regimen II* be three daily TBI fractions of 3.3 Gy each (d): $D = nd = 9.9$ Gy. Although we realize that some degree of lung shielding was used in each regimen, we have chosen not to incorporate this in the LQM, as we are simply using the two TBI regimens for demonstrative purposes only.

Let us consider the effects of these regimens, first on the bone marrow and then on the lung.

Assuming $\alpha/\beta = 10$ Gy for bone marrow:

Regimen I:

$$\text{BED}_{\text{BM}} = E_{\text{BM}} + nd\left(1 + \frac{d}{\alpha/\beta}\right)$$

$$= 12\text{Gy}\left(1 + \frac{2\text{Gy}}{10\text{Gy}}\right) = 14.4\text{Gy}_{10}$$

where the subscript 10 denotes that an α/β of 10 Gy was used.

Regimen II:

$$\text{BED}_{\text{BM}} = 9.9 \text{ Gy}\left(1 + \frac{3.3 \text{ Gy}}{10 \text{ Gy}}\right) = 13.2 \text{ Gy}_{10},$$

i.e., one would predict 9% more BED to the bone marrow from regimen I.

Turning to the lung (L), and assuming $\alpha/\beta = 3$ for lung:

$$\text{BED}_{\text{L}} = nd\left(1 + \frac{d}{\alpha/\beta}\right)$$

Regimen I:

$$\text{BED}_{\text{L}} = 12 \text{ Gy}\left(1 + \frac{2\text{Gy}}{10\text{Gy}}\right) = 20 \text{ Gy}_3$$

Regimen II:

$$\text{BED}_{\text{L}} = 9.9 \text{ Gy}\left(1 + \frac{3.3 \text{ Gy}}{3 \text{ Gy}}\right) = 20.8 \text{ Gy}_3,$$

resulting in 4% less BED to the lung from regimen I.

8.5 Dose Effect Factor and Therapeutic Gain Factor

If we consider hyperfractionated TBI (regimen I) to be the "standard" treatment, then a *dose effect factor* (DEF) can be defined for bone marrow as:

$$\text{DEF}_{\text{BM}} = \frac{\text{BED}_{\text{BM}}(\text{regimen I})}{\text{BED}_{\text{BM}}(\text{regimen II})}$$

$$= \frac{14.4 \text{ Gy}_{10}}{13.2 \text{ Gy}_{10}} = 1.09$$

Similarly, for lung (L):

$$\mathrm{DEF}_L = \frac{\mathrm{BED}_L(\text{regimen I})}{\mathrm{BED}_L(\text{regimen II})} = \frac{20\ \mathrm{Gy}_3}{20.8\ \mathrm{Gy}_3} = 0.96$$

If we assume one of the major dose-limiting tissues for TBI to be lung and we are trying to inflict as much bone marrow damage (including leukemic cell sterilization) with as little damage to lung as possible, then a term *therapeutic gain factor* (TGF) could be useful in comparing two TBI regimens where:

$$\mathrm{TGF} = \frac{\mathrm{DEF}_{BM}}{\mathrm{DEF}_L} = \frac{1.09}{0.96} = 1.14$$

The LQM would suggest that regimen I (hyperfractionated TBI) has an attractive TGF of 1.14 compared to regimen II (three fractions of 3.3 Gy each), which is a consequence of greater bone marrow kill and induction of less lung damage by regimen I as compared to regimen II.

Similar calculations carried out for kidney, the other major dose-limiting normal tissue, give, using $\alpha/\beta = 2$, a DEF_K of 0.92, and therefore, $\mathrm{TGF} = \mathrm{DEF}_{BM}/\mathrm{DEF}_K = 1.09/0.92 = 1.18$. The LQM would predict that regimen I has a preferable TGF of 1.18 as compared to regimen II, which is a consequence of greater kidney damage by regimen II.

If we consider bone marrow cell kill and both lung *and* kidney damage, then an overall TGF might be useful in comparing regimen I to regimen II.

$$\text{Overall TGF} = 1.14\ (\mathrm{BM} + \mathrm{L}) \times 1.18\ (\mathrm{BM} + \mathrm{K})$$
$$= 1.35$$

which would suggest that the hyperfractionated TBI regimen offer the better differential between leukemic cell kill and long-term organ toxicity.

8.6 Influence of Dose Fractionation

The above LQM formulae have not taken into account the influence of dose fractionation, i.e., time between fractions. Of note is that there were 6 h between fractions in regimen I compared to a full day in regimen II. The biologically effective dose (BED) relationship used above, $\mathrm{BED} = E/\alpha = nd[1 + d/(\alpha/\beta)]$ needs to be modified to account for differences in fractionation schemes. Repair may not be complete in the 6 h between fractions 1 and 2, 3 and 4, and 5 and 6 in regimen I, although full repair is likely in the 18 h between fractions 2 and 3, and 4 and 5. An *incomplete-repair factor* h_M (where M refers to the number of fractions/day) can be obtained from the literature

(THAMES and HENDRY 1987), provided an estimate can be made of repair half-times for the late-reacting tissues, namely, lung and kidney. The LQM equation needs to be modified to account for b.i.d. fractionation:

$$\mathrm{BED} = \frac{E}{\alpha} = nd\left(1 + \frac{d(1 + h_M)}{\alpha/\beta}\right)$$

The effect of *dose fractionation* is more significant for late-reacting tissue such as lung and kidney where the α/β is small, whereas little repair is thought to take place in clonogenic cells of the bone marrow between fractions (KIMLER et al. 1984). The relative effectiveness (RE), previously noted as $[1 + d/(\alpha/\beta)]$, has now been replaced by $[1 + d(1 + h_M)(\alpha/\beta)]$. The h_M values depend upon the tissue repair half-times ($T_{1/2}$) chosen, which have a range in animals for both lung and kidney. Values taken from the literature for $T_{1/2}$ in animals for lung fibrosis would be of the order of 1.5 h, but it is possible that these half-times may be significantly longer in humans (TURESSON and THAMES 1989; DE BOER and LEBESQUE 1988), possibly of the order of 3 h. Calculations of BED_L using the aforementioned values of $T_{1/2}$ and a range of time between fractions in hours are shown for regimen I in Table 8.1. Of note is that the increase in BED_L for a half-time for repair of 1.5 h in going from full repair to only 3 h between fractions is 10%, whereas when a $T_{1/2}$ of 3 h is chosen, which might be more representative of human tissues, the increase is 20%. This marked dependence of BED_L on repair half-times and fractionation interval for the lung for regimen I is illustrated in the computer-generated data in Fig. 8.1. Similar data sets can be obtained for BED_K, using a $T_{1/2}$ of 2 h from the animal literature and a time of 4 h which might be more applicable to human

Table 8.1. BED for lung for regimen I (six fractions of 2 Gy in 3 days) ($\alpha/\beta = 3$)

Half-time for repair ($T_{1/2}$, hours)	Time between fractions (hours)	BED_L (Gy_3)
	3	22 (↑10%)
	4	21.3
1.5	6	20.5
Animal	8	20.2
	Full repair	20
	3	24 (↑20%)
	4	23.2
3	6	22
Human?	8	21.3
	Full repair	20

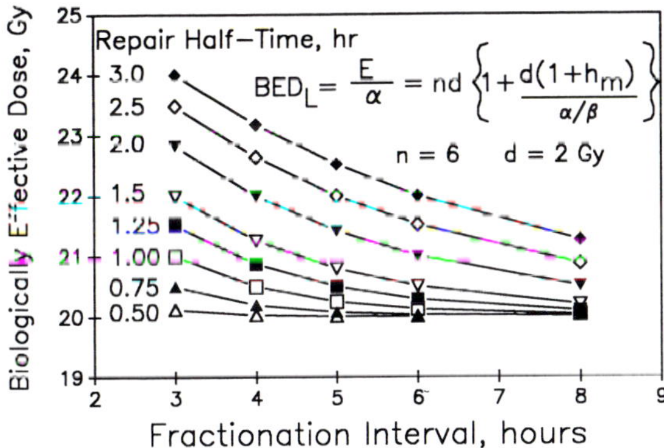

$$BED_L = \frac{E}{\alpha} = nd\left\{1 + \frac{d(1+h_m)}{\alpha/\beta}\right\}$$

Fig. 8.1. Computer-generated curves demonstrating the dependence of the BED on repair half-times in the lung and the interval between fractions in a regimen of six fractions of 2 Gy each given over 3 days. h_M represents the incomplete-repair factor obtained from Table 6.3 in THAMES and HENDRY (1987)

Table 8.2. BED for kidney for regimen I (six fractions of 2 Gy in 3 days) ($\alpha/\beta = 2$)

Half-time for repair ($T_{1/2}$, hours)	Time between fractions (hours)	BED_L (Gy_2)	
	3	28.3	($\uparrow$18%)
	4	28	
2	6	25.5	
Animal	8	24.8	
	Full repair	24	
	3	31.1	($\uparrow$30%)
	4	30	
3	6	28.3	
Human?	8	27	
	Full repair	24	

kidney (Table 8.2). The increase in BED_K from full repair to only 3 h between fractions is 18% for a $T_{1/2}$ of 2 h, whereas the increased dose and, presumably, kidney damage is more marked at 30% when half-time likely to be seen in human tissues are used in the calculations.

The expanded LQM formula was used to calculate values of BED_L and BED_K for both regimens I and II to investigate how the TGF was impacted by the possibility of incomplete repair in regimen I due to only 6 h between fractions, compared to regimen II, when full repair was expected as the fractions were given on a daily basis. Due to the lack of human data on repair half-times of lung and kidney, values from the animal literature were again used, that is, a $T_{1/2}$ of 1.5 h for lung and 2 h for kidney. Using these values and applying values of h_M from the literature, a BED_L of 20.5 Gy_3 and BED_K of 25.5 Gy_2 were obtained; this

compares to values of 19.9 Gy_3 and 24 Gy_2, respectively, when the influence of dose fractionation was not incorporated or h_M was assumed to be 0, that is, full repair. DEF_M remained as 1.09, $DEF_L = 20.5 \div 20.8 = 0.99$, and $DEF_K = 25.5 \div 26.2 = 0.97$. This gave a TGF for bone marrow compared to lung of 1.10 and a TGF of bone marrow to kidney of 1.12, resulting in an overall TGF of 1.23, again suggesting that the hyperfractionated regimen I retained its overall advantage in terms of the differential response of leukemic cell kill to possible damage to lung and kidney.

8.7 Influence of Dose Rate

There is evidence in both animals and humans supporting improved tissue tolerance to TBI when the *dose rate* is lowered, and this is particularly true for dose rates below 0.15 Gy/min. Again, this effect, like fractionation, is more marked for late-reacting tissues with small α/β values and curvier survival curves than for tissues, such as bone marrow, with large α/β values. To account for the effect of a particular dose rate on the LQM equation, a term called the *continuous-repair factor g* has been introduced:

$$BED = \frac{E}{\alpha} = nd\left(1 + \frac{gd}{\alpha/\beta}\right)$$

The continuous-repair factor *g*, which depends on time of exposure of the TBI as well as the half-times of repair of different tissues, appears to have a much greater influence on BED than does the incomplete-repair factor (h_M) when single-fraction TBI is being considered. It is the general consensus that, once TBI has been hyperfractionated, there is little extra benefit, as far as lung toxicity is concerned, to reducing the dose rate below 8–10 cGy/min, and, in the study from Italy that we have just used to demonstrate the LQM, the dose rates used were in the range of 2.9–8.5 cGy/min, a range in which there is unlikely to be any significant impact of dose rate, once the TBI has been fractionated. Moreover, the information on dose rate in many publications does not distinguish between instantaneous dose rate and mean dose rate, that is, considering the overall duration of the session, including any breaks in delivery of TBI.

We have proposed the use of the LQM with modifications in an attempt to give clinicians a straightforward but possibly oversimplistic mathematical method for comparing TBI regimens. It is entirely possible that a low dose rate single-fraction TBI, favored by many institutions in Europe, is more effective in terms of leukemic cell kill than a fractionated TBI regimen, but, as there is no agreement on the best mathematical model for comparing regimens, we have presented the LQM for consideration. A randomized trial was activated in 1987 at the Institut Gustave-Roussy comparing single-dose 10-Gy TBI (restricting the dose to the lung to 8 Gy) to a hyperfractionated schedule (11 fractions of 1.35 Gy, three fractions/day, 9 Gy to the lungs). Although such a controlled trial is urgently needed, it is possible that heterogeneity of patients within the arms of the study in terms of stage of remission and type of leukemia may thwart the best intentions of trying to elucidate the optimum TBI regimen (COSSET et al. 1989).

8.8 Chemotherapeutic Agents and TBI

We have tried using the LQM to compare the differential effect of various TBI regimens on acute- and late-reacting tissues; however, it would be desirable if the LQM were flexible enough to accommodate any modifying effect of chemotherapeutic agents, either used in the conditioning regimen or to which the children have been previously exposed. We will limit ourselves to three target cells, namely, bone marrow, lung, and kidney, and to two drugs, namely, cyclophosphamide and cisplatin. As far as bone marrow is concerned, the effects of cyclophosphamide as well as radiation may be considered as acute effects. Regarding the lung, both cyclophosphamide and radiation need only be considered in terms of late effects, that is, pneumonitis and pulmonary fibrosis. Finally, regarding kidney toxicity in children, both cyclophosphamide and cisplatin, together with radiation, cause late effects, that is, nephritis (the hemolytic-uremic syndrome is seen more commonly in adults). Although penumonitis and lung fibrosis are seen more frequently in the pediatric clinic than radiation nephritis, increasing numbers of reports of renal dysfunction are appearing the literature (TARBELL et al. 1988; BERG and BOLME 1989).

As far as bone marrow kill is concerned, it is clear that the addition of cyclophosphamide to single-dose TBI, at least in mice, causes more bone marrow kill when given after the TBI (YAN et al. 1991). Regarding damage to the lung or BED_L in our LQM, there appears to be fairly good agreement in the animal literature that there is less enhancement of lung damage by cyclophosphamide when given after the TBI (YAN et al. 1991; COLLIS and STEEL 1983). It

would be desirable if we could modify the α/β used in the LQM to account for the additional damage caused to lung by cyclophosphamide; however, TRAVIS et al. (1990) could detect no difference in α/β in mice when cyclophosphamide was given before fractionated TBI. Can we infer from these data that the target cells are the same for cyclophosphamide and radiation and that cyclophosphamide does not impact on the repair of radiation damage to lung? If the repair half-times of lung following each fraction of radiation were adversely affected by the addition of cyclophosphamide, then this would certainly impact negatively on the BED_L calculated using the LQM and imply that longer times should be allowed between TBI fractions than are currently used in order to minimize lung damage.

We previously noted that increasing numbers of reports in the literature are describing renal dysfunction in children who are survivors of BMT. In a group of 44 children with ALL and stage IV neuroblastoma, 11 developed renal dysfunction 4–7 months following BMT (TARBELL et al. 1988). Six of 17 children with ALL who had been exposed to prior drug regimens as well as cyclophosphamide followed by TBI developed renal dysfunction, although none of them required dialysis. Five of seven patients with neuroblastoma developed renal dysfunction, and their preparative regimens had included cisplatin as well as cyclophosphamide followed by fractionated TBI. Two of the patients underwent renal biopsies, and findings were consistent with radiation nephropathy. Cisplatin tends to be more damaging to renal tubules, whereas radiation can damage both tubules and glomeruli. In this study and others (BERG and BOLME 1989), renal biopsies revealed significantly more damage to glomeruli than to tubular structures. It is likely that young children are more susceptible than adults to radiation damage to the kidney, especially as many of them will have been heavily pretreated with a host of chemotherapeutic agents prior to their conditioning regimen. There is conflicting information in the animal literature regarding the tolerance of the kidney to radiation following prior exposure to cisplatin. STEWART et al. (1988) showed little effect on α/β of prior cisplatin exposure, following *local* kidney irradiation, implying that there was no reduction in repair and no modification of the x-ray response by the cisplatin. However, a modifying effect might have been seen if TBI had been used, as the tolerance of the kidney is likely to be lower than following local irradiation. MOULDER et al. (1988) showed in rats that the renal tolerance to TBI alone was of the order of 15 Gy but only about 12 Gy when cisplatin was given to the animals 4 months before the TBI. It would be prudent in children undergoing BMT to consider kidney shielding, especially if they have been pretreated with a drug such as cisplatin with known nephrotoxicity. In a study from the Medical College of Wisconsin using hyperfractionated TBI of 14 Gy in T lymphocyte-depleted BMTs, significant renal toxicity was seen, particularly in their pediatric leukemia patients, which necessitated the introduction of partial kidney shielding (LAWTON et al. 1989).

In summary, we have presented the LQM as a means of describing through the biologically effective dose (BED) concept the principles of TBI and hope that the model will be helpful to clinicians in comparing different TBI regimens described in the literature. We realize that there are shortcomings in the model, and the conflicting data in the animal literature regarding changes in α/β for kidney and lung due to chemotherapeutic agents make it hazardous to recommend any modifications in α/β. However, it is likely that agents such as cyclophosphamide and cisplatin significantly modify the radiation tolerance of lung and kidney, resulting in less or slower repair of radiation damage. From a practical standpoint, this implies the use of longer times between radiation fractions than are currently used (4–6 h, based on animal data), especially if half-times of repair are significantly longer in humans. Addressing the long-term toxicity problems by partial shielding of either lung or kidney can potentially lead to the protection of nests of leukemic cells and possible relapse, despite efforts to compensate for this bone marrow protection.

Acknowledgment. I am indebted to Dr. Bruce Kimler for the generation of the curves in Fig. 8.1.

References

Barendsen GW (1982) Dose fractionation, dose rate and iso-effects: relationships for normal-tissue responses. Int J Radiat Oncol Biol Phys 8: 1981–1997

Berg U, Bolme P (1989) Renal function in children following bone marrow transplantation. Transplant Proc 21: 3092–3094

Collis CH, Steel GG (1983) Lung damage in mice from cyclophosphamide and thoracic irradiation: the effect of timing. Int J Radiat Oncol Biol Phys 9: 685–689

Corvo R, Frassoni F, Franzone P et al. (1989) Irradiazione corporea totale frazionata e iperfrazionata nel condiziona-mento del trapianto di midollo osseo allogenico nella leucemia linfatica acuta. Risultati. Radio Med (Torino) 78: 367–372

Cosset JM, Baume D, Pico JL et al. (1989) single-dose versus hyperfractionated total body irradiation before allogeneic bone marrow transplantation. a non randomized comparative study of 54 patients at the Institut Gustave-Roussy. Radiother Oncol 15: 151–160

DeBoer RW, Lebesque JV (1988) Radiobiological implications of fractionated low dose rate irradiation. Int J Radiat Oncol Biol Phys 14: 1054–1056

Fowler JF (1989) The linear quadratic formula and progress in fractionated radiotherapy. Br J Radiol 62: 679–694

Kimler BF, Park CH, Yakar D, Mics RM (1984) Lack of recovery from radiation-induced sublethal damage in human hematopoietic cells. Br J Cancer 49 [Suppl VI]: 221–225

Kimler BF, Park CH, Yakar D (1985) Radiation response of human hemopoietic cells (normal and leukemic) assayed by in vitro colony formation. Int J Radiat Oncol Biol Phys 11: 809–816

Lawton CA, Barber-Derus S, Murray KJ, Casper JT, Ash RC, Gillin MT, Wilson JF (1989) Technical modifications in hyperfractionated total body irradiation for T-lymphocyte depleted bone marrow transplant. Int J Radiat Oncol Biol Phys 17: 319–322

Moulder JE, Fish BL, Holcenberg JS, Cheng M (1988) Effect of total-body irradiation with bone marrow transplantation on toxicity of cisplatin. In: Interaction of radiation therapy and chemotherapy. NCI Monogr 6: 29–33

Stewart FA, Luts A, Oussoren Y, Begg AC, Dewit L, Bartelink H (1988) Renal damage in mice after treatment with cisplatin and X-rays: comparison of fractionated and single-dose studies. In: Interaction of radiation therapy and chemotherapy. NCI Monogr 6: 23–27

Tarbell NJ, Guinan EC, Niemeyer C, Mauch P, Sallan SE, Weinstein HJ (1988) Late onset of renal dysfunction in survivors of bone marrow transplantation. Int J Radiat Oncol Biol Phys 15: 99–104

Thames HD, Hendry JH (1987) Fractionation in radiotherapy. Taylor and Francis, London

Travis EL, Pouzet M-T, Yan R, Fang M-A (1990) Radiation response of mouse lung previously treated with cyclophosphamide: single dose and fractionation response. Third International Conference on the Interaction of Radiation Therapy and Systemic Therapy, 9–12 March 1990. The Asilomar Conference Center, Monterey, California, pp 4–2 through 4–2C

Turesson I, Thames HD (1989) Repair capacity and kenetics of human skin during fractionated radiotherapy: erythema, desquamation, and telangiectasia after 3 and 5 years' follow-up. Radiother Oncol 15: 169–188

van Dyk J, Mah K, Keane TJ (1989) Radiation-induced lung damage: dose-time-fractionation considerations. Radiother Oncol 14: 55–69

Yan R, Peters LJ, Travis EL (1991) Cyclophosphamide 24 hours before or after total body irradiation: effects on lung and bone marrow. Radiother Oncol 21: 149–156

9 Role of Radiation Therapy in Non-Hodgkin's Lymphoma in the Child

SARAH S. DONALDSON

CONTENTS

9.1 Introduction 123
9.2 Clinical Presentation, Pathology, Management,
    Staging................................ 123
9.3 Localized Disease 126
9.4 Advanced Disease...................... 126
9.5 Central Nervous System................. 127
9.6 Lymphoma of Bone...................... 128
9.7 Emergency Indication for Radiation Therapy ... 128
9.8 Transplantation – Immunosuppression........ 129
9.9 Future................................ 130
    References............................ 130

9.1 Introduction

Non-Hodgkin's lymphoma (NHL) is not a single disease entity, but a heterogeneous collection of neoplasms of lymphoreticular cell origin which can be classified on the basis of clinical features, histopathologic features, and immunophenotype. It shares few features with the majority of NHLs seen in adults and is much more closely related to childhood acute lymphoblastic leukemia (ALL). The identification of the similarities between childhood NHL and childhood ALL led to the application of systemic antileukemic chemotherapy in an attempt to reduce the incidence of distant dissemination. Today, systemic chemotherapy is the mainstay of therapy for children with NHL. The role of radiation therapy in the primary management of childhood NHL has changed over the past 5–10 years such that there are now specific indications for its use in the management of a child afflicted with NHL. It is for this reason that it is important to review briefly the important aspects of clinical presentation, histopathological features, workup, and staging. Without an understanding of these aspects of management, appropriate treatment will not be delivered.

SARAH S. DONALDSON, MD., FACR, Professor of Radiation Oncology, Department of Radiation Oncology, Room A-083, Stanford University School of Medicine, Stanford, CA 94305, USA

9.2 Clinical Presentation, Pathology, Management, Staging

Pediatric NHL can arise in any of various sites containing lymphoid tissue, including lymph nodes, Peyer's patches, Waldeyer's ring, and thymus, and in various extralymphatic sites as well. The presenting symptoms relate to the tissue or organ involved. These tumors are among the most rapidly progressive malignancies, and the duration of symptoms is usually quite brief, often less than 4–6 weeks. Painless, rapidly progressive lymphadenopathy is common. Children with upper torso adenopathy frequently have an anterior mediastinal mass as well (Fig. 9.1), with or without a pleural effusion. Mediastinal disease often presents with symptoms of respiratory embarrassment from paratracheal and tracheobronchial compression by lymphoma (Fig. 9.2). Signs of superior vene cava obstruction are frequently seen in this setting (LINK 1985). The abdomen is the primary site in approximately 30%–40% of children; one-third of children with abdominal NHL present with the primary involvement of the

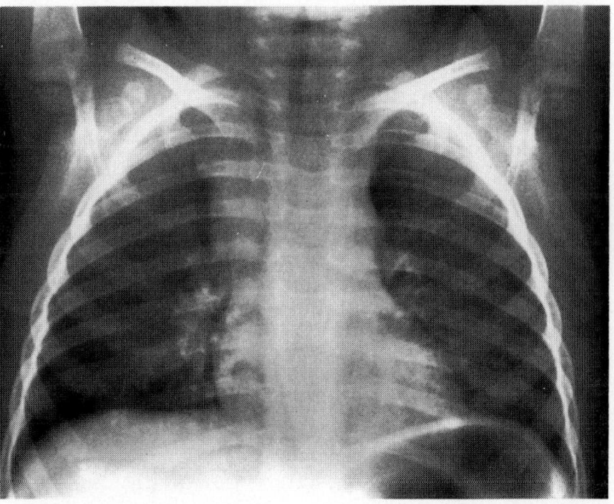

Fig. 9.1. Posteroanterior chest radiograph of a child presenting with respiratory embarrassment. There is extensive paratracheal and tracheal bronchial lymphadenopathy extending down to the carina, with a suggestion of subcarinal adenopathy as well. No pleural effusion is seen in this case

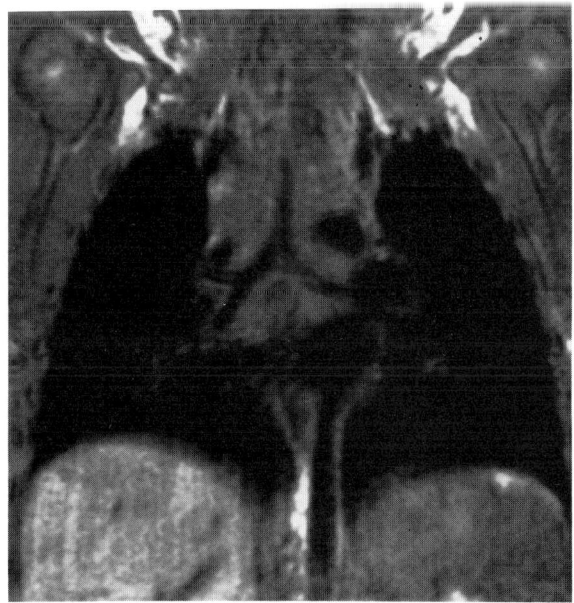

Fig. 9.2. A magnetic resonance image of the case shown in Fig. 9.1, further clarifying the mediastinal and pericarinal adenopathy. Because of the lack of pleural fluid or peripheral adenopathy, a mediastinal biopsy was undertaken to determine the diagnosis

Table 9.1. Relationship between histopathologic pattern, immunophenotype, and sites of involvement

Histologic type	Immunopheno-type	Site of involvement
Lymphoblastic	T cell	Anterior mediastinum,
	Pre-B cell	Upper torso, lymph nodes, skin
Undifferentiated Burkitt	B cell	
		Jaw, abdomen, orbit, paraspinal
Non-Burkitt		Abdomen, bone marrow, nasopharynx, lymph nodes
Large cell (histiocytic)	B cell T cell Non-T, non-B cell	Variable

gastrointestinal tract (JENKIN et al. 1969; NELSON et al. 1977). These patients present with abdominal pain and vomiting, with or without a palpable right lower quadrant mass; these symptoms are often the result of an ileocecal intussusception caused by a lymphomatous intraluminal mass. Many with abdominal lymphomas present with ascites and metabolic abnormalities, occasionally with renal failure from direct renal infiltration and/or ureteral obstruction. Between 10% and 15% have disease involving the Waldeyer's ring structures and paranasal sinuses with or without associated cervical lymph node involvement. These children present with symptoms of sinusitis or mass effect. Primary involvement of the bones of the face, particularly of the orbit and maxilla, is most commonly seen with endemic Burkitt's lymphoma in Africa. Less common primary sites include skin and bone. Primary central nervous system (CNS) lymphoma is rare and occurs among those with immunodeficiency syndromes and in patients receiving immunosuppressive therapy.

Modern histopathological classification systems correlate with immunophenotype and the site of presentation (Table 9.1). Virtually all childhood NHLs have a diffuse pattern (as opposed to a follicular or nodular pattern) and are high grade. They can be subdivided into three groups: lymphoblastic, undifferentiated, and large cell (LINK 1985). The dis-

tinction between Burkitt's and non-Burkitt's variants of undifferentiated lymphoma is controversial and these two entities are more alike than different; thus a distinction is not particularly useful. The lymphoblastic lymphomas are predominantly T-cell neoplasms, although a small percentage are derived from early B-cell precursors so that immunophenotype cannot always be predicted accurately from histology. The undifferentiated lymphomas (Burkitt's and non-Burkitt's types) are virtually all B-cell tumors. The large cell lymphomas are heterogeneous immunologically; most are transformed B cells, few are T cell derived, and a rare case is derived from the histiocyte/macrophage lineage and qualifies as a "true histiocytic lymphoma."

With appropriate management the majority of children with NHL can be cured. Optimal care is best delivered at a major center where pediatric oncologists, radiotherapists, surgeons, pathologists, immunologists, diagnostic radiologists, and nurse specialists cooperate in the management of each child.

Prompt diagnosis is essential because of the rapid cell turnover times and aggressive biology. In general the least invasive procedures should be used to gain representative tissue for pathology, immunophenotyping, and cytogenetics. Workup should involve a careful review of the peripheral blood smear, bone marrow aspirate, and biopsy. If a pleural effusion is present, thoracentesis may provide diagnostic material for cytologic and immunologic studies. Children presenting with respiratory symptoms or superior vena cava obstruction should not be subjected to general anesthesia with endotracheal intubation, because of possible edema formation in an already compromised airway (HALPERN et al. 1983). Ascitic fluid may contain malignant cells allowing for rapid diagnosis and obviating a tissue biopsy. Children with massive abdominal disease usually present with precarious renal function and metabolic derangement; thus avoidance of laparotomy and general anesthesia is recommended. It is essential to make a confirmed diagnosis before initiating treatment since correct therapy depends upon histological classification and response to treatment may be rapid. Staging studies should be completed expeditiously as the evolution of childhood NHL is rapid. Surgical staging can generally be avoided. Essential studies include: a careful physical examination with attention to all sites of palpable disease; a complete blood count, platelet count and differential; bone marrow aspirate; and a lumbar puncture (with cytocentrifuge examination of the CSF). Serum lactate dehydrogenase (LDH) may be useful as it correlates with tumor burden. Serum uric acid, electrolytes, creatinine, calcium, and phosphorous are important in children with bulky tumors. Imaging studies should include posteroanterior and lateral roentgenograms of the chest and a bone scan. Computed tomography (CT) or magnetic resonance imaging (MRI) is helpful in determining extent of disease in children with paranasal sinus involvement. Myelography or MRI of the spine should be performed if clinically indicated. However, extensive radiographic evaluation should be avoided since it contributes little information not obvious from physical examination and may delay the initiation of therapy.

Two clinical staging systems are widely accepted for childhood NHL and are shown in Tables 9.2 and 9.3. The staging system for Burkitt's lymphoma utilized by the National Cancer Institute (NCI) (Table 9.2) classifies patients according to tumor burden, which correlates with prognosis (ZIEGLER 1981). The stages A, B, and AR carry a favorable prognosis, while the prognosis is less good in patients with bulky unresectable and widely disseminated stage C or D disease. This system, useful for Burkitt's lymphoma,

Table 9.2. National Cancer Institute system for the clinical staging of Burkitt's lymphoma

Stage	Extent of tumor
A	Single extra-abdominal site
B	Multiple extra-abdominal sites
C	Intra-abdominal tumor
D	Intra-abdominal tumor with involvement of multiple extra-abdominal sites
AR	Stage C but with > 90% of tumor surgically resected

Table 9.3. St. Jude Children's Research Hospital staging scheme for non-Hodgkin's lymphoma[a]

Stage I	A single tumor (extranodal) or single anatomic area (nodal), with the exclusion of mediastinum or abdomen
Stage II	A single tumor (extranodal) with regional node involvement
	Two or more nodal areas on the same side of the diaphragm
	Two single (extranodal) tumors with or without regional node involvement on the same side of the diaphragm
	A primary gastrointestinal tract tumor, usually in the ileocecal area, with or without involvement of associated mesenteric nodes only[b]
Stage III	Two single tumors (extranodal) on opposite sides of the diaphragm
	Two or more nodal areas above and below the diaphragm
	All the primary intrathoracic tumors (mediastinal, pleural, thymic)
	All extensive primary intra-abdominal disease[b]
	All paraspinal or epidural tumors, regardless of other tumor sites
Stage IV	Any of the above with initial CNS or bone marrow involvement[c]

[a] About one-third of all children with NHL will present with limited stage I or II disease.
[b] A distinction is made between apparently localized gastrointestinal tract lymphoma and more extensive intra-abdominal disease because of their quite different patterns of survival after appropriate therapy. Stage II disease typically is limited to a segment of the gut plus or minus the associated mesenteric nodes only, and the primary tumor can be completely removed grossly by segmental excision. Stage III disease typically exhibits spread to para-aortic and retroperitoneal areas by implants and plaques in the mesentery or peritoneum, or by direct infiltration of structures adjacent to the primary tumor. Ascites may be present, and complete resection of all gross tumor is not possible.
[c] If marrow involvement is present initially, the number of abnormal cells must be 25% or less in an otherwise normal marrow aspirate with a normal peripheral blood picture.

is not applicable for patients who present with extra-abdominal tumors. The St. Jude Children's Research Hospital system (SJCRH) (Table 9.3) assigns stage on the basis of primary site as well as extent of disease (MURPHY 1978). In this system patients with mediastinal disease as well as those with massive unresectable abdominal tumors are considered to have stage III disease while those with localized gastrointestinal tumors are classified more favorably as having stage II disease. Thus, children fall into two broad categories: those with localized disease unfavorable sites (stages I and II in the SJCRH system), which includes about one-third of patients, and those with unfavorable sites or disseminated disease (stages III and IV). This latter group accounts for the majority of treatment failures.

9.3 Localized Disease

Children presenting with localized disease in favorable sites (stages I and II in the SJCRH system and stages A, B, and AR in the staging of Burkitt's lymphoma) have a high likelihood of cure when treated with modern therapy, which includes a variety of systemic chemotherapy regimens. The majority of these children have nonlymphoblastic histology, usually small non-cleaved cell Burkitt's and non-Burkitt's tumors. Most present with nasopharynx, oropharynx, or submandibular–cervical lymph node chain disease or have localized, completely resectable tumors of the gastrointestinal tract.

Murphy and colleagues demonstrated that children with localized NHL could be treated successfully with a 15-month chemotherapy regimen of reduced intensity combined with low-dose involved-field radiation (MURPHY et al. 1983). Investigators from the Children's Cancer Study Group (CCSG) reported successful therapy for 90% of children with localized NHL utilizing the COMP regimen (Cyclophosphamide, vincristine, intermediate dose methotrexate, and prednisone) for 18 months along with radiotherapy; in a follow-up randomized study the same investigators demonstrated that 6 months of treatment was as efficacious as 18 months for those with localized non-lymphoblastic NHL (ANDERSON et al. 1983; JENKIN et al. 1984; MEADOWS et al. 1989). Until this time, all regimens utilized radiation therapy in conjunction with systemic chemotherapy.

Prior to the advent of routine chemotherapy usage, there were a small percentage of children with supradiaphargmatic Ann Arbor stage I–II disease who were cured with radiotherapy alone (GLATSTEIN et al. 1974). In addition, approximately 80% of children with favorable presentation of localized of gastrointestinal tract lymphoma were cured with surgical resection followed by whole abdominal radiotherapy (NELSON et al. 1977; JENKIN et al. 1969). However, the majority of children with tumor in other primary sites, even those with apparently localized disease, developed recurrent disease after radiotherapy alone.

In an attempt to further reduce intensity and toxicity, collaborators from the Pediatric Oncology Group (POG) then embarked upon a randomized study testing the role of radiation therapy in favorable and early-stage patients. They used three cycles of CHOP (cyclophosphamide, adriamycin, vincristine, prednisone) followed by 24 weeks of daily oral 6-mercaptopurine and weekly methotrexate for stage I–II patients, with one-half of the study group receiving 27 Gy of involved-field radiotherapy and the other half receiving no radiotherapy. Among 129 patients, there was no difference in 4-year event-free survival, survival, or local control in the irradiated group as compared with nonirradiated population (LINK et al. 1990). The event-free survival was 88% for the combined modality group vs. 83% for the chemotherapy alone group ($P = 0.44$); survival was 93% for both groups. In addition there was no difference in the pattern of relapse (local and systemic failure) according to treatment received. However, there were more episodes of mucositis, infection, and myelosuppression among those receiving the combined modality program. The POG study did not use CNS prophylactic therapy for children with localized NHL outside of the head and neck region. Thus, the POG study demonstrated conclusively that nine out of ten children with localized NHL can be cured using a chemotherapy regimen of modest intensity and short duration without radiotherapy.

9.4 Advanced Disease

Children with advanced-stage NHL (stages III and IV in the SJCRH system, and stages C and D in the NCI staging system for Burkitt's lymphoma) have a less favorable prognosis. The majority of these children have either T-cell mediastinal lymphoblastic lymphoma or massive abdominal B-cell small non-cleaved cell tumors, while a minority present with advanced-stage large cell lymphoma. Specific therapy is based upon histopathology and immunology. The CCSG investigators showed the LSA_2L_2 regimen (a ten drug multiagent protocol) to be excellent therapy for advanced lymphoblastic lymphoma, but not for advanced nonlymphoblastic lymphoma (ANDERSON et al. 1983). The reverse was true for the COMP program. Since there are many similarities between advanced stage NHL and ALL, NHL therapy is today modeled after that for the biologically related acute leukemia. Thus, children with advanced-stage lymphoblastic lymphoma (the majority of whom have T-cell markers and mediastinal disease) are treated on regimens designed for patients with high-risk, T-cell ALL. Approximately three-quarters of these children with advanced lymphoblastic lymphoma remain in remission beyond 3 years (WEINSTEIN et al. 1983; DAHL et al. 1985). Patients with advanced, small non-cleaved cell lymphoma and those with B-cell ALL benefit from intensive chemotherapy using cyclophosphamide and methotrexate (MURPHY et al. 1986; ANDERSON et al. 1983; MAGRATH et al. 1984; SULLIVAN and RAMIREZ, 1985). The large cell lymphomas represent a small proportion of pediatric lymphomas. They are clinically and immunologically heterogeneous and most treatment regimens have been similar to that used in adults. Anthracycline-based regimens without cyclophosphamide are effective against large cell lymphoma (WEINSTEIN et al. 1984).

The role of radiotherapy has been studied in randomized trials among children with advanced-stage and Burkitt's lymphoma, and has not been found to be beneficial in terms of remission induction or overall disease control (MURPHY and HUSTU 1980; ZIEGLER 1977). Some investigators continue to recommend irradiation in sites of bulky disease so as to prevent local recurrence (JEREB et al. 1981); however, current randomized trials do not routinely include radiotherapy.

9.5 Central Nervous System

Primary lymphomas of the CNS are rare and usually observed in children with inherited or acquired immunodeficiency syndromes and in patients receiving immunosuppressive therapy (PATTENGALE et al. 1979). CNS lymphoma often presents as meningeal disease, although some patients (particularly those with small non-cleaved cell lymphoma) may present with spinal cord compression or cranial nerve palsy. Prophylactic therapy to the CNS to prevent meningeal relapse is an important component of therapy for children with NHL as CNS involvement occurs in about 30% of children with NHL. The risk of CNS relapse is a function of the effectiveness of the initial systemic management. Current effective systemic regimens certainly reduce the risk, which at one time approached 50% when CNS prophylaxis was omitted (WATANABE et al. 1973; HUTTER et al.1975). In general, CNS prophylaxis for children with NHL has been modeled after prophylactic regimens for children with ALL. For children with localized NHL arising outside of the head and neck, CNS prophylaxis does not appear necessary (LINK et al. 1990). However, for patients with advanced-stage lymphoblastic disease, CNS relapse does require treatment. The risk of primary meningeal relapse is also high in those with advanced small non-cleaved lymphoma. Meningeal relapse is quite unusual among those with large cell lymphoma unless there is prior bone marrow involvement (LEVITT et al. 1980). The majority of children will receive adequate prophylaxis from intrathecal therapy and will not require cranial radiotherapy. Intensive intrathecal chemotherapy with methotrexate and cytarabine, supplemented with systemic infusions of methotrexate and cytarabine, provides effective CNS prophylaxis for children with advanced small non-cleaved cell lymphoma. Children with mediastinal T-cell lymphoblastic lymphoma have been treated with CNS regimens effective for those with high-risk T-cell ALL, utilizing cranial irradiation and intrathecal chemotherapy. Preliminary data from POG indicate that intensive intrathecal chemotherapy with methotrexate, cytarabine, and hydrocortisone may be sufficient prophylactic therapy for children with lymphoblastic lymphoma and that cranial irradiation may be unnecessary (AMYLON et al. 1988). Intrathecal chemotherapy (methotrexate or cytarabine) has not been shown to be of benefit in preventing CNS disease in African Burkitt's lymphoma (ZEIGLER and BLUMING, 1971). In American Burkitt's lymphoma, CNS relapse often occurs in the setting of widespread tumor involvement and the efficacy of preventive CNS therapy has been difficult to assess.

The need for cranial radiation as CNS prophylaxis has been widely discussed (MANDELL et al. 1987; MURPHY and BLEYER, 1987). The current approach is to omit cranial radiation when effective intrathecal chemotherapy is given in conjunction with aggressive systemic combination chemotherapy, in an attempt to reduce the risk of leukoencephalopathy (MANDELL et al. 1987). When cranial irradiation is routinely used, doses of 18–24 Gy in 1.8- to 2-Gy fractions have been employed.

However, children with overt CNS lymphoma at diagnosis, children with CNS relapse, and children with leukemic transformation prior to diagnosis do require irradiation to control CNS disease (LOEFFLER et al. 1985; FREEMAN et al. 1986; MURPHY and BLEYER 1987). There is a low cure rate of leptomeningeal lymphoma with intrathecal chemotherapy alone and a relatively high rate of CNS relapse with intrathecal chemoprophylaxis alone in patients who have features of both lymphoma and leukemia (>25% blasts in the bone marrow) at diagnosis. The POG investigators gave LSA$_2$L$_2$ therapy, including maintenance intrathecal methotrexate but not CNS irradiation, to children with T-cell leukemia (which commonly presents with a lymphomatous pattern of presentation) and observed a 26% incidence of sustained CNS relapse (PULLEN et al. 1982). The combination of cranial radiotherapy with intrathecal methotrexate in the LSA$_2$L$_2$ regimen lowers the CNS relapse rate to below 7% (VECCHI et al. 1981). As in CNS leukemia, CNS lymphoma may be treated with systemic chemotherapy as well as cranial irradiation plus intrathecal therapy or cranial–spinal irradiation (CSI). Many investigators favor CSI (WILLOUGHBY 1983; LAND et al. 1985). Fortunately, overt CNS lymphoma is a rare problem today. Such patients should be treated in pediatric centers, preferably on studies evaluating treatment regimens. As HIV infections become more prevalent and more children with pediatric AIDS are seen, the frequency of primary CNS lymphomas is likely to increase in the childhood population.

9.6 Lymphoma of Bone

Primary NHL of bone is usually of large cell histology and often mimics the more common Ewing's sarcoma of bone in children. It often presents as a painful extremity lesion with or without an associated soft tissue mass. Frequently there is regional lymph node adenopathy detected on lymphography.

The role of radiation therapy for primary NHL of bone is unclear. Traditionally radiotherapy has been used in the treatment of both children and adults (LOEFFLER et al. 1986; HOWAT et al. 1987; FURMAN et al. 1989). Radiation doses of 40 Gy to the entire bone, with a cone down to a total of 50 Gy to the lesion have been recommended. Doses in excess of 60 Gy are associated with complications. However, systemic chemotherapy is now recommended for all such patients and those with lymphoma at other sites. The role of radiotherapy has been questioned in the era of effective systemic chemotherapy (HADDY et al. 1988; COPPES et al. 1991). In the Joint Center for Radiation Therapy experience there were no local recurrences among the 11 irradiated patients, but two developed second malignant tumor within the XRT field (LOEFFLER et al. 1986). The NCI has studied patients with local and advanced stages of lymphoma with bone involvement treated with chemotherapy alone, omitting radiotherapy. They had few bone recurrences but the patient numbers were small and overall survival was moderate (HADDY et al. 1988). The POG study of early-stage NHL is omitting radiation therapy for those children with isolated bone primaries. These children are being followed carefully for their patterns of failure as well as event-free survival and survival. In the University of Florida experience, chemotherapy alone for primary NHL of bone has been associated with local failure at

the site of the primary tumor (MENDENHALL et al. 1987).

9.7 Emergency Indications for Radiation Therapy

The most common emergency situations for external beam radiotherapy are superior venacaval syndrome (Fig. 9.3), acute airway compromise, cardiac tamponade, and CNS involvement with spinal cord compression and/or cranial nerve palsies. These clinical syndromes may evolve rapidly and often the patient is found to be symptomatic before diagnosis has been confirmed. In this situation where administration of systemic chemotherapy must be delayed, local-field radiation is indicated. Response is often dramatic with lymphoblastic lymphoma, with doses as low as 6 Gy in 3–4 days adequate to relieve acute symptoms. Large cell lymphomas may require slightly higher doses before response is appreciated. Because of the rapid response to radiation, a histologic diagnosis may be lost if all of the diagnostic tissue is included within a radiation portal. In this situation it is desirable, when treating the mediastinum for airway compromise for example, to leave abnormal palpable disease in the neck or a portion of the mediastinal disease out of the radiotherapy field, and

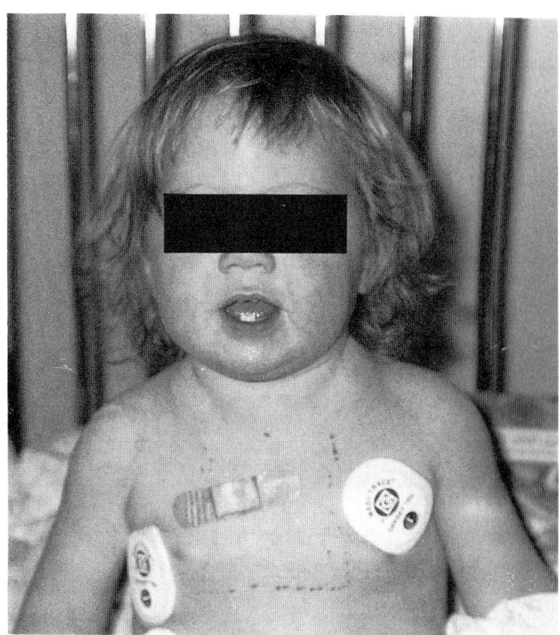

Fig. 9.3. A child presenting with typical features of superior vene cava obstruction. There is obvious periorbital edema, facial plethora, full neck, venous distension, and a prominent venous pattern visible over the anterior chest. The child's x-ray and thoracic MRI are shown in Fig. 9.1 and 9.2. The black marks on the chest demonstrate the configuration of the emergency radiotherapy fields

readily available for biopsy. Systemic prednisone and/or dexamethasone should also be avoided, for many lymphomas may respond to only a few doses of steroids and the opportunity for diagnostic tissue to be biopsied may be lost. Radiotherapy may be used as an adjunct to chemotherapy to maximize the rate of response for a newly diagnosed patient or one who fails to achieve a complete remission after induction chemotherapy. Finally, radiation may be useful for palliation of pain or mass effect.

Children who present with cranial nerve paresis present special problems. Emergent therapy is indicated to enhance reversal of cranial nerve deficits – most commonly afflicted is cranial nerve VII. It is rare that intrathecal chemotherapy will reverse cranial nerve dysfunction; however, the addition of whole brain irradiation (or base of skull radiotherapy) does enhance the likelihood of a response and may provide reversal of cranial nerve paresis (PARYANI et al. 1983). For children who present with cranial nerve palsy at the time of diagnosis, the addition of radiation is associated with improved disease-free survival, as compared to those for whom radiation is not given (53% vs 29%) (INGRAM et al. 1991). Responses may be seen after 10–12 Gy; however, durable responses require doses in the range of 24 Gy.

For patients with diffuse undifferentiated Burkitt's type lymphoma, a hyperfractionated regimen of three fractions per day is more likely to result in rapid tumor regression than is conventional fractionation (NORIN and ONYANGO, 1977). This is theorized because of the very rapid growth fraction and short potential doubling time, reported to be about 24 h in Burkitt's tumor. In the course of treatment for Burkitt's lymphoma, one must be alert to possible tumor lysis syndrome, which can result in uric acid nephropathy and renal failure requiring dialysis. Careful management of hydration with close monitoring of electrolyte balance and serum uric acid is essential during initiation of chemotherapy or radiotherapy.

9.8 Transplantation – Immunosuppression

Because failure to obtain a complete remission and relapse after complete remission are omnious signs in children with NHL of any histologic subtype, an approach with massive doses of chemotherapy–radiotherapy with or without the infusion of allogeneic or autologous bone marrow to "rescue" the patient from myelotoxicity is now being investigated (APPELBAUM et al. 1987; PHILLIP et al. 1986, 1988; BRAINE et al. 1987). Total body irradiation is often included in the preparatory regimen, most commonly with multifraction schemes of 12–13 Gy given in 3–4 days. For infants and toddlers this may require sedation and/or anesthesia 2–3 times a day. The success of bone marrow transplantation and salvage treatment for patients with recurrent disease has prompted interest in the use of such myeloablative therapy in the treatment of "high-risk" patients in first complete remission (e.g., children with CNS involvement at diagnosis). Such approaches are currently under study. Total body irradiation should be reserved for treatment in centers with a bone marrow transplant team as the treatment of any one individual is labor intensive and requires complex physics consultation and dosimetric calculations as well as special expertise in conducting the daily treatment.

We now recognize that children with primary immunodeficiency syndromes have several defects of T- or B-cell immunity or both, and have an increased susceptibility to infection as well as a high incidence of cancer, most commonly NHL. NHL occurs in children with ataxia telangiectasia, Wiskott-Aldrich Syndrome, common variable immunodeficiency, and severe combined immunodeficiency. The lymphomas are very heterogeneous, with representation from all major histologic subtypes (KERSEY et al. 1987). The lymphomas arise commonly from B lymphocytes, although occasionally T-cell lymphomas are seen. The CNS is a frequent primary tumor site.

Children afflicted with human immunodeficiency virus (HIV) are now being reported to be at high risk for development of lymphomas. This observation underscores the necessity for routine serologic studies for HIV in all newly diagnosed children with lymphoma, particularly those with B-cell lymphoma. The tumors are mostly high-grade undifferentiated or immunoblastic or Burkitt's-like lymphomas. The initial lesions tend to be polyclonal but later evolve into overt histologic, phenotypically and clinically malignant high-grade monoclonal B cell lymphomas, similar to those seen in transplant patients (LIPPMAN et al. 1988; GILL and LAVINE 1988). These tumors may be radiosensitive (EPSTEIN et al. 1988); however, the outlook is grim and survival measured in months (Italian Cooperative Group for AIDS-Related Tumors 1988).

Success in organ transplantation has now demonstrated an increased risk of malignant tumors, including NHL, among those patients receiving immunosuppressive therapy for extended periods. A disproportionate number of lymphomas are seen in recipients of extrarenal organs–cardiac allograft recipients, hepatic allograft recipients, bone marrow recipients, pancreatic recipients, heart–lung recipients, and lung allograft recipients. These lymphomas are thought to reflect the use of more intensive immunosuppression to prevent and/or treat rejection or graft versus host disease. After bone marrow transplantation, lymphomas are particularly likely to occur with the use of mismatched T-cell-depleted marrow (KERSEY et al. 1987). The incidence of NHL is particularly high after the use of cyclosporine therapy; many of these lymphomas regress with reduction or cessation of cyclosporine.

Second cancers, including lymphoma, have now been reported after successful treatment of other tumors, most notably Hodgkin's disease (COLEMAN et al. 1982; KRIKORIAN et al. 1979). These tumors appear related to the prior therapy, and in the case of development of NHL, appear correlated with chemotherapy administration rather than that of radiotherapy. The actuarial risk of developing a second cancer following successful treatment of Hodgkin's disease is less among the pediatric population than their adult counterpart (COLEMAN et al. 1982).

9.9 Future

In the past decade, remarkable advances have occurred in our understanding of the biology, management, and treatment of children with NHL. These advances have been translated into spectacular improvements in prognosis. Much of the improvement has accompanied more successful implementation of systemic chemotherapy, along with more precise and limited use of radiotherapy. However, improved treatment is still required for subsets of patients such as those with CNS disease.

Innovative approaches with cell-differentiating agents, hematopoietic growth factors, monoclonal antibodies, new drug combinations, and improvements in bone marrow transplantation hold promise for the outlook of those children with very advanced lymphoma and those who develop recurrent disease.

References

Amylon M, Murphy S, Pullen J for the Pediatric Oncology Group (1988) Treatment of lymphoid malignancies according to immune phenotype: preliminary results in T-cell disease. Proc Am Soc Clin Oncol 7: 225

Anderson JR, Wilson JF, Jenkin RDT et al. (1983) Childhood non-Hodgkin's lymphoma. The results of a randomized therapeutic trial comparing a 4 drug regimen (COMP) with a 10-drug regimen (LSA$_2$-L$_2$). N Engl J Med 308: 559–565

Applebaum FR, Sullivan KM, Buckner CD et al. (1987) Treatment of malignant lymphoma in 100 patients with chemotherapy, total body irradiation, and marrow transplantation. J Clin Oncol 5: 1340–1347

Braine HG, Santos GW, Kaizer H et al. (1987) Treatment of poor prognosis non-Hodgkin's lymphoma using cyclophosphamide and total body irradiation regimens with autologous bone marrow rescue. Bone Marrow Transplant 2: 7–14

Coleman CN, Kalpan HS, Cox R et al. (1982) Leukemias, non-Hodgkin's lymphomas and solid tumors in patients treated for Hodgkin's disease. Cancer Surv 1: 733–744

Coppes MJ, Patte C, Couanet D et al. (1991) Childhood malignant lymphoms of bone. Med Pediatr Oncol 19: 22–27

Dahl GV, Rivera G, Pui C-H et al. (1985) A novel treatment of childhood lymphoblastic non-Hodgkin's lymphoma: early and intermediate use of teniposide plus cytarabine. Blood 66: 1110–1114

Epstein LG, Di Carlo FJ, Joshi VV et al. (1988) Primary lymphoma of the central nervous system in children with acquired immunodeficiency syndrome. Pediatrics 82: 355–363

Freeman CR, Shustik C, Brisson M-L et al. (1986) Primary malignant lymphoma of the central nervous system. Cancer 58: 1106–1111

Furman WL, Fitch S, Hustu HO, Callihan T, Murphy S (1989) Primary lymphoma of bone in children. J Clin Oncol 7: 1275–1280

Gill PS, Levine AM (1988) HIV-related malignant lymphoma: clinical aspects, treatment, and pathogenesis. Cancer Invest 6: 413–416

Glatstein E, Kim H, Donaldson SS et al. (1974) Non-Hodgkin's lymphoma: VI. Results of treatment in childhood. Cancer 34: 204–211

Haddy TB, Keenan AM, Jaffe ES, Magrath IT (1988) Bone involvement in young patients with non-Hodgkin's lymphoma: efficacy of chemotherapy without local radiotherapy. Blood 72: 1141–1147

Halpern S, Chatten J, Meadows AT et al. (1983) Anterior mediastinal masses: anesthesia hazards and other problems. J Pediatr 102: 407–410

Howat AJ, Thomas H, Waters KE, Campbell PE (1987) Malignant lymphoma of bone in children. Cancer 59: 335–339

Hutter JJ, Favara BE, Nelson M, Holton LP (1975) Non-Hodgkin's lymphoma in children. Correlation of CNS disease with initial presentation. Cancer 36: 2132–2137

Ingram LC, Fairclough DL, Furman WL et al. (1991) Cranial nerve palsy in childhood acute lymphoblastic leukemia and non-Hodgkin's lymphoma. Cancer 67: 2262–2268

Italian Cooperative Group for AIDS-Related Tumors (1988) Malignant lymphoma in patients with or at risk for AIDS in Italy. J Natl Cancer Inst 88: 855–860

Jenkin RDT, Sonley MJ, Stephens CA et al. (1969) Primary gastrointestinal tract lymphoma in childhood. Radiology 92: 763–767

Jenkin RDT, Anderson JR, Chilcote RR et al. (1984) The treatment of localized non-Hodgkin's lymphoma in children: a report from the Children's Cancer Study Group. J Clin Oncol 2: 88–97

Jereb B, Wollner N, Kosloff C, Exelby P (1981) The role of

local radiation in the treatment of non-Hodgkin's lymphoma in children. Med Pediatr Oncol 9: 157–166

Kersey JH, Shapiro RS, Heinitz KJ et al. (1987) Lymphoid malignancy in naturally occurring and post bone marrow transplantation immunodeficiency disease. In: Good RA, Lindenlaub E (eds) The nature, cellular and biochemical basis and management of immunodeficiencies. FK Schattaeur Stuttgart (Symposia Medica Haechst 21, pp 289–294)

Krikorian JG, Burke JS, Rosenberg SA et al. (1979) Occurrence of non-Hodgkin's lymphoma after therapy for Hodgkin's disease N Engl J Med 300: 452–458

Land VJ, Thomas PRM, Boyett JM et al. (1985) Comparison of maintenance treatment regimens for first central nervous system relapse in children with acute lymphocytic leukemia: a Pediatric Oncology Group Study. Cancer 56: 81–87

Levitt L, Dawson D, Rosenthal D, Moloney W (1980) CNS involvement in the non-Hodgkin's lymphomas. Cancer 45: 545–552

Link MP (1985) Non-Hodgkins lymphoma in children. Pediatr Clin North Am 32: 699–720

Link MP, Donaldson SS, Berard CW, Shuster JJ, Murphy SB (1990) Results of treatment of childhood localized non-Hodgkin's lymphoma with combination chemotherapy with or without radiotherapy. N Engl J Med 322: 1169–1174

Lippman SM, Volk JR, Spier CM et al. (1988) Clonal ambiguity of human immunodeficiency virus-associated lymphomas. Similarity to post-transplant lymphomas. Arch Pathol Lab Med 112: 128–132

Loeffler JS, Ervin TJ, Mauch P, Skarin A, Weinstein HJ, Canellos G, Cassady JR (1985) Primary lymphoma of the central nervous system: pattern of failure and factors that influence survival. J Clin Oncol 3: 490–494

Loeffler JS, Tarbell NJ, Kozakewich H, Cassady JR, Weinstein HJ (1986) Primary lymphoma of bone in children: analysis of treatment results with adriamycin, prednisone, oncovin (APO) and local radiation therapy. J Clin Oncol 4: 496–501

Magrath IT, Janus C, Edwards BK et al. (1984) An effective therapy for both undifferentiated (including Burkitt's) lymphomas and lymphoblastic lymphomas in children and young adults. Blood 63: 1102–1111

Mandell LR, Wollner N, Fuks Z (1987) Is cranial radiation necessary for CNS prophylaxis in pediatrics NHL? Int J Radiat Oncol Biol Phys 13: 359–363

Meadows AT, Sposto R, Jenkin RDT et al. (1989) Similar efficacy of 6 and 18 months of therapy with four drugs (COMP) for localized non-Hodgkin's lymphoma of children: a report from the Children's Cancer Study Group. J Clin Oncol 7: 92–99

Mendenhall NP, Jones JJ, Kramer BS et al. (1987) The management of primary lymphoma of bone. Radiother Oncol 9: 137–145

Murphy SB (1978) Current concepts in cancer: childhood non-Hodgkin's lymphoma. N Engl J Med 299: 1446–1448

Murphy SB, Bleyer WA (1987) Cranial irradiation is not necessary for central-nervous-system prophylaxis in pediatric non-Hodgkin's lymphoma. Int J Radiat Oncol Biol Phys 13: 467–468

Murphy SB, Hustu HO (1980) A randomized trial of combined modality therapy for childhood non-Hodgkin's lymphoma. Cancer 45: 630–637

Murphy SB, Hustu HO, Rivera G, Berard CW (1983) End results of treating children with localized non-Hodgkin's lymphoma with a combined modality approach of lessened intensity. J Clin Oncol 1: 326–330

Murphy SB, Bowman WP, Abromowitch M et al. (1986) Results of treatment of advanced-stage Burkitt's lymphoma and B-cell (SIg+) acute lymphoblastic leukemia with high-dose fractionated cyclophosphamide and coordinated high-dose methotrexate and cytarabine. J Clin Oncol 4: 1732–1739

Nelson DF, Cassady JR, Traggis D et al. (1977) The role of radiation therapy in localized resectable intestinal non-Hodgkin's lymphoma in children. Cancer 39: 89–97

Norin T, Onyango J (1977) Radiotherapy in Burkitt's lymphoma. Conventional or suprafractionated regimen – early results. Int J Radiat Oncol Biol Phys 2: 399–406

Paryani SB, Donaldson SS, Amylon MD, Link MP (1983) Cranial nerve involvement in children with leukemia and lymphoma. J Clin Oncol 1: 542–545

Pattengale PK, Taylor CR, Panke T et al. (1979) Selective immunodeficiency and malignant lymphoma of the central nervous system. Acta Neuropathol (Berl) 48: 165–169

Philip T, Pinkerton R, Hartmann O et al. (1986) The role of massive therapy with autologous bone marrow transplantation in Burkitt's lymphoma. Clin Haematol 15: 205–217

Philip T, Hartmann O, Biron P et al. (1988) High-dose therapy and autologous bone marrow transplantation in partial remission after first-line induction therapy for diffuse non-Hodgkin's lymphoma. J Clin Oncol 6: 1118–1124

Pullen DJ, Sullivan MP, Falletta JM et al. (1982) Modified LSA$_2$-L$_2$ treatment in 53 children with E-rosette-positive T-cell Leukemia: Results and prognostic factors (a Pediatric Oncology Group Study). Blood 60: 1159–1168

Sullivan MP, Ramirez I (1985) Curability of Burkitt's lymphoma with high–dose cyclophosphamide–high-dose methotrexate therapy and intrathecal chemoprophylaxis. J Clin Oncol 3: 627–636

Vecchi V, Pession A, Serra L et al. (1981) Non-Hodgkin's lymphoma in children: results of treatment with the modified LSA$_2$-L$_2$ protocol. Med pediatr Oncol 9: 438–491

Watanabe A, Sullivan MP, Sutow WW, Wilbur JR (1973) Undifferentiated lymphoma, non-Burkitt's type: meningeal and bone marrow involvement in children. Am J Dis Child 125: 57–61

Weinstein HJ, Cassady JR, Levey R (1983) Long-term results of the APO protocol (vincristine, doxorubicin [adriamycin], and prednisone) for treatment of mediastinal lymphoblastic lymphoma. J Clin Oncol 1: 537–541

Weinstein HJ, Lack EE, Cassady JR (1984) APO therapy for malignant lymphomas of large cell "histiocytic" type of childhood: analysis of treatment results for 29 patients. Blood 64: 422–426

Willoughby MLN (1983) Treatment of overt CNS leukemia. In: Mastrangeo R, Poplack DG, Riccardi R (eds) Central nervous system prevention and treatment. Martinus Nijhoff, Boston, p 113

Ziegler J, Bluming A (1971) Intrathecal chemotherapy in Burkitt's lymphoma. Br Med J III: 508–512

Ziegler JL (1977) Treatment results of 54 American patients with Burkitt's lymphoma are similar to the African experience. N Engl J Med 297: 75–80

Ziegler JL (1981) Burkitt's lymphoma. N Engl J Med 305: 735–745

10 Effects of Therapy on Central Nervous System Functions in Children

K. KIAN ANG, ALBERT J. VAN DER KOGEL, and EMMANUEL VAN DER SCHUEREN

CONTENTS

10.1 Introduction 133
10.2 Clinical Manifestations of Iatrogenic Toxicity. . 134
10.2.1 Syndromes of Cerebral Toxicity 134
10.2.2 Myelopathy 139
10.2.3 Cognitive Impairment 140
10.2.4 Second Tumors 143
10.3 Experimental Studies 144
10.3.1 Determinants of Radiation Tolerance 144
10.3.2 Effects of Combining Chemotherapy and
       Radiation 145
10.3.3 Effects of Treatment on Behavior 145
10.4 Summary 146
     References 146

10.1 Introduction

The main indications for administering therapy to the central nervous system (CNS) in children are: treatment of primary CNS tumors, prophylaxis of intracranial relapse in childhood acute lymphoblastic leukemia (ALL), and, less frequently, treatment of skull base and paraspinal neoplasms (e.g., parameningeal rhabdomyosarcoma). Multimodality treatment is applied in most of these diseases. In children with primary CNS tumors, for example, radiation is usually combined with surgical resection and, in certain lesion types (e.g., medulloblastoma and germinoma), cytotoxic drugs may also be added. In ALL, on the other hand, radiation is routinely combined with systemic and intrathecal chemotherapy. As the survival of the majority of these children has gradually improved, late therapy sequelae have been

K. KIAN ANG, M.D. Ph.D., Professor and Deputy Chairman, Department of Radiotherapy, The University of Texas M.D. Anderson Cancer Center, 1515 Holcombe Blvd., Houston, Texas 77030, USA
ALBERT J. VAN DER KOGEL, Ph.D., Professor of Experimental Radiotherapy, Institute of Radiotherapy, University of Nijmegen, Geert Grooteplein 32, P.O. Box 9101, NL-6500 HB Nijmegen, The Netherlands
EMMANUEL VAN DER SCHUEREN, M.D., Professor and Head, Department of Radiotherapy, Academisch Zuikenhuis, St. Rafael's Kliniek, Kapucijnenvoer, B-3000 Leuven, Belgium

reported more frequently and concerns over the quality of life in long-term survivors have increased. Therefore, it is important to examine carefully iatrogenic toxicity in order to determine the scope of the problem and to identify major factors affecting the frequency of various types of complication. Concurrently, studies should be conducted to elucidate mechanisms of CNS injury. Such information will contribute to the optimization of treatment for most common childhood malignancies.

The purpose of this chapter is to review available clinical data on iatrogenic neurotoxicity and therapy-induced second malignancies. First, clinical manifestations of iatrogenic toxicity are discussed. We focus on late effects observed after treatment of primary CNS tumors and those associated with prophylactic therapy in childhood ALL. Effects of treatment on the neuroendocrine system are reviewed in another chapter. Then, recent experimental data and their clinical relevance are presented.

It became apparent from reviewing published clinical reports that the definition of "adverse effects" has changed gradually over the years because of refinement of the methods used to assess iatrogenic neurotoxicity. In earlier reports, deleterious effects usually meant overt neurologic deficits. Subsequently, in the late 1960s and early 1970s, attempts were made to quantify therapy-induced cognitive malfunction according to classification systems based on global description of daily functioning ability, such as "partially disabled either physically or mentally" or "impairment of intellect but are capable of being taught a trade," as proposed, for example, by BOUCHARD (1966) and BLOOM et al. (1969). More recently, many sophisticated specialized neuropsychometric and intelligence tests have been developed for grading cognitive skills and behavioral disorders in infants and children. In addition, advances in imaging techniques have made it possible to detect subtle structural changes in the brain; the relevance of these slight morphologic alterations, however, is still unclear. The change in the assessment methods makes it rather difficult to compare results of published series directly. To facilitate presentation and to partially circumvent the problem of changing definition we separate neurotoxicity into two groups, i.e., (a) overt functional deficits and (b) impairment of cognitive skills and learning disorders. Overt functional deficits are readily recognized by the child or parents and are detectable by routine neurologic evaluation. This group of sequelae is usually the consequence of histologically identifiable structural damage to the CNS (demyelination, necrosis). The type of symptoms and signs and the extent of the deficits depend on the site and size of the injury. On the other hand, the magnitude of impairment in cognitive skills is more cumbersome to quantify because of a wide spectrum of interindividual variations in the general population. The substrate of this neurotoxicity entity is unclear. It may reflect interference with postnatal CNS development resulting in disharmonious brain functions.

Radiation-induced neurotoxicities are best documented because a large number of children who have survived their disease are available for close follow-up and the manifestation after a fairly well defined latent period facilitates the diagnosis. The experience with chemotherapy is rather limited and the number of long-term survivors is still small. The functional repercussions of surgery have not been assessed systematically. Surgical complications have often been accepted as a "package deal" necessary to resect the disease. When gross resection cannot be accomplished, other therapy (e.g., radiation) is added. In general, neuropsychological evaluations are not performed until completion of the entire treatment. Therefore, it is difficult to discern the relative contribution of each therapy component to the development of cognitive impairment and behavioral disorders.

10.2 Clinical Manifestations of Iatrogenic Toxicity

10.2.1 Syndromes of Cerebral Toxicity

Traditionally, radiation-induced cerebral toxicity is defined on the basis of its temporal manifestation because of a lack of clear understanding of the underlying pathogenetic mechanisms. Arbitrarily, reference is made to acute, subacute, or late effects when symptoms and signs manifest within a few weeks, from 2 to 6 months, and more than 6 months from the start of therapy, respectively. This classification system, particularly the distinction between subacute effects and late toxicities, needs revision because lesions with overlapping time distributions are being recognized. For instance, there is firm evidence that the classical "late" radiation necrosis can occur at the latter part of the first 6-month period, especially after irradiation with high doses per fraction (SAFDARI et al. 1985). In addition, with the increasing role of chemotherapy in the management of malignancies, the vast majority of children and an increasing number of adults with cancer now receive combined treatments. Several chemotherapeutic agents used have been found to be toxic to the CNS by themselves. Consequently, more and more iatrogenic neurotoxicity observed is likely to result from adverse effects of drug–radiation interactions. A typical example is the association between delayed necrotizing leukoencephalopathy and high-dose chemotherapy (intravenous and intrathecal methotrexate) plus whole brain irradiation (BLEYER and GRIFFIN 1980).

In this section, we attempt to summarize various clinical entities according to the time of onset relative to the commencement of therapy. The clinical presentation and course, diagnosis, histopathology, and, when available, dose–response of these syndromes are discussed. In general terms most acute lesions are induced by chemical toxicity, while most of the clinically significant delayed complications (i.e., after latencies of at least 5–6 months) are secondary to radiation. After combined treatments, a complex spectrum of lesions emerges, with radiation enhancing chemical toxicity and vice versa. For example, acute chemical toxicity may be enhanced by radiation-induced modifications of the blood–brain barrier. An increased permeability of the blood–brain barrier has been produced experimentally with radiation doses in the therapeutic range (STORM et al. 1985; D'AVELLA et al. 1991).

10.2.1.1 Acute Cerebral Edema

Acute cerebral edema presents as an abrupt, reversible neurologic deterioration often with signs of intracranial hypertension manifesting within the first few weeks of radiotherapy. The symptoms and signs vary according to the segment of the CNS irradiated. This type of side-effect was observed in patients with intracerebral metastases who received whole brain irradiation with high incremental doses over a short duration. The pathologic substrate of this transient syndrome is not well known. It is thought to be the consequence of local edema, which is usually ameliorated by administration of corticosteroids. When severe, however, it may result in cerebral herniation

Young and co workers (1974) reported acute reactions in 49% of patients who received 15 Gy in two fractions as opposed to 15% of patients treated with 30 Gy in 15 fractions. Symptoms and signs observed included headache, nausea, vomiting, temperature elevation, and, in a few patients, cerebral herniation. Severe complications occurred primarily in patients with elevated intracranial pressure before commencement of radiotherapy. In a group of 54 patients who received a single dose of 10 Gy for cerebral metastases, reported by Hindo and associates (1970), four patients died within 2 days. It was difficult to assess the causative role of radiation because the patients who died shortly after irradiation had had severe neurologic problems before therapy. Conventional irradiation with 2 Gy or less per fraction to doses as high as 70–80 Gy rarely produces acute reactions in patients without preceding intracranial hypertension (Salazar et al. 1976; Linstadt et al. 1991).

Acute cerebral edema can occur a few hours after administration of high-dose cyclophosphamide through hyponatremia as a consequence of induction of inappropriate ADH secretion. This side-effect can be prevented by a diuretic such as furosemide (DeFronzo et al. 1973).

10.2.1.2 Acute Encephalopathy

Acute encephalopathy has been noted after administration of a number of cytotoxic agents such as L-asparaginase, methotrexate, and cytosine arabinoside (ara-C). Lethargy, somnolence, or confusion was observed about 1 week after *L-asparaginase* therapy in ~ 25% of children (Wesiss et al. 1974). More serious brain dysfunction resulting from thrombotic stroke has been associated with L-asparaginase therapy (Priest et al. 1980). The overall incidence of this complications is about 2%–3% (Clavell et al. 1986; Priest et al. 1982). The clinical features in these children include headaches, obtundation, hemiparesis, and seizures. Computed tomography performed a few days after the event reveals high-density lesions in more than 50% of children examined. The majority of children have full recovery of motor functions. However, of the 18 patients reported in the series of Priest and colleagues, five had mild residual hemiparesis and two had recurrent seizures.

Acute somnolence, fatigue, confusion, disorientation, seizures, or intracranial hypertension developing during or within a few hours after *high-dose intravenous methotrexate* (IV MTX) were reported in ~ 4% of children with osteosarcoma (Jaffe et al. 1985; Walker et al. 1986) and in two adults with lymphomas (Martino et al. 1984). This neurologic dysfunction appears to be transient. This form of encephalopathy has not been observed in children with leukemia or lymphoma (Bleyer and Poplack 1985).

Two types of neurotoxicity have been associated with the administration of *high-dose ara-C*, defined as ~3 g/m^2 every 12 h for 6–12 doses. The first, rather unique toxicity is cerebellar degeneration characterized by varying degrees of ataxia, dysarthria, and nystagmus. These signs appear 5–7 days after the first dose, worsen over the following 2–3 days, then stabilize over 2–6 days. Spontaneous complete recovery occurs during the next 1–2 weeks in the majority of patients (Lazarus et al. 1981; Salinsky et al. 1983; Winkelman and Hines 1983). The incidence of this complication is about 10%. Histologically, it is characterized by loss of Purkinje cells in the depths of cortical sulci with relative preservation of those at the crests of folia and those in the most posterior inferior portion of the cerebellum, diffuse microglial reaction, and antegrade degeneration of cerebellar cortoconuclear projections (Winkelman and Hines 1983). The second type of toxicity observed occasionally is cerebral dysfunction presenting as somnolence, confusion, seizures, lateral rectus palsy, and personality changes (Nand et al. 1986; Lazarus et al. 1981; Ventura et al. 1986). This transient cerebral dysfunction usually develops within 2 weeks of therapy.

Transient acute encephalopathy has also been noted in ~ 10% of patients after administration of *ifosfamide* (Pratt et al. 1990). Two to three days after commencement of therapy patients present with somnolence, confusion, and occasionally convulsions which subside rapidly after termination of treatment.

Acute encephalopathy has also been noted after administration of biologic response modifiers such as interferon -α and -β and interleukin-2 (Allen 1992). Symptoms and signs include reduced consciousness, worsening of focal neurologic deficit, and seizures.

10.2.1.3 Subacute Somnolence Syndrome and Focal Neurologic Abnormality

The subacute somnolence syndrome was recognized by Druckmann (1929), who observed a period of marked somnolence in 3% of children irradiated for ringworm of the scalp. In this group of children, the somnolence appeared 6–8 weeks after irradiation, persisted for up to 14 days, and then subsided spontaneously. The somnolence syndrome has also been observed in about 70% of children given prophylactic CNS therapy consisting of cranial irradiation (24 Gy in 12–16 fractions) and intrathecal methotrexate (IT MTX) for ALL (FREEMAN et al. 1973; PARKER et al. 1978). It is characterized primarily by drowsiness, nausea, and malaise without focal neurologic abnormality; these symptoms develop 3–8 weeks after cranial irradiation and persist for 1–5 weeks. However, anorexia, irritability, fever, dysphasia, ataxia, or papilledema may occur in some patients. Cranial irradiation of 18 Gy in 12 fractions induces anorexia, low-grade fever, and/or drowsiness of shorter duration (2–7 days) in 65% of children (OCHS et al. 1991). Electroencephalograms (EEGs) of these children nearly always show a diffuse slowing. The pathophysiology and histopathology of this syndrome are unknown. It is speculated that the syndrome is the result of temporary disturbance in myelin metabolism.

RIDER (1963) described a severe transient subacute neurologic dysfunction occurring in two patients who received 55 Gy in 16 and 27 fractions, respectively, for extracranial lesions. Symptoms and signs appeared 10 weeks after completion of irradiation and consisted of nausea, vomiting, cerebellar ataxia, dysarthria, dysphagia, and horizontal nystagmus. Recovery began 4–6 weeks after the onset of neurologic deterioration and was complete after 6–8 weeks. A similar clinical condition was observed in 25 of 51 patients with malignant gliomas treated with whole brain irradiation to 50 Gy (1.7–1.8 Gy fractions) and a 10-Gy boost dose followed by chemotherapy with BCNU at 8-week intervals (HOFFMAN et al. 1979). Neurologic deterioration manifested within 18 weeks after irradiation. Spontaneous improvement occurred in 7 of these 25 patients. Because the latent period of this syndrome corresponds with the turnover time for myelin, it was postulated that demyelination might be the underlying cause.

10.2.1.4 Subacute Cerebral Necrosis

Subacute cerebral necrosis has been reported in patients treated with very high doses of systemic chemotherapy with bone marrow rescue (DICHIRO et al. 1987; HUSAIN and GARCIA 1976). Chemonecro-

sis generally occurs within weeks to months after therapy. Its incidence is not well known because it usually occurs in patients with advanced disease with short life expectancy. The course of chemonecrosis is usually fatal. Histologically, it is characterized by a prominent vascular fibrinoid necrosis and discrete foci of coagulation necrosis distributed symmetrically with a predilection for gray matter (BURGER and BOYKO 1991).

Extensive parenchymal necrosis in a vascular distribution has also been reported after intracarotid chemotherapy with high-dose BCNU (BURGER et al. 1981; FOO et al. 1986; KLEINSCHMIDT-DEMASTERS 1986). Such lesions are characterized by a predilection for the gray matter in the distribution of the injected vessels. When intra-arterial chemotherapy is administered in conjunction with radiation, the lesions occur in the vascular distribution of the injected artery but have the histologic features of delayed radiation necrosis (MAHALEY et al. 1986). This observation suggests that interactions between radiation and certain cytotoxic drugs precipitate necrosis.

10.2.1.5 Delayed Necrotizing Leukoencephalopathy

A serious but fortunately much less frequent form of subacute late neurotoxicity is delayed necrotizing leukoencephalopathy, first reported by KAY and associates (1972). This syndrome typically manifests in children with ALL or primary brain tumors, 4–12 months after treatment with cranial irradiation plus methotrexate. It presents with the insidious onset of dementia, drooling, dysarthria, or dysphagia. The dementia usually progresses and is frequently accompanied by other neurologic signs such as spasticity, ataxia, seizures, and hemiplegia. In severe cases, the neurologic deterioration evolves progressively to coma, decerebration, and death. Most patients survive with signs of neurologic damage, though some have apparently recovered completely (FUSNER et al. 1977; WENDLING et al. 1978). A similar syndrome of varying severity has been noted in adults surviving intensive chemotherapy and elective cranial irradiation for small cell lung cancer (FRYTAK et al. 1989); LEE et al. 1986). The latent period in adults, however, ranges from 12 to 18 months.

GANJI and co-workers (1979) demonstrated that children with overt leukoencephalopathy had an elevated myelin basic protein concentration in the cerebrospinal fluid (> 4 mg/ml). In the early phase of leukoencephalopathy, CT demonstrates white matter abnormality mainly at the centrum ovale of the cerebral hemispheres, which presents as periventricular hypodensity, first around the frontal horns, then the occipital horns, and subsequently the entire ventricular system. The hypodense areas do not enhance after intavenous contrast administration. The late stage is marked by the presence of ventricular and subarachnoid dilatation with or without calcification in the central white matter (DiChiro et al. 1979).

Histologically, leukoencephalopathy is characterized by demyelination, axonal swelling, and fragmentation progressing to coagulation necrosis and gliosis (Hendin et al. 1974; Liu et al. 1978; Price and Jamieson 1978; Rubinstein et al. 1975). Initially, multifocal areas of coagulation necrosis usually associated with mineralized cellular debris are present in the deep white matter of the cerebral hemispheres. In the advanced stage, the white matter is reduced to a thin gliotic calcified layer. The cortical gray matter and basal ganglia are spared (Liu et al. 1978).

Bleyer and Griffin (1980) found after careful survey of literature data that the risk of leukoencephalopathy is proportional to the treatment intensity. Leukoencephalopathy has not been observed after cranial irradiation alone in the dose range of 18–24 Gy. The incidence of leukoencephalopathy after IT MTX to cumulative doses of >50 mg or IV MTX alone to cumulative doses of >18 g/m^2 is about 1%–2% (Fusner et al. 1977; Rosen et al. 1979). With two treatment modalities, cranial irradiation and IT MTX, the reported incidence ranges from 2% to 10% (Aur et al. 1977; Bleyer 1977). When three treatment modalities, cranial irradiation plus IV and IT MTX, are used, the incidence of leukoencephalopathy increases to 45% (Maurer et al. 1976). The risk of leukoencephalopathy also increases with increasing cumulative methotrexate and radiation doses. Systemic methotrexate > 400 mg, IT MTX > 150 mg, and cranial radiation dose >35 Gy are associated with a high incidence of leukoencephalopathy (Price and Jamieson 1978; Rubinstein et al. 1975).

With progressive refinement of CNS prophylaxis, the incidence of this form of neurotoxicity has decreased considerably. Clinically significant leukoencephalopathy was not observed in 49 children who received either 18 Gy CRT plus 16 doses of IT MTX (cumulative dose: 192 mg/m^2) or high-dose IV MTX (15 g/m^2) plus 15 doses of IT MTX (180 mg/m^2) and were followed for at least 5 years. None of these children had elevated levels of myelin basic protein in the CSF (Ochs et al. 1991).

10.2.1.6 Delayed Diffuse White Matter Abnormality

Diffuse white matter changes were first noted by Mikhael (1979) in an attempt to correlate the pattern of changes on CT scans and radiation dose. This abnormality emerges with the routine use of CT and magnetic resonance imaging (MRI) in the follow-up evaluation of patients; it presents as diffuse low-density lesions involving one or both cerebral hemispheres discernible several months after whole brain irradiation. Following partial cerebral irradiation, white matter alterations may extend beyond the high-dose volume. Such lesions are now best identified by T2-weighted MR images, which confirm the predilection for the periventricular regions (Constine et al. 1988; Curran et al. 1987; Tsuruda et al. 1987). Symptoms and signs associated with diffuse white matter abnormality vary from mild lassitude through personality change to marked, incapacitating dementia. Gradual memory loss progressing to severe dementia was observed in patients with pronounced ipsilateral or diffuse bilateral white matter changes (Burger et al. 1991; Constine et al. 1988).

The pathologic substrate for this entity has not been identified. Histopathologic findings are often limited to diffuse white matter pallor and reactive astrocytosis with a variable degree of edema (Burger et al. 1991). Precise dose-response data are not yet available. In adults, this syndrome generally occurs after whole brain doses of more than 50 Gy. In children, less pronounced white matter abnormality is observed after whole brain doses of 30–35 Gy (Packer et al. 1986).

10.2.1.7 Late Focal Necrosis

The most recognized late effect of therapeutic or incidental brain irradiation is frank necrosis, which tends to be more severe in the white matter (Kramer 1972; Sheline et al. 1980). Onset of this generally progressive, irreversible process in usually between 6 months and 2 years after high-dose irradiation. Radiation necrosis usually presents as a single focus within the supratentorial region. Occasionally, multiple lesions with a periventricular predilection have been observed (Safdari et al. 1984). Radiation necrosis produces an expansile and destructive lesion that becomes symptomatic because of a considerable mass effect. The clinical presentation includes focal neurologic deficits, seizures, and symptoms and signs of intracranial hypertension. The type and severity of focal neurologic deficits depend on the area and volume of brain affected.

Generally, CT reveals a single or, less frequently, multiple low-density white matter lesions with irregular contrast enhancement at the affected region, often associated with a more diffuse surrounding edema and a variable degree of mass effect (MIKHAEL 1979; VALK et al. 1988). Differentiation from disease recurrence may be difficult in patients who have been irradiated for intracerebral tumors. Positron emission tomography scan with radioactive fluorodeoxyglucose may be useful in distinguishing necrotic area from tumor by the absence of metabolic activity (DICHIRO et al. 1988; VALK et al. 1988).

Histologically, focal necrosis has a few dominant features. It is characterized by loss of myelin, swelling of axons, and a variable, invasion of foamy macrophages or reactive astrocytes. Gliosis occurs at the edge of the lesions. Usually necrotic blood vessels are seen within these lesions, but it is often difficult to find changes in larger vessels feeding into the area showing focal necrosis. Peculiar to iatrogenic radiation-induced necrosis is the presence of eosinophilic amorphous zones in the white matter that extend as tongues into the deeper layers of overlying gray matter (BURGER and BOYKO 1991).

Focal necrosis has rarely been observed after a total dose of <60 Gy when administered in ~ 2-Gy fractions (SHELINE et al. 1980). The threshold dose for fraction sizes of 1.8–2 Gy was estimated at ~ 58 Gy (LEIBEL and SHELINE 1991). The fraction size is a strong determinant of the dose–incidence relationship. Most of the reported cases of focal necrosis have occurred when radiation has been given in > 2.2 to 2.5-Gy fractions (SHELINE et al. 1980; WIGG et al. 1981).

10.2.1.8 Cerebrovasculopathies

The first type of therapy-induced vasculopathy reported is *mineralizing microangiopathy* associated with dystrophic calcification (PRICE and BIRDWELL 1978). The form of vasculopathy affects smaller blood vessels of the gray matter, mainly the putamen of the lenticular nuclei and cerebral cortical sulci. The lesion is recognizable on skull x-rays or CT scans as calcification in the region of the basal ganglia more than 10 months after completion of therapy. The neuropsychological repercussions of mineralizing microangiopathy may be minimal. In the series of Price and Birdwell, only 4 of 28 patients diagnosed

with mineralizing microangiopathy had neurologic symptoms and signs such as headache, focal seizures, ataxia, gait abnormality, and transient abnormal EEGs.

Histologically, mineralizing microangiopathy is characterized by calcium deposition primarily in small arteries, arterioles, capillaries, and venules, without inflammation (PRICE and BIRDWELL 1978). Lumina of smaller vessels are totally occluded by precipitated mineralized debris. Varying amounts of mineralized necrotic brain tissues surround the affected vessels.

In a postmortem study, PRICE and BIRDWELL (1978) found evidence of mineralizing microangiopathy in 28 of 114 (25%) children who survived ≥ 10 months after cranial irradiation (24 Gy) and IT MTX. In the series of MCINTOSH and associates (1977), calcifications in the region of the basal ganglia were identified on CT scans in 10 of 29 children who were in their first complete remission for ≥ 9 months after therapy. Cytosine arabinoside and high-dose methotrexate appear to promote development of this lesion (MCINTOSH et al. 1977). Calcifications were found in 10 of 16 children who received a cumulative dose of 0.4–5.5 g/m^2 of ara-C intravenously but in none of nine patients who received no ara-C. Regarding the 16 children treated with ara-C, calcifications were noted in 9 of 11 who also received a cumulative dose > 4.5 g/m^2 of IV MTX in contrast to one of five who received less than this amount. Children under 10 years appear to be more susceptible to this type of injury.

Another type of *late vasculopathy* initially described as a rare complication after moderate to high doses of radiation for the treatment of medulloblastomas or gliomas in children (PAINTER et al. 1975) has recently been reported by other investigators (ALLEN et al. 1991; CHUNG et al. 1992; EPSTEIN et al. 1992). The vascular lesions develop after very long latencies, varying from 2 years to more than 20 years after treatment of childhood brain tumors. There is a large variation in neurologic symptoms and signs, which often resemble those of hemorrhagic or ischemic infarcts. Narrowing of large vessels similar to radiation-induced extracerebral vasculopathies or vascular abnormalities similar to arteriovenous malformations (AVMs) were seen on neurodiagnostic imagings. These changes may sometimes be confused with progressive tumor growth. It is important to recognize this form of late effect to eliminate the danger of inappropriate treatment. The similarity with AVMs was confirmed in histopathologic studies showing large concentrations of abnormally structured blood vessels and the typical radiation-associated hyaline degenerations, formation of plaques and thrombi, and telangiectasia. These so-called late delayed lesions seem very similar to the vascular damage that develops in the rat spinal cord more than 1 year after irradiation (VAN DER KOGEL 1991a). Close follow-up of long-term survivors of childhood brain tumors is necessary to determine the incidence of this late effect and to identify possible predisposing factors for this type of late vasculopathy.

A milder form of vascular alteration, presenting as a fusiform aneurysmal dilatation of the supraclinoid carotid artery, was observed after radical microsurgical excision of childhood craniopharyngiomas (SUTTON et al. 1991). In a series of 31 children who underwent surgery between 1982 and 1990, nine were found to have fusiform aneurysmal dilatation of the carotid artery 6 months to 3 years after surgical procedures. One patient died of tumor recurrence and the remaining eight were alive and stable with a mean follow-up period of 3.7 years. None of these eight patients have had any symptoms or experienced hemorrhage as a consequence of the aneurysmal dilatation of the carotid artery, which is believed to have resulted from surgical manipulation.

10.2.2 Myelopathy

Several types of lesion described for the brain have counterparts in the spinal cord. In children many of the spinal cord injuries have been described after CNS treatment or prophylaxis for ALL with intrathecal chemotherapy and moderate doses of radiation (~24 Gy).

10.2.2.1 Acute Paraplegia

The development of acute paresis or paralysis has been mainly described after chemotherapy, most frequently with IT ara-C but also with IT MTX (reviewed by HAHN et al. 1983). The incidence of this side-effect is likely to be low because literature data are limited to case reports. The most common variety is flaccid paraplegia, often with pain and anesthesia, that develops within a day after IT chemotherapy. Recovery has occurred in the majority of affected patients. In some cases, however, the paralysis has ascended to cause respiratory failure, cardiac arrest, and death. Less frequently, a progressive spastic–ataxic paraparesis has become apparent

several weeks after a series of IT treatments. Although most authors ascribe these complications to direct neurotoxic effects of MTX and ara-C, it is possible that some of the symptoms and signs are caused by the preservatives and diluents of the drugs. Histopathologic changes are confined to the white matter and are characterized by diffuse microvacuolation, axonal swelling, and loss of myelin (BREUER et al. 1977).

10.2.2.2 Subacute Lhermitte Sign

The development of paresthesias, commonly described as Lhermitte sign, is a common side-effect of radiotherapy of a long spinal cord segment, such as mantle field irradiations for patients with Hodgkin's disease. The sign is observed after a latent period of 1–2 months and usually subsides within a few months. The occurrence of Lhermitte sign is rarely associated with permanent myelopathy, as it is induced by total doses of 35–40 Gy, which are well below those reported to result in radiation myelopathy (see below). The induction of Lhermitte sign has also been reported in connection with chemotherapy, notably cisplatin (LIST and KUMMET 1990). This usually mild side-effect resembles early somnolence syndromes after combined radio- and chemotherapy for brain tumors. The pathogenesis is likely demyelination or an interference with the turnover of myelin sheaths.

10.2.2.3 Delayed Myelopathy

The development of progressive myelopathy is one the most dreaded complications of *radiation treatment*. In attempts to avoid this complication, ultraconservative therapy approaches are frequently applied, which may compromise tumor control probability. Neurologic signs and symptoms of myelopathy are those of a progressive ascending myelopathy, often with signs of Brown-Séquard (ipsilateral paralysis and loss of discriminatory and joint sensation, and contralateral loss of pain and temperature sensation). The latent period is minimally 5–6 months, similar to radiation-induced focal necrosis in the brain. The histopathology is comparable to delayed necrotizing leukoencephalopathy or focal necrosis, with predilection for the white matter.

The dose–incidence relationship is reasonably well established in adults. A literature review by

SCHULTHEIS and STEPHENS (1992) indicates that a total dose of 45 Gy in 22–25 fractions results in ≤0.2% incidence of myelopathy. A realistic estimate of the ED_5 (less than 5% complications) for 2-Gy fractions is between 57 and 61 Gy. There are no firm clinical data to support the general belief that the radiation tolerance of the spinal cord is much lower in children than in adults, as only very few cases of childhood radiation myelopathy have been reported (SUNDARESAN et al. 1978). However, those few cases were observed after doses of about 40 Gy delivered in < 2 Gy per fraction. Therefore, it is reasonable to assume a lower tolerance in clinical practice and thus apply an approximately 5%–10% dose reduction in children.

Progressive delayed (5–6 months) demyelination of the cord has also been described after IT and IV *ara-C* administration (DUNTON et al. 1986). There are clinical data indicating that the risk of myelopathy in children is increased when intensive chemotherapy, such as combined intrathecal and intravenous MTX and ara-C, is administered concurrently with radiation (RANEY et al. 1992). Quantitative assessment in a rodent model, for example, showed that intrathecal ara-C reduces the radiation tolerance dose of the cervical spinal cord by about 20% (VAN DER KOGEL and SISSINGH 1985). Thus, it appears that ara-C and radiation are synergistic in causing spinal cord white matter injury.

10.2.3 Cognitive Impairment

Iatrogenic intellectual deterioration has received more attention in recent years. As mentioned earlier, it is difficult to quantify treatment-induced decline in intelligence because of the wide spectrum of interindividual variations in the general population. In children with brain tumors, the complexity is amplified by the presence of confounding factors known to affect cognitive functions such as destruction of nervous tissues by the neoplasm, presence of sensory and motor abnormalties, and intracranial hypertension. Lack of standardized methods to account for these variables might be responsible for the contradictory findings reported in the past. To facilitate discussion, we distinguish cognitive deficits observed in long-term survivors of ALL from those identified in children surviving primary brain tumors. This distinction is important because of critical differences in clinical and treatment characteristics between the two groups. First, children

with ALL have no cerebral dysfunction prior to CNS prophylaxis whereas those with primary brain tumors have preexisting confounding factors of varying degree. Second, the therapy for ALL is generally more uniform than treatment for primary brain tumors. Third, the intensity of CNS treatment is less in leukemia patients than in children with brain tumors.

10.2.3.1 Cognitive Functions in Survivors of Childhood ALL

The cognitive functioning of children cured of ALL has been studied extensively. Results of numerous retrospective studies undertaken to assess the adverse effects of *cranial irradiation* on cognitive function have been reported during the last two decades. The common caveats of these retrospective analyses include evaluation of patients treated during different periods, relatively short follow-up times, small sample sizes, and absence of pretreatment baseline data. In addition, most of the children treated with cranial irradiation also received intrathecal chemotherapy. Nevertheless, several conclusions can be derived from these studies. In summarizing the conclusions, the results of studies that involved a relatively larger number of patients and those that were designed to assess risk factors are discussed in detail.

There is evidence that the combination of cranial irradiation to a dose of 24 Gy delivered in 1.5 to 2-Gy fractions and IT MTX produces a mild, diffuse cerebral malfunction. This conclusion was drawn from the results of a relatively large retrospective study (COPELAND et al. 1988). The five groups of children enrolled in this study were: (a) newly diagnosed cases of leukemia or lymphoma who received triple intrathecal chemotherapy consisting of MTX, ara-C, and hydrocortisone ($n = 29$); (b) newly diagnosed cases of solid tumors or Hodgkin's disease who received no CNS treatment ($n = 21$); (c) long-term survivors (≥ 5 years) of leukemia or lymphoma who received triple intrathecal chemotherapy ($n = 24$); (a) long-term survivors of leukemia or lymphoma who received 24 Gy cranial irradiation and triple intrathecal chemotherapy ($n = 25$); and (e) long-term survivors of solid tumors or Hodgkin's disease who received no CNS treatment ($n = 25$). Cognitive test batteries administered included the Wechsler Intelligence Scale for Children–Revised (WISC-R, which measures Full-Scale, Verbal, and Performance IQs), the Wide Range Achievement Test

(WRAT, which evaluates reading, spelling, and arithmetic abilities), and the Peabody Individual Achievement Test (which assesses reading skills). The results showed that the IQ scores of all five groups of children were within the average normative range. However, children who received 24 Gy cranial irradiation and triple intrathecal chemotherapy scored slightly but consistently lower on Full-Scale IQ, Performance IQ, Arithmetic, Block Design, Coding, Similarities, and Picture Completion than those in other therapy groups.

There exists a relationship between the dose of prophylactic cranial irradiation and the late cognitive sequelae (HALBERG et al. 1992). A recent retrospective study assessed neuropsychological functioning of three groups of childhood cancer patients. The first two study groups consisted of children treated for ALL between 1971 and 1984 who received either 24 Gy cranial irradiation in 12 fractions ($n = 19$) or 18 Gy cranial irradiation in 10 fractions ($n = 16$). Both groups of children also received IT MTX (with cranial irradiation in 30 and after cranial irradiation in five) as additional CNS prophylaxis. The third group consisted of 12 children treated for Wilms' tumor during the same period; these children did not receive CNS therapy and were selected as controls in order to account for the possible disrupting effect that a significant illness could have on development. Each individual was administered the WISC-R test and WRAT. All participants were off therapy for at least 70 months at the time of neuropsychological assessment. It was found that the mean IQ and WRAT scores of all groups were within the average range (> 90). Direct comparison between the groups revealed that children who received 18 Gy cranial irradiation performed at the same level as controls. However, those who received 24 Gy performed significantly worse than the other two groups on all measures. Children who received 24 Gy scored on average 12 points less than those receiving 18 Gy. This study established that the threshold dose of cranial irradiation (when administered in conjuction with IT MTX) for inducing a mild, diffuse information-processing deficit is between 18 Gy in 10 fractions and 24 Gy in 12 fractions.

It appears that CNS therapy at age < 5 years is associated with a higher risk for developing cognitive impairment. In HALBERG et al.'s series (1992), eight of nine irradiated patients who had IQ scores of < 90 received cranial radiotherapy before they were 5 years old. This finding supports a previously reported observation that younger children tend to develop more severe neuropsychological dysfunction after

CNS prophylaxis (EISER and LANSDOWN 1977; JANNOUN 1983).

A recent report indicates that the sequence of IT MTX administration relative to cranial irradiation is a determinant of neuropsychological toxicity (BALSOM et al. 1991). In this retrospective study, two groups of patients were tested by WISC-R or the Wechsler Adult Intelligence Scale 2–11 years after receiving CNS prophylaxis. Both groups of children received six doses of IT MTX ($12\,mg/m^2$, max. $15\,mg$, per dose) and 24 Gy cranial irradiation (delivered in 2-Gy fractions), but in a different sequence. The control group received four doses of IT MTX during and two doses of IT MTX after cranial irradiation ($n = 45$), whereas the second (pre-RT) group was given two doses of IT MTX before and four doses of IT MTX during cranial irradiation ($n = 27$). Multiple regression analysis revealed that the Full-Scale IQ of the pre-RT group was 7.1 points higher than that of the control group, but the difference was not statistically significant ($P = 0.10$). Further analysis showed that the difference was due entirely to female patients. Among all the girls in the study, the Full-Scale IQ of the pre-RT group was 15.9 points higher than that of the control group ($P = 0.02$). The difference was even larger (28.5 points) and highly significant ($P = 0.0001$) in girls who were treated at less than 5 years of age. These findings are consistent with the results of a rodent study showing that the radiation-induced myelopathy can be ameliorated with methotrexate infused via the lateral cerebral ventricle beginning 7 days prior to irradiation (GEYER et al. 1988).

The neuropsychological toxicity of chemotherapy has not been evaluated adequately until recently. A comprehensive prospective trial addressed the relative toxicity of *parenteral methotrexate* versus cranial irradiation (OCHS et al. 1991). In this study, patients who achieved complete remission with induction chemotherapy were randomized to received either cranial irradiation (RT group) or IV MTX group) as CNS prophylaxis. Patients in the RT group received 18 Gy cranial irradiation in 12 fractions plus five concurrent doses of IT MTX; those in the MTX group received a total of 15 intravenous infusions of $1\,g/m^2$ methotrexate (first three at weekly intervals then every 6 weeks) and IT MTX. Patients in the RT group received a total of 192 mg/m^2 of IT MTX and those in the MTX group, 180 mg/m^2. Neuropsychological tests administered were the Wechsler Preschool Scale, Primary Scale of Intelligence, or WISC-R depending on the age, and the WRAT. Patients were tested immediately after remission induction, then at yearly intervals until cessation of therapy, and subsequently every other year over the next 5 years. The results showed that means for tests of intelligence or academic achievements did not differ between the two groups. With the exception of final arithmetic scores, means for tests of intelligence or academic achievements were not significantly different from the means of a normative population. However, statistically significant decreases in Full-Scale IQ, Verbal IQ and arithmetic achievement were found within both groups. Clinically important decreases ($\geq$15 points) on one or more neuropsychological measures occurred in 14 of 23 patients in the RT group and in 16 of 26 children in the MTX group. General follow-up evaluations revealed that 15 patients in the RT group had somnolence syndrome, and four developed cerebral calcifications late in their clinical course. In the MTX group, 15 had abnormal EEGs and six had early, transient white matter hypodensities on CT scans. There was no correlation between these changes and the neuropsychological test results. It was concluded that 18 Gy cranial irradiation and parenteral methotrexate are associated with comparable decreases in neuropsychological functions. The lack of a deficit pattern suggests, however, that other factors such as school absences and delayed development due to illness may have contributed to decreased cognitive functions.

10.2.3.2 Cognitive Deficits in Survivors of Childhood Brain Tumors

Literature data on cognitive deficits in survivors of childhood brain tumors are rather imprecise and conflicting because the methodology to discern the relative contributions of various factors is still in the developmental stage. Most articles report results of retrospective studies in a limited number of children with heterogeneous risk factors. Some conclusions and general impressions, particularly with regard to risk factors, are summarized.

It has been observed in numerous studies that a significant proportion of children surviving brain tumors have impaired intellectual, academic, and emotional status. Quantitative data were obtained by KUN and co-workers (1983), who conducted neuropsychological testing in 30 children (19 male and 11 female) who underwent treatment for primary brain tumors between 1979 and 1981. The age of the study population ranged from 2 to 16 years (median: 6) and the site of the primary tumor was supratentorial in 15 patients and infratentorial in the remaining 15. Nine patients were evaluated after surgery and 21 after postoperative radiotherapy. The radiation treatment was delivered in 1.5 1.8 Gy per fraction to total doses ranging from 50 to 54 Gy for partial brain irradiation or from 40 to 58 Gy for whole brain irradiation. Patients underwent a routine neurologic examination and neuropsychological assessments by methods appropriate for their age. The routine examination revealed that 24 children functioned at a normal or near normal level while six (two in the surgery group and four in the postoperative radiotherapy group) had significant impairment. Intellectual evaluations were successful in 23 patients (seven patients could not be assessed because of severe visual problems or language barrier) and revealed a median Full-Scale IQ of 97. However, the score was <70 in two children, 70–79 in two, and 80–89 in four. Two of the nine children tested before irradiation had below normal scores. The results of a second evaluation in ten children, performed 10–26 months after the first test, showed that the intellectual performance improved in two, deteriorated in three, and was stable in five. Social-emotional adjustment was assessed in 21 patients. Median scores on the Personality Inventory for Children tests were within the normal range in all categories but a strong tendency toward psychotic symptomatology was observed. The data suggest that children with supratentorial primaries and those receiving cranial irradiation tend to have more severe impairment. Potential selection bias, however, cannot be excluded.

The results of a prospective study suggest that young age at the time of treatment is a risk factor (MULHERN and KUN 1985). Twenty-six children (12 male and 14 female) who underwent treatment between 1980 and 1984 were assessed in this study. The age of the study population ranged from 2 to 16 years (median 7.8) and the site of the primary tumor was supratentorial in 15 patients and infratentorial in the remaining 11. Twenty-three patients underwent craniotomy during which gross total resection of the tumor was accomplished in 17 patients. All children received radiotherapy delivered in schedules similar to those used in the first study discussed earlier (KUN et al. 1983). Neuropsychological evaluations were carried our before and 6 months after radiotherapy. Deficits in selective attention were noted in 27% of children at initial evaluation and in 15% of children at second assessment. The proportion of children < 6 years of age manifesting attention deficits was greater than that of children $\geq$ 6 years

(63% vs 11% at initial assessment, and 33% vs 6% at second evaluation). In children ≥ 6 years of age, all intellectual parameters were within the normal range at both evaluations. The scores of younger children were also within the normal range at initial assessment. However, the mean memory score was significantly lower than in the normative sample at second evaluation. Overall, 63% of younger children, as opposed to 11% of older children, displayed clinical deterioration on one or more intellectual parameters ($P < 0.01$).

Two studies have recently been undertaken to evaluate the intellectual performance of children who have received whole brain irradiation. In the initial retrospective study, PACKER and co-workers (1988) assessed the intellectual performance of 24 children treated for primitive neuroectodermal tumor. They were treated with surgery, radiation, and, in some cases, also with systemic chemotherapy (CCNU, vincristine, and prednisone) between 1975 and 1984. The radiation treatment component consisted of ~ 40 Gy fractionated craniospinal irradiation plus boost irradiations to the primary tumor site to a median cumulative dose of 52 Gy (range: 45–65 Gy) for patients older than 2 years. Younger patients received 18–20 Gy craniospinal irradiation followed by boost irradiations to cumulative doses of 45–46 Gy. Nineteen children (79%) were found to function well in everyday activities. Neuropsychological tests revealed a median Full-Scale IQ of 97 (within the normal range) for the 17 patients assessed. Only three children had a Full-Scale IQ of < 80. Factors associated with poor performance and lower Full-Scale IQ were preoperative obtundation (mean IQ: 67) and the need for permanent shunt (mean IQ: 73). Younger age at diagnosis and complicated postoperative course also appeared to be associated with lower Full-Scale IQ.

In the subsequent prospective study, the intellectual performance of 18 children with primary brain tumors treated with postoperative whole brain irradiation and chemotherapy consisting of cisplatin, CCNU, or vincristine (13 patients) between 1983 and 1986 was evaluated and compared to that of the control group consisting of 14 children with cerebellar astrocytomas who underwent surgical resection only (PACKER et al. 1989). The radiotherapy regimens were 36 Gy whole brain irradiation plus 18–20 Gy boost dose for children older than 3 years and 24 Gy whole brain irradiation plus 24–26 Gy boost dose for children between 1.5 and 3 years. The mean baseline Full-Scale IQ of both groups was 105. There was no change in the Full-Scale IQ over the 2-year period in the control group; three children had Full-Scale IQs between 70 and 80 and one child required special education. In contrast, the Full-Scale IQ of the study group decreased to 97 and 91, 1 and 2 years after treatment, respectively. The decline in IQs at 2 years inversely correlated with age at diagnosis (children < 7 years of age had a median IQ of 82, as opposed to 102 for older patients). Two years after therapy, two children had IQs < 70 and seven had IQs > 100. Smaller declines were observed in Performance and Verbal IQs. Twelve patients (67%) required special education. This study demonstrated that cranial irradiation (whole brain plus boost) in combination with chemotherapy had little effect on the intellectual performance of children older than 7 years but decreased the Full-Scale IQ of younger children by ~ 25 points.

10.2.4 Second Tumors

The risk of developing a second malignancy becomes evident as more children survive the index cancer. The overall likelihood that survivors of childhood cancer will develop a second malignancy is estimated to be about 10 times higher than that in age-matched controls (OLSEN 1986). Factors contributing to this increased incidence include prior treatment, genetic predisposition, and environmental factors.

An update of The Late Effects Study Group (a consortium of 12 pediatric oncology institutions from the United States, Canada, and Europe) revealed 292 patients with second malignancies diagnosed between 1972 and 1983 (MEADOWS et al. 1985). Further analysis showed that the second tumors were located in tissues previously exposed to radiation in 198 (68%) patients. The most common tumor was bone sarcoma in patients who received irradiation with or without chemotherapy, whereas it was acute leukemia in those who received chemotherapy without irradiation. It was also noted that 73 of the 292 patients who developed second primaries had diseases known to be associated with increased incidence of cancer such as retinoblastoma and neurofibromatosis. This study thus demonstrates the contribution of prior therapy and genetic predisposition in the pathogenesis of second malignancies.

Recently, several investigators have studied the features of iatrogenic neural tumors in humans. The most extensive study was that conducted by RON and associates (1988) in 10,834 Israeli children who received low-dose irradiation (mean radiation dose of 1.5 Gy) for tinea capitis between 1948 and 1960.

Sixty neural tumors were observed in this population, which corresponds to a 30-year cumulative risk of 0.8% ± 0.2%. The estimated relative risks compared with 10834 matched controls and 5392 siblings who were not irradiated were 6.9 for all tumors and 8.4 for neural neoplasms of the head and neck. The most frequently occurring neural neoplasms were meningiomas, gliomas, and nerve sheath tumors. The relative risk varied with type of second primary. It was 9.5 for meningiomas, 2.6 for gliomas, 18.8 for nerve sheath tumors, and 3.3 for other neural neoplasms. A dose–response relationship was found in this study. The estimated relative risk was 3.4 for children receiving < 1.3 Gy as opposed to 20 for those irradiated to 2.5 Gy.

Second brain tumors have also been observed in children who received cranial irradiation (18–24 Gy) and IT MTX as CNS prophylaxis for ALL and those who received high-dose irradiation (generally from 40 to 60 Gy) for primary CNS neoplasms. General criteria applied for defining a neoplasm as treatment induced are: a long latent period, a location within the radiation portals, and a tumor histologically distinct from the primary lesion. Two types of tumor predominating in these clinical settings are gliomas and meningiomas. SHAPIRO and colleagues (1989) reported seven cases and found through a literature survey 30 more cases of malignant gliomas that occurred after radiation with or without chemotherapy (IT MTX). The primary diseases were CNS tumors, ALL, tinea capitis, and Hodgkin's disease. A wide range of radiation doses were delivered. The majority of patients received therapy for primary tumors at < 18 years of age. Consequently, the mean age at diagnosis of secondary gliomas was 24 years. The latent period between treatment and subsequent diagnosis of gliomas ranged from 1 to 26 years. The distribution appears bimodal, with one peak at 5–8 years and another at 21–28 years.

SOFFER and associates (1989) presented features of three patients with secondary intracranial meningiomas they observed along with those of 29 other cases reported in the literature. The primary diseases were CNS tumors, ALL, and vascular malformations. All but one patient received irradiation at a young age (mean age: 9.4 years). The mean latent period between initial treatment and diagnosis of meningiomas was 19.8 years (range: 2 to 47 years), which is shorter than the mean latency of meningiomas induced by low radiation doses used in the treatment of tinea capitis.

The relative risk of developing secondary cranial tumors after therapy has recently been evaluated by BRADA and co-workers (1992). These investigators assessed the risk of second brain tumors in a cohort of 334 patients with pituitary adenoma treated with conservative surgery and radiation (median dose: 45 Gy). Five patients developed a second brain tumor (astrocytoma in two, meningioma in two, and meningeal sarcoma in one) after a follow-up of 3760 person years. The estimated cumulative risk of developing a second brain tumor was 1.3% (95% confidence interval: 0.4%–3.9%) over the first 10 years and 1.9% (0.7–5.0%) over 20 years. The estimated relative risk of developing brain tumor compared with the incidence in the normal population was 9.4 (3.1–21.9).

Second brain tumors have also been observed in two children with ALL who received chemotherapy without radiation (REGELSON et al. 1965; TEFFT et al. 1968). It has not been possible to estimate the relative risk of drug-induced second CNS tumors because the number of long-term chemotherapy survivors is still limited.

10.3 Experimental Studies

10.3.1 Determinants of Radiation Tolerance

The basic strategy for radiation treatment of malignant diseases is to maximize the therapeutic differential between effects on tumors and surrounding normal tissues. From radiobiologic principles, this is generally achieved by dose fractionation and optimal distribution of these dose fractions in time. In adults, a reduction in the dose per fraction results in a substantial increase in the CNS tolerance provided the time interval between irradiations is long enough to allow cellular repair processes to proceed, whereas lengthening the overall duration of radiotherapy has a negligible impact. Recent experimental data indicate that these general time–dose fractionation features of adult CNS tolerance may not be applicable in infants and young children. The most critical factors determining the radiation tolerance of the CNS are briefly reviewed.

The effect of age on the *dose–incidence* relationship has recently been addressed in a rodent model. It was found that the ED_{50} (i.e., the dose for induction of paresis in 50% of animals) for a single radiation exposure (single dose) for 1-week-old rats is approximately 10% less than that for 3-week-old or adult animals (19.5 vs 21.5 Gy) (RUIFROK et al. 1992). This indicates that the CNS of very young individuals is slightly more sensitive to radiation-induced injury.

The impact of *fraction size* on the tolerated dose has been investigated extensively. Early clinical studies, followed by animal investigations in the rat spinal cord, showed a steep rise in tolerance when doses per fraction were decreased. In the linear-quadratic model of dose fractionation, the fractionation sensitivity is expressed as the α/β ratio. Low α/β ratios (i.e., 2–4 Gy) reflect a strong dependency of radiation tolerance on fraction size. For the endpoint of delayed white matter necrosis in brain and cord, α/β values are generally around 2 Gy for adult CNS, both in humans and in animals (LEIBEL and SHELINE 1991; VAN DER KOGEL 1991a). However, recent studies have revealed a lower fractionation sensitivity in 1-week-old rats, reflected in an α/β ratio of 4.5 Gy (Ruifrok et al. 1992). The lower single dose tolerance and higher α/β ratio suggest a reduced spinal cord tolerance to fractionated irradiations, but this lower tolerance may be compensated by proliferation during a course of several weeks (see below).

The importance of *time between fractions* has recently drawn much interest because of the occurrence of an unexpectedly high incidence of radiation myelopathy associated with the use of an accelerated radiation regimen delivering three irradiations per day (DISCHE 1991). The time between fractions was kept at a minimum of 6 h based on the initial results of a rodent study showing a half-time ($T_{1/2}$) of repair of ~ 1.5 h (ANG et al. 1987). The subsequent experimental study on repair kinetics in adult rat spinal cord by ANG et al. (1992) showed the presence of a slow repair component with a $T_{1/2}$ of 3.8 h. The higher than expected incidence of myelopathy after three fractions a day can be at least partly attributed to incomplete repair between fractions. So, it is important to account for the reduction in tolerance when two or more fractions are delivered per day. Recent studies on repair kinetics in the 1-week-old rat spinal cord showed a half-time of repair of 1.5 h, with no indication of a slow repair component (RUIFROK et al. 1993a). This observation would suggest more flexibility in using accelerated schedules for very young individuals and predict a possible large sparing associated with the use of continuous low-dose-rate irradiation. However, extrapolation from this experimental observation to the clinic should be done with extreme caution.

There is clear evidence that *extending the time intervals between fractions beyond 24* h does not lead to a further gain in the tolerance of adult CNS when the overall treatment time is in the range of 6–8 weeks. A recent split-dose experiment in 1 to 3-week-old rats, however, showed that lengthening the inter-

val between two irradiations from 1 to 6 weeks results in an increase in tolerance doses by 20%–30% (RUIFROK et al. 1993a).

10.3.2 Effects of Combining Chemotherapy and Radiation

Experimental data on the effects of chemotherapy on the radiation tolerance of the CNS are relatively scarce. The influence of age has not been addressed systematically. Cytotoxic agents found to modify CNS tolerance in adult rodents are ara-C and mitotane. Intrathecal ara-C at a dose of 100 mg/kg given *before* irradiation reduces the isoeffective radiation doses for white matter necrosis by ~ 20%, but has no detectable modifying effect when administered after irradiation (VAN DER KOGEL and SISSINGH 1985). Intraperitoneal administration of high-dose ara-C (9 g/kg) 2 h before irradiation also reduces the isoeffective radiation doses for white matter necrosis by ~ 20% (MENTEN et al. 1989). Oral mitotane given at a dose of 300 mg/kg daily for 5 days *before* irradiation reduces the tolerance by ~ 40%; administration of the agent after irradiation results in a tolerance reduction of ~ 15% (GLICKSMAN et al. 1982).

Methotrexate administered intrathecally (4 mg/kg) or infused into the lateral cerebral ventricle through a pump (which maintains a mean CSF concentration of 1.6×10^{-6} molar) before irradiation was found to result in a slight radioprotection, i.e., a 6%–9% increase in the isoeffective doses for white matter necrosis (VAN DER KOGEL and SISSINGH 1985; GEYER et al. 1988). In contrast, MTX given during or after irradiation had no detectable modifying effect (GEYER et al. 1988). These findings have recently been supported by clinical data in children with ALL receiving IT MTX and cranial irradiation in a different sequence (BALSOM et al. 1991).

Agents investigated and found to have no modifying effect are: AZQ (ANG et al. 1986), actinomycin, BCNU, and vincristine (reviewed by VAN DER KOGEL 1991b).

10.3.3 Effects of Treatment on Behavior

A rodent model has recently been developed to study the effects of therapy on spontaneous behavior in individual animals (MULLENIX et al. 1990). Briefly, a pair of rats, one experimental and one matched control, were placed simultaneously into a Plexiglas box containing a clear separation partition with small holes and tested during the first 15 min of exploration of the novel environment. A computer pattern recognition system automatically recorded and classified individual behavioral acts displayed during exploration. Analysis was based on comparison of behavioral initiations, total time, and time structure. The initial study revealed that a permanent gender-specific change in the time structure of behavior was induced by a combination of prednisolone, methotrexate, and radiation treatment but not by radiation alone. The effects observed consisted of abnormal clustering and dispersion of acts in a pattern indicative of disrupted development of sexually dimorphic behavior. This model would be useful in screening the relative neurotoxicity of various treatment modalities.

10.4 Summary

Long-term survival rates of children with cancer have improved considerably during the last few decades. As a consequence, an increasing number of late complications are being observed. Iatrogenic neurotoxicities, in general, affect the quality of life rather dramatically because they compromise self-care ability and interfere with the individual's integration in society. Therefore, it is essential to assess the frequency and study the pathogenesis of various treatment-induced CNS malfunctions so that future therapy refinement can also be directed at reducing the incidence and severity of neurotoxicities.

Side-effects of ionizing radiation have been studied extensively. The features of various radiation-induced complications are presented in this chapter. With greater insight into factors governing CNS radiation tolerance, the incidence of brain necrosis and myelopathy has recently been reduced, e.g., by delivering radiation in small dose fractions (1.8–2 Gy). There is clear evidence that cranial irradiation to doses of 50–60 Gy results in an observable decline in intellectual performance in about one-third of children. Children who receive radiotherapy to the whole brain at young age are most likely to be affected.

The morbidity of chemotherapy is being monitored. Several agents, such as methotrexate and cytosine arabinoside, have been found to be neurotoxic when administered intrathecally or given intravenously in high doses. These agents, administered concurrently with radiation, such as in CNS prophylaxis of children with ALL, have resulted in increased neurotoxicity. Modifications in radiation and drug dose and in the sequence of combined treatment have already diminished the treatment toxicity without reducing its efficacy in this subset of children. Studies are in progress to assess effects of treatment on behavior and to elucidate the pathogenesis of radiation- and drug-induced injury; hopefully, these studies will lead to the development of strategies effective in diminishing neurotoxicity.

Relative to the general population, long-term survivors of childhood cancers have been found to have an increased risk for developing new cancers. The higher incidence of second tumors in this population could be due to many factors. Previous radiation, chemotherapy, and genetic predisposition are perhaps the main contributors. Systematic follow-up of cohorts of patients treated with well-defined therapy schemes is essential to estimate the relative oncogenic effect of various agents.

References

Allen JC (1992) Complications of chemotherapy in patients with brain and spinal cord tumors. Pediatr Neurosurg 17: 218–224

Allen JC, Miller DC, Budzilovich GN, Epstein FJ (1991) Brain and spinal cord hemorrhage in long term survivors of malignant pediatric brain tumors – a possible late effect of therapy. Neurology 41: 148–150

Ang KK, van der Kogel AJ, van der Schueren E (1986) Effect of combined AZQ and radiation on the tolerance of the rat spinal cord. J Neurooncol 3: 349–352

Ang KK, Thames HD, van der Kogel AJ, van der Schueren E (1987) Is the rate of repair of radiation-induced sublethal damage in rat spinal cord dependent on the size of dose per fraction? Int J Radiat Oncol Biol Phys 13: 557–562

Ang KK, Jiang GL, Guttenberger R, Thames HD, Stephens LC, Smith CD, Feng Y (1992) Impact of spinal cord repair kinetics on the practice of altered fractionation schedules. Radiother Oncol 25: 287–294

Balsom WR, Bleyer WA, Robison LL et al. (1991) Intellectual function in long-term survivors of childhood acute lymphoblastic leukemia: protective effect of pre-irradiation methotrexate? A Children's Cancer Study Group study. Med Pediatr Oncol 19: 486–492

Bleyer WA, Griffin TW (1980) White matter necrosis, mineralizing micrangiography, and intellectual abilities in survivors of childhood leukemia: associations with central nervous system irradiation and methotrexate. In: Kagan JA, Gilbert AR (eds) Radiation damage to the nervous system, Raven, New York, pp 155–174

Bleyer WA, Poplack DG (1985) Prophylaxis and treatment of leukemia in the central nervous system and other sanctuaries. Semin Oncol 12: 131–148

Bloom HJG, Wallace ENK, Henk JM (1969) The treatment and prognosis of medulloblastoma in children: a study of 82 verified cases. AM J Roentgenol 105: 43–62

Bouchard J (1966) Radiation therapy for tumors and disease of the nervous system. Lea & Febiger, Philadelphia

Brada M, Ford D, Ashley S et al. (1992) Risk of second brain tumour after conservative surgery and radiotherapy for pituitary adenoma. Br Med J 304: 1343–1346

Breuer AC, Pitman SW, Dawson DM, Schoene WC (1977) Paraparesis following intrathecal cytosine arabinoside. Cancer 40: 2817–2822

Burger P, Boyko OP (1991) Radiation injury to the nervous system. In: Gutin P, Liebel S, Sheline G (eds) The pathology of central nervous system radiation injury. Raven, New York, pp 191–209

Burger PC, Kamenar E, Schold SC (1981) Encephalomyelopathy following high-dose BCNU therapy. Cancer 48:1318–1327

Chung E, Bodensteiner J, Hogg JP (1992) Spontaneous intracerebral hemorrhage: a very late delayed effect of radiation therapy. J. Child Neurol 7: 259–263

Clavell LA, Gelber RD, Cohen HJ et al. (1986) Four-agent induction and intensive asparaginase therapy for treatment of childhood acute lymphoblastic leukemia. N Engl J Med 315: 657–663

Constine LS, Konski A, Ekholm S (1988) Adverse effects of brain irradiation correlated with MR and CRT imaging. Int J Radiat Oncol Biol Phys 15: 319–330

Copeland DR, Dowell RE Jr, Fletcher JM et al. (1988) Neuropsychological effects of childhood cancer treatment. J Child Neurol 3: 53–62

Curran WJ, Heckt-Leavitt C, Schut L, Zimmerman RA, Nelson DF (1987) Magnetic resonance imaging of cranial radiation lesions. Int J Radiat Oncol Biol Phys 13: 1093–1098

d'Avella D, Cicciarello R, Albiero F et al. (1991) Quantitative study of blood-brain barrier permeability changes after experimental whole-brain radiation. Neurosurgery 30: 30–34

DeFronzo R, Braine H, Colvin OM (1973) Water intoxication in man after cyclophosphamide therapy. Ann Intern Med 78: 861–869

DiChiro G, Arimitsu T, Brooks RA, Morgenthaler DG, Johnson GS, Jones AE, Keller MR (1979) Computed tomography profiles of periventricular in hydrocephalus and leukoencephalopathy. Radiology 130: 661–666

DiChiro G, Oldfield E, Wright DC et al. (1987) Cerebral necrosis after radiotherapy and/or intraarterial chemotherapy for brain tumors: PET and neuropathologic studies. Am J Neuroradiol 8: 1083–1091

DiChiro G, Oldfield E, Wright DC (1988) Cerebral necrosis after radiotherapy and/or intraarterial chemotherapy for brain tumors: PET and neuropathologic studies. Am J Roentgenol 150: 189–197

Dische S (1991) Accelerated treatment and radiation myelitis. Radiother Oncol 20: 1–2

Druckmann A (1929) Schlafsucht als Folge der Röntgenbestrahlung. Beitrag zur Strahlenempfindlichkeit des Gehirns. Strahlentherapies 33: 382–384

Dunton SF, Nitschke R, Spruce WE, Bodensteiner J, Krous HF (1986) Progressive ascending paralysis following administration of intrathecal and intravenous cytosine arabinoside. Cancer 57: 1083–1088

Eiser C, Lansdown R (1977) Retrospective study of intellectual development in children treated for acute lymphoblastic leukemia. Arch Dis Child 52: 525–529

Epstein MA, Packer RJ, Rorke LB, Zimmerman RA, Goldwein JW, Sutton LN, Schut L (1992) Vascular malformation with radiation vasculopathy after treatment of chiasmatic/hypothalamic glioma. Cancer 70: 887–893

Foo SH, Choi IS, Berenstein A et al. (1986) Supraophtalmic intracarotid infusion of BCNU for malignant glioma. Neurology 36: 1437–1444

Frytak S, Shaw NJ, O'Neill BP (1989) Leukoencephalopathy in small cell lung cancer patients receiving prophylactic cranial irradiation. Am J Clin Oncol 12. 27–33

Fusner J, Poplack DG, Pizzo PA, DiChiro G (1977) Leukoencephalopathy following chemotherapy for rhabdomyosarcoma; reversibility of cerebral changes demonstrated by computed tomography. J Pediatr 91: 77–79

Gangji D, Reaman GH, Cohen SR, Bleyer WA, Ladisch S, Poplack DG (1979) Elevated basic myelin protein in the cerebrospinal fluid of acute lymphoblastic leukemia patients with leukoencephalopathy. Proc Am Assoc Cancer Res Am Assoc Clin Oncol 20: 353

Geyer JR, Taylor EM, Milstein JM, Shaw CM, Hubbard BA, Geraci JP, Thornquist M, Bleyer WA (1988) Radiation methotrexate, and white matter necrosis: laboratory evidence for neural radioprotection with preirradiation methotrexate. Int J Radiat Oncol Biol Phys 15: 373–375

Glicksman AS, Bliven SF, Leith JT (1982) Modification of radiation damage in rat spinal cord by mitotane. Cancer Treat Rep 66: 1545–1547

Hahn AF, Feasby TE, Gibert JJ (1983) Paraparesis following intrathecal chemotherapy. Neurology 33: 1032–1038

Halberg FE, Kramer JH, Morre IM, Wara WM, Matthay KK, Ablin AR (1992) Prophylactic cranial irradiation dose effects on late cognitive function in children treated for acute lymphoblastic leukemia. Int J Radiat Oncol Biol Phys 22: 13–16

Hendin B, DeVivo DC, Torach R, Lell M, Ragab AH, Vietti TJ (1974) Parenchymatous degeneration of the central nervous system in childhood leukemia. Cancer 33: 468–482

Hindo WA, DeTrana FA, Lee MS, Hendrickson FR (1970) Large dose increment irradiation in treatment of cerebral metastases. Cancer 26: 138–141

Hoffman WF, Levin VA, Wilson CB (1979) Evaluation of malignant glioma patients during the postirradiation period. J Neurosurg 50: 624–628

Husain MM, Garcia JH (1976) Cerebral "radiation necrosis": vascular and glial features. Acta Neuropathol (Berl) 36: 381–385

Jaffe W, Takaue Y, Anzai T, Robertson R (1985) Transient neurologic disturbances induced by high-dose methotrexate treatment. Cancer 56: 1356–1360

Jannoun K (1983) Are cognitive and educational development affected by age at which prophylactic therapy is given in acute lymphoblastic leukemia? Arch Dis Child 58: 953–958

Kay HEM, Knapton PJ, O'Sullivan JP et al. (1972) Encephalopathy in acute leukemia associated with methotrexate therapy. Arch Dis Child 47: 344–353

Kleinschmidt-Demasters BK (1986) Intracarotid BCNU leukoencephalopathy. Cancer 57: 1276–1280

Kramer S (1972) Radiation effect and tolerance of the central nervous system. Front Radiat Ther Oncol 6: 332–345

Kun LE, Mulhern RK, Crisco JJ (1983) Quality of life in children treated for brain tumors. J Neurosurg 58: 1–6

Lazarus HM, Herzig RH, Herzig G, Phillips GL, Roessmann U, Fishman DJ (1981) Central nervous system toxicity of high-dose systemic cytosine arabinoside. Cancer 48: 2577–2582

Lee JS, Umsawasdi T, Lee Y (1986) Neurotoxicity in long-term survivors of small cell lung cancer. Int J Radiat Oncol Biol Phys 12: 313–321

Leibel SA, Sheline GE (1991) Tolerance of the brain and spinal cord to conventional irradiation. In: Gutin PH, Leibel SA, Sheline GE (eds) Radiation injury to the nervous system. Raven, New York, pp 239–256

Linstadt DE, Edwards MSB, Prados M, Larson DA, Wara

WM (1991) Hyperfractionated irradiation for adults with brain stem gliomas. Int J Radiat Oncol Biol Phys 20. 757–760

List AF, Kummet TD (1990) Spinal cord toxicity complicating treatment with cisplatin and etoposide. Am J Clin Oncol 13: 256–258

Liu HM, Maurer HS, Vongsrivut S, Conway JJ (1978) Methotrexate encephalopathy. A neuropathologic study. Hum Pathol 9: 635–648

Mahaley MS Jr, Whaley RA, Blue M, Bertsch L (1986) Central neurotoxicity following intrcarotid BCNU chemotherapy for malignant gliomas. J Neurooncol 3: 297 314

Martino RL, Benson AB, Merritt JA, Brown JJ, Lesser JR (1984) Transient neurologic dysfunction following moderate-dose methotrexate for undifferentiated lymphoma. Cancer 54: 2003–2005

McIntosh S, Fischer DB, Rothman S, Rosenfield N, Lobel JS, O'Brien RT (1977) Intracranial calcifications in childhood leukemia; and association with systemic chemotherapy. J Pediatr 91: 909–913

Meadows AT, Baum E, Fossati-Bellani F et al. (1985) Second malignant neoplasms in children: an update from the Late Effects Study Group. J Clin Oncol 3: 532–538

Menten J, Landuyt W, van der Kogel AJ, Ang KK, van der Schueren E (1989) Effects of high dose intraperitoneal cytosine arabinoside on the radiation tolerance of the rat spinal cord. Int J Radiat Oncol Biol Phys 17: 131–134

Mikhael MA (1979) Radiation necrosis of the brain: correlation between patterns on computed tomography and dose of radiation. J Comput Assist Tomogr 3: 241–249

Mulhern RK, Kun LE (1985) Neuropsychologic function in children with brain tumors. III. Interval changes in the six months following treatment. Med Pediatr Oncol 13: 318–324

Mullenix PJ, Kernan WJ, Tassinari MS, Schunior A, Waber DP, Howes A, Tarbell NJ (1990) An animal model to study toxicity of central nervous system therapy for childhood acute lymphoblastic leukemia: effects on behavior. Cancer Res 50: 6461–6465

Nand S, Messmore HL, Patel R, Fisher SG, Fisher RI (1986) Neurotoxicity associated with systemic high-dose cytosine arabinoside. J Clin Oncol 4: 571–575

Ochs J, Mulhern R, Fairclough D et al. (1991) Comparison of neuropsychologic functioning and clinical indicators of neurotoxicity in long-term survivors of childhood leukemia given cranial radiation or parenteral methotrexate: a prospective study. J Clin Oncol 9: 145–151

Olsen JH (1986) Risk of second cancer after cancer in childhood. Cancer 57: 2250–2254

Packer RJ, Zimmerman RS, Bilaniuk LT (1986) Magnetic resonance imaging in the evaluation of treatment related central nervous system damage. Cancer 58: 635–640

Packer RJ, Sposto R, Atkins TE et al. (1987) Quality of life in children with primitive neuroectodermal tumor (medulloblastoma) of the posterior fossa. Pediatr Neurosci 13: 169–155

Packer RJ, Sutton LN, Atkins TE et al. (1989) A prospective study of cognitive function in children receiving whole-brain radiotherapy and chemotherapy: 2-year results J Neurosurg 70: 707–713

Painter MJ, Chutorian AM, Hilal SK (1975) Cerebrovasculopathy following irradiation in childhood. Neurology 25: 189–194

Pratt C, Goren MP, Meyer WH, Singh B, Dodge RK (1990) Ifosfamide neurotoxicity is related to previous cisplatin treatment for pediatric solid tumors. J Clin Oncol 8: 1399–1401

Price RA, Birdwell DA (1978) The central nervous system in childhood leukemia. Cancer 42: 717–728

Price RA, Jamieson PA (1978) The central nervous system in childhood leukemia. II. Subacute leukoencephalopathy. Cancer 35: 306–318

Priest JR, Ramsay NKC, Latchaw RE et al. (1980) Thrombotic and hemorrhagic strokes complicating early therapy for childhood acute lymphoblastic leukemia. Cancer 46: 1548–1554

Priest JR, Ramsay NKC, Steinherz PG et al. (1982) A syndrome of thrombosis and hemorrhage complicating L-asparaginase therapy for childhood acute lymphoblastic leukemia. J Pediatr 100: 984–989

Raney B, Tefft M, Heyn R, Newton W, Morris-Jones P, Haeberlen V, Maurer H (1992) Ascending myelitis after intensive chemotherapy and radiation therapy in children with cranial parameningeal sarcoma. Cancer 69: 1498–1506

Regelson W, Bross IDJ, Hananian J, Nigogosyan G (1965) Incidence of second primary neoplasms in children. Cancer 18: 58–72

Rider WD (1963) Radiation damage to the brain. A new syndrom. J Can Assoc Radiol 14: 67–69

Ron E, Modan B, Boice JD Jr, Alfandary E, Stovall M, Chetrit A, Katz L (1988) Tumors of the brain and nervous system after radiotherapy in childhood. N Engl J Med 19: 1033–1039

Rubinstein LJ, Herman MM, Long TF, Wilbur JR (1975) Disseminated necrotizing leukoencephalopathy; a complication of treated central nervous system leukemia and lymphoma. Cancer 35: 291–305

Ruifrok ACC, van der Kogel AJ (1993) The effect of intraspinal cytosine arabinoside on the re-irradiation tolerance of the cervical spinal cord of young and adult rats. Eur J Cancer 29A(12): 1766–1770

Ruifrok ACC, Kleiboer BJ, van der Kogel AJ (1992) Radiation tolerance and fractionation sensitivity of the developing rat cervical spinal cord. Int J Radiat Oncol Biol Phys 24: 505–510

Ruifrok ACC, Kleiboer BJ, van der Kogel AJ (1993a) Repair kinetics of radiation damage in the developing rat cervical spinal cord. Int J Radiat Biol 63: 501–508

Ruifrok ACC, Thames HD, van der Kogel AJ (1993b) Age-dependent retreatment tolerance of the rat cervical spinal cord. Proceedings of the 41st Annual Meeting of the Radiation Research Society, Dallas, p 62

Safdari GH, Boluix B, Gros C (1984) Multifocal brain radionecrosis masquerading as tumor dissemination. Surg Neurol 21: 35–41

Safdari H, Fuentes JM, Dubois JB, Alirezai M, Castan P, Vlahovitch B (1985) Radiation necrosis of the brain: time of onset and incidence related to total dose and fractionation of radiation. Neuroradiology 27: 44–47

Salazar OM, Rubin P, McDonald JV, Feldstein ML (1976) High dose radiation therapy in the treatment of glioblastoma multiforme: a preliminary report. Int J Radiat Oncol Biol Phys 1: 717–727

Salinsky MC, Levine RL, Aubuchon JP, Schutta HS (1983) Acute cerebellar dysfunction with high-dose ara-C therapy. Cancer 51: 426–429

Schultheiss TE, Stephens LC (1992) Invited review: permanent radiation myelopathy. Br J Radiol 65: 737–753

Shapiro S, Mealey J Jr, Sartorius C (1989) Radiation-induced intracranial malignant gliomas. J Neurosurg 71: 77–82

Sheline GE, Wara WM, Smith V (1980) Therapeutic irradiation and brain injury. Int J Radiat Oncol Biol Phys 6: 1215–1228

Soffer D, Gomori JM, Seigal T, Shalit MN (1989) Intracranial meningiomas after high-dose irradiation. Cancer 63: 1514–1519

Storm AJ, van der Kogel AJ, Nooter K (1985) Effect of X-irradiation on the pharmacokinetics of methotrexate in rats: alteration of the blood-brain barrier. Eur J Cancer Clin Oncol 21: 759–764

Sundaresan N, Gutierrez FA, Larsen MB (1978) Radiation myelopathy in children. Ann Neurol 4: 47–50

Sutton LN, Gusard D, Bruce DA, Fried A, Packer RJ, Zimmerman RA (1991) Fuisform dilatations of the carotid artery following radical surgery of childhood craniopharyngiomas. J Neurosurg 74: 695–700

Tefft M, Vawter GF, Mitus A (1968) Second primary neoplasms in children. Am J Roentgenol 103: 800–822

Tsuruda JS, Kortman KE, Bradley WG, Wheeler DC, Jan Dalsam W, Bradley TP (1987) Radiation effects on cerebral white matter: MR evaluation. Am J Radiol 149: 165–171

Valk PE, Budinger TF, Levin VA (1988) PET of malignant cerebral tumors after interstitial brachytherapy. Demonstration of metabolic activity and correlation with clinical outcome. J Neurosurg 69: 830–838

van der Kogel AJ (1991a) Central nervous system radiation injury in small animal models. In: Gutin PH, Leibel SA, Sheline GE (eds) Radiation injury to the nervous system. Raven, New York, pp 91–111

van der Kogel AJ (1991b) The nervous system: radiobiology and experimental pathology. In: Scherer E, Streffer C, Trott KR (eds) Radiopathology of organs and tissues. Springer, Berlin Heidelberg New York, pp 191–212

van der Kogel AJ, Sissingh HA (1985) Effects of intrathecal methotrexate and cytosine arabinoside on the radiation tolerance of the rat spinal cord. Radiother Oncol 4: 239–251

Ventura GJ, Keating MJ, Castellanos AM, Glass JP (1986) Reversible bilateral lateral rectus muscle palsy associated with high-dose cytosine arabinoside and metopantrane therapy. Cancer 58: 1633–1635

Walker RW, Allen JC, Rosen G, Caparros B (1986) Transient cerebral dysfunction secondary to high-dose methotrexate. J Clin Oncol 4: 1845–1850

Weiss HD, Walker MD, Wiernik PH (1974) Neurotoxicity of commonly used neoplastic agents. N Engl J Med 291: 75–81

Wendling LR, Bleyer WA, DiChiro G, McIlvanie SK (1978) Transient severe periventricular hypodensity after leukemia prophylaxis with cranial irradiation and intrathecal methotrexate. J Comput Assist Tomogr 2: 502–505

Wigg DR, Koschel K, Hodgson GS (1981) Tolerance of the mature human central nervous system to photon irradiation. Br J Radiol 54: 787–79

Winkelman MD, Hines JD (1983) Cerebellar degeneration caused by high-dose cytosine arabinoside: a clinicopathological study. Ann Neurol 14: 520–527

Young DF, Posner JB, Chu F (1974) Rapid-course radiation therapy of cerebral metastases: results and complications. Cancer 34: 1069–1076

11 Hodgkin's Disease

Nancy Price Mendenhall

CONTENTS

11.1   Introduction 151
11.2   Epidemiology and Etiology 151
11.3   Pathology 153
11.4   Patterns of Involvement and Spread 153
11.5   Diagnosis and Staging.................. 154
11.5.1 Biopsy Technique 154
11.5.2 Staging System....................... 154
11.5.3 Staging Evaluation.................... 154
11.6   Radiotherapy 156
11.6.1 Treatment Volume.................... 156
11.6.2 Dose 156
11.6.3 Technique.......................... 157
11.7   Treatment Results 165
11.7.1 Radiotherapy Alone................... 165
11.7.2 Chemotherapy Alone 166
11.7.3 Combined Modality Therapy 166
11.8   Complications of Treatment 166
11.8.1 Radiotherapy 166
11.8.2 Chemotherapy 170
11.8.3 Combined Modality Therapy 170
11.9   Management of Recurrent Disease 171
11.10 New Directions..................... 171
       References 171

11.1 Introduction

Hodgkin's disease (HD) is a disease of lymph nodes that has a predictable pattern of spread. The disease is unique in several respects. Most of the patients affected with this cancer are older children or young adults, and most are cured and will survive either to lead normal lives or to develop late sequelae of treatment. HD is usually very sensitive to both radiation and chemotherapy, which allows for many effective treatment approaches with either a single treatment modality or different combined modality regimens. The patterns of failure and toxicities of different treatment approaches vary, and the toxicities of both radiotherapy and various chemotherapy regimens are dose related. Because HD is one of the few malig-

Nancy P. Mendenhall, M.D., Professor and Chair, Department of Radiation Oncology, University of Florida Health Science Center, P.O. Box 100385, Gainesville, FL 32610–0385, USA

nancies in which there is a realistic chance of salvage in the event of first treatment failure, it is possible to choose a treatment option initially that produces a lower complication rate even though the risk of relapse may be higher. In this disease, perhaps more than in any other malignancy today, the clinician usually must choose among many treatment options and has the responsibility to consider not only the survival result, but also the late effects of the treatment choice (Donaldson 1984, 1990).

11.2 Epidemiology and Etiology

Approximately 7900 new cases of HD occur in the United States each year (Boring et al.1993), about half in patients between the ages of 15 and 30 years. About 10% of patients are less than 15 years of age (Donaldson et al.1976; Jenkin et al.1975). The disease is rare before the age of 4 years; only 2%–3% of all HD patients are in this age group. It gradually increases in incidence through the adolescent and young adult years to peak in the mid 20s. Before adolescence there is a strong male predominance beginning with a male to female ratio of 19:1 in patients less than 4 years old (Kung 1991). The male–female ratio decreases to 1.2:1 in the adolescent years (Jenkin et al. 1975; Norris et al. 1975; Parker et al. 1976) (Table 11.1).

The cause of HD is unknown. Although most cases of HD are neither obviously clustered nor temporally associated with a known infectious illness, evidence of case clustering has been reported that may be consistent with prior exposure to a common etiologic environmental factor. Schwartz et al. (1978) reported a cluster of ten cases of HD and three cases of non-Hodgkin's lymphoma (NHL) in a rural town of 1250 people over a 24-year period. The cases closely surrounded a large grain elevator storing navy beans. Lymphocytes of town residents compared with lymphocytes of nonresidents showed increased levels of transformations when challenged with navy bean extracts; a phytohemagglutinin from

Table 11.1. Age and gender distribution in children with HD

Institution, accrual dates	No. of pts.	Male – female ratio according to age range (yr)			
		0–5	6–10	11–15	0–15
Mayo Clinic, 1935–1970[a]	116	11:2	35:9	34:25	80:36
Princess Margaret Hospital, 1958–1973[b]	109	8:4	13:9	42:33	63:46
Stanford University School of Medicine, 1962–1974[c]	105	5:4	23:7	35:31	63:42
Total	330	24:10 (2.4)	71:25 (2.8)	111:89 (1.2)	206:124 (1.7)

[a] Norris et al. (1975)
[b] Jenkin et al. (1975)
[c] Parker et al. (1976)

the navy bean was isolated that had the ability to stimulate lymphocytes. SCHWARTZ et al. hypothesized that HD might result from altered immunity in the setting of chronic immune stimulation by a mitogenic substance in the environment. Clustering also is reported from Germany (DÖRKEN 1975), New South Wales (CORBETT and O'NEILL 1988), Wales and England (ALEXANDER et al. 1991), California (GLASER 1990), Washington State (ROSS and DAVIS 1990), Israel (ABRAMSON et al. 1980), Bahrain (HAMADEH et al. 1981), Newfoundland (BUEHLER 1983), Greater Manchester (MANGOUD et al. 1985), and Boston (GREENBERG et al. 1983).

In one study of 1803 newly diagnosed cases of HD, the young adult peak was attributable to the nodular sclerosing subtype of HD. The nodular sclerosing subtype appeared to have a different geographic distribution than the other subtypes of HD (ALEXANDER et al. 1991), and HD patients in the 50- to 79-year age range were more likely to have a lower socioeconomic status and to live in an urban area, whereas patients in the 0- to 24-year age range were more likely to have a higher socioeconomic status. In another study, a pattern of small, widely dispersed clusters was observed, rather than a large-scale cluster aground a single point source exposure, suggesting exposure to a ubiquitous environmental agent (GLASER 1990). In a study of HD in Washington State, the hypothesis of a viral etiologic component was tested by looking for spatial clustering of HD cases with varied assumptions of no latency period, different latency intervals, and different age-at-exposure intervals. Assuming no latency period or a latency period of less than 15 years revealed no evidence of clustering. However, in patients diagnosed after the age of 40, evidence suggestive of clustering in the childhood and teenage years was found, raising the possibility that exposure to a virus or other environ-

mental factor during a specific age interval was an etiologic factor (ROSS and DAVIS 1990).

Epstein-Barr virus (EBV) is known to be associated with other malignancies, such as endemic Burkitt's lymphoma and undifferentiated nasopharyngeal carcinoma (GAFFEY and WEISS 1990). Apparently, patient age at the time of exposure is important in these other illnesses. Infection with EBV during adolescence and early adulthood results in a clinical syndrome of infectious mononucleosis, whereas infection during childhood is associated with Burkitt's lymphoma; the time of exposure in association with nasopharyngeal carcinoma is less critical (DE-THÉ 1982). One argument against a causative relationship between EBV and HD is the fact that EBV is a common infection and HD is an uncommon malignancy. Additionally, many patients with serum antibody evidence of prior EBV infection do not develop HD, and no serum antibody evidence of prior infection can be identified in many patients with HD. However, new molecular techniques that are capable of identifying sequences of EBV genome incorporated into the DNA of human cells have demonstrated evidence of prior EBV infection in most patients with HD (KNECHT et al. 1991; PALLESEN et al. 1991; SAMOSZUK and RAVEL 1991). In one study (SHIBATA et al. 1991), multiple genotypes of EBV were found in mononucleosis patients, but only one EBV genotype was evident in patients with HD. In another study, the pattern of gene expression in patients with HD was similar to that seen in patients with undifferentiated nasopharyngeal carcinoma, but different from the pattern observed in patients with NHL (HERBST et al. 1991). One of the genes identified in the Reed-Sternberg cells is a gene coding for latent membrane protein, believed to be responsible for inducing cell transformation, and thus carrying the potential for being an etiologic agent in HD

(HERBST et al. 1991; PALLESEN et al. 1991). Some studies have shown that the EBV DNA is present primarily in Reed-Sternberg cells rather than in the normal inflammatory background cells (UHARA et al. 1990), but others have also reported the presence of EBV in some B and T lymphocytes in HD patients (WEISS 1991) and in other nonneoplastic cells (COATES et al. 1991). Molecular evidence of prior EBV infection is found less frequently in some histologic subtypes and presentations of HD than others (JARRETT et al. 1991; PALLESEN et al. 1991; WEISS 1991). An interesting hypothesis is that Reed-Sternberg cells may be natural hybridomas, formed when retroviral antigens expressed by the mononuclear HD cell attract reactive B and/or T cells that fuse with the HD cell rather than attack it (SINKOVICS 1991). Alternatively, the true Reed-Sternberg cell may be derived from an immature lymphoid cell that is infected with EBV, which activates antigen production characteristic of a mature activated lymphocyte, thus causing the apparent dissociation of phenotype and genotype in these cells (STEIN et al. 1991). Either hypothesis explains the origin of the Reed-Sternberg cell and is consistent with the theory that HD is a rare consequence of a latent infection with EBV virus, developing in the setting of a sustained host response to chronic tissue-based antigenic stimulation (MUELLER 1991).

11.3 Pathology

The diagnosis of HD is based on the finding of Reed-Sternberg cells in the midst of an appropriate inflammatory background of eosinophils, plasma cells, and normal lymphocytes. The lineage of the Reed-Sternberg cell is in question, although it is believed to be of the monocyte line. There are four basic histologic subtypes characterized by an increasing number of Reed-Sternberg cells and a decreasing number of normal-appearing inflammatory cells: lymphocyte predominant, nodular sclerosis, mixed cellularity, and lymphocyte depleted. The diagnosis of HD is usually easy for the hematopathologist, but even expert hematopathologists frequently disagree as to the histologic subtype. Although treatment is not predicated on histologic subtype, patterns of presentation correlate with subtype. Most patients with large mediastinal masses have the nodular sclerosis subtype. The mixed-cellularity subtype is most frequently associated with subclinical disease in the abdomen (identified at laparotomy) and, in some series, with

recurrence of the disease in pelvic lymph nodes (MAUCH et al. 1988). A high proportion of patients with limited peripheral disease have lymphocyte predominant HD.

Immunophenotyping and flow cytometry are important tools for excluding other lymphoid malignancies from the differential diagnosis, although neither technique will definitively identify HD, which has a heterogeneous phenotype. A subset of the lymphocyte-predominant histologic subtype has an immunophenotype consistent with B lymphocytes and contains evidence of EBV viral genome much less frequently than other histologic subtypes of HD (JARRETT et al. 1991; PALLESEN et al. 1991; WEISS 1991).

11.4 Patterns of Involvement and Spread

Hodgkin's disease is a disease of lymph nodes and usually remains within lymph nodes, with extranodal extension occurring only in the presence of bulky disease. The pattern of lymph node involvement is highly nonrandom. When a single nodal site is involved (stage I), it is in the low neck or supraclavicular area in approximately 70% of cases, the mediastinum in 10%, the axillae in 10%, and the inguinal and femoral nodes in the remaining 10%. When more than one but fewer than five sites are involved, the pattern of involvement is almost exclusively that of contiguous nodal groups. One apparent exception is the common involvement of the low neck or supraclavicular nodes and the spleen and/or upper abdominal (celiac, porta hepatic, splenic hilar, and upper para-aortic) nodes; the low neck and upper abdominal nodes are directly related through the thoracic duct.

Preauricular nodes may be involved in the presence of bulky upper neck nodes. Epitrochlear, popliteal, occipital, mesenteric, internal iliac, and presacral nodes are rarely involved in HD, even in advanced stages. The disproportionate involvement of nodes in the low neck and supraclavicular area is consistent with a viral component of origin in which the lymph nodes draining infected mucosal sites are most commonly involved. The pattern of contiguously involved lymph node groups when fewer than five sites are involved is most consistent with a single site of origin and spread through lymphatic channels. When more than four sites are involved, the pattern of involvement is less predictable and less likely to be confined to lymph nodes (KAPLAN 1980). Extranodal involvement most commonly comprises direct extension to the lung from adjacent mediastinal masses; pulmonary nodules, usually associated with large mediastinal masses or hilar adenopathy; or liver, bone, or bone marrow involvement, usually associated with extensive involvement of the spleen. Central nervous system involvement is extremely rare even in advanced disease. Direct extension into bone and the spinal canal occurs, however, with bulky disease, usually in the low neck area. Involvement of Waldeyer's ring is rare, even in the presence of bulky upper neck adenopathy, and makes the diagnosis suspect.

11.5 Diagnosis and Staging

11.5.1 Biopsy Technique

The differential diagnosis in children and young adults with adenopathy includes infection, particularly cat-scratch fever, and other malignancies such as NHL, leukemia, lymphoepithelioma, and rhabdomyosarcoma, as well as HD. Lymph nodes involved by HD are usually nontender, firm but not rock-hard, rubbery, and plump. The history may be confusing because adenopathy in HD may wax and wane. Most patients have had a trial of antibiotic therapy before biopsy. When biopsy is performed, it is preferable to remove the largest, most clinically suspicious node rather than a smaller, more superficial node as there are often enlarged, but histologically normal, nodes associated with HD. The entire lymph node should be removed if possible, because some processes are focal, and knowledge of the pattern of involvement within the lymph node may be useful to the pathologist. The histology must be reviewed by an expert hematopathologist, because HD may be confused with benign processes and NHL. If HD or NHL is suspected, biopsy material is always sent for flow cytometry and immunophenotyping in addition to histologic study.

11.5.2 Staging System

The Ann Arbor staging system is used (Table 11.2) (American Joint Committee on Cancer 1988). A useful modification is the distinction between stage III_1 disease, which includes only involvement of the upper abdomen (the spleen, splenic hilar, celiac, and porta hepatic nodes), and III_2 disease, which includes lower abdominal involvement (para-aortic and pelvic nodes) (DESSER et al. 1977). In all stages, spleen

Table 11.2. Staging system[a]

Stage	Description
I	Involvement of single lymph node region (I) or localized involvement of a single extralymphatic organ or site (I_E).
II	Involvement of two or more lymph node regions on the same side of the diaphragm (II) or localized involvement of a single associated extralymphatic organ or site and its regions on the same side of the diaphragm (II_E). Note: The number of lymph node regions involved may be indicated by a subscript (e.g., II_3).
III	Involvement of lymph node regions on both sides of the diaphragm (III), which may also be accompanied by localized involvement of an associated extralymphatic organ or site (III_E), by involvement of the spleen (III_S), or both (III_{E+S}).
IV	Disseminated (multifocal) involvement of one or more extralymphatic organs, with or without associated lymph node involvement, or isolated extralymphatic organ involvement with distant (non regional) nodal involvement.

[a]American Joint Committee on Cancer (1988)

involvement is indicated by the subscript S and extranodal extension by the subscript E.

All patients are also classified as to whether constitutional symptoms are present; if one or more of these symptoms is present, a postscript of B is added to the stage, and if not, a postscript of A is added. The constitutional symptoms are strictly defined as unexplained weight loss of greater than 10% of normal body weight in a period of no more than 6 months before diagnosis, fever greater than 101°F, and night sweats. Other symptoms noted to occur in patients with HD, but not classified as B symptoms, include pruritus and alcohol-induced pain. The pruritus, most frequently generalized and severe, is often the reason for which the patient seeks medical attention. Alcohol-induced pain is rare, but striking when present; it is usually localized to sites of disease and may be the first indication of disease recurrence.

11.5.3 Staging Evaluation

A thorough history is obtained with emphasis on the presence of B symptoms, other constitutional symptoms, general performance status, and symptoms indicative of sites of disease such as cough, shortness of breath, chest pain, back pain, and bone pain. The past medical history is explored for evidence of prior infection, specifically mononucleosis and a history of warts (MAUCH et al. 1983). A child's remaining growth potential is assessed based on age, parental stature, and Tanner stage.

A thorough physical examination is performed, documenting abnormalities in Waldeyer's ring , the condition of the teeth, the presence and size of any abnormal lymph nodes in all potential node-bearing sites, and the status of the liver and spleen. A routine cardiopulmonary examination is performed, and the axial skeleton is percussed to elicit any bony tenderness.

Routine laboratory studies include complete blood cell count, platelet count, sedimentation rate, liver function studies, renal profile, and baseline thyroid function studies.

Routine imaging studies include chest roentgenography and computed tomography (CT) of the chest, abdomen, and pelvis. Lymphangiography is a standard part of the imaging evaluation in adults but is often difficult to perform in children and is no longer carried out in children in many centers. The primary advantage of lymphangiography is its capacity to identify filling defects and architectural changes indicative of HD in normal-sized lymph nodes that would not be apparent on pelvic CT. However, lymphangiograms reliably show only the pelvic and para-aortic nodes and thus cannot identify IIIA1 disease; additionally, they are technically difficult to perform and difficult for the inexperienced radiologist to interpret. In studies comparing the accuracy of CT and lymphangiograms for identifying abdominal and pelvic disease, the results are mixed (CASTELLINO et al. 1984; JONSSON et al. 1983; MAGNUSSON et al. 1982; MANSFIELD et al. 1991; SOMBECK et al. 1993). Lymphangiograms aid in treatment planning for patients receiving pelvic irradiation and in follow-up for the early detection of pelvic lymph node recurrences. Additional imaging studies that are useful in certain settings include magnetic resonance imaging (MRI) in the chest to delineate hilar adenopathy and pericardial extension, gallium scanning, and MRI in the abdomen to distinguish unfilled bowel and vessels from retroperitoneal, porta hepatic, and celiac adenopathy.

Despite the use of modern abdominal imaging techniques, the inaccuracy of clinical staging is 25%–45% (Table 11.3). Laparotomy for pathologic staging includes removal of the spleen, multiple wedge and needle biopsies of the liver, and multiple biopsies of abdominal and pelvic lymph nodes. Because chemotherapy is effective in eliminating subclinical disease, the role of laparotomy with splenectomy is in question. The major complication arising from splenectomy is an increased rate of infection, specifically from encapsulated organisms such as *Pneumococcus*, leading to pneumonia, sepsis, and meningitis. The rate of such infections even before the development of prophylactic presplenectomy vaccination with Pneumovax was quite low, estimated at 5%–10% (Table 11.4). Since the routine administration of Pneumovax before splenectomy and prophylactic antibiotic therapy after splenectomy, most major institutions treating children with HD report few serious infections.

The risk of such infections is correlated with the presence of advanced or recurrent disease and possibly with the use of extensive chemotherapy (ABRAHAMSEN et al. 1990; BACCARANI et al. 1986; DONALDSON and KAPLAN 1982; SCHIMPFF et al. 1975). The main advantage of laparotomy is knowledge of the presence and extent of abdominal and pelvic disease, which may influence the radiation treatment volume and the amount of chemotherapy delivered. Additional advantages of laparotomy include an opportunity for oophoropexy in female patients and, because the spleen is removed, a significant decrease in the amount of lung and kidney irradiated. Larger volumes of these organs are necessarily exposed to radiation when the spleen must be irradiated .

Table 11.3. Incidence of stage change with laparotomy

Institution, accrual dates	Patients	Age range (yr)	Patients with stage change at laparotomy		
			Up-staged	Down-staged	Total changed (%)
Children's Hospital of Western Ontario, 1970–1986[a]	39	≤ 18	5	12	17 (44)
Stanford University Medical Center, 1970–1983[b]	53	≤ 14	14	7	21 (40)
Pediatric Oncology Group, 1986–1991[c]	203	≤ 21	52	4	56 (28)

[a] SCHNEEBERGER and GIRVAN (1988)
[b] DONALDSON and LINK (1987)
[c] MENDENHALL et al. (1993)

Table 11.4. Risk of serious infection after splenectomy for IID[a]

Institution, date of report	Patients	Patients with serious infection (%)		Patients dead of infection (%)	
Collected series, 1972[b]	1170	16	(< 1)	6	(< 1)
Baltimore Cancer Research Center, 1975[c]	92	6	(< 7)	3	(3)
Children's Cancer Study Group, 1976[d]	200	18	(9)	8	(4)
Stanford University Medical Center, 1982[e]	146	16	(11)	< 4	(< 3)
Intergroup Hodgkin's Disease in Childhood Study, 1984[f]	234	4	(1.7)	0	(0)
University of Chicago, 1985[g]	239	2	(< 1)	1	(< 1)
Bologna, 1986[h]	342	5	(1.8)	3	(1)
Joint Center for Radiation Therapy, 1988[i]	315	8	(2)	2	(< 1)
University of Florida, 1992[a]	133	9	(7)	1	(< 1)

[a] JOCKOVICH et al. (1994)
[b] DESSER and ULTMANN (1972)
[c] SCHIMPFF et al. (1975)
[d] CHILCOTE et al. (1976)
[e] DONALDSON and KAPLAN (1982)
[f] HAYS et al. (1984)
[g] CORNBLEET et al. (1985)
[h] BACCARANI et al. (1986)
[i] MAUCH et al. (1988)

11.6 Radiotherapy

11.6.1 Treatment Volume

Treatment initially was given only to the site of involvement, but early attention to the patterns of failure after localized treatment showed that most failures occurred outside the irradiated volume in adjacent nodal sites, leading to the concept of "complementary field" or adjacent nodal area irradiation to eliminate subclinical disease (PETERS 1966). Standard radiation treatment volumes include the following:

– *Involved field* irradiation includes the entire nodal area (not just the particular node).
– *Extended field* irradiation includes the involved nodal area and the clinically uninvolved contiguous nodal areas at risk for subclinical disease (KAPLAN 1980).
– *Mantle field* irradiation includes the neck, supraclavicular, infraclavicular, axillary, mediastinal, hilar, and inferior mediastinal lymph nodes. This field is extended to include the entire cardiac silhouette and half or all the lung parenchyma when indicated.
– *Total nodal* irradiation treats all nodal areas usually involved in HD including mantle, para-aortic, spleen (if present), pelvic, inguinal, and femoral lymph node fields.
– *Subtotal or modified total nodal* irradiation is identical to total nodal irradiation but does not include the pelvic, inguinal, and femoral lymph nodes.
– *Inverted Y* irradiation treats the femoral, inguinal, pelvic, and para-aortic nodes ± spleen and/or splenic pedicle.
– *Liver* irradiation treats the liver in a separate field or in combination with a para-aortic node field.
– *Preauricular field* irradiation treats a small volume encompassing the preauricular nodes.
– *Waldeyer's ring field* irradiation includes the pre- and postauricular nodes, the occipital nodes, and the lymphoid structures in the base of tongue, tonsillar fossae, and nasopharynx; this treatment is rarely necessary in HD.
– *Comprehensive lymphatic* (total nodal, comprehensive lymphoid) irradiation includes mantle, Waldeyer's ring, whole abdominal, pelvic, inguinal, and femoral irradiation. This field is used rarely in HD but more often in non-Hodgkin's lymphoma, where mesenteric node involvement is common.

11.6.2 Dose

Early studies demonstrated increased control rates in HD with doses of 25 Gy or higher (PETERS 1966). The relationship between tumor control and radiation dose was first described as linear (KAPLAN 1980) and later as a sigmoid curve (FLETCHER and SHUKOVSKY 1975). Recent retrospective studies have failed to demonstrate increased control rates with

Table 11.5 Local control (in field) of stage I–III HD in children (≤ 18 years old) treated with radiotherapy alone (*n* = 40)[a]

Dose (Gy)	Sites controlled/sites treated	
	Clinically negative sites	Clinically positive sites
< 25	10/10	1/1
25–29.99	36/36	5/5
30–34.99	72/72	9/9
35–39.99	76/76	45/49 (92%)
≥ 40	9/9	13/14 (93%)
Total	203/203 (100%)	73/78 (94%)

[a] Courtesy of W. Mark McCollough, M.D. Patients treated at University of Florida from October 1964 to February 1986; analysis March 1988

doses above 30 Gy, providing evidence for a sigmoid dose-response relationship in HD (Hanks et al. 1983; Schewe et al. 1988; Thar et al. 1979). The rates of local control in stage I and II pediatric (less than 16 years old) patients treated for HD at the University of Florida with radiotherapy alone or in conjunction with chemotherapy are correlated with radiation dose in Table 11.5. Doses of 25–30 Gy for subclinical disease and 30–35 cGy for clinically evident disease are usually adequate for local control when radiotherapy is used alone.

When radiotherapy is used in conjunction with chemotherapy, the doses of radiation may be reduced. When a complete response is achieved with six cycles of chemotherapy, a dose of 15–25 Gy is sufficient (Behrendt et al. 1987; Dionet et al. 1988; Donaldson and Link 1987; Jenkin et al. 1982; Prosnitz et al. 1985, 1988). Response to chemotherapy is predictive of the likelihood of local control. At the University of Florida, local recurrences were observed only in patients who did not demonstrate a complete response to chemotherapy (Table 11.6). If less than a complete response is achieved with chemotherapy, it is unclear whether the dose of radiation can be reduced, so standard doses (30–35 Gy for clinically evident disease and 25–30 Gy for subclinical disease) are recommended. The minimum dose of radiation necessary to ensure a high probability of local control in conjunction with two to four cycles of chemotherapy is unknown. The Pediatric Oncology Group is investigating the efficacy of 25 Gy to involved sites after a complete response to four cycles of chemotherapy.

11.6.3 Technique

The treatment technique for HD is difficult and varies even among centers with extensive experience in the management of HD. The technique used at the University of Florida is discussed in this chapter. Other appropriate treatment techniques are described in other sources (Kaplan 1980). The national Patterns of Care study demonstrated that the likelihood of relapse or death in patients treated with radiation therapy for HD varies with the institution and that relapse and death rates, which are associated with inadequate field margins, are significantly higher in community practices than in academic institutions (Hanks et al. 1983). Therefore, if radiotherapy is used to treat a child with HD, it should be delivered in an academic center that has experience with this treatment.

11.6.3.1 Standard Mantle

The mantle field includes the lymph nodes in the upper, mid, and lower cervical chains, and the

Table 11.6. Local control (in field) according to chemotherapy response in children (≤ 18 years old) with HD treated with combined modality therapy (n = 27)[a]

Stage	Local control in radiotherapy field correlated with chemotherapy response			
	Excluded[b]	No response	Partial response	Complete response
I	0	No data	No data	1/1
II	1	0/2	1/1	6/6
III	1[c]	0/1	3/6	4/4
IV	1	No data	0/1	2/2
Total		0/3	4/8	13/13

[a] Courtesy of W. Mark McCollough, M.D. Patients treated at University of Florida from October 1964 to February 1986; analysis March 1988 [b] Excluded if patient died less than 2 years after treatment or disease recurred out of field with no evidence of local recurrence [c] Received radiotherapy before chemotherapy

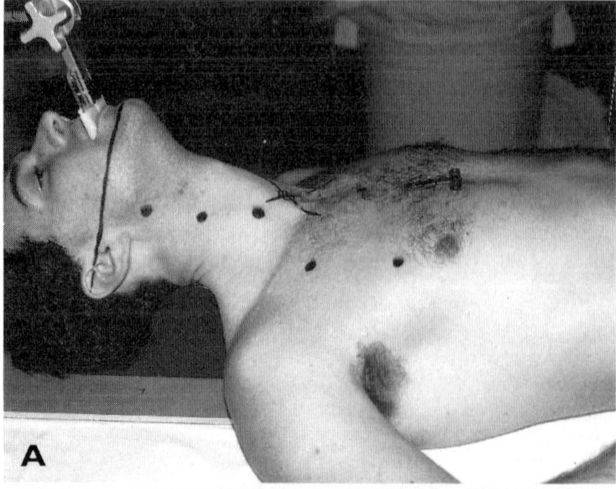

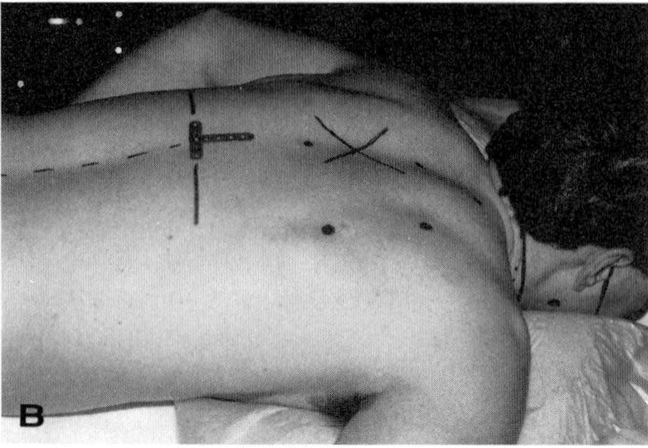

Fig. 11.1. A The first step in simulation of the mantle field is to establish a reproducible treatment position. The patient is aligned on the simulation table with a midline laser, neck extension is positioned with a bite block, and arms are placed akimbo. The superior border of the mantle is set so that the beam will pass through the mandible and mid tragus, and the inferior border is placed according to the presence and extent of mediastinal disease. Points for dose calculations with the Clarkson technique are marked with radiopaque dots before taking the simulation film. For a standard mantle, these points include the upper, mid, and lower neck; the mid and low axilla; the central axis, which usually falls at approximately the suprasternal notch; the spinal cord; the mid and inferior mediastinum; and the anterior pericardium. **B** A customized body mold is fabricated for the posterior mantle field to assure reproducible positioning of the patient. The arms are placed akimbo. The inferior border of the mantle is determined by the presence and extent of mediastinal disease, and the superior border is set so that the beam will exit at approximately the thyroid notch, flashing across the trapezius muscle. This technique avoids irradiation of the posterior fossa or mandible, but does require the addition of an anterior upper neck boost (see Fig. 11.2J)

submental, supraclavicular, infraclavicular, mid and low axillary, mediastinal, hilar, and internal mammary areas. The mantle is treated with anterior and posterior fields. For treatment of the anterior field, the patient is supine with elbows flexed to 90° and hands resting on iliac crests (Fig.11.1A). [In some centers, the arms are elevated and the hands are

placed on the vertex of the head in an attempt to raise axillary and infraclavicular lymph nodes superiorly (and laterally) and thereby to irradiate less lung.] A bite block and head holder secure reproducible neck extension and immobility. The patient is leveled and aligned on the simulation table with a midline laser.

For treatment of the posterior field (Fig.11.1B), the patient is prone in a customized upper torso mold. The arms are abducted to 90°, and the hands are placed on the iliac crests. The treatment volume is the same as for the anterior mantle with two exceptions. The upper border is set at simulation so that the radiation beam exits through the thyroid notch, and the upper neck nodes, the posterior fossa, and the oral cavity are not treated through the posterior portal; an anterior upper neck boost is required to achieve a sufficient upper neck dose (Fig.11.2J). In addition, the infraclavicular nodes are not included in the posterior field unless clinically involved; therefore, the lung blocks extend cephalad to just below the clavicles. (This technique spares additional lung, but can only be used if the fields are weighted 3:2 in favor of the anterior portal so that the infraclavicular nodes will receive a sufficient dose from the anterior portal alone.)

The treatment of a 14-year-old boy with pathologic stage IIIA$_S$ disease is shown in Fig.11.2. The standard mantle, used when patients have nonbulky or no mediastinal disease, includes a 2-cm margin below the clavicles, a 1-cm margin of lung in the axillary fields, a 2-cm margin around the hila, and any visible tumor, and a 1.5-cm margin lateral to the posterior vertebral bodies. Blocks are added to shield the larynx (anteriorly), mandible (anteriorly), humeral heads, and spinal cord (posteriorly). The hila are blocked (Fig.11.2G,I) during the last few treatments because the dose to this area is substantially higher than in the mediastinum because of increased transmission through lung parenchyma.

11.6.3.2 Special Mantle Techniques for the Patient with Bulky Mediastinal Disease

Two techniques are used to extend the mantle volume to include the cardiac silhouette, hemilung, or whole lung: the split-course technique and the thin lung transmission block. When there is large mediastinal adenopathy present and the patient is treated with radiotherapy alone, treatment begins with equally weighted fields including the entire treatment volume at 1 Gy per day and continues to an uncorrected lung dose of 15 Gy for elective lung treatment. Mantle treatment is then interrupted for 2 weeks (during which a para-aortic field may be treated) to allow for tumor regression. Mantle irradiation resumes with standard mantle blocks which are based on the tumor shrinkage that occured with the initial 2 weeks of treatment and the 2 weeks of para-aortic treatment. This approach results in a lower rate of pneumonitis than is produced by continuous-course irradiation (THAR and MILLION 1980), has not been associated with an inferior control rate when compared with continuous-course therapy, and allows for substantial reduction in the high-dose volume.

In the patient who is receiving irradiation after chemotherapy, the choice between the two techniques for delivering lung or cardiac irradiation is based on the chemotherapy response. If there is a complete or good partial response to chemotherapy, use of a thin lung transmission block is preferred (Fig.11.3, 11.4). A thin block is designed of sufficient thickness that heart and lung receive the prescribed heart and lung dose over the time required to deliver the full mantle treatment. If the response is poor and little of the lung can be shielded, the split-course method is used so that the high-dose mantle volume can be reduced if there is an early response to irradiation.

11.6.3.3 Preauricular Field

When there is disease in the mid or upper neck, there is a small risk of disease in the preauricular nodes. A small field encompassing the preauricular node area is treated with 5 or 6 MeV electrons (Fig. 11.2 K). This field overlaps the upper border of the mantle by 1 cm. The usual dose for elective treatment is 20 Gy in ten fractions.

11.6.3.4 Waldeyer's Ring

The Waldeyer's ring field is rarely used in HD as there is little risk for disease in the extranodal lymphoid tissue in the nasopharynx, tonsil, and base of tongue. Occasionally the disease in the upper neck is difficult to encompass with a standard mantle, even in conjuction with preauricular fields. The Waldeyer's ring field includes the preauricular, postauricular, parotid, upper cervical, transverse spinal, jugulodigastric, and submental nodes. Because the surface contour and depths of nodes at risk vary, electrons are not used. This field is generally used only if there is bulky disease within this treatment volume. If the bulky upper neck disease is unilateral, the fields may be weighted so that the uninvolved side receives only the dose judged adequate for subclinical disease. Although this technique reduces the already low risk of xerostomia, asymmetric growth may occur if small children are treated with this technique. Differences in dose of as little as 5 Gy may produce detectable changes in subsequent follow-up (see Figs. 11.5, 11.6).

11.6.3.5 Para-aortic Field

The standard para-aortic field is treated through equally weighted anterior and posterior portals. The lateral borders are 2 cm lateral to the transverse processes (usually, the field is about 9 cm wide). The inferior border is at the bottom of the fourth lumbar vertebra. It is important to ascertain the kidney location. Usually the medial third of each kidney is included in the para-aortic field; when the dose to the para-aortic field is between 30 and 35 Gy, and only one-third of the total kidney volume is irradiated, the risk of renal complications is negligible.

Because of radiation beam divergence, a gap is placed between the para-aortic field and the mantle field (Fig. 11.2F, L–M). In most institutions, the length of the gap is calculated so that the divergent mantle and para-aortic field beams will meet at the depth of the para-aortic nodes. Care must be taken in planning the match; if the gap is placed over an area of potential disease anterior or posterior to the para-aortic nodes (e.g., internal mammary nodes) and the gap is calculated for the fields to match at the para-aortic nodes or another midline structure such as the spinal cord, the anterior or posterior nodes can be missed or undertreated. At the University of Florida, an empiric gap of 1.5 cm on the skin between the inferior border of the mantle and the superior border of the para-aortic field has been used in all patients treated since the early 1970s; this approach has resulted in no cases of transverse myelitis and only a single failure in the area of the gap. An alternative method, which is used at the University of Florida in patients at high risk for disease in the usual area of the gap, is to treat an "extended" field which includes both the mantle and para-aortic fields (see Fig. 11.3) (FARAH et al. 1988).

11.6.3.6 Spleen Field

The spleen is treated in a separate field, separated from the para-aortic field by a 1-cm gap on the skin,

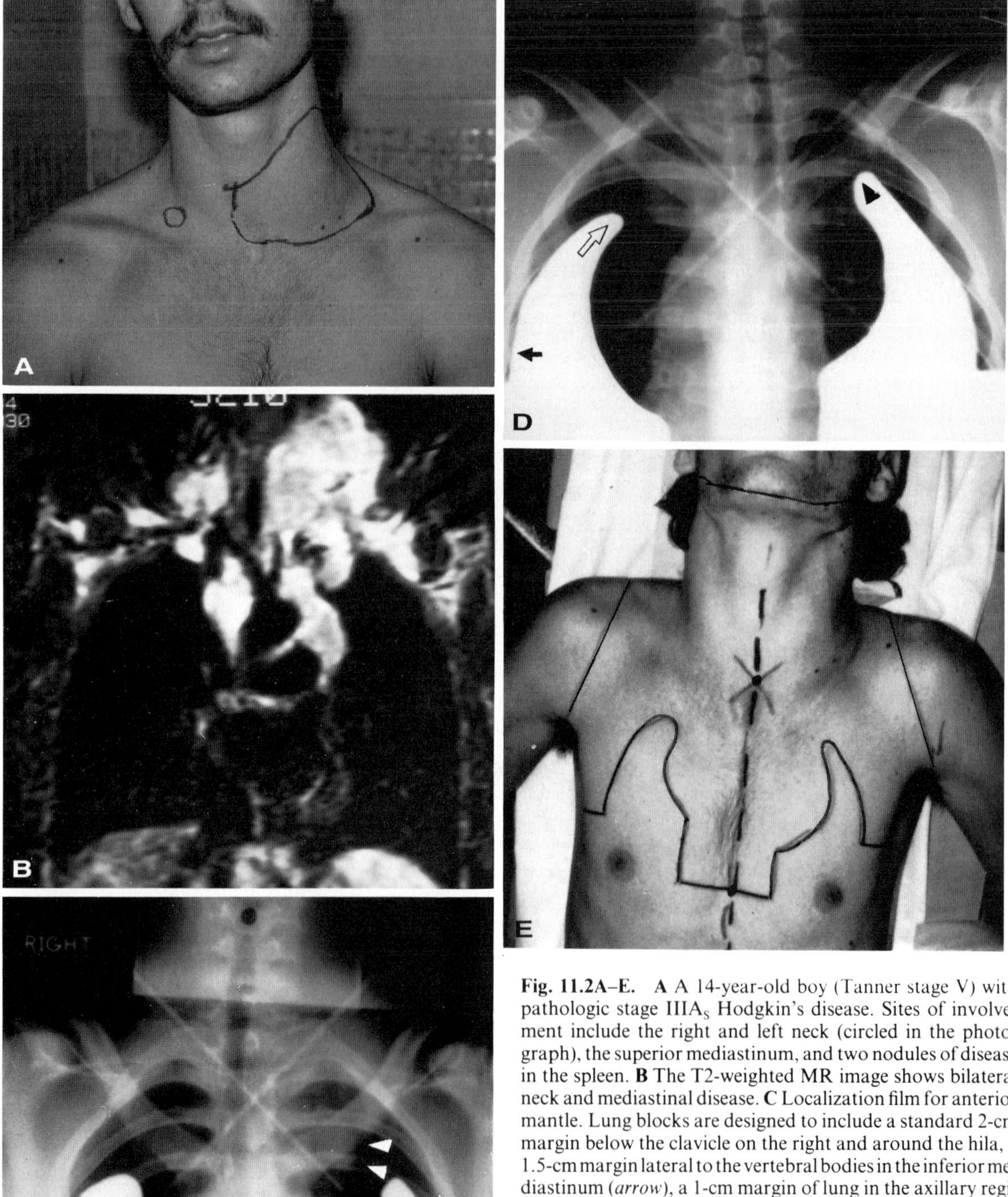

Fig. 11.2A–E. **A** A 14-year-old boy (Tanner stage V) with pathologic stage IIIA$_S$ Hodgkin's disease. Sites of involvement include the right and left neck (circled in the photograph), the superior mediastinum, and two nodules of disease in the spleen. **B** The T2-weighted MR image shows bilateral neck and mediastinal disease. **C** Localization film for anterior mantle. Lung blocks are designed to include a standard 2-cm margin below the clavicle on the right and around the hila, a 1.5-cm margin lateral to the vertebral bodies in the inferior mediastinum (*arrow*), a 1-cm margin of lung in the axillary regions (*black arrowhead*), and a 2-cm margin around the mediastinal tumor, visible in the left infraclavicular area (*white arrowheads*). **D** Localization film for the posterior mantle. Lung blocks are designed with the same margins on the inferior mediastinum, hila, axillae (*arrow*), and the tumor (*open arrow*) as the anterior mantle except for coverage of the infraclavicular nodes (*arrowhead*), which is achieved entirely with the anterior mantle field. This technique requires 3:2 anterior field weighting to ensure an adequate dose to the infraclavicular nodes while minimizing the dose to the lung. **E** Lines drawn on skin delineate the anterior mantle field and guide placement by hand of the shoulder, mandibular, and laryngeal blocks. In this patient, the laryngeal block was applied after the administration of 15 Gy because of the bulky neck disease

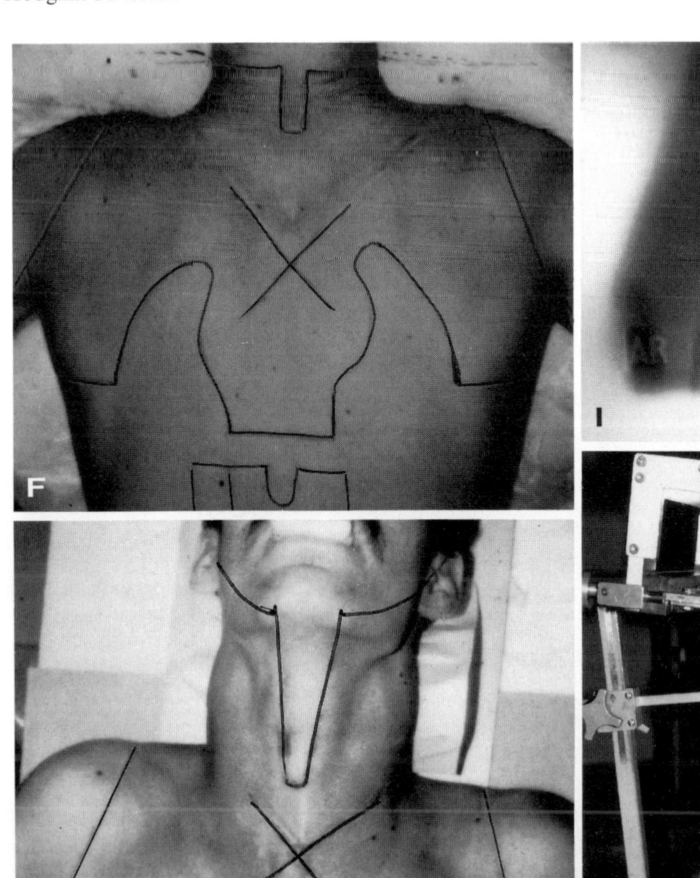

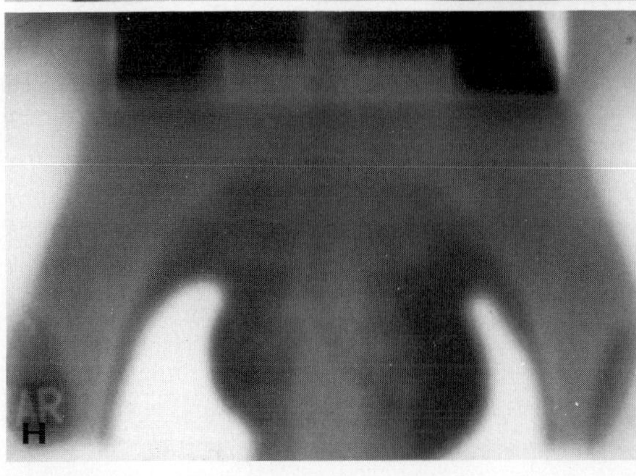

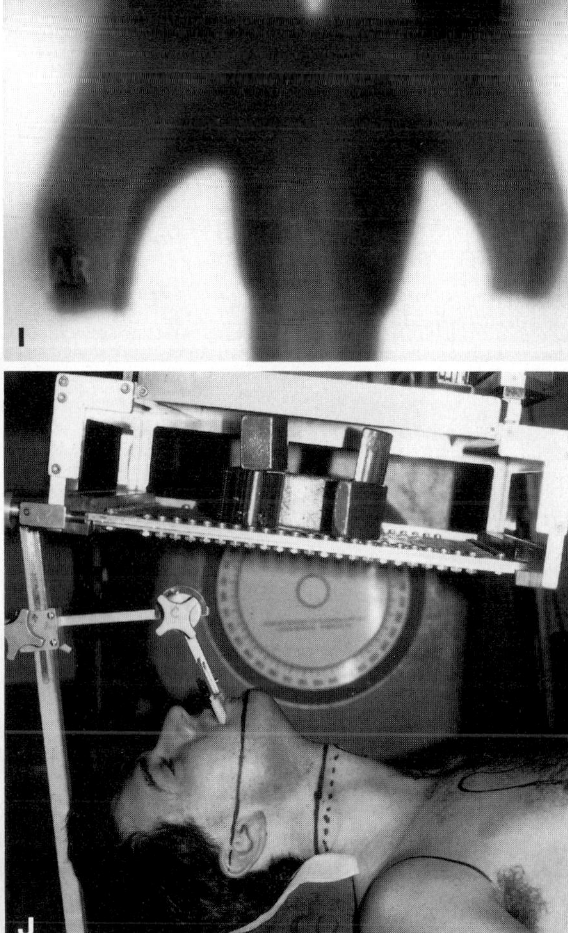

Fig. 11.2F–J. (*Cont.*) **F** Lines drawn on the skin delineate the posterior mantle field and guide placement by hand of the shoulder blocks, the spinal cord block, and the superior field border. Note the 1.5-cm skin gap between the mantle and para-aortic fields. This technique provides adequate protection for the spinal cord when the specified mantle and para-aortic doses do not exceed 30–35 Gy, the mantle weighting is 3:2 in favor of the anterior field, the para-aortic fields are weighted 1:1, and a 2 × 1 cm spinal cord block is used on the posterior para-aortic field. **G** Lines drawn on the skin delineate the anterior mantle field after the addition of a full midline-laryngeal block and bilateral hilar blocks. **H** Port film of anterior mantle field demonstrating adequate axillary, inferior mediastinal, infraclavicular, and tumor margins as well as adequate shoulder blocks. **I** Port film of anterior mantle field demonstrating adequate laryngeal and shoulder blocking and adequate shielding of the hila during the final mantle treatments; margins are adequate except in the left axilla. **J** The boost for the anterior neck dose is delivered with a complete 2-cm midline block. The lower border of the anterior neck boost field overlaps the exit border of the posterior field by 1 cm.

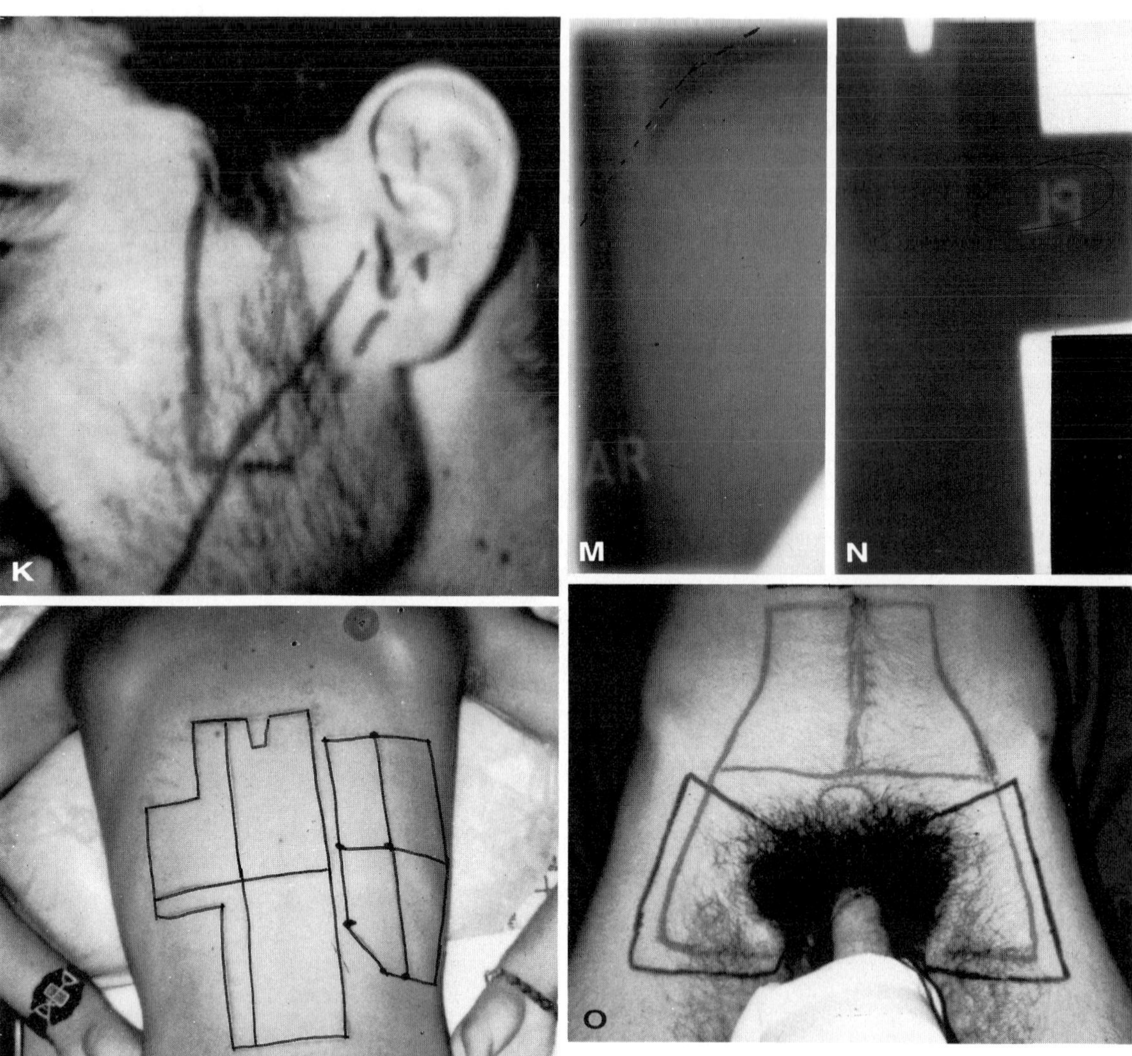

Fig. 11.2 K–O. (*Cont.*) **K** Preauricular field used when there is upper neck adenopathy. Treatment is given with low-energy electrons, usually 6 MeV. **L** Lines drawn on the skin delineate the posterior liver, para-aortic, and splenic pedicle fields. **M** Port film of the anterior liver field. A small block to shield lung is permissible (*broken line*). **N** Port film of the posterior para-aortic and splenic field. The film label was inadvertently placed over the surgical clip marking the splenic pedicle. **O** Lines drawn on the skin delineate the anterior pelvic field as well as anterior fields used to boost the dose to the femoral nodes using an electron beam. With this technique, the femoral nodes are not included in the posterior field, so electron boost fields are required (see Fig. 11.4B). A special testicular block (beneath the sheet) is used to shield the testicles during the anterior and posterior para-aortic and pelvic treatments (see Fig. 11.9). The testicular shield is difficult to use with small children

or in a single combined field that includes the para-aortic area and spleen (Fig. 11.7). The advantage of the separate field is greater ease in daily setup, less transmitted and scattered irradiation to normal tissues (which are beneath the block on the combined field), and the possibility of preferential weighting of the dose to the posterior portal (3:2 in favor of the posterior) as the spleen is usually a posterior structure. The advantage of the combined field is the lack of dose inhomogeneity in the gap area.

11.6.3.7 Splenic Hilar Nodes

In the patient who has a laparotomy, splenic hilar nodes may be left behind after splenectomy, so a splenic hilar field is usually treated. This field may be separated from the para-aortic field by 1 cm or in-cluded as part of the para-aortic field (Fig. 11.2 L–N). This field cannot be designed unless the surgeon has marked the location of the splenic hilum with clips at laparotomy. The anterior and posterior fields are equally weighted.

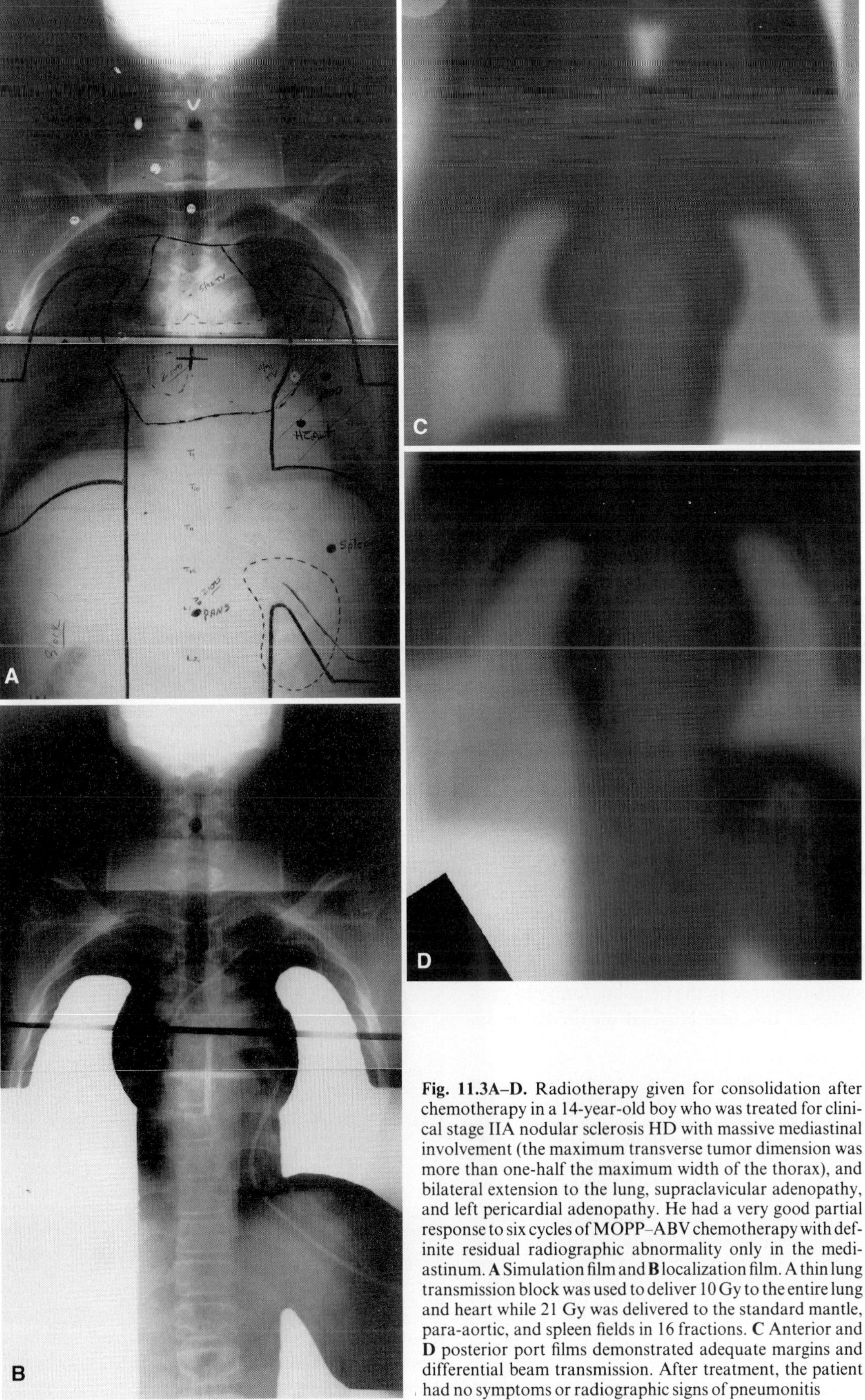

Fig. 11.3A–D. Radiotherapy given for consolidation after chemotherapy in a 14-year-old boy who was treated for clinical stage IIA nodular sclerosis HD with massive mediastinal involvement (the maximum transverse tumor dimension was more than one-half the maximum width of the thorax), and bilateral extension to the lung, supraclavicular adenopathy, and left pericardial adenopathy. He had a very good partial response to six cycles of MOPP–ABV chemotherapy with definite residual radiographic abnormality only in the mediastinum. **A** Simulation film and **B** localization film. A thin lung transmission block was used to deliver 10 Gy to the entire lung and heart while 21 Gy was delivered to the standard mantle, para-aortic, and spleen fields in 16 fractions. **C** Anterior and **D** posterior port films demonstrated adequate margins and differential beam transmission. After treatment, the patient had no symptoms or radiographic signs of pneumonitis

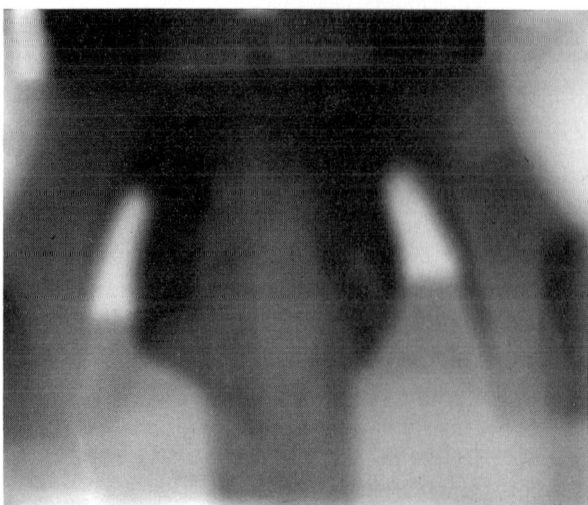

Fig. 11.4. Port film for anterior mantle field in a patient who originally had stage IVA HD with a large mediastinal mass and multiple bilateral pulmonary nodules, was treated with chemotherapy alone, and had recurrences in the mediastinal and para-aortic lymph nodes. Combined modality therapy with six cycles of chemotherapy and total nodal irradiation was used for salvage. The entire lung was treated with radiotherapy to a dose of 15 Gy in 21 fractions through a two-tiered transmission block while the mediastinum received 35 Gy. This patient did not develop pneumonitis and remains free of disease recurrence and pulmonary complications 3 years after salvage treatment

11.6.3.8 Pelvic Field

The anterior pelvic portal includes the common iliac, external iliac, inguinal, and femoral nodes (Figs. 11.2O, 11.8A). The iliac crests and midline structures are shielded. Because the posterior field does not include the inguinal or femoral nodes, additional treatment to these nodes is given with electrons through anterior fields (Fig. 11.8B). The pelvic fields are weighted 3:2 in favor of the anterior field. The position of the common and external iliac nodes varies with reference to the bony anatomy, so optimal design of this field is based on the lymphan-

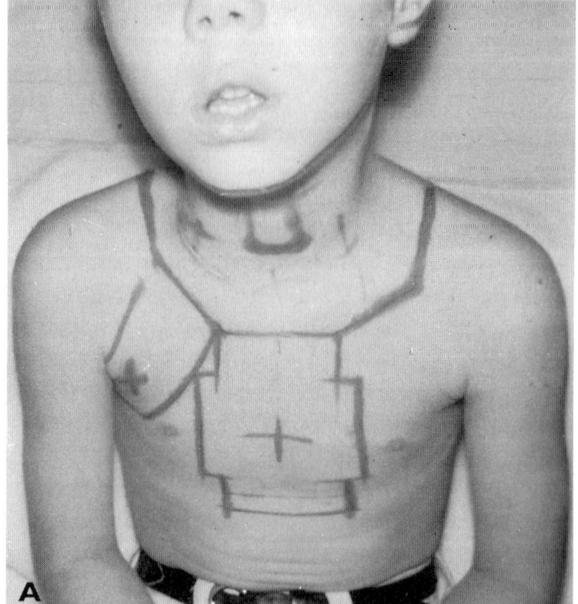

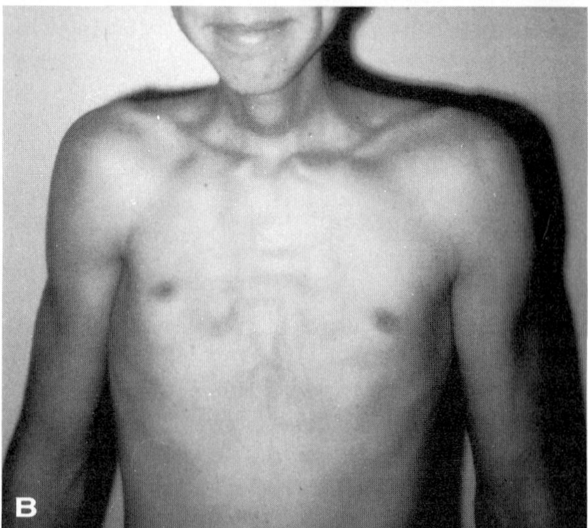

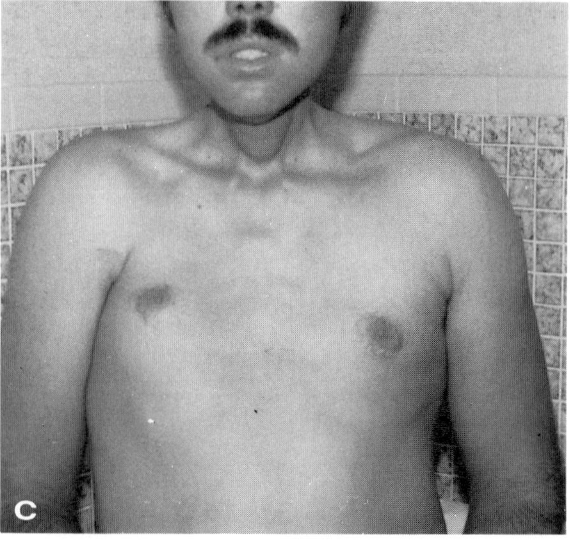

Fig. 11.5. A Treatment fields for a 6-year-old boy with stage IA HD who had a 3.5 × 5 cm mass in the right lower neck. The dose to the neck was 40 Gy given in 20 fractions; the axilla received 37 Gy tumor dose at 4.4 cm in 20 fractions, and the mediastinum, 38 Gy tumor dose at 6.25 cm in 20 fractions. All fields were anterior, and all were treated once a day, 5 days a week, with cobalt-60. **B** The patient at age 15, demonstrating significant hypoplasia in the neck and pectoral area. The right nipple is displaced because of relative hypoplasia in the right infraclavicular and axillary area. **C** The patient at age 29 has persistent significant hypoplasia in the neck and pectoral areas. He also developed a thyroid adenoma, leading to subtotal thyroidectomy at age 27, and aortic valve stenosis with atrial dilatation and chest pain and lightheadedness on exertion

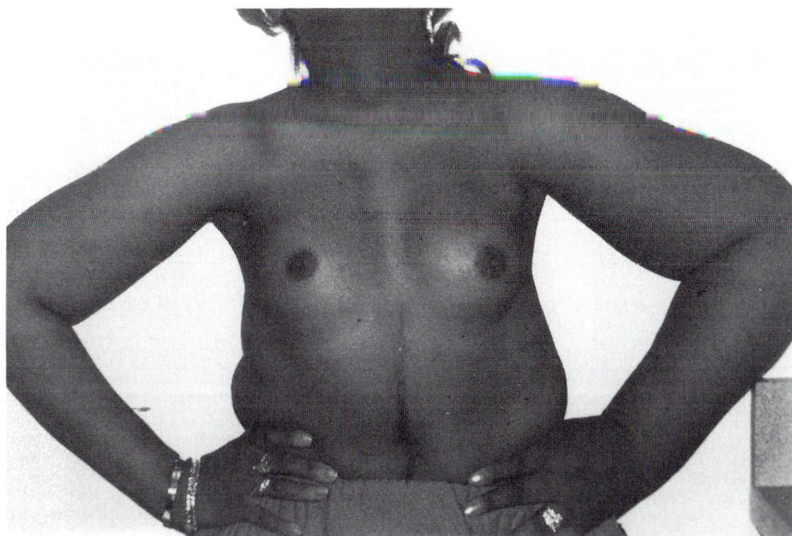

Fig. 11.6. Patient at age 29 who was treated for HD at age 8. She had pathologic stage IIB mixed cellularity HD with bilateral involvement of the neck and axillae. She received 46 Gy to the mediastinum, neck, and left axilla and 37.6 Gy to the right axilla, as well as 37.60 Gy to the splenic pedicle, para-aortic, and pelvic nodes. Although she was cured of HD, the sequelae of radiotherapy include ovarian ablation, mild kyphosis and scoliosis, bone and soft tissue hypoplasia in the irradiated areas, and edema of the left upper extremity

giogram. To preserve fertility in male patients, a special testicular shield is used to reduce scattered irradiation from treatment of the pelvic (and para-aortic) field (Fig. 11.9). In female patients, ovarian ablation uniformly occurs unless the overies are transfixed to a midline position and shielded. At oophoropexy, clips should be placed on the proximal and distal ends of the ovaries for optimal shield design (see Fig. 11.8).

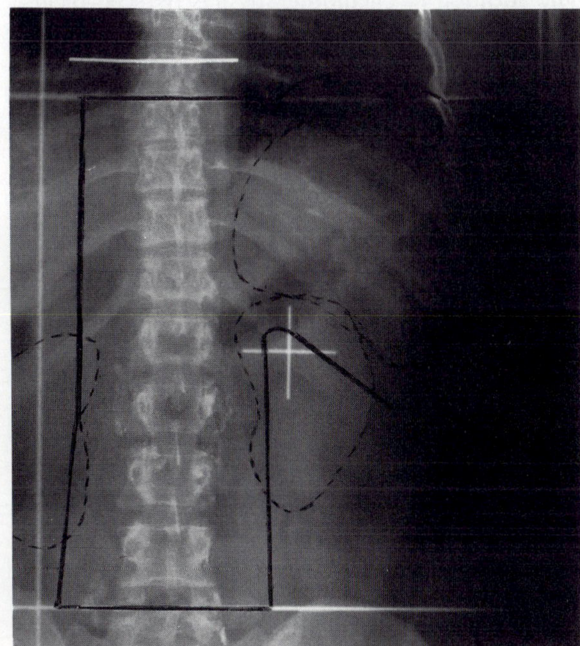

Fig. 11.7. Typical anterior spleen field in conjunction with para-aortic field. A 2-cm spinal cord block is added by hand on the posterior spleen–para-aortic field

11.7 Treatment Results

11.7.1 Radiotherapy Alone

Results of radiotherapy alone from various institutions treating children with HD are shown in Table 11.7. Relapse rates for series treating stage III disease, series from cooperative groups, and series using limited radiation treatment volumes are higher, but ultimate survival rates are similar because of the high rate of salvage after treatment failure for early-stage disease. With single institutions, prognostic factors within stage I and II as well as stage III disease (such as B symptoms, large mediastinal adenopathy, more than four sites of involvement, more than four nodules of spleen involvement, IIIA2 disease) have been identified which predict for higher relapse rates with radiotherapy alone (HOPPE et al. 1980, 1982; MAUCH et al. 1985; PROSNITZ et al. 1985; THAR et al. 1979). In stage I and II disease, freedom-from-relapse rates from single institutions treating with extended fields range from 70% to 90%; survival rates are 85%–100%. Because of impaired musculoskeletal development after doses greater than 30 Gy, only children who have achieved most of their growth potential are treated with radiation alone today.

11.7.2 Chemotherapy Alone

The results of several institutions treating children with HD with chemotherapy alone are shown in Table 11.8. Relapse-free survival and survival rates in patients with early-stage disease treated with

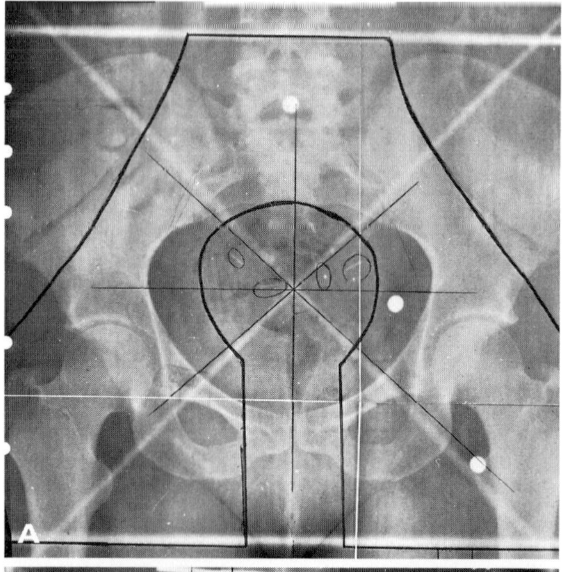

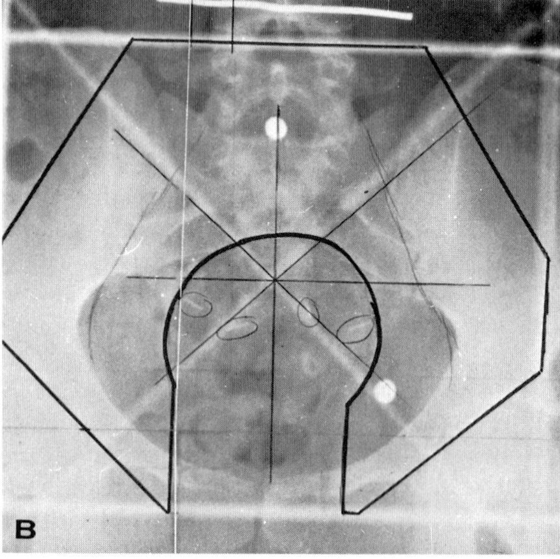

Fig. 11.8. A Simulation film of anterior pelvic field in a female patient. Metallic clips (*circled*) indicate the medial and lateral borders of each ovary. The round radiopaque markers are points for Clarkson calculations. **B** Simulation film of posterior pelvic field in a female patient. The femoral nodes are not included in the posterior field, but receive a boost dose through anterior electron beam fields (see Fig. 11.2O). This technique reduces the dose of radiation to the femoral heads

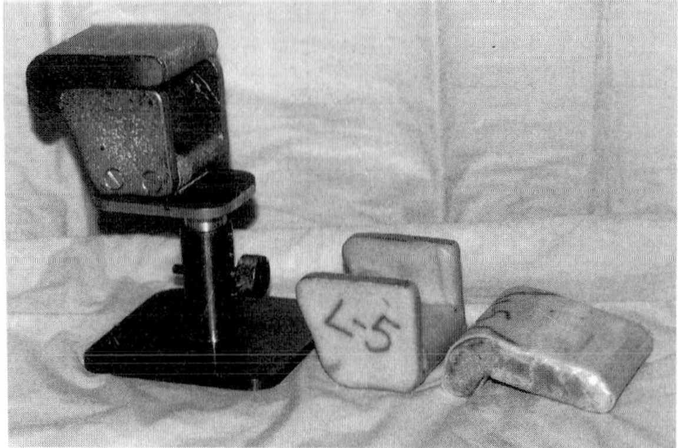

Fig. 11.9. Testicular shields. The two-piece testicular shield is used for both anterior and posterior field treatments. The shield is placed on a stand when the patient is supine and directly on the table when the patient is prone. The shields on the table have been coated with wax to decrease irradiation of the scrotal skin by low-energy electrons scattered from the shield

11.7.3 Combined Modality Therapy

Because of the dose-related toxicities observed after treatment with either radiotherapy or chemotherapy alone and the differing patterns of relapse, combined modality therapy has been used in an effort not only to improve relapse-free and overall survival rates, but also to decrease late effects of therapy. The addition of chemotherapy has reduced recurrence rates after radiation alone (HAGEMEISTER et al. 1991) and allowed reduction in radiation dose (DONALDSON and LINK 1987); the inclusion of radiotherapy in treatment regimens has likewise allowed reduction in the number of courses of chemotherapy (SCHELLONG et al. 1986, 1988, 1989). The results of combined modality therapy in children with HD are shown in Table 11.9. The majority of children with HD are treated with combined modality therapy.

11.8 Complications of Treatment

11.8.1 Radiotherapy

chemotherapy alone exceed 90% although most series report several fatal treatment complications. Because of concern about dose-related chemotherapy toxicity and a predictable pattern of involved-field recurrence after chemotherapy alone, treatment with chemotherapy alone is usually reserved for children with small-volume disease who have not achieved their growth potential.

Complications of radiotherapy are related to total dose, dose per treatment, the volume of tissue treated, tolerance of the normal tissues in the treatment volume, and age of the patient. Commonly recognized complications of radiotherapy with standard doses and techniques currently employed include a 25%–50% rate of subsequent thyroid dysfunction (HANCOCK SL et al. 1991), an increased risk of dental

Table 11.7. Results of treatment of children with HD with radiotherapy alone

Institution, accrual dates	No. of Patients	Age (yr)	Stage	Dose (Gy)	RF[a]/EF[b]/DF[c]	Absolute
Involved Field						
United Kingdom Children's Cancer Study Group, 1982–1988[d]	59	≤ 15	CSI	35	85[a] (3)	98 (3)
Intergroup Study of Hodgkin's Disease in Children, 1977–1981[e]	39	≤ 18	PSI/II	35–40	41[a] (5)	95 (5)
Memorial Sloan-Kettering, 1970–1981[f]	51	≤ 19	PSI/IIA	36	71[a] (10)	93 (10)
St. Bartholomew's, 1970–1985[g]	28	≤ 15	CSI	35–40	79[a] (10)	96 (10)
Extended Field						
Stanford University Medical Center, 1970–1985[g]	48	≤ 15	PSI/II	40–44	82[a] (10)	86 (10)
Intergroup Study of Hodgkin's Disease in Children, 1977–1981[e]	58	≤ 18	PSI/II	35	67[a] (5)	96 (5)
Hospital for Sick Children, Toronto, 1969–1977[h]	52	≥ 17	PSI-IIIB	35	54[a] (10)	89 (10)
Children's Hospital of Philadelphia, 1970–1980[i]	11	≤ 18	PSI-IIA	36–40	70[a] (10)	100 (10)
Mayo Clinic, 1970–1976[j]	19	≤ 16	PSI-IIA	≥ 30	90[c] (4)	95 (4)
Joint Center for Radiation Therapy, 1969–1977[k]	49	≤ 16	PSI-IIA	36–40	88[l]	98[l]
Institute Gustave-Roussy, 1972–1976[m]	30	≤ 15	CSI-II	40	63[c] (7)	93 (7)

[a] Relapse-free survival or freedom from relapse
[b] Event-free survival
[c] Disease-free survival
[d] BARRETT et al. 1990
[e] GEHAN et al. 1990
[f] JEREB et al. 1984
[g] DONALDSON et al. 1990
[h] JENKIN and BERRY 1980
[i] LANGE and LITTMAN 1983
[j] DEARTH et al. 1980
[k] MAUCH et al. 1983
[l] Not an actuarial probability; relapse-free survival calculated by a direct method.
[m] BAYLE-WEISGERBER et al. 1984

problems unless good dental hygiene is maintained, a 1%–2% rate of both acute and late pulmonary and cardiac problems, a 1% rate of abdominal complications, a probable increase in second malignancy rate, and musculoskeletal hypoplasia in small children treated with standard doses of radiation (35–40 Gy).

Most complications associated with irradiation are related to the mantle treatment volume. The major acute pulmonary complication of radiotherapy is pneumonitis, usually seen after hemilung or whole-lung irradiation in patients with clinical evidence of pulmonary involvement or a high risk of subclinical pulmonary or pleural involvement in the presence of large mediastinal or hilar disease.

Occasionally, pneumonitis is associated with the cessation of steroids when chemotherapy is given after irradiation. The risk of pneumonitis can be decreased with the use of a thin lung transmission block (Fig. 11.3) or split-course treatment, techniques that alter the dose per treatment and the overall time during which the radiation is delivered (CARMEL and KAPLAN 1976; THAR and MILLION 1980). In patients with bulky mediastinal disease given standard radiotherapy and elective lung irradiation, the risk of pneumonitis is on the order of 10%–15%. Management in symptomatic patients should be immediate and aggressive with steroids, observation in the hospital, and supportive therapy because this

Table 11.8. Results of treatment of children with HD with chemotherapy alone

Institution, accrual dates	No. of patients	Age (yr)	Clinical stage	Chemotherapy regimen	Survival (yr) RF[a]/DF[b]/NFR[c]		AS[d]		Fatal nonneoplastic complications	Second malignancies (leukemia)
Uganda Cancer Institute, 1967–1977[e]	48	≤16	I–IIIA IIIB–IV	MOPP×6	No data		75% (5)[f] 60% (5)[f]		1	1
Combined series, South Africa, 1969–1979[g]	27	≤14	I–II III–IV	MVOPP×6	11/11[c] 5/16[c]	(5) (5)	90% (10) 40% (10)		1	1
Netherlands Cancer Institute, 1975–1984[h]	21	≤15	I/III[i]	MOPP×6	19/21[b]		100% (5)		0	0
Combined series, Australia and New Zealand, 1978–1987[j]	38 15	≤16	I/II III/IV	MOPP×6 or ChlVPP×6	92%[a]	(5)	94% (5)		2	0
Jordan University Medical School, 1979–1987[k]	14 14	≤12	I–II III–IV	MOPP×4–6 MOPP×6–9	92%[a]	(5)	100% (5)		0	0

[a] Relapse-free survival or freedom from relapse
[b] Disease-free survival
[c] No. free from relapse/no. treated in patients with ≥2 year follow-up
[d] Absolute survival
[e] OLWENY et al. (1978)
[f] Calculations based on complete responders
[g] JACOBS et al. (1984)
[h] BEHRENDT et al. (1987)
[i] Small volume < 4 cm
[j] EKERT et al. (1988)
[k] MADANAT (1989)

complication can be fatal. If the patient has received chemotherapy, other sources for pneumonia should be ruled out with lung biopsy after steroids have been administered. Pulmonary fibrosis may occur, but is usually confined to the apices of the lung and paratracheal parenchyma and rarely results in impairment of pulmonary function (SMITH et al. 1989).

With optimal treatment technique and dose, the risk of cardiac dysfunction is low (GREEN et al. 1987; MEFFERD et al. 1989). Acute pericarditis occurs 6 weeks to 1 year after irradiation; the risk is related to treatment technique (delivery of most of the dose through an anterior portal), dose per fraction, total dose, and volume of heart irradiated (CARMEL and KAPLAN 1976; COSSET et al. 1988, 1991). Pericardial effusions often are asymptomatic and resolve without therapy; if the patient is symptomatic, steroids may be administered and the effusion tapped. Constrictive pericarditis can occur in subsequent years of follow-up and is probably related to the same factors as acute pericarditis. Part of the pericardium may be removed surgically if the patient is symptomatic. Other cardiac events such as myocardial infarction appear to be increased in successfully treated patients and may be related to acceleration of atherosclerotic plaque formation in the coronary vessels within the treatment field. However, many of

the patients in whom cardiac events have been observed have other risk factors including type IV hyperlipidemia, history of smoking, familial history of cardiac disease, obesity, hypertension, and diabetes. All patients with HD should be counseled against smoking and screened periodically for hyperlipidemia and hypertension.

An additional complication rarely observed is transverse myelitis, which in most cases is related to suboptimal radiotherapy technique in matching fields. A more frequent neurologic side-effect of mantle irradiation is Lhermitte's sign, a transient effect probably related to damage and regeneration of myelin. With Lhermitte's sign, the patient reports a shock-like sensation radiating down the legs, usually precipitated by walking, jogging, or simple flexion of the cervical spine. Lhermitte's sign usually appears within 6 weeks to 3 months of irradiation and may last from several weeks to more than 6 months. It occurs in about 20% of patients receiving mantle irradiation and does not herald any permanent neurologic sequelae.

Thyroid dysfunction after mantle irradiation is most often hypothyroidism, but hyperthyroidism has been reported. Thyroid function studies are performed routinely after radiotherapy, usually at yearly intervals in the asymptomatic patient, and thyroid

Table 11.9. Results of treatment of children with HD with combined modality therapy

Institution, accrual dates	No. of patients	Age (yr)	Stage	RT volume/ dose (Gy)	Chemotherapy regimen	% Projected survival (years of follow-up)		Fatal nonneoplastic complications	Second malignancies (leukemia)
						Cause-specific	Absolute		
Netherlands Cancer Institute 1975–1984[a]	16	≤15	CSI-III[b]	IF/25	MOPP×6	14/16[c]	100 (5)	None	None
Stanford University Medical Center, 1970–1983[d]	27 28	≤14	PSI/II PSIII/IV	IF/15–25	MOPP×6	96[e] (10) 84[e] (10)	100 (10) 78 (10)	No data	4 (3)
Intergroup Study of Hodgkin's Disease in Children, 1977–1981[f]	97	≤18	PSI-II	IF/35–40	MOPP×6	95[e] (5)	93 (5)	No data	5 (3)
Institut Gustave-Roussy, Villejuif, and Hôpital Saint-Louis, Paris, 1965–1976[g]	178	≤15	CSI-II	IF or EF/40	MOPP×3 or 6	85[h] (10)	93 (10)	8	No data
Royal Marsden Hospital and St. Bartholomew's Hospital, London, 1974–1982[i]	80	≤16	CSI-IVB	IF/25–30	ChlVPP×3 or 6	82[e] (5)	94 (5)	1	No data
Hôpital Saint-Louis, Paris, 1972–1980	72	≤19	CSI-IIB	IF/40	MOPP×3 or 6 or ChlVPP ×3	88[e] (12)	92 (12)	2	1
French Society of Pediatric Oncology and Hôpital Saint-Louis, Paris, 1982–1987[k]	88	≤18	CSI-IIA	IF/20[l]	ABVD×4 + ABVD×2 + MOPP×2	94[h] (4)	No data	No data	No data
	49		CSI-IIB, CSIII	IF+PA+ S/20[l]	MOPP×3 + ABVD×3	93[h] (4)	95 (4)	No data	No data
	20		IV	IF+PA+ S/20[l]	MOPP×3 + ABVD×3	54[h] (4)	No data	No data	No data
Stanford University Medical Center, 1982–1986[m]	34	≤17	II-IV	IF/15–25	Alternating ABVD and MOPP×6	94[e] (2)	92 (2)	No data	4 (3)
Children's Cancer Study Group, 1984–1987[n]	64	≤18	III/IV	IF/21	ABVD×12	87[o] (3)	87 (3)	2	1
Hospital for Sick Children, Toronto, 1969–1979[p]	57	≤17	Unfavorable CSI-IV	MTNI/ 20–30	MOPP×6	80[e] (10)	85[e] (10)	3	4
Children's Hospital of Philadelphia, 1970–1980[q]	34	≤18	IIB-IVB	IF/20–36	COPP×6	60[e] (5)	86 (5)	1	0

IF, involved field; EF, extended field; PA, para-aortic field; S, spleen field; MTNI, modified total nodal irradiation

[a] BEHRENDT et al. (1987)
[b] Large volume >4 cm
[c] Number free from relapse/number treated in patients with ≥ 2 years' follow-up
[d] DONALDSON and LINK (1987)
[e] Relapse-free survival or freedom from relapse
[f] GEHAN et al. (1990)
[g] BAYLE-WEISGERBER et al. (1984)
[h] Disease-free survival
[i] ROBINSON et al. (1984)
[j] CRAMER and ANDRIEU (1985)
[k] DIONET et al. (1988)
[l] 40 Gy for < 70% response in 16/157 (10%) patients
[m] MEFFERD et al. (1989)
[n] FRYER et al. (1990)
[o] Event-free survival
[p] JENKIN et al. (1990)
[q] LANGE and LITTMAN (1983)

hormone replacement is instituted before symptoms develop.

Prophylactic daily fluoride applications and regular dental care prevent dental complications in most patients; the risk of xerostomia or subsequent dental problems is very low unless a Waldeyer's ring field was treated.

The most frequent abdominal complication after radiotherapy for HD is bowel adhesion, which is rare in patients who have not had abdominal surgery (e.g., staging laparotomy). With doses of 35 Gy or less, and daily doses of no more than 2 Gy, the risk is 1% or less (COIA and HANKS 1988). No significant risk of renal, liver, or intrinsic bowel complications exists.

Permanent gonadal injury can be avoided in most male patients with special testicular shielding (see Fig. 11.9) during irradiation, which reduces scattered (indirect) irradiation, primarily the result of treatment of the pelvic, para-aortic, and spleen fields. Without special testicular shielding, the oligospermia rate is at least 50% after pelvic irradiation (ORTIN et al. 1990). In male patients receiving greater than 40 Gy to the pelvic nodes after laparotomy, a small incidence of hydrocele was noted, but no cases occurred with pelvic doses less than 40 Gy.

The ovaries are less sensitive to scattered irradiation than the testicles, but require special protection if the pelvic nodes are irradiated. Protection of the ovaries is much more difficult than testicular shielding. An oophoropexy can be performed at laparotomy; if laparotomy was not performed, or if the ovaries have moved after laparotomy, they can be transfixed through a laparoscopy procedure (WILLIAMS and MENDENHALL 1992). The incision is approximately 2 cm and the internal organs suffer little trauma, so simulation and treatment can be started within 1 or 2 days of the procedure. Even with oophoropexy and careful shielding, the ovaries receive a substantial amount of scattered irradiation and are at some risk for temporary or permanent ablation with pelvic irradiation. The only cases of ovarian failure observed in the Stanford series were associated with more than three cycles of MOPP chemotherapy and pelvic irradiation with no ovarian shielding or suboptimal ovarian shielding (ORTIN et al. 1990). The success in preserving ovarian function when pelvic irradiation is administered varies (BRAMSWIG et al. 1989) and is highly technique dependent (see Fig. 11.8).

In addition to the complications listed above, which can occur in patients of all ages, pediatric patients with HD are also at risk for impaired development of bone and soft tissues within the field of irradiation. Characteristic changes after mantle irradiation include shortening of the interclavicular distance and a skinny neck (Figs. 11.5, 11.6). Visible and palpable soft tissue defects are also apparent within the para-aortic and spleen fields. If prepubertal breast tissue is irradiated to full dose, it likewise will not develop appropriately. Doses in excess of 40 Gy also place the child at risk for significant subsequent fibrosis and possible arm or leg edema (Fig. 11.6). Musculoskeletal hypoplasia is clearly related to the dose administered and to the age and developmental status of the child at the time of treatment. Doses of 25 Gy or less in adolescents, 20 Gy in 6- to 10-year-old children, and 15 Gy in children less than 6 years old cause no significant hypoplasia (DONALDSON and LINK 1987).

Second malignancies are noted in survivors of HD. In one series, the probability of developing any second malignancy was 2% at 5 years, 5% at 10 years, and 9% at 15 years, and most second solid malignancies occurred in previously irradiated fields (MEADOWS et al. 1989). As many young patients requiring mediastinal irradiation are women, particular follow-up care should be addressed to the risk for later breast cancer. The true incidence of second malignancy will not be realized until large cohorts of children cured of HD pass through the sixth through eighth decades of life, when most adult malignancies appear.

11.8.2 Chemotherapy

The rate of fatal sepsis with modern administration of chemotherapy is about 1%. Chemotherapy regimens such as MOPP that are based on alkylating agents carry two major toxicities of concern: acute leukemias and other second malignancies, and sterility. The major risks of the antibiotic-based regimens such as ABVD are cardiac (LIPSCHULTZ et al. 1991) and pulmonary (MEFFERD et al. 1989).

11.8.3 Combined Modality Therapy

Acute leukemia has been linked to the alkylating agents in MOPP and occurs in approximately 6% of children receiving six cycles of MOPP (DONALDSON and LINK 1987) and involved-field radiotherapy. Data in adults suggest that the risk is related to dose and possibly age and stage, and possibly is enhanced in the postsplenectomy patient (KALDOR et al. 1990;

MEADOWS et al. 1989; MENDENHALL et al. 1989). Most studies addressing possible enhancement of the leukemia risk by the addition of radiotherapy to the combined modality regimen have not demonstrated a significant increase in leukemia risk; in addition, leukemias are seen only rarely after radiotherapy, most usually in the event of a treatment failure that is managed with MOPP chemotherapy. Most often, leukemia occurs between 2 and 8 years after exposure to the alkylating agent, but later occurence of leukemia is occasionally reported.

The rate of male sterility after six cycles of MOPP (ORTIN et al. 1990) or other alkylating agents (BRAMSWIG et al. 1989) approaches 100%. Occasionally, the azoospermia is transient, as a few men have recovered normal sperm counts more than 10 years after chemotherapy (ORTIN et al. 1990; MENDENHALL et al. 1991). The male sterility risk is dose related and is only about 50% after two cycles of MOPP (DACUNHA et al. 1984). The high risk of sterility with six cycles of MOPP applies to both pre- and postpubertal male patients (ORTIN et al. 1990). Peripheral neuropathy is a common, but usually transient, side-effect related to vincristine.

In 20 asymptomatic children treated with six cycles of alternating ABVD/MOPP and low-dose (15–25 Gy) involved-field radiotherapy, a comparison of pre- and posttreatment pulmonary function studies showed that more than 50% of children had a reduced or abnormal carbon monoxide diffusing capacity, and 40% had restrictive or obstruction changes in lung volume and spirometry (MEFFERD et al. 1989). The abnormalities in pulmonary function were observed after bleomycin doses as low as 36 units/m^2 (the equivalent of one dose). On cardiac nuclear gated angiograms, 14% of patients had a low resting ejection fraction or decreased response to exercise. Twenty-one percent had abnormal results on thyroid function studies. The authors concluded that the risks of thyroid and cardiac dysfunction were low, but the pulmonary risks were high and warranted close attention.

11.9 Management of Recurrent Disease

The management of recurrent disease is highly individualized. Factors that affect prognosis and choice of therapy include extent of disease at presentation and recurrence, site of recurrence, prior therapy, and disease-free interval (MAUCH et al. 1980; MENDENHALL et al. 1991; ROACH et al. 1990; VINCIGUERRA et al. 1986). Treatment approaches depend on extent of disease and prior therapy and include radiotherapy or chemotherapy alone in selected cases (FOX et al. 1987; MAUCH et al. 1987; ROACH et al. 1987), combined modality treatment, and high-dose chemotherapy (with or without radiotherapy) plus bone marrow transplantation.

11.10 New Directions

The challenges in Hodgkin's disease are to develop less toxic, but equally efficacious, treatment approaches in early- and intermediate-stage disease (HORNING et al. 1988) and to develop more effective treatment regimens for patients with advanced and recurrent disease.

In the past two decades, significant progress has come from the recognition that most toxicity is dose related and that with the use of combined modality therapy, the doses of both radiation and chemotherapy agents can be reduced significantly without reducing efficacy.

Significant progress in reducing treatment failure has also been made through combining different chemotherapy regimens and radiotherapy. Future directions include the search for better and less toxic agents, development of better methods of controlling and delivering treatment, attempts to understand the causes of treatment failure, and efforts to address these causes with specific therapies.

References

Abrahamsen AF, Borge L, Holte H (1990) Infection after splenectomy for Hodgkin's disease. Acta Oncol 29: 167–170

Abramson JH, Goldblum N, Avitzur M, Pridan H, Sacks MI, Peritz E (1980) Clustering of Hodgkin's disease in Israel: a case-control study. Int J Epidemiol 9: 137–144

Alexander FE, Ricketts TJ, McKinney PA, Cartwright RA (1991) Community lifestyle characteristics and incidence of Hodgkin's disease in young people. Int J Cancer 48: 10–14

American Joint Committee on Cancer (1988) Manual for staging of cancer, 3rd edn. J.B. Lippincott, Philadelphia, pp 255–257

Baccarani M, Fiacchini M, Galieni P, Gherlinzoni F, Fanin R, Fasola G, Mazza P, Tura S (1986) Meningitis and septicaemia in adults splenectomized for Hodgkin's disease. Scand J Haematol 36: 492–498

Barrett A, Crennan E, Barnes J, Martin J, Radford M (1990) Treatment of clinical stage I Hodgkin's disease by local radiation therapy alone: a United Kingdom Children's Cancer Study Group study. Cancer 66: 670–674

Bayle-Weisgerber C, Lemercier N, Teillet F, Asselain B, Gout M, Schweisguth O (1984) Hodgkin's disease in children. Results of therapy in a mixed group of 178 clinical and pathologically staged patients over 13 years. Cancer 54: 215–222

Behrendt H, van Bunningen BNFM, van Leeuwen EF (1987) Treatment of Hodgkin's disease in children with or without radiotherapy. Cancer 59: 1870–1873

Boring CC, Squires TS, Tong T (1993) Cancer statistics, 1993. CA 43: 7–26

Bramswig JH, Heimes U, Heiermann E, Schlegel W, Schellong G (1989) Postpubertal gonadal function in 138 patients treated for Hodgkin's disease (HD) during childhood and adolescence. Proc Am Soc Clin Oncol 8: 279 (abstract # 1088)

Buehler SLK (1983) The epidemiology of Hodgkin's disease in Newfoundland. Diss Abstr Int (Sci) 44: 1792–B

Carmel RJ, Kaplan HS (1976) Mantle irradiation in Hodgkin's disease: an analysis of technique, tumor eradication, and complications. Cancer 37: 2813–2825

Castellino RA, Hoppe RT, Blank N, Young SW, Neumann C, Rosenberg SA, Kaplan HS (1984) Computed tomography, lymphography, and staging laparotomy: correlations in initial staging of Hodgkin disease. AJR 143: 37–41

Chilcote RR, Baehner RL, Hammond D, Investigators and Special Studies Committee of the Children's Cancer Study Group (1976) Septicemia and meningitis in children splenectomized for Hodgkin's disease. N Engl J Med 295: 798–800

Coates PJ, Slavin G, D'Ardenne AJ (1991) Persistence of Epstein-Barr virus in Reed-Sternberg cells throughout the course of Hodgkin's disease. J Pathol 164: 291–297

Coia LR, Hanks GE (1988) Complications from large field intermediate dose infradiaphragmatic radiation: an analysis of the Patterns of Care outcome studies for Hodgkin's disease and seminoma. Int J Radiat Oncol Biol Phys 15: 29–35

Corbett S, O'Neill BJ (1988) A cluster of cases of lymphoma in an underground colliery. Med J Aust 149: 178–179, 181–182, 184–185

Cornbleet MA, Vitolo U, Ultmann JE et al. (1985) Pathologic stages IA and IIA Hodgkin's disease: results of treatment with radiotherapy alone (1969–1980). J Clin Oncol 3: 758–768

Cosset JM, Henry-Amar M, Girinski T, Malaise E, Dupouy N, Dutreix J (1988) Late toxicity of radiotherapy in Hodgkin's disease. The role of fraction size. Acta Oncol 27: 123–129

Cosset JM, Henry-Amar M, Pellae-Cosset B, Carde P, Girinski T, Tubiana M, Hayat M (1991) Pericarditis and myocardial infarctions after Hodgkin's disease therapy. Int J Radiat Oncol Biol Phys 21: 447–449

Cramer P, Andrieu J-M (1985) Hodgkin's disease in childhood and adolescence: results of chemotherapy-radiotherapy in clinical stages IA-IIB. J Clin Oncol 3: 1495–1502

da Cunha MF, Meistrich ML, Fuller LM et al. (1984) Recovery of spermatogenesis after treatment for Hodgkin's disease: limiting dose of MOPP chemotherapy. J Clin Oncol 2: 571–577

Dearth JC, Gilchrist GS, Burgert EO Jr, Telander RL, Cupps RE (1980) Management of stages I to III Hodgkin disease in children. J Pediatr 96: 829–836

Desser RK, Ultmann JE (1972) Risk of severe infection in patients with Hodgkin's disease or lymphoma after diagnostic laparotomy and splenectomy. Ann Intern Med 77: 143–146

Desser RK, Golomb HM, Ultmann JE et al. (1977) Prognostic classification of Hodgkin disease in pathologic stage III, based on anatomic considerations. Blood 49: 883–893

De-Thé G (1982) Epidemiology of Epstein-Barr virus and associated diseases in man. In: Roizman B (ed) The herpesviruses, vol 1. Plenum, New York, pp 25–103

Dionet C, Oberlin O, Habrand JL et al. (1988) Initial chemotherapy and low-dose radiation in limited fields in childhood Hodgkin's disease: results of a joint cooperative study by the French Society of Pediatric Oncology (SFOP) and Hôpital Saint-Louis, Paris. Int J Radiat Oncol Biol Phys 15: 341–346

Donaldson SS (1984) Editorial: Is involved field irradiation alone optimal therapy for a child with Hodgkin's disease? Med Pediatr Oncol 12: 322–324

Donaldson SS (1990) Hodgkin's disease in children. Semin Oncol 17: 736–748

Donaldson SS, Kaplan HS (1982) Complications of treatment of Hodgkin's disease in children. Cancer Treat Rep 66: 977–989

Donaldson SS, Link MP (1987) Combined modality treatment with low-dose radiation and MOPP chemotherapy for children with Hodgkin's disease. J Clin Oncol 5: 742–749

Donaldson SS, Glatstein E, Rosenberg SA, Kaplan HS (1976) Pediatric Hodgkin's disease. II. Results of therapy. Cancer 37: 2436–2447

Donaldson SS, Whitaker SJ, Plowman PN, Link MP, Malpas JS (1990) Stage I–II pediatric Hodgkin's disease long-term follow-up demonstrates equivalent survival rates following different management schemes. J Clin Oncol 8: 1128–1137

Dörken H (1975) Hodgkin's disease: an epidemiological study on 140 children – urban/rural relation, profession of parents, domestic animal contact. Arch Geschwulstforsch 45: 283–298

Ekert H, Waters KD, Smith PJ, Toogood I, Mauger D (1988) Treatment with MOPP or ChlVPP chemotherapy only for all stages of childhood Hodgkin's disease. J Clin Oncol 6: 1845–1850

Farah R, Ultmann J, Griem M et al. (1988) Extended mantle radiation therapy for pathologic stage I and II Hodgkin's disease. J Clin Oncol 6: 1047–1052

Fletcher GH, Shukovsky LJ (1975) The interplay of radiocurability and tolerance in the irradiation of human cancers. J Radiol Electrol 56: 383–400

Fox KA, Lippman SM, Cassady JR, Heusinkveld RS, Miller TP (1987) Radiation therapy salvage of Hodgkin's disease following chemotherapy failure. J Clin Oncol 5: 38–45

Fryer CJ, Hutchinson RJ, Krailo M et al. (1990) Efficacy and toxicity of 12 courses of ABVD chemotherapy followed by low-dose regional radiation in advanced Hodgkin's disease in children: a report from the children's Cancer Study Group. J Clin Oncol 12: 1971–1980

Gaffey MJ, Weiss LM (1990) Viral oncogenesis: Epstein-Barr virus. Am J Otolaryngol 11: 375–381

Gehan EA, Sullivan MP, Fuller LM et al. (1990) The intergroup Hodgkin's disease in children: a study of stages I and II. Cancer 65: 1429–1437

Glaser SL (1990) Cluster investigations: spatial clustering of Hodgkin's disease in the San Francisco Bay area. Am J Epidemiol 132 [Suppl 1]: S167–S177

Green DM, Gingell RL, Pearce J, Panahon AM, Ghoorah J (1987) The effect of mediastinal irradiation on cardiac function of patients treated during childhood and adolescence for Hodgkin's disease. J Clin Oncol 5: 239–245

Greenberg RS, Grufferman S, Cole P (1983) An evaluation of space-time clustering in Hodgkins's disease. J Chronic Dis 36: 257–262

Hagemeister FB Fuller LM, Velasquez WS et al. (1991) Two cycles of MOPP and radiotherapy: effective treatment for stage IIIA and IIIB Hodgkin's disease. Ann Oncol 2: 25–31

Hamadeh RR, Armenian HK, Zurayk HC (1981) A study of clustering of cases of leukemia, Hodgkin's disease and other lymphomas in Bahrain. Trop Geogr Med 33: 42–49

Hancock SL, Cox RS, McDougall IR (1991) Thyroid diseases after treatment of Hodgkin's disease. N Engl J Med 325: 599–605

Hancock BW, Vaughan Hudson G, Vaughan Hudson B, Haybittle JL, Bennett MH, MacLennan KA, Jelliffe AM (1991) British National Lymphoma Investigation randomized study of MOPP (mustine, oncovin, procarbazine, prednisolone) against LOPP (Leukeran substituted for mustine) in advanced Hodgkin's disease – long term results. Br J Cancer 63: 579–582

Hanks GE, Kinzie JJ, White RL, Herring DF, Kramer S (1983) Patterns of Care outcome studies. Results of the National Practice in Hodgkin's disease. Cancer 51: 569–573

Hays DM, Ternberg JL, Chen TT et al. (1984) Complications related to 234 staging laparotomies performed in the Intergroup Hodgkin's Disease in Childhood study. Surgery 96: 471–478

Herbst H, Dallenbach F, Hummel M, Niedobitek G, Pileri S, Müller-Lantzsch, Stein H (1991) Epstein-Barr virus latent membrane protein expression in Hodgkin and Reed Sternberg cells. Proc Natl Acad Sci USA 88: 4766–4770

Hoppe RT, Rosenberg SA, Kaplan HS, Cox RS (1980) Prognostic factors in pathological stage IIIA Hodgkin's disease. Cancer 46: 1240–1246

Hoppe RT, Coleman CN, Cox RS, Rosenberg SA, Kaplan HS (1982) The management of stage I–II Hodgkin's disease with irradiation alone or combined modality therapy: the Stanford experience. Blood 59: 455–465

Horning SJ, Hoppe RT, Hancock SL, Rosenberg SA (1988) Vinblastine, bleomycin, and methorexate: an effective adjuvant in favorable Hodgkin's disease. J Clin Oncol 6: 1822–1831

Jacobs P, King HS, Karabus C, Hartley P, Werner D (1984) Hodgkin's disease in children. A ten-year experience in South Africa. Cancer 53: 210–213

Jarrett RF, Gallagher A, Jones DB et al. (1991) Detection of Epstein-Barr virus genomes in Hodgkin's disease: relation to age. J Clin Pathol 44: 844–848

Jenkin D, Chan H, Freedman M et al. (1982) Hodgkin's disease in children: treatment results with MOPP and low-dose, extended-field irradiation. Cancer Treat Rep 66: 949–959

Jenkin D, Doyle J, Berry M et al. (1990) Hodgkin's disease in children: treatment with MOPP and low-dose, extended field irradiation without laparotomy – late results and toxicity. Med Pediatr Oncol 18: 265–272

Jenkin RDT, Berry MP (1980) Hodgkin's disease in children. Semin Oncol 7: 202–211

Jenkin RDT, Brown TC, Peters MV, Sonley MJ (1975) Hodgkin's disease in children. Cancer 35: 979–990

Jereb B, Tan C, Bretsky S, He S, Exelby P (1984) Involved field (IF) irradiation with or without chemotherapy in the management of children with Hodgkin's disease. Med Pediatr Oncol 12: 325–332

Jockovich M, Mendenhall NP, Sombeck MD, Talbert JL, Copeland EM III (1994) Long-term complications of laparotomy in Hodgkin's disease. Ann Surg 219: 615–624

Jonsson K, Karp W, Landberg T, Mortensson W, Tennval J, Tylen U (1983) Radiologic evaluation of subdiaphragmatic spread of Hodgkin's disease. Acta Radiol Diag 24: 153–159

Kaldor JM, Day NE, Clarke EA et al. (1990) Leukemia following Hodgkin's disease. N Engl J Med 322: 7–13

Kaplan HS (1980) Hodgkin's disease, 2nd edn. Harvard University Press, Cambridge, Mass

Knecht H, Odermatt BF, Bachmann E et al. (1991) Frequent detection of Epstein-Barr virus DNA by the polymerase chain reaction in lymph node biopsies from patients with Hodgkin's disease without genomic evidence of B- or T-cell clonality. Blood 78: 760–767

Kung F (1991) Hodgkin's disease in children 4 years of age or younger. Cancer 67: 1428–1430

Lange B, Littman P (1983) Management of Hodgkin's disease in children and adolescent toxics. Cancer 51: 1371–1377

Lipschultz SE, Colan SD, Gelber RD, Perz-Atayde AR, Sallan SE, Sanders SP (1991) Late cardiac effects of doxorubicin therapy for acute lymphoblastic leukemia in childhood. N Engl J Med 324: 808–814

Madanat FF (1989) MOPP therapy in children with Hodgkin's disease. Am J Pediatr Hematol Oncol 11: 407–410

Magnusson A, Hagberg H, Hemmingsson A, Lindgren PG (1982) Computed tomography, ultrasound and lymphography in the diagnosis of malignant lymphoma. Acta Radiol Diag 23: 29–35

Mangoud A, Hillier VF, Leck I, Thomas RW (1985) Space-time interaction in Hodgkin's disease in Greater Manchester. J Epidemiol Community Health 39: 58–62

Mansfield CM, Fabian C, Jones S et al. (1991) Comparison of lymphangiography and computed tomography scanning in evaluating abdominal disease in stages III and IV Hodgkin's disease. A Southwest Oncology Group study. Cancer 66: 2295–2299

Mauch P, Ryback ME, Rosenthal D, Weichselbaum R, Hellman S (1980) The influence of initial pathologic stage on the survival of patients who relapse from Hodgkin's disease. Blood 56: 892–897

Mauch P, Weinstein H, Botnick L, Belli J, Cassady JR (1983) An evaluation of long-term survival and treatment complications in children Hodgkin's disease. Cancer 51: 925–932

Mauch P, Goffman T, Rosenthal DS, Canellos GP, Come SE, Hellman S (1985) Stage III Hodgkin's disease: improved survival with combined modality therapy as compared with radiation therapy alone. J Clin Oncol 3: 1166–1173

Mauch P, Tarbell N, Skarin A, Rosenthal D, Weinstein H (1987) Wide-field radiation therapy alone or with chemotherapy for Hodgkin's disease in relapse from combination chemotherapy. J Clin Oncol 5: 544–549

Mauch P, Tarbell N, Weinstein H et al. (1988) Stage IA and IIA supradiaphragmatic Hodgkin's disease: prognostic factors in surgically staged patients treated with mantle and para-aortic irradiation. J Clin Oncol 6: 1576–1583

Meadows AT, Obringer AC, Marrero O et al. (1989) Second malignant neoplasms following childhood Hodgkin's disease: treatment and splenectomy as risk factors. Med Pediatr Oncol 17: 477–484

Mefferd JM, Donaldson SS, Link MP (1989) Pediatric Hodgkin's disease: pulmonary, cardiac, and thyroid function following combined modality therapy. Int J Radiat Oncol Biol Phys 16: 679–685

Mendenhall NP, Shuster JJ, Million RR (1989) The impact of stage and treatment modality on the likelihood of second malignancies and hematopoietic disorders in Hodgkin's disease. Radiother Oncol 14: 219–229

Mendenhall NP, Taylor BW Jr, Marcus RB Jr, Million RR (1991) The impact of pelvic recurrence and elective pelvic irradiation on survival and treatment morbidity in early-stage Hodgkin's disease. Int J Radiat Oncol Biol Phys 21: 1157–1165

Mendenhall NP, Cantor AB, Williams JL et al. (1993) With modern imaging techniques, is staging laparotomy necessary in pediatric Hodgkin's Disease? A Pediatric Oncology Group study. J Clin Oncol 11: 2218–2225

Mueller N (1991) An epidemiologist's view of the new molecular biology findings in Hodgkin's disease. Ann Oncol 2 [Suppl 2]: 23–28

Norris DG, Burgert EO, Cooper HA, Harrison EG Jr (1975) Hodgkin's disease in childhood. Cancer 36: 2109–2120

Olweny CLM, Katongole-Mbidde E, Kiire C, Lwanga SK, Magrath I, Ziegler JL (1978) Childhood Hodgkin's disease in Uganda. A ten year experience. Cancer 42: 787–792

Ortin TTS, Shostak CA, Donaldson SS (1990) Gonadal status and reproductive function following treatment for Hodgkin's disease in childhood: the Stanford experience. Int J Radiat Oncol Biol Phys 19: 873–880

Pallesen G, Hamilton-Dutoit SJ, Rowe M, Young LS (1991) Expression of Epstein-Barr virus latent gene products in tumour cells of Hodgkin's disease. Lancet 337: 320–322

Parker BR, Castellino RA, Kaplan HS (1976) Pediatric Hodgkin's disease. I. Radiographic evaluation. Cancer 37: 2430–2435

Peters MV (1966) Prophylactic treatment of adjacent areas in Hodgkin's disease. Cancer Res 26: 1232–1243

Prosnitz LR, Cooper D, Cox EB, Kapp DS, Farber LR (1985) Treatment selection for stage IIIA Hodgkin's disease patients. Int J Radiat Oncol Biol Phys 11: 1431–1437

Prosnitz LR, Farber LR, Kapp DS, Scott J, Bertino JR, Fischer JJ, Codman EC (1988) Combined modality therapy for advanced Hodgkin's disease: 15-year follow-up data. J Clin Oncol 6: 603–612

Roach M III, Kapp DS, Rosenberg SA, Hoppe RT (1987) Radiotherapy with curative intent: an option in selected patients relapsing after chemotherapy for advanced Hodgkin's disease. J Clin Oncol 5: 550–555

Roach M III, Brophy N, Cox R, Varghese A, Hoppe RT (1990) Prognostic factors for patients relapsing after radiotherapy for early-stage Hodgkin's disease. J Clin Oncol 8: 623–629

Robinson B, Kingston J, Costa RN, Maplas JS, Barrett A, McElwain TJ (1984) Chemotherapy and irradiation in childhood Hodgkin's disease. Arch Dis Child 59: 1162–1167

Ross A, Davis S (1990) Point pattern analysis of the spatial proximity of residences prior to diagnosis of persons with Hodgkin's disease. Am J Epidemiol 132 [Suppl 1]: S53–S62

Samoszuk M, Ravel J (1991) Frequent detection of Epstein-Barr viral deoxyribonucleic acid and absence of cytomegalovirus deoxyribonucleic acid in Hodgkin's disease and acquired immunodeficiency syndrome-related Hodgkin's disease. Lab Invest 65: 631–636

Schellong G, Waubke-Landwehr A-K, Langermann H-J, Riehm H-J, Brämswig J, Ritter J (1986) Prediction of splenic involvement in children with Hodgkin's disease. Significance of clinical intraoperative findings. A retrospective statistical analysis of 154 patients in the German Therapy Study DAL-HD-78. Cancer 57: 2049–2056

Schellong G, Brämswig JH, Schwarze EW et al. (1988) An approach to reduce treatment and invasive staging in childhood Hodgkin's disease: the sequence of the German DAL Multicenter studies. Bull Cancer 75: 41–51

Schellong G, Hörnig I, Schwarze EW, Wannenmacher M (1989) Risk factor adapted treatment of Hodgkin's lymphoma in childhood: strategies and results of three consecutive multicenter studies in the Federal Republic of Germany. Recent Results Cancer Res 117: 205–213

Schewe KL, Reavis J, Kun LE, Cox JD (1988) Total dose, fraction size, and tumor volume in the local control of Hodgkin's disease. Int J Radiat Oncol Biol Phys 15: 25–28

Schimpff SC, O'Connell MJ, Greene WH, Wiernik PH (1975) Infections in 92 splenectomized patients with Hodgkin's disease. A clinical review. Am J Med 59: 695–701

Schneeberger AL, Girvan DP (1988) Staging laparotomy for Hodgkin's disease in children. J Pediatr Surg 23: 714–717

Schwartz RS, Callen JP, Silva J Jr (1978) A cluster of Hodgkin's disease in a small community: evidence for environmental factors. Am J Epidemiol 108: 19–25

Shibata D, Hansmann M-L, Weiss LM, Nathwani BN (1991) Epstein-Barr virus infections and Hodgkin's disease: a study of fixed tissues using the polymerase chain reaction. Hum Pathol 22: 1262–1267

Sinkovics JG (1991) Hodgkin's disease revisited: Reed-Sternberg cells as natural hybridomas. Crit Rev Immunol 11: 33–63

Smith LM, Mendenhall NP, Cicale MJ, Block ER, Carter RL, Million RR (1989) Results of a prospective study evaluating the effects of mantle irradiation on pulmonary function. Int J Radiat Oncol Biol Phys 16: 79–84

Sombeck MD, Mendenhall NP, Kaude JV, Torres GM, Million RR (1993) Correlation of lymphangiography, computed tomography, and laparotomy in the staging of Hodgkin's disease. Int J Radiat Oncol Biol Phys 25: 425–429

Stein H, Herbst H, Anagnostopoulous I, Niedobitek G, Dallenbach F, Kratzsch HC (1991) The nature of Hodgkin and Reed-Sternberg cells, their association with Epstein-Barr virus and their relationship to anaplastic large-cell lymphoma. Ann Oncol 2 [Suppl 2]: 33–38

Thar TL, Million RR (1980) Complications of radiation treatment of Hodgkin's disease. Semin Oncol 7: 174–183

Thar TL, Million RR, Hausner RJ, McKetty MHB (1979) Hodgkin's disease, stages I and II. Relationship of recurrence to size of disease, radiation dose, and number of sites involved. Cancer 43: 1101–1105

Uhara H, Sato Y, Mukai K et al. (1990) Detection of Epstein-Barr virus DNA in Reed-Sternberg cells of Hodgkin's disease using the polymerase chain reaction and in situ hybridization. Jpn J Cancer Res 81: 272–278

Vinciguerra V, Propert KJ, Coleman M et al. (1986) Alternating cycles of combination chemotherapy for patients with recurrent Hodgkin's disease following radiotherapy. A prospectively randomized study by the Cancer and Leukemia Group B. J Clin Oncol 4: 838–846

Weiss LM (1991) Epstein-Barr virus and Hodgkin's disease. A correlative in situ hybridization and polymerase chain reaction study. Am J Pathol 139: 1269–1265

Williams RS, Mendenhall NP (1992) Laparoscopic oophoropexy for preservation of ovarian function before pelvic node irradiation. Obstet Gynecol 80: 541–543

12 Neuroblastoma

J. ROBERT CASSADY

CONTENTS

12.1   Introduction 175
12.2   Epidemiology 175
12.3   Etiology. 176
12.4   Natural History and Evaluation 176
12.5   Pathology. 178
12.6   Prognostic Features and Staging. 178
12.7   Therapy. 180
12.7.1 General Comments 180
12.7.2 Surgery 181
12.7.3 Chemotherapy 183
12.7.4 Radiation Therapy 184
12.7.5 Bone Marrow Transplantation 188
12.8   Results 190
12.9   Prevention/Early Diagnosis 191
12.10   Future Goals 191
        References 191

12.1 Introduction

Neuroblastoma (NB), an enigmatic disease with protean manifestations, represents the most common non-central nervous system solid tumor of childhood. Approximately 450 new cases (~ 8% of all childhood tumors) are diagnosed annually in the United States (YOUNG et al. 1978; KRAMER et al. 1983; MICHAELIS and KAATSCH 1986).

Although recognized for decades as the tumor which most frequently undergoes spontaneous regression, substantial overall improvements in survival have only begun to be achieved by improved surgical techniques and other nonsurgical approaches in the past two decades. NB serves as a paradigm for demonstrating the possible influence of age on both prognosis and radiation sensitivity, phenomena that have negatively impacted pediatric radiation oncology when incorrectly extrapolated to

J. ROBERT CASSADY, M.D., Professor and Head, Department of Radiation Oncology, The University of Arizona, Health Sciences Center, 1501 North Campbell Ave., Tucson, AZ 85724, USA

other tumors such as Wilms' tumor and rhabdomyosarcoma.

12.2 Epidemiology

Like many pediatric malignancies, NB occurs with greater frequency in males (~1.25:1.0) for unknown reasons (GREEN 1985). Careful fetal, infant, and early childhood autopsy studies demonstrate that the clinical incidence of this tumor is much lower than its apparent pathologic occurrence rate. Thus, clinically, 10–15 cases are diagnosed annually for every one million children less than 15 years old, whereas pathologically a rate of one case per 50–200 has been documented (BECKWITH and PERRIN 1963; GUIN et al. 1969). Although usually ascribed to "spontaneous regression," the true cause for this discrepancy is not known.

Neuroblastoma is the most common tumor of any type appearing in the first year of life and progressively decreases in frequency with increasing age, becoming rare after 7–8 years (BADER and MILLER 1979; KAYE et al. 1986; EVANS et al. 1987; KRETSCHMAR 1991). The rapidly decreasing incidence figures with age are consistent with the theory that NB is a congenital tumor arising in fetal neural crest tissue. Pertinent consequences of this observation relate to tumor growth rate and age of presentation and their relation to necessary follow-up time to ascertain recurrence (vide infra) (COLLINS 1955). The median age at diagnosis is 24 months (GREEN 1985).

Tumor deposits have been noted at virtually every body site; however, the disease tends to present at autonomic nervous system sites of neural crest tissue and the majority of cases originate in the adrenal and periadrenal regions. Figure 12.1 shows primary site locations in 1667 cases. The site of presentation is also a function of age, with infants more frequently presenting with cervicomediastinal disease than children older than 13 months (PIZZO et al. 1989). A significant number (6.5%) of patients (often infants) present with metastases with no obvious primary.

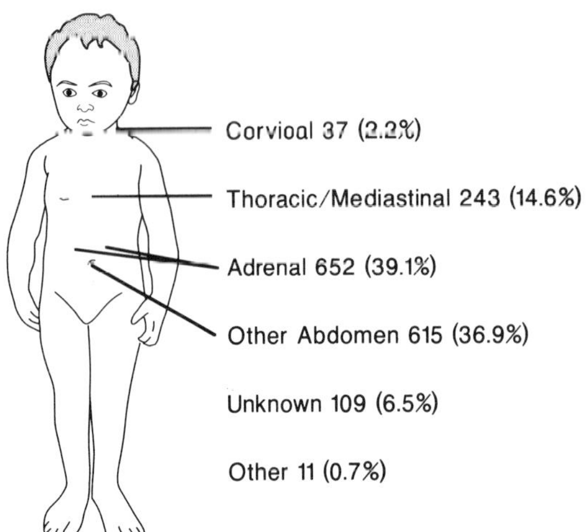

Fig. 12.1. Primary site of presentation for NB. Data collected from several representative series, including ROSEN et al. (1984), BERTHOLD et al. (1986), and GREEN (1985)

12.3 Etiology

The etiology of NB is unknown. Associations are recognized with a variety of conditions, including neurofibromatosis (KNUDSON and AMROMIN 1966; WITZLEBEN and LINDY 1974), fetal alcohol and hydantoin syndromes (SHERMAN and ROIZEN 1976; RAMILO and HARRIS 1979; SEELER et al. 1979) nesidioblastosis (GROTTING et al. 1979), Beckwith-Wiedemann syndrome (EMERY et al. 1983), and, perhaps, Hirschsprung's disease (HOPE et al. 1965; GAISIE et al. 1979). A very rare familial neuroblastoma syndrome characterized by young age at presentation, autosomal dominant transmission, and multiple primaries has been reported (CHATTEN and VOORHESS 1967; LEAPE et al. 1978; MANCINI et al. 1982; FELICI et al. 1990). KNUDSON and MEADOWS (1980) have postulated that infants with stage IVS (vide infra) NB represent a multifocal hereditary equivalent of retinoblastoma.

Chromosomal abnormalities have been frequently noted, the most common being deletion of chromosome 1 (1p32) or monosomy of chromosome 1 (1p-). Chromosome 17 abnormalities have also been reported (BRODEUR et al. 1981; SCHWAB 1988).

The presence of double minutes (DM) and homogeneously staining regions (HSR) in NB cells has been regularly reported (BALABAN-MALENBAUM and GILBERT 1980; EMANUEL et al. 1985; IKEGAKI et al. 1986; SCHWAB 1988) Gene amplification of the N-*myc* (v-*myc*) gene, normally located at the 2p22–24 region, accounts for these findings, which are seen primarily in biologically aggressive, advanced-stage

disease (SCHWAB 1988). The N-*myc* copy number of a tumor appears to remain relatively constant over time, uninfluenced by therapy. Although prognostically relevant (vide infra), the relationship of these findings to tumor causation or progression is not known (BRODEUR et al. 1984; SEEGER et al. 1985).

12.4 Natural History and Evaluation

Children with NB may present with a wide range of symptoms and signs (JAFFE 1976; ROSEN et al. 1984; KRETSCHMAR 1991) (Table 12.1). Unlike the case of many childhood malignancies, the majority of children with NB (~ 60%) present with distant metastatic disease and many others have regional nodal disease. In addition to the common finding of an abdominal mass, children (especially those older than 24 months) frequently present with systemic symptoms of fever, lethargy, malaise, and generalized pain from widespread metastases (GREEN 1985). If the disease is far advanced, symptoms of bleeding from disseminated intravascular coagulopathy may be present (SCOTT and MORGAN 1983).

Children may present with paresis or paralysis from a paraspinal tumor which goes through the neural foramen ("dumbbell tumor") into the spinal canal (TRAGGIS et al. 1977; ADAM and HOCHHOLZER 1981). Less commonly, children may present with heterochromia iridis and Horner's syndrome from a cervical/supraclavicular primary (JAFFE et al. 1975). Severe diarrhea may be the primary complaint, presumably due to tumor release of a vasoactive intestinal peptide (VIP)-like substance (SWIFT et al. 1975). As this tumor is well recognized to produce a variety of catecholamines, children occasionally present with hypertension and its symptoms (KEDAR et al. 1981; WEINBLATT et al. 1983). Very infrequently, children, usually with early-stage disease and thoracic or paraspinal primaries, present with opsoclonus, polymyoclonus, and ataxia (SOLOMAN and CHUTORIAN 1968). Although not proven, this syndrome has been postulated to be due to an antitumor

Table 12.1. Presenting Symptoms in NB (271 patients) (data from GREEN 1975)

Symptom	No.	%
Mass or swelling	150	55.0
Pain	86	32.0
Fever/weight loss	84	31.0
Neurologic	36	13.0
Respiratory	11	4.1

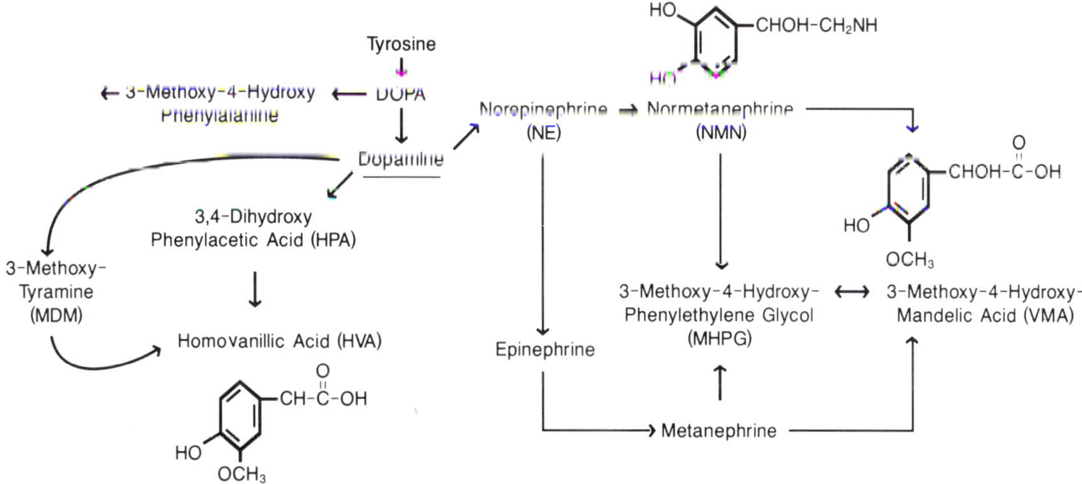

Fig. 12.2. Catecholamine metabolic pathway. Levels of VMA, NE, MHPG, and HVA may all be elevated in children with NB, especially those with disseminated disease

autoimmune-type phenomenon with cross-reactivity against cerebellar tissue. Young children, usually with stage IVS disease (vide infra), present with generalized bluish skin nodules ("blueberry muffin" – also seen in histiocytosis or infantile acute mono- myelogenous leukemia) and/or moderate or severe respiratory distress from massive hepatic involvement and limitation of diaphragmatic excursion (D'ANGIO et al. 1971; EVANS et al. 1980, 1981; KRETSCHMAR 1991).

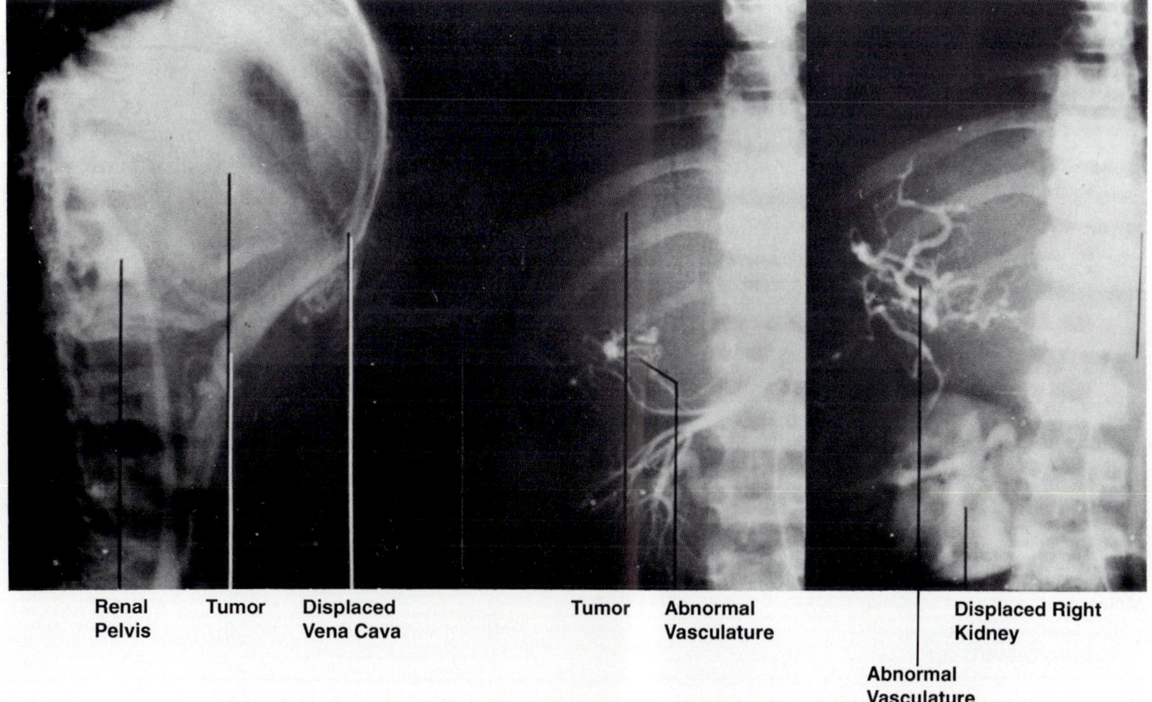

Fig. 12.3. Typical suprarenal NB demonstrating displacement of ipsilateral kidney downwards with the superior pole of the kidney displaced laterally. Retroperitoneal primary extension and model disease frequently encases the great vessels and extends superiorly in the chest cavity. Note the anteriorly displaced vena cava. (DE VITA et al. 1982)

More localized symptoms from metastatic disease may be present, and unexplained atraumatic bilateral orbital ecchymoses are usually found to be related to disseminated NB. Why these and other bony metastases are so frequently symmetrical is not known.

In addition to a thorough history and physical examination, 24-h urine catecholamine levels should be measured. Levels of vanillylmandelic acid (VMA), norepinephrine, homovanillic acid (HVA), and 3-methoxy-4-hydroxyphenyl-ethylene glycol may all be elevated (Fig. 12.2) (Kaser and Studnitz 1961; GITLOW et al. 1970; LAUG et al. 1978).

Imaging studies should include an isotopic bone scan and CT and/or MRI of the primary site (Fig. 12.3). Should the primary be extra-abdominal, imaging of the adrenal and perirenal areas should be considered as multiple primary tumors may occur. Although signs of intraparenchymal metastatic lung disease are rare (usually occurring only in older children), a chest x-ray frequently demonstrates displacement of the posterior paraspinous pleura due to posterior nodal or primary extension. Bone marrow aspiration and biopsy are mandatory, as are the usual CBC and serum electrolytes, and hepatic and renal studies. A myelogram may be indicated in patients with neurologic signs or symptoms, as may plain films of symptomatic bones.

Meta-iodobenzylguanidine is a norepinephrine analog which can be labeled with radioactive iodine and, as it is absorbed and stored by NB tissue, imaging and therapeutic trials using this material have gained recent prominence. It may demonstrate lesions (usually bony) not visualized by other techniques. Therapeutically a minor palliative role has usually been reported (VOUTE et al. 1985; MOYES et al. 1989; KLINGEBIEL et al. 1991).

12.5 Pathology

Neuroblastomas belongs to the group of "small round blue cell tumors" of infancy and childhood. Classically, scanty cytoplasm is present and the nucleus is hyperchromatic (Table 12.2). Tumor cells may cluster in a tubular fashion with dense neurofibrils in the center (Homer-Wright rosette). Hemorrhage, calcification, and lymphocytic infiltration may be present. At the other end of the spectrum, the ganglioneuroma may contain large differentiated ganglion cells set in a matrix of nerve fibrils. Intermediate mixtures in all possible combinations exits.

SHIMADA et al. (1984) have developed a pathologic grouping system based on cellular differentiation and the quantity of stroma present (Fig. 12.4). Combined with age and the mitosis–karyorrhexis index (nuclear characteristics) prognosis could be determined with relative accuracy.

More recently, BRODEUR et al. (1984) and SEEGER et al. (1985) have correlated the average number of N-*myc* copies, separated into three groups, with stage and prognosis (Table 12.3, Fig. 12.5). The N-*myc* copy number parallels the biologic virulence of NB. Most patients with more than three copies have stage III or IV disease.

12.6 Prognostic Features and Staging

An array of features have been correlated with prognosis (CASSADY 1990). All investigators agree on the independent prognostic value of age at diagnosis and anatomic extent of disease (BRESLOW and McCANN 1971). It has frequently been noted that median age increases with increasing stage (excepting IVS).

Table 12.2. Immunohistochemical findings in small cell tumors of soft tissue[a]

	Cytokeratin	Vimentin	Desmin	Neurofilament	LCA[b]	NSE[b]	S-100
Malignant Lymphoma	0	+/–	0	0	+	0	0
Neuroblastoma/ neuroepithelioma	0	+/–	0	+/–	0	+	0
Ewing's sarcoma	0	+	0	0	0	0	0
Melanoma	0	+	0	0	0	0	+
Embryonal rhabodomyosarcoma	0	+	+	0	0	0	0

[a] It is frequently extremely difficult to distinguish the various "small blue round cell tumors" of childhood by light microscopy and by simple morphology. Immunohistochemical techniques developed in the past decade have provided significantly improved discrimination, especially when combined with clinical parameters including patient age and other pathologic techniques including electron microscopy. An accurate diagnosis is obviously crucial in formulating an appropriate therapeutic plan.
[b] LCA, leukocyte common antigen; NSE, neuron-specific enolase

Fig. 12.4. Shimada histopathologic grouping for prognosis (SHIMADA 1984) based on an analysis of 295 patients, 73 of whom had Evans-D'Angio stage IV disease – a disproportionately good stage distribution. Note that children with a "good prognosis" include those with stroma-rich tumors which are mixed and well differentiated and a subset of the much larger stroma-poor group that are more differentiated

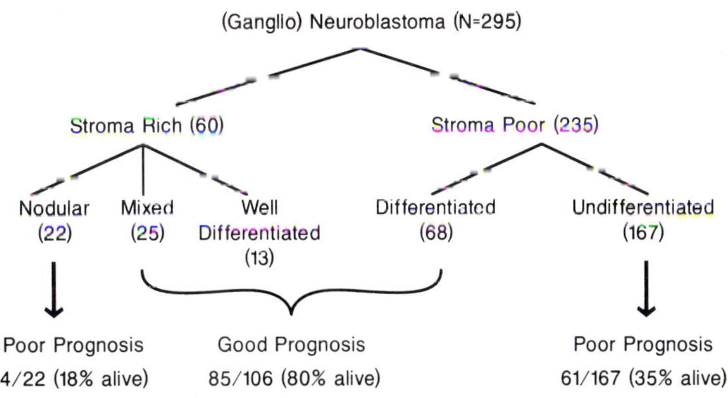

Other features that have been correlated with prognosis include pathology (Shimada system) (SHIMADA et al. 1984), assays of neuron-specific enolase (ZELTZER et al. 1985), serum ferritin (Hann et al. 1985), quantitative ratios of VMA/HVA levels (LAUG et al. 1978), tumor site of origin (CARLSEN et al. 1986), degree of maturation (BECKWITH and MARTIN 1968), N-*myc* copy number (BRODEUR et al. 1984; SEEGER et al. 1985) and extent of surgical resection. Multivariate analysis has most frequently identified age, stage, serum ferritin, and Shimada pathology as

significant variables, although the latter features may not be duplicated in all hands (CASSADY 1990).

Four principal staging systems have been developed for this condition: the initial and widely used system of Evans and D'Angio (EVANS et al. 1971), the system developed at St. Jude, in which the importance of lymph node involvement was stressed (HAYES et al. 1983), a modification of the St. Jude system developed by the Pediatric Oncology Group (POG) (NITSCHKE et al. 1988), and finally, an International system which hopefully combines the best aspects of earlier systems and will allow better definition of true risk factors (BRODEUR and SEEGER 1988; BRODEUR et al. 1988; SMITH et al. 1989; American Joint Committee on Cancer 1983). In the St. Jude system, the special (IVS) group identified by Evans and D'Angio has not been separately identified. These staging systems are depicted in Table 12.4. Approximate distribution of children by Evans-D'Angio stage is illustrated in Table 12.5.

Table 12.3. Correlation of N-MYC copy number with Evans-D'Angio stage (data from BRODEUR et al. 1984)

No. of copies	Stage I	II	III	IV	IVS
1	8	14	7	21	5
3–10	0	2	5	8	0
>10	0	0	8	11	0

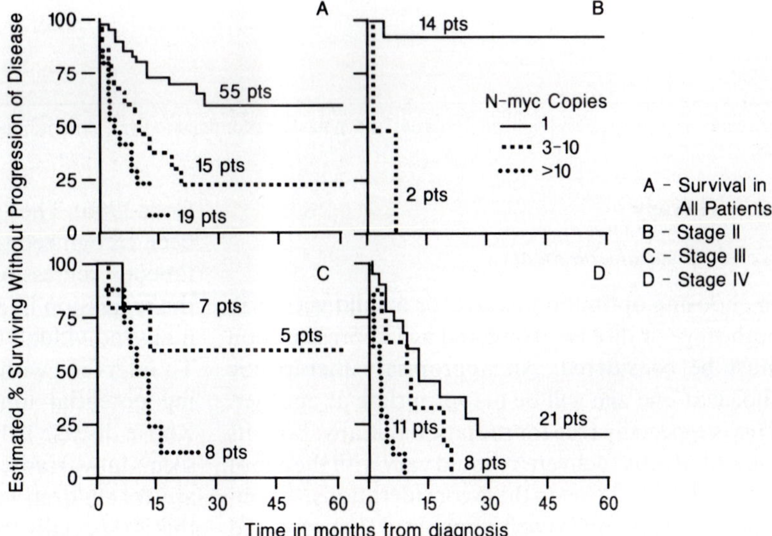

Fig. 12.5. Relationship of N-*myc* copy number to prognosis and stage. *Panel A* represents survival data in all patients (Evans/D'Angio stage II–IV) while *panels B–D* represent data in individual stages. The relative paucity (2 pts.) of patients with >3 copies with stage II disease is notable, as is their frequency in stage IV. (Data from SEEGER et al. 1985)

Table 12.4. The four principle staging systems for NB

St. Jude Children's Research Hospital (SJCRH)	Pediatric Oncology Group (POG)	Evans-D'Angio system	International staging system
Stage I: Localized tumor completely resected. *Stage IIA:* Localized tumor completely resected but with pathologic evidence of microscopic tumor through the capsule. *Stage IIB:* Localized unresectable or partially resected tumor. *Stage IIIA:* Disseminated disease with no bone or bone marrow involvement [stage IIIA: dissemination to regional nodes only]. *Stage IIIB:* Disseminated disease with one localized bone lesion but no bone marrow involvement. *Stage IIIC:* Disseminated disease with bone marrow and/or generalized bone involvement.	*Stage A:* Complete gross resection of primary tumor, with or without microscopic residual. Intracavitary lymph nodes, not adherent to but removed with the primary, must be histologically free of tumor. Nodes adherent to or within the tumor resection may be positive for tumor without restaging patient to stage C. If primary is in abdomen or pelvis, liver must be histologically free of tumor. *Stage B:* Grossly unresected primary tumor. Nodes and liver as in stage A. *Stage C:* Complete or incomplete resection of primary. Intracavitary nodes that are not adherent to the primary are histologically positive for tumor. Liver as in stage A. *Stage D:*[a] Any of dissemination of disease beyond intracavitary modes, that is, extracavitary nodes, liver, skin, bone marrow, or bone.	*Stage I:* Tumors confined to the organ or structure of origin. *Stage II:* Tumors extending in continuity beyond the organ or structure of origin but not crossing the midline. Regional lymph nodes on the homolateral side may be involved. *Stage III:* Tumors extending in continuity beyond the midline. Regional lymph nodes bilaterally may be involved. *Stage IV:* Remote disease involving skeleton, parenchymatous organs, soft tissues, distant lymph node groups, and so on. *Stage IVS:* Patients who would otherwise be stage I or II, but have remote disease confined only to one or more of the following sites: liver, skin, or bone marrow (without radiographic evidence of bone metastases on complete skeletal survey).	*Stage I:* Localized tumor confined to the area of origin; complete gross excision, with or without microscopic residual disease; identifiable ipsilateral and contralateral lymph nodes negative microscopically. *Stage 2A:* Unilateral tumor with incomplete gross excision; identifiable ipsilateral and contralateral lymph nodes negative microscopically. *Stage 2B:* Unilateral tumor with complete or incomplete gross excision; with positive ipsilateral regional lymph nodes; identifiable contralateral lymph nodes negative microscopically. *Stage 3:* Tumor infiltrating across the midline with or without regional lymph node involvement; or, unilateral tumor with contralateral regional lymph node involvement; or, midline tumor with bilateral regional lymph node involvement. Stage 4: Dissemination of tumor to distant lymph nodes, bone, bone marrow, liver, and/or other organs (except as defined in stage 4S). *Stage 4S:* Localized primary tumor as defined for stage 1 or 2 with dissemination limited to liver, skin, and/or bone marrow.

[a] Patients with ipsilateraly confined primaries and metastases confined to liver, skin or bone marrow (*not* bone) have been designated Ds.

12.7 Therapy

12.7.1 General Comments

In choosing optimum therapy for a child with NB, both stage or disease extent and age at presentation must be considered. An appropriate therapeutic choice at one age will be inappropriate at another. This is especially true for radiation therapy: both its use and the dose delivered should vary with the age of the child. In addition to these considerations, "spontaneous regression" is well recognized (EVERSON and Cole 1966). The "special" or IVS category of NB has been recognized to frequently undergo such "spontaneous regression," perhaps similar in nature to the regression in occult fetal NB that must occur in many individuals based on neonatal autopsy studies. To intervene with overly aggressive treatment having potential long-term consequences in a child whose disease is likely to disappear spontaneously seems unwarranted. Therefore, to some degree, therapy for children with NB must be individualized, and this is especially true for those in the first year of life.

Table 12.5. Incidence of Evans-D'Angio stage at presentation ($n = 390$) (data from Berthold et al. 1986 and Rosen et al. 1984)

Evans-D'Angio stage	No.	%
I	32	8.2
II	56	14.4
III[a]	85	21.8
IV	181	46.4
IVS	36	9.2

[a] The interseries variation in the frequency of stage III was notable. In Rosen et al., 14.4% of children were stage III, whereas in Berthold et al., 25% were stage III.

12.7.2 Surgery

Surgery plays a central role in diagnosis, staging, and treatment of NB. Sixty percent of children with NB present with metastatic disease. In many of these children, diagnosis will be made by bone marrow studies or a combination of examination, imaging studies, and biochemical marker studies. On occasion, biopsy of a metastatic site (i.e., lymph node or skin nodule) will be necessary to establish the diagnosis. In children with metastatic disease, evidence for the role of surgery either initially or at "second (or third) look" in obtaining cure is uncertain but suggestive (see Sect. 12.7.5) (August et al. 1984; Philip et al. 1987; Hartmann et al. 1987).

Children with regionally limited disease and no evidence of nonadherent lymph node disease are cured in a high proportion of cases by gross resection of tumor with no other adjuvant therapy (Table 12.6). Nitschke et al. (1988), reporting for the POG, has demonstrated an 89% actuarial 2-year disease-free survival in 101 children with POG stage A disease grossly resected with no planned additional therapy. Of 49 children actually followed for 2 years, 40 were disease free. In addition to resection, these children also had surgical staging, with routine liver biopsy (39/50) in those with abdominal primaries and lymph node sampling (37) or search (56) in 93 of the 101 patients. In 83 children in whom pathology of resection margins could be assessed, 33 had positive microscopic margins. These 33 children fared equally well. Only one relapse has occurred beyond the first year of follow-up. Four of nine children relapsed at locoregional sites (2/4 NED off therapy for relapse) and four neonates developed distant relapse in a pattern suggesting metachronous Evans-D'Angio IVS disease (4/4 NED off therapy for relapse).

This work confirms earlier nonprospective studies and reaffirms that gross surgical resection should

Table 12.6. Results of surgery as sole therapy for NB

Author	No. of pts.	Stage	Other primary therapy	Age		Relapse	Local or Regional	Site of relapse		Salvage	% Survival	Comments
								L&D	Distant			
Nitschke et al. (1988)	101	All pts. POG stage A E/D stage: I 84 II 10 III 7	0	55 (< 1 yr)	46 (> 1 yr)	9	4	0	5	2/4 local 4/5 distant (3 deaths)	89% NED at 2 yr (SE 5%) 49 followed for > 2 yr	5 pts. lost to follow up 4 young pts. failed with metachronous IVS pattern
Matthay et al. (1989)	156	E/D stage II	0 (75 pts.) XRT 66 C 8	116 (< 2 yr)	39 (> 2 ye)	14 (8 with S only)	7 (S only)	1 (with S only)	6 (2 with S only)	8 (6 with S only) 5/7 locoreg. salvage	98% at 6 yr with S only. 95% at 6 yr with S + other therapy	Excellent ability to salvage relapse
Adam and Hochholzer (1981)	18 (all thoracic)	E/D stage I	0 (1/2 were < 3 yr)	?	?	0	0	0	0	0	100%	Interesting data on some patients who were older with incomplete resection treated with S+XRT±C with late relapse

Abbreviations: POG, Pediatric Oncology Group; E/D, Evans-D'Angio; L, local; D, Ddistant; Ned, no evidence of disease; S, surgery; XRT, radiation therapy; C, chemotherapy

be the sole initial therapy for most of these children (HAYES et al. 1983; BERTHOLD et al. 1986; NITSCHKE et al. 1988). Six children in this study underwent surgical sacrifice of one kidney to accomplish gross resection. Controversy exists as to the relative merits of this approach versus partial resection with organ retention and careful follow-up, reserving additional therapy for documented tumor progression. Alternatively, the less-favored approach of partial resection, organ retention, and low-dose regional irradiation can be followed. At this time, this author would favor organ retention and postsurgical multiagent chemotherapy for a short period for these children (HAYES et al. 1983; 1984; NITSCHKE et al. 1983).

For unresectable but regionally limited tumors without nodal metastases (POG stage B), initial biopsy and/or partial resection with subsequent postchemotherapy surgical re-resection has yielded excellent results (ZUCKER and MARGULIS 1979; HAYES et al. 1983; GREEN et al. 1985).

MATTHAY et al. (1989) recently reviewed 156 patients with Evans-D'Angio stage II disease and raised serious questions about the need for any adjuvant nonsurgical therapy in this group. Although the study was not randomized and therefore potentially biased, the 6-year disease-free survival rate for 75 children receiving surgery alone was not significantly different from the rate for those receiving radiation and/or chemotherapy. Of perhaps equal importance, five of seven patients whose disease progressed after surgery alone were salvaged with additional treatment. Thus survival (at 6 years) was equivalent in both groups (S=98%; $S \times C$ 95%). No difference in progression-free survival was seen in 40 children with untreated gross residual disease when compared with 59 with gross residual disease who received radiation + chemotherapy. As POG stage B patients are not comparable to those with Evans-D'Angio stage II, 10%–15% of whom have positive nodes, extrapolation is not possible. However, a significant fraction of POG stage B patients are, in fact, also Evans-D'Angio stage II, and for this group, surgery alone appears appropriate.

As in Evans-D'Angio stage I patients, the long-term functional and structural morbidity of surgical resection alone versus more limited surgery and chemotherapy ± radiation therapy for certain subsets of Evans-D'Angio stage II patients (i.e., those with spinal canal disease or renal encasement) is not known, and it is possible that improved results (not survival) might be possible by use of combined therapy in some patients.

The role of second- and/or third-look surgery in children with POG stage C and D disease in controversial (HAASE et al. 1989). The former group will be discussed in Sect. 12.7.4.

Relapse or progression at the primary site in children with initially unresectable metastatic NB (not stage IVS) managed primarily with aggressive multiagent chemotherapy is not uncommon (ROSEN et al. 1984). No evidence exists suggesting a benefit to overly aggressive but nevertheless incomplete resection attempts ("tumor insult") in these children. Should no additional regional treatment (surgery or radiation therapy) be delivered following postsurgical chemotherapy, the first site of relapse or progression is frequently locoregional. However, it is debatable whether additional locoregional therapy in children not undergoing attempted bone marrow transplantation (vide infra) alters ultimate prognosis, as opposed to relapse pattern. The role of surgery in determining the degree of locoregional tumor extension and nodal disease is, however, well recognized.

Although primary resection is recommended and usually possible in children presenting with Evans-D'Angio stage IVS [POG stage D(S)], who, by definition, must have ipsilaterally confined and therefore not extensive primaries, it is uncertain what role primary resection plays in the overall favorable prognosis of these children with or without aggressive systematic management. HAAS et al. (1988) have claimed no benefit to complete resection.

Also controversial is the role of extensive surgery in children who present with primaries that are both intra- and extraspinal ("dumbbell tumors") (TRAGGIS et al. 1977; PUNT et al. 1980; HAYES et al. 1984). Most current investigators recommend dual surgical approaches directed at both extra- and intraspinal disease resection, perhaps combined with multiagent adjuvant chemotherapy. Although prognosis for survival is excellent in this group, it will be of interest and important to compare and contrast the long-term functional results of this dual surgical approach without localized radiation therapy with the results in patients treated in the past with less aggressive surgery and often without laminectomy but with regional low or intermediate dose radiation therapy (JACOBSON et al. 1983; ROSEN et al. 1984).

Surgical placement of a temporary graft (Silastic patch) in the anterior abdomen of children with stage IVS disease may be necessary to alleviate life-threatening respiratory compromise caused by rapid and massive hepatomegaly. Although frequently unsuccessful, such attempts may be life-saving (SCHNAUFER and KOOP 1975).

12.7.3 Chemotherapy

Neuroblastoma is a chemosensitive but often chemoincurable disease. However, modern multiagent and kinetically based regimens have recently been demonstrated to have curative potential in certain relatively favorable subsets of patients with disseminated disease and, when used in conjunction with autologous or allogeneic bone marrow transplant, may effect cure in a minority of previously doomed older patients with metastatic disease (JAFFE 1976; HAYES et al. 1977; FINKLESTEIN et al. 1979; GREEN et al. 1981; FRANTZ et al. 1982; ROSEN et al. 1984; KRETSCHMAR et al. 1984; KUSHNER and HELSON 1987; PAUL et al. 1991).

Many classes of agents have demonstrated efficacy. Alkylating agents, usually in combination, are the mainstay of all current regimens; however, platinum derivatives, vinca alkaloids, anthracycline antibiotics, epipodophylline derivatives, and, rarely, antimetabolites have all been utilized and shown activity (CASTLEBERRY 1990).

Four current, relatively effective multiagent regimens are shown in Table 12.7.

It has been proposed that chemotherapy lacks a role in POG stage A, except perhaps for organ salvage purposes. As the impact of radiation therapy is at best controversial in the initial management of POG stage B children, with a recognized potential for undesirable late consequences, many investigators recommend initial subtotal resection followed by combination chemotherapy and then second-look surgery (HAYES et al. 1984; GREEN et al. 1985). However, results reported by MATTHAY et al. (1989; vide supra) from the Children's Cancer Study Group (CCSG) indicate that some (perhaps the majority) of these children are being treated unnecessarily by chemotherapy. It is uncertain why these results are substantially better than historical data, although stage migration and selection are likely (KINNIER-WILSON and DRAPER 1974). Utilization of the recently proposed International staging system might resolve many of these difficulties (BRODEUR and SEEGER 1988).

Chemotherapy has been demonstrated to have curative potential in a minority of children with regionally extensive and/or lymph node-positive disease (Evans-D'Angio stage III, POG stage C). Although HAYES et al. (1983) demonstrated control in 7/13 infants with SJCRH stage III disease using surgery and chemotherapy alone, results were substantially worse for older children (4/23) (HAYES et al. 1983). A recent randomized POG study has confirmed earlier single-institution studies confirming the value of regional irradiation added to surgery and chemotherapy (CASTLEBERRY et al. 1991).

Among children with disseminated disease, three groups exist for whom cure is possible in a substantial fraction of cases by means of conventional, multiagent chemotherapy without resort to transplant approaches.

Table 12.7. Response rates for current chemotherapy regimens for advanced stage IV NB[a]

Author	Regimen	Complete and partial response		
		%	No.	Comments
FINKLESTEIN et al. (1979)	Cyclophosphamide, vincristine, DTIC ± adriamycin ("COD ± (Adriamycin")	80	48/60	
KUSHNER and HELSON (1987)	Vincristine, adriamycin, cyclophosphamide, 5-FU, ara-C, Hydroxyurea (N4SE)	88	29/33	70% CR + good partial response
PHILIP et al. (1987)	Cisplatin, VM-26, cyclophosphamide, adriamycin, vincristine (PE/CADO)	97	34/35	68% CR + good partial response
FRANTZ et al. (1982)	Vincristine, adriamycin, nitrogen mustard, cyclophosphamide, cisplatin, DTIC (MADDOC)	74	20/27	Median survival ~32 mo

[a] Note the relatively consistent use of alkylating agents, adriamycin, and vinca alkaloids.

The excellent prognosis of children with Evans-D'Angio stage IVS [POG stage D(S)] disease has been noted. In fact, many of these infants (>90% are less than 13 months old at diagnosis) will do well following initial diagnosis and resection of the primary tumor without any additional systemic (or local) therapy (PUNT et al. 1980; ROSEN et al. 1984; HAAS et al. 1988). However, many will also require intervention, and initial management is controversial (ROSEN et al. 1984). In D'Angio and Evans' original series, although an 84% survival at 2 years was documented, 21/25 or 80% received therapeutic intervention at some time (D'ANGIO et al. 1971). Similarly, the POG reported that four of ten "untreated" children required intervention with multiagent chemotherapy (KRETSCHMAR 1991). The occasionally advocated position of withholding cytotoxic therapy in this group despite clinical progression is to be decried and has probably led to the unnecessary demise of some children. In general, systemic therapeutic approaches (as opposed to low-dose local irradiation of the liver, etc.) are recommended for nonstable progressive disease. The overall outcome should be excellent, with more than 75%–80% of these children being cured (EVANS et al. 1981; KRETSCHMAR 1991).

Two subgroups of children with POG stage D (Evans-D'Angio stage IV) disease have a survival probability of 50% or more. ROSEN et al. (1985) reported six children who had stage IV disease solely by virtue of distant node-positive disease. Three of these children were long-term survivors after aggressive chemoradiotherapy. A favorable outcome in this distinctly uncommon group of patients has also been commented on by others.

A more common group comprises infants less than 13 months of age at diagnosis who present with POG stage D or Evans-D'Angio stage IV disease. KRETSCHMAR et al. (1984) and subsequently PAUL et al. (1991) have reported survival of more than 70% of this group initially treated with VAM-DTIC or MADDOC, and these excellent results have been maintained with substantially longer follow-up intervals. The CCSG and investigators at St. Jude have reported survival results of 40%–50% in this group with somewhat less aggressive regimens, while results similar to these published from Boston have been reported from New York (FINKLESTEIN et al. 1979; KUSHNER and HELSON 1987).

Unfortunately, the three above-mentioned groups represent a minority of all children with NB who present with disseminated disease. Although children older than 6 years of age at diagnosis were

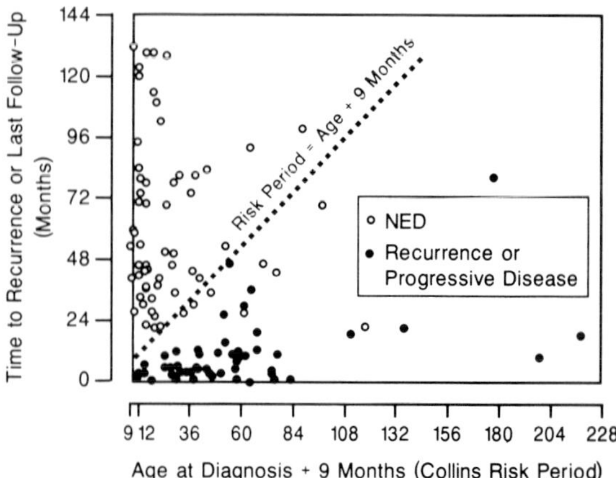

Fig. 12.6. Collin's risk period (age at diagnosis +9 months) for 118 patients with NB. Collin's risk period provides an excellent measure of follow-up time necessary to ascertain cure in NB. Almost all reported recurrences in NB fall within this period. (Data on this figure are from the series reported by ROSEN et al.1984)

reported by the CCSG to have a 50% survival at 2.5 years, these older children have uniformly relapsed in subsequent follow-up and demonstrate the relevance and importance of Collins' risk period (Fig. 12.6) in follow-up of children with NB (COLLINS 1955; FINKLESTEIN et al. 1979). Several investigators have called attention to the problem of late recurrence in this condition, especially in older patients (SCHWEISGUTH 1968; HINTON and BUSCHKE 1968; DELORIMIER et al. 1969; HELSON et al. 1972; KONRAD et al. 1973; JAFFE 1976; DANNECKER et al. 1983; FIORILLO et al. 1984).

In a comprehensive review of 56 children with stage IV disease managed at Boston's Dana Farber Cancer Institute and Children's Hospital, 4 of 46 children less than 13 months of age at diagnosis were 2+ year disease-free survivors. Three of these children had only nodal disease (vide supra) and the fourth has subsequently relapsed and died prior to passing Collins' risk-period (ROSEN et al. 1984). Similar results are regularly found in the literature if the previously discussed favorable subsets are removed. Thus the potential for cure using conventional chemotherapy is at best remote for this group, who constitute 40%–50% of all patients with NB.

12.7.4 Radiation Therapy

Radiation therapy (RT) has played a role in both curative and palliative management of NB for many decades. An apparent beneficial effect to its use postoperatively has been reported from nonrandomized single-institution studies by many authors, including FARBER (1940), WITTENBORG (1950), LINGLEY et al. (1967), PEREZ et al. (1967), and, in the past decade, ROSEN et al. (1984) and JACOBSON et al. (1983). More recently, the benefit of its use has been confirmed in a randomized study of POG stage C patients (CASTLEBERRY et al. 1991).

The place of RT in the initial curative management of patients with NB has changed rapidly in the past decade, coincidentally with improved surgery and chemotherapy and an improved knowledge of the natural history of the disease. It is clear that virtually all children with Evans-D'Angio stage I and the majority of (or perhaps all) children with Evans-D'Angio stage II disease are currently best managed without initial postsurgical RT (NITSCHKE et al. 1988; MATTHAY et al. 1989). Although subgroups of children may be identified in these two groups in whom the functional outcome of initial management may be improved by reduced surgery and the use of chemotherapy and/or irradiation, the size of these subgroups will be small. A proportion of children in both of the aforementioned groups will develop local and/or distant relapse after initial surgical management, and in these children radiation may well play a curative role. Similarly, future studies may identify children in both stages with a sufficiently high relapse rate after surgery alone to justify additional treatment with chemotherapy and/or irradiation. Recent demonstration of relapse in six of seven children with Evans-D'Angio stage II disease with more than three copies of N-*myc* may indicate such a group (MATTHAY et al. 1989).

The reason for the substantial difference between results in children older than 1 year with stage II disease reported in four earlier large series (survival: 39/83=47%) (BRESLOW and MCCANN 1971; KINNIER-WILSON and DRAPER 1974; EVANS et al. 1976a,b, 1982) and recent CCSG results in 75 children of all ages with stage II disease (including 32 with known residual disease) who received only surgery (89% 2+ year relapse-free and 98% overall survival) is not known and therefore of concern (MATTHAY et al. 1989). Perhaps improved staging whereby children are currently downstaged relative to historical results and/or patient selection accounts for these differences as it is clear that surgical treatment alone does not.

Although the staging systems are not comparable, the foregoing considerations also applies to children with POG stage B disease. The necessity of chemotherapy (or radiation therapy) in this latter group is unknown as many of these children will have Evans-D'Angio stage I or stage II disease where current data fail to support the need for any initial postsurgical adjuvant therapy. GREEN et al. (1985) reported on 47 patients with POG stage B disease, of whom 43 had completed therapy with adequate follow-up. An initial aggressive chemotherapy approach produced complete responses in 26, and a further six were rendered disease free by delayed surgery. Of the 11 patients with residual tumor, four achieved freedom from disease following chemotherapy (cisplatin plus VM-26) and surgery. Of the 36 patients achieving complete response (26 + 6 + 4), four patients relapsed. At the time of the report only 4 of the 47 patients had died. Five patients received investigator-elected RT at unspecified times (3/5 remain disease free). Despite the much more aggressive treatment employed, these results appear somewhat less favorable than those reported by the CCSG in their stage II patients, pointing to the difficulties in attempting comparison of two staging systems (MATTHAY et al. 1989).

Improved results have been obtained with Evans-D'Angio stage III patients and perhaps those stage II patients (~10%–15%) with noncontiguous positive lymph nodes. Routine use of wide-field, intermediate-dose RT in older patients (>13 months) with POG stage C disease has been reported to be of benefit by CASTLEBERRY et al. (1991) in a randomized study. In 57 patients, both the incidence of complete remission [22/29 (76%) vs 13/28 (46%)] and the number of patients in continuous remission after 2 years [17/29 (59%) vs. 9/28 (32%)] were improved in patients receiving routine RT. Survival was also significally improved [24/33 (73%) vs 12/29 (41%)]. Both local and distant relapses were seen in both groups.

Although an alteration in relapse site and slight prolongation of time to relapse may result from the use of regional RT in combination with multiagent chemotherapy and surgery in older children with Evans-D'Angio stage IV (POG stage D) disease, no convincing long-term survival benefit is apparent except in those children who are stage IV solely by virtue of nodal metastases (ROSEN et al. 1984, 1985). Similarly, RT plays at best a minor role in the curative treatment of infants with stage IV disease and children with Evans-D'Angio stage IVS [POG D (S)] tumors. Localized low-dose treatment to the liver has been utilized with benefit in occasional stage IVS children with respiratory/abdominal distress from progressive growth of hepatic metastatic disease. When utilized, a radiation dose of 4.5–7.5 Gy to partial liver volumes has generally been adequate (EVANS 1980; HALPERIN and COX 1986; KUSHNER and

CHEUNG 1988). PESCHEL et al. (1981) have described possible chemical alterations in renal function levels in three infants as a result of delivery of 12–14 Gy. However, with currently available chemotherapeutic regimens, use of RT in this group of children will only very rarely be needed.

In contrast, use of total body irradiation (TBI) at higher dose levels and treatment of residual or persistent primary NB with additional RT have apparently had a beneficial effect in children undergoing bone marrow transplantation for NB (AUGUST et al. 1984; PHILIP et al. 1987). GRAHAM-POLE (personal communication) and GEE and GRAHAM-POLE (1990) have reported six progression-free survivors among ten children transplanted in first remission who received local irradiation, whereas there were only 14 such survivors among 40 who did not. Of 50 children who received 12 Gy TBI, 18 (36%) have remained progression free, in contrast to 4 of 24 (17%) who received only 9 Gy. While neither of these differences achieves statistical significance, when combined with the negative selection for children who received local boost irradiation (those with residual bulk tumor), they are very suggestive.

12.7.4.1 Radiation Dose

Several features of NB make an analysis of dose-response (local control) with RT difficult. These features include the well-known ability of the disease to spontaneously regress and/or mature and the well-recognized difference in biologic aggressiveness between tumors occurring in infants and children less than 18 months of age, children with early-stage disease, and older children with advanced disease. It is also difficult to assess local control results in older children with Evans-D'Angio stage IV (POG stage D) disease, in whom metastases are poorly controlled and reseeding of previously controlled tumor sites is a real possibility. Although potentially helpful in providing insight into better treatment techniques such as hyperfractionation, in vitro data with cultured NB are suspect and not totally relevant to the clinical situation in view of the inability to develop primary cultures in several favorable classes of patients. Thus, more so than in most tumor types, the possibility of clonal selection and nonrepresentational in vitro sampling must be raised as a real concern in NB models (REYNOLDS et al. 1980; WHELDON et al. 1986a,b, 1987).

Clinically, it is well recognized that radiation doses of 9–18 Gy nearly always effect local control of residual microscopic disease and gross tumors in infants and limited volume disease in early-stage older children (LINGLEY et al. 1967; PEREZ et al. 1967; STELLA et al. 1970; EVANS et al. 1982; JACOBSON et al. 1983; ROSEN et al. 1984; GREEN 1985; HALPERIN and COX 1986). Local control rates published in several series treating children in these groups are listed in

Table 12.8. Local control of NB by radiation therapy (where possible, children have been separated by both age and stage)

Services	No. of pts.	Stage (Evans-D'Angio)	Age < 1 yr	Age > 1 yr	Dose (Gy)	No. controlled/ no. Rxed	Comments
ROSEN et al. (1984)	28	II	9	19	14–15 for < 1 yr 18–28 for > 1 yr	9/9 < 1 yr 17/19 > 1 yr	3 older (< 7 yr) children received radiation doses of 40 Gy
	16	III	9	7	14–15 < 1 yr 25–35 > 1 yr	8/9 < yr 5/7 > 1 yr	Combined with intensive chemotherapy and surgery, VAM-DTIC, and MADDOC
JACOBSON et al. (1983)	7	II	4	3	12–40	7/7	
	13	III	4	9	12–40 (10 <20)	10/13 all failures > 1 yr	All failures had local component
EVANS et al. (1984)	11	II	?	?	12–24	8/11 all failures > 1 yr	All failures had local component
	13	III	?	?	12–24	7/13 all failures > 1 yr	All failures had local component
HALPERIN and COX (1986)	7	II	?	?	14.8–26.5	7/7	All patients < 20 mo age at diagnosis
	13	III	?	?	12–48.4	9/13 all failures > 1 yr	
NINANE et al. (1982)	24	II	?	?	20–35	19/24 "3-yr survivors"	No child < 1 yr died of tumor-related causes. True local failures are not identified

Abbreviations: VAM-DTIC, vincristine, doxorubicin, nitrogen mustard, DTIC; MADDOC, nitrogen mustard, dosorubicin, *d*-cisplatin, DTIC, vincristine, cyclophosphamide

Table 12.8 and approach 100% (STELLA et al. 1970). Although it is recognized that rapid tumor shrinkage usually occurs soon after institution of irradiation in these children, it is also clear from NITSCHKE et al. (1988) and MATTHAY et al.'s (1989) recent report as well as other single-institution reports that residual microscopic and gross tumor may be biologically inactive and ultimately regress, much as a juvenile hemangioma in an infant will (KNUDSON and MEADOWS 1980; CASSADY 1984). Therefore, while the upper limit for radiation dose can be set at that level which will regularly effect local control for these patients, the lower dose at which recurrences or progression become a difficulty is not known and in many instances may be O Gy.

Equally difficult to establish is the radiation dose that will regularly accomplish long-term local control in older children with biologically aggressive tumors. Local failure in this group is a frequent site of first relapse. BERTHOLD et al. (1986) reported that 33% of 96 patients with relapsed NB failed locally, and most of these were in Evans-D'Angio stage IV patients greater than 1 year of age. ROSEN et al. (1984) noted that local failure represented a major component of first relapse in 24 of 39 (62%) children with Evans-D'Angio stage IV disease. Thirty-two children (82%) had some component of local failure. Although radiation therapy (25–30 Gy) appeared to alter relapse patterns [6/15 major component (XRT) vs 6/7 (O XRT)], the great majority of patients in both treatment groups had uncontrolled local tumor at death. Data from transplant centers where local irradiation has been delivered to bulk sites, including the primary, appear to show a decrease in the proportion of relapsing patients failing locally; however, even with such treatment, local failure may occur (AUGUST et al. 1984; IKEDA et al. 1991; MATTHAY et al. 1991).

Combined with these known examples of local failure is the realization that more than 50% of these patients will relapse even with aggressive therapy and transplant attempts and time to death will be short (generally less than 3 years). Thus, given the general validity of the Collins' hypothesis in NB and the older ages of many of these children, many will die before an adequate time to assess local control has passed.

Recognizing these problems, it is clear that the dose necessary to obtain a high rate of local control is unknown. Doses in excess of 25 Gy are necessary for reasonable local control results in children (>1 year) with Evans-D'Angio stage III or POG stage C disease, most of whom have had extensive surgical

resections and thus have minimal or at most modest amounts of disease to treat (CASTLEBERRY et al. 1991). HAASE et al. (1989) have recently demonstrated the apparent importance of total or near-total resection in children with stage III disease, although analysis for possible selection bias in those achieving gross resection is not possible from the published data.

ROSEN et al. (1984) identified a substantial risk of local failure in Evans-D'Angio stage IV children, even if they had been irradiated with doses of 30–35 Gy. As normal tissue tolerances (in particular kidney, gastrointestinal tract, liver, and spinal cord) limit external beam approaches for the volumes of tissue that it is frequently necessary to treat, reliance on second- or third-look surgery combined with innovative irradiation approaches [intraoperative radiation therapy (IORT), intraoperative interstitial implants, IORT plus hyperthermia or stereotaxic radiosurgery attempts using the spine as a fixation point] may be necessary for further dose elevation with acceptable toxicity in the future. At present, suboptimal control of already disseminated disease usually makes local control of lesser importance.

12.7.4.2 Radiation Volume

As patients with NB requiring RT usually have advanced disease, the volume of tissue that needs to be treated will usually be large. Regional nodal sites should be encompassed in children with POG stage C disease as well as generous margins around the primary, encompassing likely occult extension and possible microscopic postsurgical residual disease (CASTLEBERRY et al. 1991). A shrinking field approach should generally be followed and *initial* volumes should usually encompass initial tumor extent (rather than postsurgical residual disease) for this reason.

For situations requiring irradiation in children with biologically less aggressive disease (e.g., hepatic treatment in a stage IVS patient who is chemoresistant), margins generally can be much more restricted and, in the IVS case, it is not necessary to treat the entire hepatic tumor volume.

12.7.4.3 Palliation

Many children with stage IV (or D) disease fail initial treatment, frequently displaying development of bony or soft tissue metastases requiring palliation for relief of pain, lumen competency, pressure phenomena, etc. Especially in this generally chemo-resistant setting, radiation has outstanding efficacy.

Two approaches are possible. External beam radiation fields directed at the symptomatic site [orbit(s), bone, etc.] with delivery of 12–30 Gy in 2- to 3-Gy fractions will usually produce prompt relief of pain. Major mass reduction usually requires doses at the higher end of the stated range, and mass response is frequently biphasic, with an initially rapid reduction followed by a slower prolonged response. Occasionally, particularly in the treatment of bony disease, an increase in symptoms (especially pain) may occur 1–3 h after initial treatment. In virtually every instance, prompt and very gratifying symptomatic relief will then occur over the next several hours, suggesting that the increase in symptoms was from tumor cell injury and swelling.

Alternatively, should many sites be symptomatic, treatment with radioactively-tagged MIBG can be considered. This agent is a guanethidine analog which has a high affinity for the adrenal medulla and certain neurectodermal tumors, including NB. Many drugs may theoretically interfere with MIBG absorption, including amitriptyline, ephedrine, and phentermine (MOYES et al. 1989). Considerable experience has now been gained in using this agent diagnostically, where it has been shown to have high specificity and sensitivity. Therapeutic experience has been relatively limited. It has primarily been employed in palliative situations, and in this context a significant incidence of initial tumor response has occurred, unfortunately usually followed by rapid recurrence. Current trials are assessing the value of this agent when used early in advanced-stage disease (DEKRAKER et al. 1991).

12.7.5 Bone Marrow Transplantation

Although newer, more aggressive regimens combining surgery, multiagent chemotherapy, and, frequently, repeat surgery and irradiation have lengthened the median survival time, there have been only anecdotal reports of older patients (>1 year) with stage IV (stage D) disease who have been disease-free survivors beyond Collins' risk interval. In the past decade, investigators have therefore been testing bone marrow transplantation, evaluating both allogeneic and, more frequently, autologous transplantation as intensification therapy used in conjunction with standard combined therapy as described above.

Results obtained at several major centers are depicted in Table 12.9 (AUGUST et al. 1984; D'ANGIO et al. 1985; PHILIP et al. 1987; HARTMANN et al. 1987; DINI et al. 1989; GRAHAM-POLE J., personal communication; GEE and GRAHAM-POLE 1990; FRANZONE et al. 1990; ZUCKER et al. 1990; MATTHAY et al. 1991; IKEDA et al. 1991; SEEGER et al. 1991; SEEGER and REYNOLDS 1991). It is important to note that with the exception of the studies by HARTMANN et al. (1987) and PHILIP et al. (1987), results presented are selected as the total number of children from which the transplanted group comes is not known. Although selection may influence referral, HARTMANN et al. (1987) and PHILIP et al. (1987) present all stage IV patients presenting to their hospitals in a specified period. A further feature of note is the paucity of follow-up data beyond 5 years.

No clear advantage is seen for a specific pretransplantation chemotherapy induction regimen among the many used. Overall, toxicity rates of both the various induction regimens and the different transplantation approaches are high. Although small numbers preclude statistical significance in some studies, a clear collective advantage accrues to patients in whom a complete remission with near-total surgical primary removal has been possible. Patients who undergo transplantation when in partial remission or who have substantial primary residual nearly all eventually die of NB if treatment toxicity is avoided.

In better risk patients, it is unclear whether ultimate treatment failure derives from inadequate clearing of tumor cells remaining in the body or from retransplantation of NB in children undergoing autologous approaches. The similarity of failure rates between allogeneic and autologous approaches combined with a high reported failure rate in prior sites of bulk disease in some reports favors inadequate induction of remission prior to transplantation.

Although the great majority of series utilize fractionated TBI, the ultimate importance of TBI in the success of transplantation is uncertain (DINI et al. 1989). Data supporting a role for both local and systemic irradiation derive from an analysis of failure sites in certain series and from the POG study – preliminary data from the latter study demonstrate a favorable trend in unfavorably selected children receiving primary site irradiation (Fig. 12.7) and a similar slight favorable trend in children receiving 12 Gy versus 9 Gy (GRAHAM-POLE J., personal communication; GEE and GRAHAM-POLE 1990).

Both French series (LYON and PARIS) note that bone marrow predominates as the relapse site and no mention has been made of local relapse (PHILIP et al. 1987; HARTMANN et al. 1987). MATTHAY et al. (1991),

Table 12.9. Representative results from several recently published reports on bone marrow transplantation from centers in the United States and Europe

Author	No. of pts. and type	Stage		Initial regimen	Ablative regimen	Radiation therapy		Outcome				Comment
		Primary presentation	Prior relapse			1° ± bulk	TBI	Survival	Toxic deaths	Relapse	Relapse site	
AUGUST et al. (1984)	Allogeneic (4) Autologous (6)	0	10	Surgery and variable drugs	2–variable 8–Ad VM-26 Melph	10 Gy/5 Fx	4 NED 22+ to 54+ mo; 2 allog., 2 autol.	4 (2 c̄ NB)	4	4	(2) Distant (2) L&D	All > 3 yr 9/10 c̄ CR p̄ BMT
PHILIP et al. (1987)	Allogeneic (2) autologous (54)	Stage IV > 1 yr	0	PE/CAdo evaluated	VCR Melph (37)	ō	12 Gy; 2 Gy × 6 b.i.d.	39% prog-free at 24 mo	7 (19%)	12	"Majority bone marrow"	45 evaluable 8 c̄ BMT due to progression. of 23 pts with PR prior to BMT, 13% alive at 24 mo. of 14 pts with CR/VGPR prior to BMT, 40% alive at 24 mo
HARTMON et al. (1987)	Autologous (33) (of 62 seen)	All stage IV, 32 > 1 yr, 1 at 11 mo.	0	CAdo (16) OPEC (3)	BCNU VM-26 (33) Melph	2 patients unknown dose	ō	~39% NED 30 mo	4	14	1 local; 13 distant bone/BM	18/33 received 2nd autol. BMT. 2nd Rx had no clear favorable impact
SEEGER et al. 1991 SEEGER and REYNOLDS 1991 MATTHAY et al. 1991	Autologous (101)	"High risk" most c̄ stage IV > 1 year age	Possibly none	14 with 2nd or 3rd Rx C, Ad, VM-16 or VM-26, DDDP	"VAMP" (DDDP VM-26), Ad, Melph) (46) or "PEM" (55)	Yes, but unknown dose and number treated	3.33 Gy × 3 of 2 Gy × 6 given b.i.d.	43% at 24 + mo 40% at 50+ mo (39 mo median)	14 (10/46 = 22% with VAMP)	30	L+D Local – 8 Local – 10 BM – 12 Bone – 10 Liver – 5 Other – 6	6 of 7 relapses in pts. c̄ gross residual local disease. 10/18 local relapse in those with gross total resection
IKEDA et al. 1985	Autologous	"High risk"	?0	"Various"	VAMP PEM	10 Gy in 5 Fx in most	10–12 Gy (3.33 Gy × 3 (2 × 6 b.i.d.)	?	12 (9 early)	18	5/24 c̄ abd. tumor had local relapse	Data somewhat suggestive of local effect of RT and S
D'ANGIO et al. 1985	Autologous (21) Allogeneic (10)	Stage IV > 1 yr (26) Stage III (5)	?0	"Various"	VM-26 Melph ± Ad	Some	10 Gy 3.33 Gy × 3	10 CR at 3-103 + mo 7/10 > 36 + mo	9	14	–	Data with long RFS very suggestive of cure (4 > 5 + yr)

Abbreviations: Ad, adrimycin; M, Melph, melphalan; DDDP, d-cisplatin; VCR, V, and O, vincristine; E, etoposide; C, cyclophosphamide; NED, no evidence of disease; BM, bone marrow; D, distant; L, local; CR, complete remission; PR, partial remission; VGPR, very good partial remission; RFS, relapse free survival

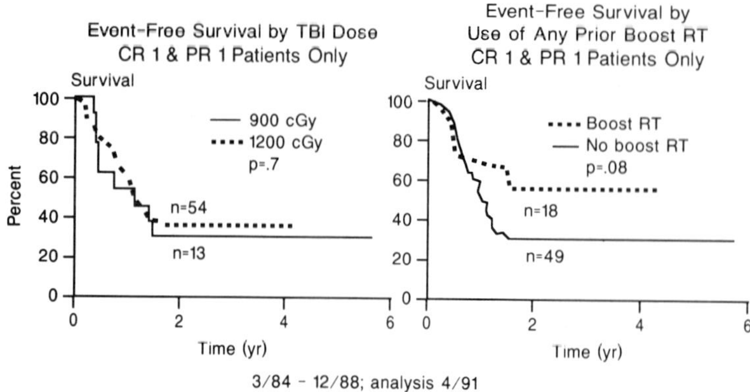

Fig. 12.7. Data demonstrating effect of total body irradiation (*TBI*) dose and boost radiation therapy (*RT*) in children undergoing bone marrow transplantation for NB. Data shown in this figure are for children transplanted in first complete (*CR*) or partial (*PR*) remission. Data previously published for children transplanted in CR1 or PR1 or after more than one relapse showed a greater trend for benefit of the higher radiation dose to the whole body (GEE and GRAHAM-POLE 1990). Data shown in this figure have been reproduced with permission from R.B. Marcus for the Pediatric Oncology Group)

Table 12.10. Effect of complete resection (initial or delayed) on survival in Evans-D'Angio stage III NB[a]

| Survival status | Age | | | | | | Histology (Shimada) | | | | | | Total | | |
| | <2 yr | | | >2 yr | | | Favorable | | | Unfavorable | | | | | |
	CR	NO	CR	CR	NO	CR	CR	NO	CR	CR	NO	CR	CR	NO	CR
Alive	11	15	7	10			9	11		5	10		18	6	
Dead	0	13	6	19			0	4		5	23		25	32	

CR, complete resection

[a] Results are from the recent series of HAASE et al. (1989) and demonstrate an apparent effect on survival of complete gross tumor removal. Note that only 6 of 38 children with Evans-D'Angio stage III disease not undergoing gross total resection survive.

from the United States, noted that 18 of 30 patients who relapsed had local recurrence (such recurrence occurred in six of the seven patients who had gross residual disease). Although local radiation therapy was utilized in some patients, its impact on local relapse could not be ascertained. IKEDA et al. (1991) noted local relapse in only 5 of 26 failures and ascribed this low incidence to pretransplantation surgical resection and radiation.

12.8 Results

More than 85%–90% of all children who present with Evans-D'Angio stage I or stage II disease should sur-

vive. In addition, a slightly smaller percentage of infants with stage IVS or stage IV disease are regularly cured today. Modern series combining aggressive surgery, chemotherapy, and radiation therapy and, in some instances, bone marrow transplantation report control of 65%–80% of cases of Evans-D'Angio stage III and POG stage C disease (ROSEN et al. 1984; KUSHNER and HELSON 1987; CASTLEBERRY et al. 1991). Representative results are depicted in Table 12.10 and Fig. 12.8.

The aforementioned groups of patients represent 55%–60% of all patients with NB. The remaining group – children greater than 1 year of age with stage IV disease – represents the current problem. With the

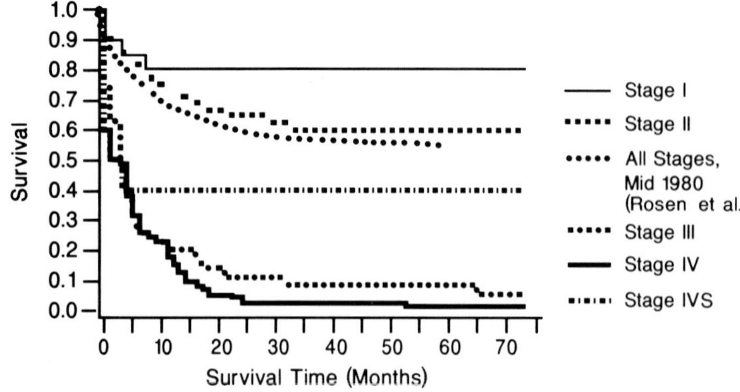

Fig. 12.8. Survival data by Evans-D'Angio stage for two large recently published series of children treated for NB (BERTHOLD et al. 1986 and ROSEL et al. 1984). ROSEN et al.'s data for all stages are shown, while the data from BERTHOLD et al. are shown by stage. Notable are differences by stage between the two series. ROSEN et al.'s data include much more uniform success for children with Evans-D'Angio stage I, II, or III disease and infants with stage IV disease; BERTHOLD et al.'s results for all stage III and stage IV patients are less successful. Intensity in both chemotherapy and radiation therapy is felt to most probably account for these differences

advent of allogeneic and autologous bone marrow transplantation, a significant fraction of these patients are possibly now being cured for the first time. When selection factors are eliminated and the entire group is evaluated optimistically, 15%–20% are today being cured (DINI et al. 1989). Collectively therefore, 55%–65% of all patients with NB should today be controlled. Recent data from ROSEN et al. (1984: 58% 2+ year survival) and BERTHOLD et al. (1986: 46% 2+ year survival) and a recent review by CRIST and KUN (1991: 55% 2+ year survival) support these results.

When in time is the child with NB cured? COLLINS, assessing this question in the case of Wilms' tumor, suggested that embryonal tumors with possible fetal origin should, if not cured, become clinically evident at a time posttreatment equal to age at diagnosis + 9 months, assuming constant growth rates. This hypothesis has been applied to NB and at present offers a conservative estimate of cure (ROSEN et al. 1984) (Fig. 12.6). Clinically these data suggest a less rapid growth rate for NB in older children, and this impression in supported by CCSG data on older patients (FINKLESTEIN et al. 1979).

Although scanty in number, several reports in the literature document late relapse (beyond 5–10 years and beyond Collins' risk period) (HINTON and BUSCHKE 1968; SCHWEISGUTH 1968; DELORIMIER et al. 1969; HELSON et al. 1972; KONRAD et al. 1973; JAFFE 1976; DANNECKER et al. 1983; FIORILLO et al. 1984). Few series report 20- or 30-year follow-up for this disease and it will be important to assess this problem in the future, especially in children with early-stage disease treated with surgery only and with microscopic or gross residual disease.

12.9 Prevention/Early Diagnosis

In the past decade, the Japanese have undertaken large-scale prevention programs in an attempt to improve outcome in children with NB through early diagnosis (SAWADA et al. 1984; NISHI et al. 1987; TAKEDA 1989; SAWADA 1990; TUCHMAN and WOODS 1990). Two programs in Kyoto and Sapporo City demonstrate an apparent three- to fourfold improvement in overall survival and a marked reduction at presentation in the percentage of patients with late-stage disease (SAWADA et al. 1984; NISHI et al. 1987). Recent evidence of an apparent decrease in all deaths from NB in Japan in the mid-1980s is encouraging (HANAWA et al. 1980). Although the findings are potentially quite exciting, from the data presented it is not possible to exclude the possibility that a marked increase in diagnosis of biologically nonaggressive tumors is occurring, thereby artificially inflating both "cure" rates and percentage of early-stage patients. Several large studies are currently underway in an attempt to assess the validity of the Japanese hypothesis as such a program, if verified, would be cost-effective and markedly improve both survival and consequences of survival (WOODS and TUCHMAN 1987; MCWILLIAMS 1987; LEMIEUX et al. 1989; TUCHMAN and WOODS 1990).

12.10 Future Goals

Better understanding of NB and better care for children with the disease will require study and improvements in several areas:

1. Better treatment for children with stage IV disease.
2. Consistent use and agreement on a common staging system. The International system seems to be an excellent beginning, and continued use of two systems by the two major collaborative groups in the United States is counterproductive.
3. Identification of risk groups which will allow separation of children best treated by surgery and observation and those requiring more intensive therapy. It would be desirable to initially control nearly 100% of children with early-stage disease rather than the 80%–90% controlled at present.
4. Better understanding of the biology of NB, which will permit understanding of why these tumors may not grow or spontaneously regress in one case and be lethal in another.
5. Ascertainment of the validity and possibly improvement of current attempts at early diagnosis while seeking ways in which NB might be prevented.
6. Both retrospective and prospective long-term follow-up studies to ascertain the true incidence of late relapse. If a significant incidence is found, it should be determined whether it is associated with a particular therapeutic plan.

References

Adam A, Hochholzer L (1981) Ganglioneuroblastoma of the posterior mediastinum: a clinicopathologic review of 80 cases. Cancer 47: 373–381

American Joint Committee (AJC) on Cancer (1983) Neuroblastoma. In: Manual for staging of cancer, 2nd edn. J.B. Lippincott, Philadelphia, pp 237–239

August CS, Serota FT, Koch PA et al. (1984) Treatment of advanced neuroblastoma with supralethal chemotherapy, radiation and allogeneic or autologous marrow reconstitution. J Clin Oncol 2: 609–616

Bader KL, Miller RW (1979) US cancer incidence and mortality in the first year of life. Am J Dis Child 133: 157

Balaban-Malenbaum G, Gilbert F (1980) Relationship between homogeneously staining regions and double minute chromosomes in human neuroblastoma cell lines. In: Evans AE (ed) Advances in neuroblastoma research. Raven, New York, pp 97–107

Beckwith JB, Martin RF (1968) Observation on the histopathology of neuroblastomas. J Pediatr Surg 3: 106–110

Beckwith JB, Perrin EV (1963) In situ neuroblastomas: a contribution to the natural history of neural crest tumors. Am J Pathol 43: 1089–1104

Berthold F, Brandeis WE, Lampert F (1986) Neuroblastoma: diagnostic advances and therapeutic results in 370 patients. Monogr Pediatr 18: 206–223

Breslow N, McCann B (1971) Statistical estimation of prognosis for children with neuroblastoma. Cancer Res 331: 2098–2103

Brodeur GM, Seeger RC (1988) International criteria for diagnosis, staging and response to treatment in patients with neuroblastoma. In: Evans AE, D'Angio GJ, Knudson AG et al. (eds) Advances in neuroblastoma research (2). Alan R Liss, New York, pp 509–524

Brodeur GM, Green AA, Hayes FA et al. (1981) Cytogenetic features of human neuroblastomas and cell lines. Cancer Res 41: 4678–4686

Brodeur GM, Seeger RC, Schwab M, Varmus HE, Bishop JM (1984) Amplification of N-*myc* in untreated human neuroblastomas correlates with advanced disease stage. Science 224: 1121–1124

Brodeur GM, Seeger RC, Barrett A et al. (1988) International criteria for diagnosis, staging and response to treatment in patients with neuroblastoma. J Clin Oncol 6: 1874–1881

Carlsen NLT, Christensen I, Schroeder H et al. (1986) Prognostic factors in neuroblastomas treated in Denmark from 1943–1980. Cancer 58: 2726–2735

Cassady JR (1984) A hypothesis to explain the enigmatic natural history of neuroblastoma. Med Pediatr Oncol 12: 64–67

Cassady JR (1990) Prognostic factors affecting the outcome of children with neuroblastoma. In: Pochedly C (ed) Neuroblastoma: tumor biology and therapy. CRC Press, Boca Raton, Ann Arbor, Boston, pp 370–379

Castleberry RP, Jr (1990) Chemotherapy of neuroblastoma. In: Pochedly C (ed) Neuroblastoma: tumor biology and therapy. CRC Press, Boca Raton, FL, pp 306–315

Castleberry RP, Kun LE, Shuster JJ et al. (1991) Radiotherapy improves the outlook for patients older than 1 year with Pediatric Oncology Group Stage C neuroblastoma. J Clin Oncol 9: 789–795

Chatten J, Voorhess ML (1967) Familial neuroblastoma. Report of a kindred with multiple disorders, including neuroblastoma in four siblings. N Engl J Med 277: 1230–1236

Collins VP (1955) Wilms' tumor: its behavior and prognosis. J La State Med Soc 107: 474–480

Crist WM, Kun LE (1991) Common solid tumors of childhood. N Engl J Med 324: 461–471

D'Angio GJ, Evans AE, Koop CE (1971) Special pattern of widespread neuroblastoma with a favorable prognosis. Lancet I: 1046–1049

D'Angio GJ, August C, Elkins W et al. (1985) Metastatic neuroblastoma managed by supralethal therapy and bone mar-
row reconstitution (BMRc). Results of a four-institution Children's Cancer Study Group Pilot Study. In: Evans AE (ed) Advances in neuroblastoma research. Alan R. Liss, New York, pp 557–563

Dannecker G, Leidig E, Treuner J, Niethammer D (1983) Late recurrence of neuroblastoma: a reason for prolonged follow-up? Am J Pediatr Hematol Oncol 5: 271–274

deKraker. J, Hoefnagel CA, Voute PA et al. (1991) Neuroblastoma (NBL) treated with ^{131}I-mIBG (abstract C-1105). Proc Am Soc Clin Oncol 10: 314

DeLorimier AA, Bragg KU, Linden G (1969) Neuroblastoma in childhood. Am J Dis Child 118: 441–450

De Vita V, Hellman S, Rosenberg S (1982) Cancer Principles and Practice of Oncology, 1st edn. of JB. Lippincott, Philadelphia.

Dini G, Philip T, Hartmann R et al. (1989) Bone marrow transplantation for neuroblastoma: a review of 509 cases. Bone Marrow Transplant 4: 42–46

Emanuel BS, Balaban G, Boyd JP et al. (1985) N-*myc* amplification in multiple homogeneously staining regions in two human neuroblastomas. Proc Natl Acad Sci USA 82: 3736–3740

Emery LG, Shields M, Shah NR, Garbes A (1983) Neuroblastoma associated with Beckwith-Wiedemann syndrome. Cancer 52: 176–179

Evans AE (1980) Staging and treatment of neuroblastoma. Cancer 45: 1799–1802

Evans AE, D'Angio GJ, Randolph JA (1971) A proposed staging for children with neuroblastoma. Children's Cancer Study Group A. Cancer 27: 374–378

Evans AE, Albo V, D'Angio GJ et al. (1976a) Factors influencing survival of children with non-metastatic neuroblastoma. Cancer 38: 661–666

Evans AE, Albo V, D'Angio GJ et al. (1976b) Cyclophosphamide treatment of patients with localized and regional neuroblastoma. A randomized study. Cancer 38: 655–660

Evans AE, Chatten J, D'Angio GJ et al. (1980) A review of 17 IV-S neuroblastoma patients at the Children's Hospital of Philadelphia. Cancer 45: 833–839

Evans AE, Baum E, Chard R (1981) Do infants with stage IV-S neuroblastoma need treatment? Arch Dis Child 56: 271–274

Evans AE, D'Angio GJ, Koop CE (1982) The role of multimodel treatment of non-metastatic neuroblastoma (abstract). Am Acad Med Section on Hematology/Oncology. New York

Evans AE, D'Angio GJ, Propert K, Anderson J, Hann H-WL (1987) Prognostic factors in neuroblastoma. Cancer 59: 1853–1859

Everson TC, Cole WH (1966) Spontaneous regression of neuroblastoma In: Everson TC, Cole WH (eds) Spontaneous regression of cancer. WB Saunders, Philadelphia, p 88–163

Farber S (1940) Neuroblastoma. Am J Dis Child 60: 749–751

Felici L, Limiento D, Giorgi PL (1990) Multifocal neuroblastoma. Med Pediatr Oncol 18: 231–233

Finklestein JZ, Klemperer MR, Evans A et al. (1979) Multiagent chemotherapy for children with metastatic neuroblastoma: a report from Children's Cancer Study Group. Med Pediatr Oncol 6: 179–188

Fiorillo A, Migliorati R, Fiore M et al. (1984) Late recurrence of disseminated neuroblastoma after 3 years of continuous remission. J Pediatr 104: 161–162

Frantz CN, Gelber RD, Belli JA et al. (1982) Aggressive treatment of neuroblastoma. In: Rayband C, Clement R, Lebreuil G (eds) Pediatric oncology. Excerpta Medica, Amsterdam p 175

Franzone P, Scarpati D, Vitale V et al. (1990) Chemoradiotherapy and autologous bone marrow transplantation in poor prognosis neuroblastoma. Radiother Oncol [Suppl 1] 102–104

Gaisie G, Oh KS, Young LW (1979) Co-existent neuroblastoma and Hirschsprung's disease – another manifestation of the neurocristopathy. Pediatr Radiol 8: 161–163

Gee AP, Graham-Pole J (1990) Use of bone marrow purging and bone marrow transplantation for neuroblastoma. In: Pochedly C (ed) Neuroblastoma: tumor biology and therapy. CRC Press, Boca Raton, FL, pp 318–332

Gitlow SE, Bertani LM, Rausen A et al. (1970) Diagnosis of neuroblastoma by qualitative and quantitative determination of catecholamine metabolites in urine. Cancer 25: 1377

Green AA, Hayes FA, Hustu HO (1981) Sequential cyclophosphamide and doxorubicin for induction of complete remission in children with disseminated neuroblastoma. Cancer 48: 2310

Green AA, Casper J, Nitschke R et al. (1985) The treatment of children with localized grossly unresectable (POG stage B) neuroblastoma. Proc ASCO 4: 245

Green DM (1985) Neuroblastoma. In: Green DM (ed) Diagnosis and management of malignant solid tumors in infants and children. Martinus Nijhoff, Boston, pp 187–256

Grotting JC, Kassel S, Dehner LP (1979) Nesidioblastosis and congenital neuroblastoma: a histologic and immunocytochemical study of a new complex neurocristopathy. Arch Pathol Lab Med 103: 642–646

Guin GH, Gilbert EF, Jones B (1969) Incidental neuroblastoma in infants. Am J Clin Pathol 51: 126–136

Haas D, Ablin AR, Miller C, Zoger S, Matthay KK (1988) Complete pathologic maturation and regression of stage IV-S neuroblastoma without treatment. Cancer 62: 818–825

Haase GM, Wong KY, deLorimer AA, Sather HN, Hammond GD (1989) Improvement in survival after excision of primary tumor in stage III neuroblastoma. J Pediatr Surg 24: 194–200

Halperin EC, Cox EB (1986) Radiation therapy in the management of neuroblastoma: the Duke University Medical Center experience 1967–1984. Int J Radiat Oncol Biol Phys 12: 1829–1837

Hanawa Y, Sawada T, Tsunoda A (1980) Decrease in childhood neuroblastoma death in Japan. Med Pediatr Oncol 18: 472–475

Hann H-WL, Evans AE, Cohen IJ, Leitmeyer JE (1981) Biologic differences between neuroblastoma stages IVs and IV: measurements of serum ferritin and E-rosette inhibition in 30 children. N Engl J Med 305: 425–429

Hann H-WL, Evans AE, Siegel SE et al. (1985) Prognostic importance of serum ferritin in patients with stages III and IV neuroblastoma: the children's Cancer Study Group experience. Cancer Res 45: 2843–2848

Hartmann O, Benhamon E, Beaujean F et al. (1987) Repeated high-dose chemotherapy followed by purged autologous bone marrow transplantation as consolidation therapy in metastatic neuroblastoma. J Clin Oncol 5: 1205–1211

Hayes FA, Green AA (1977) Neuroblastoma. In: Kelley VC (ed) Practice of Pediatrics, vol III. Harper & Row, Hagerstown Md, Chap 77, pp 1–6

Hayes FA, Green AA, Mauer AM (1977) Correlation of cell kinetic and clinical response to chemotherapy in disseminated neuroblastoma. Cancer Res 37: 3766–3770

Hayes FA, Green AA, Hustu HO et al. (1983) Surgicopathologic staging of neuroblastoma. Prognostic significance of regional lymph node metastases. J Pediatr 102: 59–62

Hayes FA, Thompson EI, Hvizala E et al. (1984) Chemotherapy as an alternative to laminectomy and radiation in the management of epidural tumor. J Pediatr 104: 221–224

Helson L, Grabstaid H, Huvos AG, D'Angio GJ, Murphy ML (1972) Neuroblastoma. Observations on long-term survivors. Clin Bull 1: 3–9

Hinton P, Buschke F (1968) Neuroblastoma in children, 42 cases. Radiol Clin Biol, pp 19–28

Hope JW, Borns PF, Berg PK (1965) Roentgenologic manifestations of Hirschsprung's disease in infancy. AJR 95: 217–229

Ikeda H, August CS, Goldwein J, Ross AJ, Evans AE, D'Angio GJ (1991) Relapse patterns in neuroblastoma (NBL) patients (pts) related to "de-bulking" (DB) treatments prior to bone marrow transplantation (BMT) (abstract C-1115). Proc Am Soc Clin Oncol 10: 317

Ikegaki N, Bukovsky J, Kennett RH (1986) Identification and characterization of the NMYC gene product in human neuroblastoma cells by monoclonal antibodies with defined specificities. Proc Natl Acad Sci USA 83: 5929–5933

Jacobson HM, Marcus RB, Thar TL et al. (1983) Pediatric neuroblastoma: postoperative radiation therapy using less than 2000 rad. Int J Radiat Oncol Biol Phys 9: 501–505

Jaffe N (1976a) Neuroblastoma: review of the literature and an examination of factors contributing to its enigmatic character. Cancer Treat Rev 3: 61–82

Jaffe N (1976b) Recrudescence of neuroblastoma after apparent cure. JNCI 57: 731–732

Jaffe N, Cassady JR, Filler RM, Petersen R, Traggis D (1975) Heterochromia and Horner syndrome associated with cervical and mediastinal neuroblastoma. J Pediatr 87: 75–77

Kaser H, Studnitz W (1961) Urine of children with sympathetic tumors. AMA J Dis Child 102: 199–204

Kaye JA, Warhol MJ, Kretschmar C et al. (1986) Neuroblastoma in adults: three case reports and a review of the literature. Cancer 58: 1149

Kedar A, Glassman M, Voorhess ML et al. (1981) Severe hypertension in a child with ganglioneuroblastoma. Cancer 47: 2077–2080

Kinnier-Wilson LM, Draper GJ (1974) Neuroblastoma: its natural history and prognosis: a study of 487 cases. Br Med J 3: 301–307

Klingebiel T, Berthold F, Treuner J et al. (1991) Meta iodobenzylguanidine (mIBG) in treatment of 47 patients with neuroblastoma: results of the German neuroblastoma trial. Med Pediatr Oncol 19: 84–88

Knudson AG Jr, Amromin GD (1966) Neuroblastoma and ganglioneuroma in a child with multiple neurofibromatosis – implications for the mutational origin of neuroblastoma. Cancer 19: 1032–1037

Knudson AG Jr, Meadows AT (1980) Regression of neuroblastoma IV-S: a genetic hypothesis. N Engl J Med 302: 1254–1255

Konrad PN, Singher J, Neerhout RC (1973) Late death from neuroblastoma. J Pediatr 82: 80–82

Kramer S, Meadows AT, Evans AE (1983) Incidence of childhood cancer experience of a decade in a population-based registry. JNCI 70: 49

Kretschmar CS (1991) Neuroblastoma. In: Moosa AR, Schimpff SC, Robson MC (eds) Comprehensive textbook of oncology, vol 2, 2nd edn. Williams and Wilkins, Baltimore, pp 1499–1513

Kretschmar CS, Frantz CN, Rosen EM, Cassady JR, Levey R, Sallan SE (1984) Improved prognosis for infants with stage IV neuroblastoma. J Clin Oncol 2: 799–803

Kushner BH, Cheung N-KV (1988) Neuroblastoma. Pediatr Ann 17: 269–284

Kushner BH, Helson L (1987) Coordinated use of sequentially escalated cyclophophamide and cell-cycle-specific chemotherapy (N4SE protocol) for advanced neuroblastoma: experience with 100 patients. J Clin Oncol 5: 1746–1751

Laug WE, Siegel SE, Shaw KNF, Landing B, Baptist MA, Gutenstein M (1978) Initial urinary catecholamine metabolite concentrations and prognosis in neuroblastoma. Pediatrics 62: 77–83

Leape LL, Lowman JT, Loveland GC (1978) Multifocal non-disseminated neuroblastoma: report of two cases in siblings. J Pediatr 92: 75–77

Lemieux B, Auray-Blais C, Gigèure R, Scriver CR (1989) Neuroblastoma screening: the Canadian experience. Med Pediatr Oncol 17: 379–381

Lingley JF, Sagerman RH, Santulli TV, Wolff JA (1967) Neuroblastoma: management and survival. N Engl J Med 277: 1227–1230

Mancini AF, Rosito P, Faidella G et al. (1982) Neuroblastoma in a pair of identical twins. Med Pediatr Oncol 10: 45–51

Matthay KK, Sather HN, Seeger RC, Haase GM, Hammond GD (1989) Excellent outcome of stage II neuroblastoma is independent of residual disease and radiation therapy. J Clin Oncol 7: 236–244

Matthay KK, Atkinson J, Reynolds CP, Selch M, Seeger RC (1991) Patterns of relapse after autologous bone marrow transplantation (BMT) for neuroblastoma (abstract C1096). Proc Am Soc Clin Oncol 10: 312

McWilliams NB (1987) Screening infants for neuroblastoma in North America. Pediatrics 79: 1048–1049

Michaelis J, Kaatsch P (1986) Cooperative documentation of childhood malignancies in the FRG. System design and five-year results. Monogr Pediatr 18: 56

Moyes J, McCready VR, Fullbrook A (eds) (1989) Neuroblastoma: MIBG in diagnosis and management. Springer, London Berlin Heidelberg

Ninane J, Pritchard J, Morris-Jones PH et al. (1982) Stage II neuroblastoma. Adverse prognostic significance of lymph node involvement. Arch Dis Child 57: 438

Nishi M, Miyake H, Takeda T et al. (1987) Effects of the mass screening of neuroblastoma in Sapporo City. Cancer 60: 433–436

Nitschke R, Humphrey GB, Sexauer CL, Smith EI (1983) Neuroblastoma: therapy for infants with good prognosis. Med Pediatr Oncol 11: 154–158

Nitschke R, Smith EI, Shochat S et al. (1988) Localized neuroblastoma treated by surgery. A Pediatric Oncology Group study. J Clin Oncol 6: 1271–1279

Paul SR, Tarbell NJ, Korf B et al. (1991) Stage IV neuroblastoma in infants: long term survival. Cancer 67: 1493–1497

Perez CA, Vietti T, Ackerman LV, Eagleton MD, Powers WE (1967) Tumors of sympathetic nervous system in children: appraisal of treatment and results. Radiology 88: 750–760

Peschel RE, Chen M, Seashore J (1981) The treatment of massive hepatomegaly in stage IV-S neuroblastoma. Int J Radiat Oncol Biol Phys 7: 549–553

Philip T, Bernard JL, Zucker JM, et al. (1987) High dose chemoradiotherapy with bone marrow transplantation as consolidation treatment in neuroblastoma: an unselected group of stage IV patients over 1 year of age. J Clin Oncol 5: 266–271

Pizzo PA, Horowitz ME, Poplack DG, Hays DM, Kun LE (1989) Solid tumors of childhood. In: DeVita VT Jr, Hellman S, Rosenberg SA (eds) Cancer: principles and practice of oncology, 3rd edn. JB Lippincott, Philadelphia, pp 1624–1631

Punt J, Pritchard J, Pincott JR, Till K (1980) Neuroblastoma: a review of 21 cases presenting with spinal cord compression. Cancer 45: 3095–3101

Ramilo J, Harris VJ (1979) Neuroblastoma in a child with the hydantoin and fetal alcohol syndrome. The radiographic features. Br J Radiol 52: 993–995

Reynolds CP, Frenkel EP, Smith RG (1980) Growth characteristics of neuroblastoma in vitro correlate with patient survival. Trans Assoc Am Physicians 93: 203–211

Rosen EM, Cassady JR, Frantz CN, Kretschmer C, Levey R, Sallan S (1984) Neuroblastoma: the Joint Center for Radiation Therapy/Dana-Farber Cancer Institute/Children's Hospital experience. J Clin Oncol 2: 719–732

Rosen EM, Cassady JR, Frantz CN et al. (1985) Stage IV-N: a favorable subset of children with metastatic neuroblastoma. Med Pediatr Oncol 13: 194–198

Sawada T (1990) Possibilities for early diagnosis by urinary screening for catecholamine metabolites. In: Pochedly C (ed) Neuroblastoma: tumor biology and therapy. CRC Press, Boca Raton, FL, pp 335–347

Sawada T, Hirayama M, Nakata T et al. (1984) Mass screening for neuroblastoma in infants in Japan. Lancet 2(II): 271–273

Sawaguchi S, Suganuma Y, Watanabe I et al. (1980) Studies of the biological and clinical characteristics of neuroblastoma. III. Evaluation of the survival rate in relation to 17 factors. Nippon Shoni Geka Gakkai Zasshi. 16: 51–66

Schnaufer L, Koop CE (1975) Silastic abdominal patch for temporary hepatomegaly in stage IV-S neuroblastoma. J Pediatr Surg 10: 73–75

Schwab M (1988) Molecular genetics of human neuroblastoma. In: Slaysen M, Voute PA (eds) Molecular biology and genetics of childhood cancer: approaches to neuroblastoma. Ellis Horwood Ltd for John Wiley, New York, pp 26–37

Schweisguth O (1968) Treatment of neuroblastoma. J Pediatr Surg 3: 183–184

Scott JP, Morgan E (1983) Coagulopathy of disseminated neuroblastoma. J Pediatr 103: 219–222

Seeger RC, Reynolds CP (1991) Treatment of high-risk solid tumors of childhood with intensive therapy and autologous bone marrow transplantation. Pediatr Clin North Am 38: 393–424

Seeger RC, Brodeur GM, Sather H et al. (1985) Association of multiple copies of the N-*myc* oncogene with rapid progression of neuroblastoma. N Engl J Med 313: 1111–1116

Seeger RC, Matthay KK, Villablanca R et al. (1991) Intensive chemoradiotherapy and autologous bone marrow transplantation (ABMT) for high risk neuroblastoma (abstract #C-1089). Proc Am Soc Clin Oncol 10: 310

Seeler RA, Israel JN, Royal JE, Kaye CI, Rao S, Abulaban M (1979) Ganglioneuroblastoma and fetal hydantoin-alcohol syndromes. Pediatrics 63: 524–527

Sherman S, Roizen N (1976) Fetal hydantoin syndrome and neuroblastoma (letter). Lancet II: 517

Shimada H, Chatten J, Newton WA Jr et al. (1984) Histopathologic prognostic factors in neuroblastic tumors: definition of subtypes of ganglioneuroblastoma and an age-linked classification of neuroblastomas. JNCI 73: 405–416

Smith EI, Haase GM, Seeger RC, Brodeur GM (1989) A surgical perspective on the current staging in neuroblastoma – the international neuroblastoma staging system proposal. J Pediatr Surg 24: 386–390

Soloman GE, Chutorian AM (1968) Opsoclonus and occult neuroblastoma. N Engl J Med 279: 475–477

Stella JR, Schweisguth O, Schlienger M (1970) Neuroblastoma, a study of 144 cases treated in the Institut Gustave-Roussy over a period of 7 years. AJR 108: 324–332

Swift PGF, Bloom SR, Harris F (1975) Watery diarrhea and ganglioneuroma with secretion of vasoactive intestinal peptide. Arch Dis Child 50: 896–899.

Takeda T (1989) History and current status of neuroblastoma screening in Japan. Med Pediatr Oncol 17: 361–363

Traggis DG, Filler RM, Druckman H, Jaffe N, Cassady JR (1977) Prognosis for children with neuroblastoma presenting with paralysis. J Pediatr Surg 12: 419–425

Tuchman M, Woods WG (1990) The scientific basis for neuroblastoma screening: facts and hypotheses. In: Pochedly C (ed) Neuroblastoma: tumor biology and therapy. CRC Press, Boca Raton, FL, pp 349–368

Voute PA, Hoefnagel CA, Marcuse HR, deKraker J (1985) Detection of neuroblastoma with ^{131}I-meta-iodobenzylguanidine In: Evans AE, D'Angio GJ, Seeger RC (eds) Advances in neuroblastoma research. Alan R. Liss, New York, pp 389–398

Weinblatt ME, Heisel MA, Siegel SE (1983) Hypertension in children with neurogenic tumors. Pediatrics 71: 947–951

Wheldon TE, O'Donoghue J, Gregor A, Livingstone A, Wilson L (1986a) Radiobiological consideration in the treatment of neuroblastoma by total body irradiation. Radiother Oncol 6: 317–326

Wheldon TE, Wilson L, Livingstone A et al. (1986b) Radiation studies on multicellular tumor spheroids derived from human neuroblastoma: absence of sparing effect of dose fractionation. Eur J Cancer Clin Oncol 22: 563–566

Wheldon TE, O'Donaghue JA, Gregor A (1987) Radiobiological rationale for hyperfractionation in the radiotherapy of neuroblastoma. Int J Radiat Oncol Biol Phys 13: 1430

Wittenborg MH (1950) Roentgen therapy in neuroblastoma. A review of 73 cases. Radiology 54: 679

Witzleben CL, Lindy RA (1974) Disseminated neuroblastoma in a child with von Recklinghausen's disease. Cancer 34: 786–790

Woods WG, Tuchman M (1987) Neuroblastoma: the case for screening infants in North America. Pediatrics 79: 869–873

Young JL Jr, Heise HW, Silverberg E, Myers MH (1978) Cancer incidence, survival and mortality for children under 15 years of age. American Cancer Society, New York, p 8

Zeltzer PM, Marangos PJ, Sather H et al. (1985) Prognostic importance of serum neuron specific enolase in local and widespread neuroblastoma. In: Evans AE, D'Angio GJ, Seeger RC (eds) Advances in neuroblastoma research. Alan R. Liss New York, pp 286–294

Zucker JM, Margulis E (1979) Radio-chemotherapy of postoperative minimal residual disease in neuroblastoma. Recent Results Cancer Res 68: 423

Zucker JM, Bernard JL, Philip T, Gentet JC, Michon J, Bouffet E for the LMCE Group (1990) High dose chemotherapy with BMT as consolidation treatment in neuroblastoma – the LMCE-1 unselected group of patients revisited with a median follow-up of 55 months after BMT (abstract #C-1139). Proc Am Soc Clin Oncol 9: 294

13 Malignant Brain Tumors Including Medulloblastoma, Embryonal Neuroectodermal Tumors, and Tumors of the Pineal Region, with a Special Discussion of the Management of Brain Tumors in Children of 3 Years and Younger

LARRY E. KUN

CONTENTS

13.1 Malignant Central Nervous System Tumors
in Children 197
13.2 Medulloblastoma 197
13.2.1 Clinical Presentation and Evaluation 198
13.2.2 Treatment. 199
13.2.3 Results of Treatment 201
13.3 CNS Embryonal Neuroepithelial Tumors. 201
13.3.1 Clinical Presentation and Evaluation 202
13.3.2 Treatment 203
13.3.3 Results of Treatment 203
13.4 Pineal Region and Intracranial
Germ Cell Tumors 204
13.4.1 Clinical Presentation and Evaluation 205
13.4.2 Treatment 206
13.4.3 Results of Treatment 208
13.5 Malignant Tumors in Infants and
Young Children 208
References 210

13.1 Malignant Central Nervous System Tumors in Children

Tumors of the central nervous system (CNS) are relatively common in children, representing 20% of all neoplasms. Approximately 1700 children below 21 years of age present with primary CNS tumors annually in the United States, 95% of which originate within the brain (WALKER et al. 1985).

Tumors of the CNS are defined by both histologic type and site of origin. The major diagnostic categories are outlined in Table 13.1. Half of all pediatric CNS tumors are astrocytic neoplasms (i.e., astrocytomas, malignant gliomas, or brain stem gliomas). Although the term "malignant" is difficult to define in the context of CNS neoplasms, the most common tumors identified as "malignant" by histology and/or biologic potential for invasion or dissemination are medulloblastomas, malignant (high-grade) gliomas, pontine gliomas, ependymomas, primitive

LARRY E. KUN, M.D., Chairman, Department of Radiation Oncology, St. Jude Children's Research Hospital, 332 North Lauderdale, P.O. Box 318, Memphis, TN 38101-0318, USA

neuroectodermal tumors (PNETs), and pineal region/germ cell tumors (Childhood Brain Tumor Consortium 1988; DUFFNER et al. 1986).

The median age at diagnosis for all CNS tumors in children is 6 years. Infants and young children less than 2 years old account for 15% of pediatric brain tumors; 30% occur in children 2–5 years old (DUFFNER et al. 1986).

The most common malignant CNS presentations are discussed within the context of the background data and rationale supporting current management recommendations and clinical investigations.

13.2 Medulloblastoma

The term "medulloblastoma" was introduced by Bailey and Cushing to describe a primitive posterior fossa tumor of childhood (BAILEY and CUSHING 1925). The tumor was thought to rise from the

Table 13.1. CNS tumors in children. [Modified from the Childhood Brain Tumor Consortium ($n = 3291$) and the SEER data base ($n = 887$) (Childhood Brain Tumor Consortium 1988; DUFFNER et al. 1986)]

Histology/site	Relative frequency
Low-grade gliomas	38%
Astrocytomas - supratentorial	18%
- cerebellar	15%
- spinal	2%
Oligodendroglioma	2%
Ganglioglioma	1%
Malignant gliomas	14%
Anaplastic astrocytoma, glioblastoma	6%
Brain stem glioma	8%
Medulloblastoma	20%
Ependymoma	11%
Craniopharyngioma	7%
Embryonal tumors – supratentorial[1]	4%
Pineal region and germ cell tumor	4%
Choroid plexus tumors	1%

[a] Includes PNETs, ependymoblastoma, cerebral neuroblastoma; pineoblastoma included with pineal region tumor

embryonal "medulloblast," hypothetically located in the external granular layer of the cerebellum and capable of differentiating along neuronal or glial lines. Although the putative "medulloblast" has never been identified, the tumor does appear to arise from the subependymal matrix cells located in the cerebellar external granular layer of the posterior medullary velum (RUBINSTEIN 1989). The tumor is characterized by small, round, blue cells typical of childhood embryonal neoplasms, with recognized differentiation primarily toward neuronal, glial (astrocytic and oligodendroglial), and, less often, muscular elements (BURGER et al. 1987).

The most common cytogenetic findings in medulloblastoma are deletion of 17p or loss of chromosome 1 (RAFFEL et al. 1990). Double minutes, associated with c-*myc* amplification, are noted in a minority of tumors (BURGER and FULLER 1991). Flow cytometry can identify medulloblastomas by dominant diploid, hyperdiploid, or tetraploid cell lines (TOMITA et al. 1988b; GAJJAR et al. 1993b; ZERBINI et al. 1993; SCHOFIELD et al. 1992).

Confusion between medulloblastoma and the more generic term "PNET" has been apparent since RORKE (1983) introduced a unifying concept of primitive embryonal tumors in children. Broadly defined, PNET includes the hypercellular, small, round, blue cell CNS tumors occurring in children that share similar histologic features, locations adjacent to the ventricular system or the subarachnoid space, and relative responsiveness to both irradiation and chemotherapy. Hypothetically, neoplastic transformation of a common primitive neuroepithelial cell within the subependymal zone anywhere in the CNS may give rise to a neoplasm which is capable of differentiating toward neuronal and/or any of the glial lines (i.e., astrocytic, ependymal, or oligodendroglial) (RORKE 1983). The concept groups together medulloblastoma (the "posterior fossa PNET") with pineoblastoma, neuroblastoma, ependymoblastoma, and undifferentiated supratentorial embryonal tumors (RORKE et al. 1985).

Debate concerning the PNET concept has centered on the value of retaining the distinct tumor types noted above, recognizing their unique clinical features and substantial variation in outcome. Questions have also been raised regarding the putative common neoplastic origin of the embryonal PNETs. RUBINSTEIN (1985) pointed out the possibility of malignant transformation at any stage of differentiation, rather than uniformly at the primitive precursor cell level. Conceptually, Rubinstein's explanation assumes that the differing maturation

Table 13.2. Revised histologic typing of CNS tumors – embryonal tumors (1993) (adapted from KLEIHUES 1993)

I. Embryonal tumors
   1. Medulloepithelioma
   2. Neuroblastoma
   3. Ependymoblastoma
   4. Primitive neuroectodermal tumors (PNETs)
     a. Medulloblastoma
     b. Cerebral (or supratentorial) PNETs

---

potentials are determined by preexistent commitments to specific differentiation pathways related to the age at which the neoplastic transformation occurs and to the anatomic site of neoplastics development (RUBINSTEIN 1985; BURGER and FULLER 1991).

The new WHO classification (Table 13.2) includes a group of *embryonal* childhood CNS tumors which maintains the distinct, clinically identified neoplasms (e.g., pineoblastoma, ependymoblastoma, neuroblastoma, and the very primitive medulloepithelioma) while recognizing a category of "primitive neuroectodermal tumors" comprising (a) medulloblastoma, the distinctive "posterior fossa PNET", and (b) a histologically similar primitive supratentorial lesion without dominant differentiation, simply identified as "supratentorial PNET" (KLEIHUES 1993).

13.2.1 Clinical Presentation and Evaluation

Medulloblastoma is predominantly a tumor of childhood. The median age of presentation is 5–6 years; 20% occur in infants less than 2 years old. Boys and girls are equally affected.

The most common site of origin of medulloblastoma is the midline cerebellar vermis. The tumor fills and usually obstructs the fourth ventricle, resulting in hydrocephalus. Medulloblastoma extends toward the brain stem along the floor of the fourth ventricle. The Chang staging system (Table 13.3) roughly indicates the degree of tumor extension and invasiveness. Most observers distinguish "low-stage" tumors (T_1, T_2, T_{3a}) from "high-stage" tumors (T_{3b}, T_4) largely by the presence of brain stem invasion or extension beyond the posterior fossa (CHANG et al. 1969; BLOOM et al. 1990; TAIT et al. 1990). Adolescents often present with tumors located within the cerebellar hemisphere; such tumors tend to be localized, with a lower frequency of brain stem involvement.

Medulloblastoma is the classic CNS tumor associated with subarachnoid seeding. Neuraxis dissemination is apparent at diagnosis in approximately

Table 13.3. Chang staging of medulloblastoma (CHANG et al. 1969), as modified by J. LANGSTON (personal communication, 1988)

T_1	Tumor less than 3 cm in diameter
T_2	Tumor greater than or equal to 3 cm in diameter
T_{3a}	Tumor greater than 3 cm in diameter with extension into the aqueduct of Sylvius and/or into the foramen of Luschka
T_{3b}	Tumor greater than 3 cm in diameter with unequivocal extension into the brain stem
T_4	Tumor greater than 3 cm in diameter with extension up past the aqueduct of Sylvius and/or down past the foramen magnum (i.e., beyond the posterior fossa)

(Note: No consideration is given to the number of structures invaded or the presence of hydrocephalus, differing from the pre-CT based Chang system. T_{3b} is generally defined by intraoperative demonstration of tumor extension into the brain stem even in the absence of unequivocal radiographic evidence.)

M_0	No evidence of gross subarachnoid or hematogenous metastasis
M_1	Microscopic tumor cells found in cerebrospinal fluid
M_2	Gross nodular seedings demonstrating in the cerebral subarachnoid space, or in the third or lateral ventricles
M_3	Gross nodular seeding in spinal subarachnoid space
M_4	Metastasis outside the cerebrospinal axis

25% of cases. Deutsch reported positive neuraxis staging in 46% of children: malignant CSF cytology in 13% (M_1 in the Chang system, Table 13.3), non-contiguous intracranial disease in 6% (M_2), and imaging evidence of spinal subarachnoid disease in 27% (M_3) (DEUTSCH 1988). Other series have found dissemination in as few as 10% of children (FLANNERY et al. 1990).

Staging is achieved by pre- and postoperative imaging and by surgical observation of local tumor extent. The presence of brain stem invasion is best determined by the neurosurgeon. Postresection tumor residual can be documented by gadolinium-enhanced magnetic resonance imaging (MRI) [or enhanced computed tomography (CT)]; this is preferably done within 1–3 days after surgery to limit confusion with postoperative changes. Neuraxis staging is mandatory in medulloblastoma. CSF cytology and spinal imaging (gadolinium-enhanced MRI or CT-based myelography) are commonly obtained at or beyond 10–14 days following surgery. There is increasing interest in obtaining spinal MR imaging prior to initial surgery. Although radionuclide bone scan and bone marrow biopsy are often required in protocol settings, their routine use may be difficult to justify.

13.2.2 Treatment

13.2.2.1 Surgery

There is increasing recognition of the importance of maximal surgical resection in medulloblastoma. Current operative techniques enable the pediatric neurosurgeon to achieve complete resection in approximately 30%–40% of cases and near-total (> 90%) removal in an additional 30%–45% (Table 13.4) (PARK et al. 1983; HUGHES et al. 1988; ZELTZER 1992; JENKIN et al. 1990a). The degree of resection correlates directly with outcome, likely reflecting both the more limited tumor extent or invasiveness of those amenable to resection and the value of macroscopic tumor excision. Operative mortality is 2% or less (JENKIN et al. 1990a; ALBRIGHT et al. 1989). Aggressive surgery is associated with significant, if

Table 13.4. Degree of surgical removal[a] and outcome (medulloblastoma)

Authors[b]	Interval	No.	Disease-free survival at 5 years					
			Total resection %*	Survival	Near-total resection %*	Survival	Limited resection %*	Survival
JENKIN et al. (1990a)	1977–87	72	39	93%	30	41%	30	48%
HUGHES et al. (1988)	1968–84	60	30	69%	48	69%	22	40%
SCHOFIELD et al. (1992)	1975–85	47	(57)[c]	80%	(57)[c]	80%	39	38%

[a] Total resection = surgically complete with negative postoperative imaging; near-total = >90% removal; limited resection = <90% resection [includes "subtotal" defined as 50%–90% removal (SCHOFIELD et al. 1992), partial removal, or biopsy only]
[b] Statistically significant differences are reported between total resection vs combined near-total and limited resection in JENKIN et al.'s and HUGHES et al.'s analyses and between combined total and near-total resection vs limited resection in SCHOFIELD et al.'s analysis
[c] Data for total and near-total resection are combined in SCHOFIELD et al.'s report
*% of all cases managed, respectively, by total, near-total, and limited resection

usually transient, symptoms and signs of cerebellar and/or brain stem dysfunction. Up to 10% of children may show the so-called posterior fossa syndrome, marked by difficulty in swallowing, ataxia, and dyspraxia; more severe instances of bulbar dysfunction demonstrate mutism, inability to swallow, and depressed respiratory drive sometimes requiring ventilatory support (WISOFF and EPSTEIN 1984). Improvement over several weeks or months is the rule, and such signs should not dissuade one from appropriate radiation therapy.

The goal of "total removal" may not, however, justify long-term neurologic disability from an overly aggressive surgical attempt. Finally, ventriculoperitoneal shunting procedures should be avoided wherever possible as they risk dissemination of tumor to sites not well treated or untreatable by radiation therapy. In practice, approximately 1/4 of children receive ventriculoperitoneal shunt in the postoperative period (ALBRIGHT et al. 1989).

13.2.2.2 Radiation Therapy

The central role of radiation therapy in management of medulloblastoma has been recognized since the 1930s (CUTLER et al. 1936). BLOOM et al.'s (1969) report established the cure of this tumor with orthovoltage craniospinal irradiation (CSI): 32% 5-year survival and 25% long-term disease control at 10+ years were achieved.

The principle of radiation therapy include (a) CSI to encompass the entire subarachnoid space and (b) high-dose irradiation to the posterior fossa primary region. The necessity of fully including the subarachnoid volume is readily apparent in the subfrontal failures reported after treatment techniques that inadequately covered the cribriform plate (JEREB et al. 1982; HALBERG et al. 1991). A recent trial of aggressive chemotherapy and partial neuraxis irradiation (i.e., including only the posterior fossa and spine) only confirms earlier data indicating inferior disease control with incomplete coverage of the subarachnoid volume (LANDBERG et al. 1980; BOUFFET et al. 1992).

Medulloblastoma is a relatively radiosensitive tumor. Studies of radiobiologic parameters in medulloblastoma cell lines indicate a surviving fraction after 2 Gy of 28%, comparable to other radiosensitive childhood tumors including neuroblastoma and markedly different from the resistant malignant gliomas (FERTIL and MALAISE 1985). Clinical analyses indicate a definite dose-response rela-

tionship for the posterior fossa; both local tumor control and survival correlate with posterior fossa dose above 50 Gy (SILVERMAN and SIMPSON 1982; PARK et al. 1983; HUGHES et al. 1988). Current protocols require 54–56 Gy to the posterior fossa with conventional fraction size of 1.5–1.8 Gy daily.

The appropriate dose to the neuraxis is less certain. Recent series indicating long-term survival rates above 50% have uniformly used doses of 35–40 Gy to the cranium and 30–35 Gy to the spine (BLOOM et al. 1990; JENKIN et al. 1990a; HALBERG et al. 1991). TOMITA and MCLONE (1986) reported excellent disease control following only 25 Gy to the neuraxis in a subset of children with "low-stage," totally resected medulloblastoma. Based in part upon the latter experience, the two U.S. pediatric cooperative groups [Pediatric Oncology Group (POG) and Children's Cancer Group (CCG)] conducted a randomized trial of conventional (36 Gy) versus reduced (23.4 Gy) CST in low-stage medulloblastoma (Chang T_1–$T_{3a}M_0$) following complete or near-total resection. The study, confined to children more than 3 years old, has shown statistically superior results with 36 Gy: 80% 3-year disease-free survival compared to 56% in the reduced-dose arm (DEUTSCH et al. 1991). The reduced-dose group has experienced a 29% rate of isolated neuraxis failure, a pattern apparent in only 1 of 52 on the full-dose arm (DEUTSCH et al. 1991). The data confirm the requirement for 36 Gy CSI in children more than 3 years old who are treated with surgery and irradiation alone.

A recent report from UCSF has again raised the question of reduced neuraxis dose, based upon 77% control following 25 Gy CSI in conjunction with limited-term chemotherapy (procarbazine, hydroxyurea) in "favorable" medulloblastoma (HALBERG et al.). The rationale for reducing the radiation dose beyond the posterior fossa is to attempt to reduce the potential neuropsychological, somatic, and endocrine changes associated with neuraxis irradiation. There is no assurance that 24–25 Gy CSI plus chemotherapy will result in less morbidity than 36 Gy CSI alone (KUN and CONSTINE 1991). The two strategies will be tested in a randomized national study (including POG and CCG) for selected cases with low-stage, resected disease, addressing both the relative efficacy and the long-term toxicities of conventional doses of radiation therapy alone compared to reduced-neuraxis-dose irradiation in conjunction with chemotherapy.

Studies of altered fractionation have been preliminarily reported in this tumor system. The radiosensitivity of medulloblastoma in cell culture and clinically apparent radioresponsiveness suggest that this tumor may be ideal for hyperfractionation, potentially improving the therapeutic ratio with reference to diminished late toxicities and/or improved tumor control (FERTIL and MALAISE 1985). Trials to date reflect attempts to diminish late neurotoxicities by maintaining conventional dose levels with hyperfractionated delivery, or to improve disease control in high-stage or metastatic medulloblastoma by delivering higher numerical doses by a hyperfractionated technique (ALLEN et al. 1992; KUN et al. 1990–91; PRADOS et al. 1994).

13.2.2.3 Chemotherapy

Chemotherapy response has been well documented in medulloblastoma. Alkylating agents (e.g., cyclophosphamide), cisplatin and carboplatin, vincristine, and etoposide have shown efficacy in phase II studies (FRIEDMAN and OAKES 1987: PACKER 1990). Prospective trials by the CCG, POG, and International Society of Pediatric Oncology (SIOP) have established a benefit for "adjuvant" chemotherapy in children with high-stage or unfavorable medulloblastoma (EVANS et al. 1990; TAIT et al. 1990; KRISCHER et al. 1991). PACKER (1990) reported impressive disease-free survival (90% at 3 years) in children with unfavorable disease characteristics using full-dose CSI with concurrent vincristine followed by cisplatin and CCNU.

A decade of trials testing preirradiation chemotherapy has provided valuable data regarding responsiveness to individual agents and multiagent regimens (ALLEN et al. 1983; PENDERGRASS et al. 1987; KOVNAR et al. 1990, 1993). In very young children, investigations of prolonged postoperative chemotherapy are easily justified within the context of the risk-benefit ration (see below). In older children, it is not clear whether preirradiation chemotherapy is beneficial (e.g., reducing overt disease at the primary site and within the subarachnoid volume to potentially microscopic levels, facilitating subsequent radiation control) or deleterious (e.g., altering the cellular kinetics to initiate accelerated repopulation by the time of radiation therapy, or inducing radiation resistance as suggested in laboratory studies (ALLEN et al. 1983; DePOOTER et al. 1991; WITHERS et al. 1988). An ongoing POG trial addresses the sequencing of the two modalities, measuring outcome and tolerance of pre versus postirradiation cisplatin and etoposide in high-stage medulloblastoma. Important is selection of a preirradiation chemotherapy regimen that allows timely and continuous subsequent irradiation (KOVNAR et al. 1990). A recent POG study in high-risk medulloblastoma documented response to an aggressive preirradiation schedule, but resulted in unacceptable delays in starting radiation therapy and interruptions during CSI (MOSICJCZUK et al. 1993).

13.2.3 Results of Treatment

Long-term survival has improved significantly over the past 3 decades (Table 13.5). Results from the 1960–1980 era indicate 5-year survival of 55%–65%; only more recent series suggest overall survival at the 70% level following contemporary, aggressive surgery and irradiation (HUGHES et al. 1988; LEFKOWITZ et al. 1988; BLOOM et al. 1990; JENKIN et al. 1990a). Late recurrence and sometimes prolonged postrecurrence survival result in a 10%–15% further decline in survival rates between the 5th and 10th posttreatment year (Table 13.5) (HUGHES et al. 1988; LEFKOWITZ et al. 1988). In analyzing "best results" with surgery and irradiation, children with complete resection and full-dose CSI have enjoyed 5-year disease-free survival at the 78%–95% level (JENKIN et al. 1990a; HALBERG et al. 1991). Early reports of 80%–90% survival in advanced medulloblastoma following irradiation and cisplatin-containing chemotherapy also remain to be verified in both single-institution and multi-institutional studies with adequate follow-up intervals (PACKER 1990).

13.3 CNS Embryonal Neuroepithelial Tumors

The embryonal CNS tumors of childhood represent a diverse and controversial group of malignant,

Table 13.5. Survival following surgery and radiation therapy – medulloblastoma

Author	Treatment interval	Number of children	Survival at 5 years	Survival at 10 years
BLOOM et al. (1969)	1950–69	90	35%	26%
HUGHES et al. (1988)	1968–84	60	68%	44%
LEFKOWITZ et al. (1988)	1970–83	44	54%	41%
BLOOM et al. (1990)	1970–81	53	53%	45%
JENKIN et al. (1990a)	1977–87	72	71%	63%

usually poorly differentiated neoplasms. The recent WHO classification identifies most of the embryonal tumors as specific clinicohistologic entities based upon site of origin, histology, immunohistochemistry, and ultrastructural characteristics (Table 13.2) (KLEIHUES 1993. BURGER and FULLER 1991; CRUZ-SANCHEZ et al. 1991). In sum, these tumors comprise approximately 5% of pediatric brain tumors, occurring most often in very young children. Among children less than 3 years old, poorly differentiated embryonal tumors accounted for 18% of malignant brain tumors in the recent POG study (DUFFNER et al. 1993).

The controversy regarding nomenclature and classification of the embryonal CNS tumors has been summarized above. The specific supratentorial *primitive neuroectodermal tumor (PNET)* was identified in 1973 by HART and EARLE as a clinically malignant cerebral tumor occurring in young children. By definition, the PNET is a predominantly undifferentiated lesion with foci of divergent differentiation toward glial, neuronal, and mesenchymal lines (CRUZ-SANCHEZ et al. 1991). Of the poorly differentiated embryonal tumors accessioned to the POG infant study mentioned above, more than 50% can be classified as PNET, lacking a dominant cell line recognizable as one of the specific embryonal tumors (DUFFNER et al. 1993).

The most primitive, if rare, embryonal tumor is the *medulloepithelioma*. The tumor is architecturally similar to primitive medullary epithelium, including primitive tubular structures; differentiation toward glial, neuronal, and mesenchymal line may be present (RUBINSTEIN 1985). Similarly infrequent is the *primitive polar spongioblastoma*. The tumor is believed to arise from migrating glial precursor cells, and is composed of immature unipolar glial cells; there may be evidence of differentiation toward astrocytic or oligodendroglial lines (RUBINSTEIN 1985).

Ependymoblastoma is a cellular, poorly differentiated neoplasm characterized by ependymal differentiation; pathognomonic is the presence of multilayered rosettes including mitotic figures, similar to the rosettes seen in retinoblastoma (Flexner-Wintersteiner rosettes) (RUBINSTEIN 1989). The tumor is typically remote from the ventricles, presumably arising from ectopic ependymal precursor cells (RUBINSTEIN 1985). Ependymoblastoma is generally felt to be a unique embryonal lesion different from the spectrum of differentiated or anaplastic ependymomas (BURGER and FULLER 1991).

Pineoblastoma is the supratentorial embryonal tumor most often described as "similar histological-ly to medulloblastoma." The tumor is usually marked by sheets of undifferentiated cells and scattered Homer-Wright (unilayered) rosettes; less often, fleurettes and Flexner-Wintersteiner rosettes more typical of retinoblastoma may be seen (HERRICK and RUBINSTEIN 1979). Pineoblastoma presents in both children and adults but like the other embryonal tumors, it is most common in the first decade and particularly in the very young (HERRICK and RUBINSTEIN 1979; BORIT et al. 1980; LINGGOOD and CHAMPMAN 1992; DUFFNER et al. 1993).

Cerebral neuroblastoma is a distinct malignant neuroepithelial tumor. The tumor varies histologically from a classical neuroblastoma pattern, including Homer-Wright rosettes, to a highly desmoplastic lesion; ganglionic differentiation is apparent in up to 25% of cases (RUBINSTEIN 1985, 1989; BENNETT and RUBINSTEIN 1984). Cerebral neuroblastoma represents a more differentiated tumor of committed neuronal lineage in comparison to the undifferentiated PNET (BERGER et al. 1983).

13.3.1 Clinical Presentation and Evaluation

The poorly differentiated embryonal tumors occur almost exclusively as intracerebral lesions. PNET may occur primarily as a spinal cord tumor (KOSNIK et al. 1978). Primary cerebellar neuroblastoma has been recognized, although its distinction from medulloblastoma is unclear (BENNETT and RUBINSTEIN 1984). The embryonal tumors are marked by rapid onset of symptoms, usually related to nonspecific increased intracranial pressure (KOSNICK et al. 1978; ASHWAL et al. 1984).

The PNET is typically cystic, often with hemorrhagic foci, and usually well demarcated from the surrounding cerebral tissue (HART and EARLE 1973; ASHWAL et al. 1984). The other embryonal tumors (medulloepithelioma, polar spongioblastoma, ependymoblastoma) also occur as deep-seated cerebral lesions, although typically more invasive in nature and poorly circumscribed. Pineoblastoma enlarges the pineal gland and presents as a mass lesion often infiltrating into the midbrain or the adjacent deep cerebral tissues, or extending through the tentorium into the posterior fossa (JOOMA and KENDALL 1983). Cerebral neuroblastoma may be cystic or solid; the tumor is circumscribed when cystic, although the solid tumors are usually infiltrative (BENNETT and RUBINSTEIN 1984).

The embryonal tumors, in general, are associated with a high likelihood of neuraxis dissemination.

Subarachnoid seeding at diagnosis or at the time of initial disease progression has been documented in 30%–35% or more of the supratentorial PNETs, ependymoblastomas, and pineoblastomas (ASHWAL et al. 1984; RUBINSTEIN 1985; HERRICK and RUBINSTEIN 1979; LINGGOOD and CHAPMAN 1992). There are few data to substantiate a different pattern of growth among the less common medulloepithelioma or polar spongioblastoma. More controversial is the incidence of neuraxis dissemination in cerebral neuroblastomas. The initial report of this entity, based largely on autopsy data, indicated subarachniod seeding in 38% of cases. (HORTEN and RUBINSTEIN 1976). A follow-up clinicohistologic study based upon referred pathology and survey data suggested a frequency of neuraxis seeding similar to that noted in the other embryonal tumors (BENNETT and RUBINSTEIN 1984). A single-institution report of a relatively small and mature group indicated a very low risk of subarachnoid failure following local therapy, particularly among cystic neuroblastomas (BERGER et al. 1983).

Extraneural metastases have been documented in PNET with a frequency of approximately 4%, primarily after CNS failure (ASHWAL et al. 1984). Extraneural and ventriculoperitoneal shunt metastases occur with surprising frequency among pineoblastomas (GURURANGAN et al. 1993; RICH et al. 1985).

Postoperative evaluation includes cranial MRI, preferably within the first few postsurgical days. Neuraxis staging (gadolinium-enhanced spinal MRI or CT-based contrast myelography and CSF cytology) is indicated for all the embryonal tumors. CSF and serum levels of β-human chrionic gonadotropin (β-hCG) and α-fetoprotein (α-FP) are necessary in pineal region tumors (PACKER et al. 1984).

13.3.2 Treatment

Management of embryonal tumors is dependent upon age, tumor type, and disease extent. For localized lesions in potentially resectable sites, the initial approach is macroscopic tumor resection. The limited available data suggest that approximately one-quarter to one-half of intracerebral lesions may be completely resectable in the case of PNET or cerebral neuroblastoma (BERGER et al. 1983; PIGOTT et al. 1990). Recent series of pediatric pineal region tumors indicate a fairly systematic approach for biopsy (see below) rather than attempted resection (JOOMA and KENDALL 1983; EDWARDS et al. 1988).

Available clinical series reporting outcome in cases of PNET, cerebral neuroblastoma, and pineoblastoma suggest responsiveness but only limited likelihood of disease control following postoperative irradiation (HERRICK and RUBINSTEIN 1979; ASHWAL et al. 1984; BERGER et al. 1983; PACKER et al. 1984a; LINGGOOD and CHAPMAN 1992). Most series report the use of CSI for CNS embryonal tumors, though there is some debate on the validity of this approach in the case of cerebral neuroblastoma. The documented rate of neuraxis dissemination in PNET and ependymoblastoma readily supports such therapy; limited data for medulloepithelioma and polar spongioblastoma lead one to pursue similar therapy in these rare tumors (HART and EARLE 1973; RUBINSTEIN 1985; ASWAL et al. 1984; KOSNICK et al. 1978; GAFFNEY et al. 1985). Lacking dose-response data in any of the embryonal tumors, one would recommend treatment to tolerance doses: CSI to 35–36 Gy in children 3–4 years of age or older, with local "boost" to the primary site to a cumulative level of 54–55 Gy.

BERGER et al. (1983) reported the UCSF experience with cerebral neuroblastoma, detailing disease control in six of six cystic lesions following often incomplete resection and local irradiation. Other data indicate a likelihood of CSF dissemination that argues strongly for CSI in most, if not all, such tumors (HORTEN and RUBINSTEIN 1976; BENNETT and RUBINSTEIN 1984). Selected use of wide local fields, especially in young children with cystic, resected lesions, may be warranted.

Preoperative chemotherapy, as utilized in the POG infant brain tumor trial (see below), has been relatively ineffective for embryonal tumors in general and pineoblastoma in particular. The progression-free survival for pineoblastomas at 2 years is only 18%, which is statistically lower than for any other histologic category (DUFFNER et al. 1993). Adjuvant chemotherapy, including alkylating agents, platinum compounds, and nitrosoureas, does appear to have improved outcome in PNET (ASHWAL et al. 1984). Limited data on pineoblastoma outside the infant setting also suggest a benefit from combined therapy (PACKER et al. 1984a).

13.3.3 Results of Treatment

Disease control rates have been disappointing in embryonal tumors. Survival beyond 2–5 years is reported in 0%–25% of cases of PNET (KOSNICK et al. 1978; ASHWAL et al. 1984; GAFFNEY et al. 1985;

PIGOTT et al. 1990). Although data are relatively limited, survival among patients with cerebral neuroblastoma has been documented at nearly 60% in two reports (BERGER et al. 1983; BENNETT and RUBINSTEIN 1984). Pineoblastomas have been among the least curable pineal region tumors in infants; combined therapy may be successful in 60% of older children (DUFFNER et al. 1993; PACKER et al. 1984a; EDWARDS et al. 1988; JAKACKI et al. 1993).

13.4 Pineal Region and Intracranial Germ Cell Tumors

Tumors of the pineal region comprise 3%–4% of pediatric intracranial neoplasms in North America. Three major tumor types account for more than 90% of pineal region lesions: germ cell, pineal parenchymal, and glial tumors. The histologic distribution is shown in Table 13.6. Germ cell tumors represent 60%–70% of hostologically verified tumors in recent pediatric series. In Japan and parts of China, up to 5%–10% of childhood brain tumors are pineal region neoplasms, and the proportion identified as germ cell tumors is as high as 85%–90% (JENNINGS et al. 1985; TAKAKURA 1984; SANO et al. 1989).

Intracranial germ cell tumors arise almost exclusively around the third ventricle, primarily in the pineal region (50%–60%) and the suprasellar region (30%–35%), less commonly in the basal ganglia or elsewhere (HO and LIU 1992; FELIX and BECKER 1990–91; JENNINGS et al. 1985). Germinomas account for more than 70% of the intracranial germ cell tumors, representing nearly half of all pineal region tumors and the vast majority of suprasellar germ cell tumors in children. Intracranial germinomas are histologically similar to seminomas. Immunohistochemical markers are strongly positive for placental alkaline phosphatase; β-hCG or α-FP may be weakly positive histochemically (FELIX and BECKER 1990–91; HO and LIU 1992). Other intracranial germ cell tumors include embryonic (embryonal carcinoma) and extraembryonic (endodermal sinus tumor, choriocarcinoma) neoplasms marked by characteristic histology and immunohistochemical staining with α-FP and/or β-hCG (FELIX and BECKER 1990–91; HO and LIU 1992). Teratomas, immature teratomas, and malignant teratomas, the latter in association with one or more of the malignant germ cell lines, are relatively common in young children. Mixed patterns, involving two or more germ cell types sometimes in association with teratoma, account for a varying proportion of intracranial germ cell tumors (EDWARDS et al. 1988; JOOMA and KENDALL 1983; JENKIN et al. 1990b; HERRICK and RUBINSTEIN 1979).

The previously used terms "pinealoma" (generically describing tumors in the pineal region that had not been histologically verified) and "ectopic pinealoma" (usually limited to germinoma in the suprasellar region) have largely been replaced by specific histologic diagnoses.

Pineal parenchymal tumors are classified as the mature appearing pineocytoma and the relatively undifferentiated pineoblastoma. Although described as circumscribed and relatively "benign" in adults, pineocytomas in young children may be associated with aggressive neuraxis and local dissemination (BORIT et al. 1980; PACKER et al.1984a). Adolescents share the less malignant characteristics seen in adults, infrequently evidencing significant local invasiveness or dissemination (DISCLAFANI et al. 1989). Pineoblastomas are categorized among the poorly differentiated embryonal tumors, discussed in the previous section.

Table 13.6. Pineal region tumors (children) – histology

Series[a]	Years	No.	Germinoma	Other GCTs		Pineal parenchymal tumors	Astro-cytoma[b]	Other lesions[c]
				Malignant	Benign			
JOOMA and KENDALL (1983)	1972–1982	19	9	4	2	2	2	
EDWARDS et al. (1988)	1974–1986	36	11	9	2	4	8	2
JENKIN et al. (1990b)	1959–1986	35	16	7	1	7	4	
Total		90	40%	22%	6%	14%	16%	2%

GCTs, germ cell types
[a] Pediatric series reporting systematic (JOOMA and KENDALL 1983; EDWARDS et al. 1988) or majority (JENKIN et al. 1990b) tissue diagnosis in pineal region tumors (excludes suprasellar neoplasms)
[b] Benign and malignant astrocytic tumors
[c] Glial, arachnoid cysts

The frequency of *glial tumors* in the pineal region varies in part with the accuracy of neuroimaging. One can now more precisely differentiate tumors arising in the pineal gland, most often germ cell or pineal parenchymal in nature, from those arising in the adjacent tectal plate or mesencephalon. Both low-grade gliomas (primarily astrocytomas, uncommonly oligodendrogliomas or ependymomas) and malignant gliomas are documented in the pineal region (EDWARDS et al. 1988; JOOMA and KENDALL 1983; JENKIN et al. 1990b). Glial and arachnoid cysts also occur in this area (EDWARDS et al. 1988).

13.4.1 Clinical Presentation and Evaluation

Tumors of the pineal region occur most commonly within the first three decades, with a peak incidence in adolescence. Pineal germinomas occur with greatest frequency in teenage boys; suprasellar germinomas tend to occur as often in girls and more uniformly throughout the two pediatric decades.

Children with pineal region tumors present with symptoms of increased intracranial pressure and obstructive hydrocephalus, usually secondary to compression of the sylvian aqueduct. Parinaud's syndrome is present to varying degrees in two-thirds of cases, typically including diminished upward gaze, light-near dissociation of pupillary response (i.e., little or no response to light, but constriction with accommodation and attempted convergence), and limited ability to converge. Precocious puberty in younger children or delayed puberty in adolescents is more often associated with suprasellar involvement, but is described with pineal lesions as well (ERLICH and APUZZO 1985).

Suprasellar tumors classically present with a triad of diabetes insipidus, visual field deficits, and accelerated or delayed sexual development. Hypopituitarism is often noted (SUNG et al. 1978; LEGIDO et al. 1989).

Magnetic resonance imaging is invaluable in defining primary tumor extent and potential subependymal infiltration around the third or lateral ventricles (KOLLIAS et al. 1991–92). A variable proportion of adolescent patients present as multiple midline germinomas, clinically noted as a primary pineal mass with associated diabetes insipidus and neuroradiologically as multiple enhancing nodules within the third ventricular region (Fig. 13.1) Spinal assessment is indicated by gadolinium-enhanced MRI or CT-based myelography. CSF cytology is recommended although it may be unreliable in germi-

nomas due to confusion with similar appearing lymphocytes (SHIBAMOTO et al. 1988). Determination of serum and CSF biochemical markers (i.e., α FP, β hCG) is helpful both in establishing tumor type and in follow-up. β-hCG may be elevated to some degree in germinomas and, less classically, pineoblastomas; significantly increased β-hCG levels more often accompany malignant teratomas or chroiocarcinomas. Elevated α-FP indicates the presence of embryonal carcinoma or endodermal sinus tumor (JOOMA and KENDALL 1983; BJORNSSON et al. 1985).

Reports of peritoneal metastasis via ventriculoperitoneal shunts are uncommon, but have been

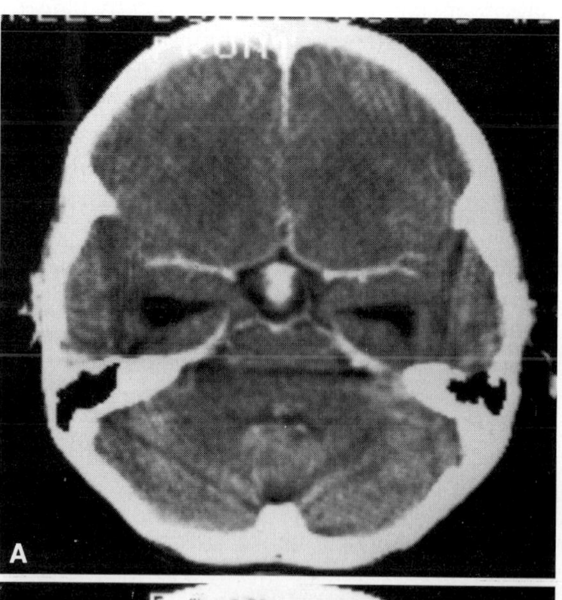
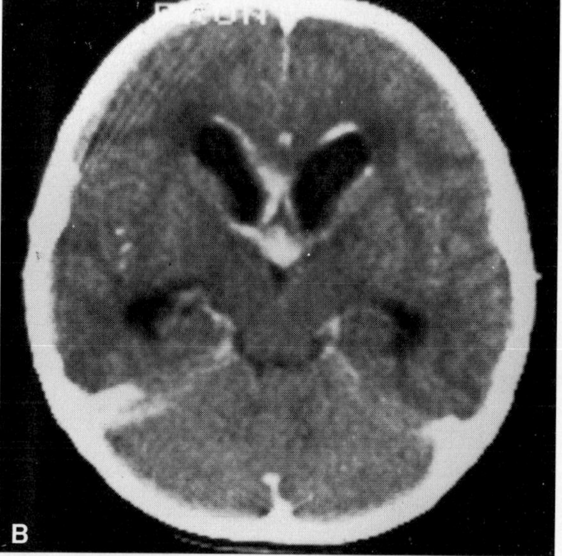

Fig. 13.1A,B. Suprasellar germinoma demonstrating primary lesion (**A**) and subependymal infiltration around the frontal horn of the lateral ventricles (**B**). There is current disease control 6 years following CSI

most often associated with pineal region neoplasms (RICH et al. 1985; GURURANGAN et al. 1993). Abdominal ultrasound or CT to rule out peritoneal seeding may be indicated if there is prolonged delay in treatment following ventriculoperitoneal shunt placement or at the time of disease recurrence.

13.4.2 Treatment

13.4.2.1 Surgery

There remains some debate regarding the role of surgery in pineal region tumors; ventriculoperitoneal shunt is often required (EDWARDS et al. 1988). Prior to the 1970s, operative mortality rates often exceeded 10%–33% in direct pineal surgery for neoplasms (LINGGOOD and CHAPMAN 1992). Empiric irradiation was recommended as a radiodiagnostic test, interpreting rapid tumor response as an indication of both radiosensitivity and tumor type, generally assumed to be germinoma. Lesions demonstrating rapid response following 20–25 Gy to local (ventricular) fields were treated by primary irradiation, often with change in treatment volume to CSI (RICH et al. 1985; DEARNALEY et al. 1990). Conversely, lesions with little immediate response at 20–25 Gy were assumed to be "resistant" or of relatively insensitive tumor type (e.g., malignant teratoma, glioma) and were handled either by higher-dose, local irradiation or by surgical intervention (RICH et al. 1985; BLOOM et al. 1990).

More recent surgical series indicate little if any operative mortality following biopsy (stereotactic or open) EDWARDS et al. 1988; PACKER et al. 1984a; LINGGOOD and CHAPMAN 1992). Operative morbidity in the current era is generally limited to transient worsening of oculomotor signs in up to 25% of cases (EDWARDS et al. 1988; PACKER et al. 1984a; LINGGOOD and CHAPMAN 1992).

The advantage in establishing the histologic tumor type seems to outweigh concerns regarding postoperative morbidity or a previously suggested potential increase in neuraxis dissemination attendant to biopsy procedures (JOOMA and KENDALL 1983; DEARNALEY et al. 1990; WARA et al. 1979). Recent studies fail to substantiate increased risk of subarachnoid dissemination in children undergoing stereotactic or open biopsy (LINSTADT et al. 1988; JENKIN et al. 1990b). Initial serum and, where possible, CSF markers may obviate the need for biopsy in lesions associated with α-FP or substantial β-hCG elevation, identified as more malignant

germ cell types requiring aggressive therapy. In the absence of such markers, biopsy is indicated to determine cell type and the appropriate therapy. Surgical resection may be definitive in gliomas or pineocytomas (STEIN 1984; LEIBEL and SHELINE 1987). Outcome appears to be improved with histologically directed therapy compared to treatment based upon "radiodiagnostic" definition of tumor type (DEARNALEY et al. 1990; JENKIN et al. 1990b; LINSTADT et al. 1988).

13.4.2.2 Radiation Therapy

Radiation therapy is highly effective for intracranial germinomas. Several mature series indicate cure rates in excess of 60%–90% for both pineal region and suprasellar germinomas (DEARNALEY et al. 1990; JENKIN et al. 1990b; LINSTADT et al. 1988). There is general agreement on radiation dose, but considerable controversy regarding the appropriate radiation volume for germinomas and, to a lesser degree, other pineal region tumors.

A dose response for intracranial germinomas is apparent at the 50 Gy level. Earlier data from SUNG et al. (1978) demonstrated local tumor control in 90% of patients following > 50 Gy compared to 53% who received lower doses. KERSCH et al. (1988) have more recently reported a similar analysis relating survival to dose: 78% survival was observed following primary irradiation to > 50 Gy compared to 58% with <50 Gy. The few local failures reported in several recent series share dose levels below 50 Gy (SHIBAMOTO et al. 1988; ABAY et al. 1981; JENKIN et al. 1990b; DATTOLI and NEWALL 1990).

The controversy regarding radiation volume is based upon the variably reported rate of subarachnoid dissemination in series detailing histologically confirmed intracranial germinomas and in series outlining results without histologic diagnosis. SUNG et al. (1978) reported a 5-year incidence of largely spinal subarachnoid seeding in 10% of pineal region tumors (primarily not histologically verified) and 37% of suprasellar tumors (primarily biopsied germinomas). The series has stood as a landmark for those recommending CSI due to its size, relatively lengthy follow-up, and actuarial analysis of patterns of failure.

The reported incidence of distant subarachnoid seeding at diagnosis is generally low. Concurrent involvement of multiple subependymal sites around the third ventricle (most often pineal and suprasellar locations) is noted in 15%–30% of cases (RICH et al.

1985; LINSTADT et al. 1988; GLANZMANN and SEELENTAG 1989). Such *multiple midline tumors* seem to be uniformly germinomas and are associated with excellent outcome following CSI or, less often, local irradiation which includes the *ventricular volume* without full cranial or spinal therapy (RICH et al. 1985; LINSTADT et al. 1988; GLANZMAN and SEELENTAG 1989). Distant subarachnoid metastasis within the spine is rare at diagnosis.

CSF cytology has been positive in up to 50% of case (JOOMA and KENDALL 1983; SHIBAMOTO et al. 1988; GLANZMANN and SEELENTAG 1989). The implication of positive cytology is unclear generally in CNS tumors; in intracranial germinomas, there is documentation of long-term disease-free survival in six of six children with positive cytology treated only to the local third ventricular volume (i.e., without CSI) (SHIBAMOTO et al. 1988).

Conflicting data regarding CNS dissemination are most apparent in several recent, relatively small series which report excellent outcome following local irradiation, usually defined as including the ventricular volume with "boost" to the primary tumor. LINSTADT et al. (1988) reported 12 of 12 patients with biopsy-proven germinomas to be free of disease after limited volume irradiation. In cases treated without histologic diagnosis, local therapy resulted in 73% relapse-free 5-year survival; three of the four patients with recurrent disease had only local failures. The 5-year actuarial risk of spinal failure was 8% in the latter group.

Shibamoto, Glanzman, and Dearnaley showed no significant difference in outcome following CSI or only wide local fields (SHIBAMOTO et al. 1988; GLANZMANN and SEELENTAG 1989; DEARNALEY et al. 1990). In contrast, KERSCH et al. (1988) reported statistically superior disease-free survival following neuraxis irradiation. An update of the Toronto experience indicates disease-free survival in ten of ten children following CSI and spinal failure in two of nine with less comprehensive irradiation (JENKIN et al. 1990b). JENKIN et al.'s (1990b) review of the literature in histologically verified intracranial germinomas found spinal seeding in 18% of 39 cases following local irradiation, comparable to the 23% incidence reported in LINSTADT et al.'s (1988) review.

There is no textbook agreement on the treatment volume for intracranial germinomas. It is the author's opinion that CSI offers a small but significant advantage in durable disease control for all histologically demonstrated germinomas. In patients with multiple midline tumors or evidence of subependymal or subarachnoid disease, there is more widespread support for CSI (SHIBAMOTO et al. 1988; DEARNALEY et al. 1990; JENKIN et al. 1990). The dose to the neuraxis may be as low as 25 Gy routinely, a level likely to limit late effects related to the neuraxis volume except in the youngest pediatric presentations.

Germinomas and the other malignant intracranial germ cell tumors are relatively sensitive to systemic chemotherapy. High response rates have been documented following drug regimens similar to those used for gonadal germ cell tumors (ALLEN et al. 1987; DEARNALEY et al. 1990; SENAN et al. 1991; KOBAYASHI et al. 1989; FINLAY et al. 1992).

The chemosensitivity of gonadal seminoma has encouraged two investigational treatment strategies for children with intracranial germinoma. ALLEN et al. (1987) reported complete responses in 10 of 11 children following initial chemotherapy (primarily using cyclophosphamide alone). Subsequent reduced-dose irradiation to limited, local volumes (30 Gy) for localized tumors and CSI (20–36 Gy) for disseminated neuraxis disease resulted in recurrence-free survival in 10/11 patients with relatively short follow-up. A more "radical" approach has been preliminarily reported for primary chemotherapy alone. FINLAY et al. (1992) noted complete response in 12 of 12 children treated with carboplatin, bleomycin, and etoposide; none had recurred at a short median follow-up (12 months), eliminating irradiation entirely to date. This approach must be considered highly investigational in a tumor long associated with excellent outcome following radiation therapy.

The malignant germ cell tumors have also shown excellent response rates to cisplatin-based chemotherapy regimens. In recurrent tumors, initial complete responses have almost systematically been followed by later disease progression (DEARNALEY et al. 1990; KOBAYASHI et al. 1989; SENAN et al. 1991. NEUWELT and FRENKEL 1984). Limited data regarding pre-irradiation chemotherapy or combined modality treatment suggest improvement in outcome for the more malignant histologic groups (i.e., choriocarcinoma, embryonal carcinoma, endodermal sinus tumors) compared to radiation therapy alone (ALLEN et al. 1987: KOBAYASHI et al. 1989). The international consortium testing chemotherapy alone reported six complete and two partial responses in children with the tumor types other than germinoma; follow-up is as yet short for the six continuously responding case (FINLAY et al. 1992).

13.4.3 Results of Treatment

Recent series indicate overall 5-year survival in pineal region tumors of 65%–80% (WARA et al. 1979; SHIBAMOTO et al. 1988; RICH et al. 1985; GLANZMANN and SEELENTAG 1989). As regards biopsy-proven germinomas, 5- and 10-year disease-free survival rates of 75%–85% are the norm following adequate radiation therapy (EDWARDS et al. 1988; JENKIN et al. 1990b; DEARNALEY et al. 1990; GLANZMANN and SEELENTAG 1989). Earlier reports indicated a less favorable outcome with suprasellar germinomas (SUNG et al. 1978). More recent data show excellent disease control (90+%) in suprasellar germinomas following biopsy and CSI (LEGIDO et al. 1989; DEARNALEY et al. 1990). The impact of radiation volume in intracranial germinomas has been discussed above; summary data are given in Table 13.7 suggesting superior results with full neuraxis irradiation. Similar differences have been documented in published reviews, yet remain unconfirmed in most single-institution reports (LINSTADT et al. 1988; LEGIDO et al. 1989; DEARNALEY et al. 1990; KERSH et al. 1988). Failures occur predominantly within the first 5 years; up to 10%–15% late recurrence has been noted between 5 and 10 years after therapy (SUNG et al. 1978; GLANZMAN and SEELENTAG 1989).

Malignant germ cell tumors other than germinomas have classically shown survival rates of 25%–33% (GRAZIANO et al. 1987; LINGGOOD and CHAPMAN 1992), but contemporary series report only 0%–20% survival for specific histologic groups (i.e., embryonal carcinoma, endodermal sinus tumor, choriocarcinoma) despite aggressive surgery and irradiation (PACKER et al. 1984b; SANO et al. 1989; JENNINGS et al.1985; DEARNALEY et al. 1990).

Data regarding more recent primary chemotherapy and systematic combined modality approaches

are still premature (FINLAY et al. 1992; SENAN et al. 1991). The responsiveness of malignant germ cell tumors to chemotherapy and the unfavorable outcome certainly suggest a role for combined therapy in such histologically documented tumors.

13.5 Malignant Tumors In Infants and Young Children

Between 10% and 15% of pediatric brain tumors occur in infants and children less than 2 years old (JOOMA et al. 1984; TOMITA and MCLONE 1985). Neonates (from birth to 2 months of age) have a unique frequency of teratomas, often presenting as huge intracranial lesions that are histologically benign but associated with extremely poor outcome (BUETOW et al. 1990). The anatomic distribution in youngsters differs from that in older children; supratentorial tumors predominate in the first 1–2 years of life compared to the more prevalent infratentorial tumors thereafter. Astrocytoma is the most common tumor, but the proportion of histologically malignant cell types (in order of frequency: medulloblastoma, ependymomas, choroid plexus tumors including carcinomas, and malignant gliomas) exceeds that seen in children beyond 3–5 years of age (TOMITA and MCLONE 1985; JOOMA et al. 1984; ZELTZER 1992).

Symptoms occurring in the very young most often include change in behavior, irritability, vomiting, or apparent decrease in vision. The elasticity of the skull, open fontanelles, and relative adaptiveness of the still immature brain often permit substantial tumor growth before clinical signs become apparent. Primary lesions tend to be quite sizeable. The frequency of overt subarachnoid metastasis at diagnosis is higher than that seen in older children: 40% with medulloblastoma or PNET, 15% with other histologic groups (TOMITA and MCLONE 1985; DUFFNER et al. 1993; EVANS et al. 1990).

Treatment in this age group is often complicated by greater operative morbidity and limited tolerance to irradiation. Operative mortality rates approached 30% less than 2 decades ago; the current rate of 5% exceeds the rare postoperative death in older children (TOMITA and MCLONE 1985; JOOMA et al. 1984). BLOOM et al. (1969) described dramatic functional consequences in the few long-term survivors of infant medulloblastoma in 1969, recommending a 10%–20% reduction in dose for children less than 2 years old based upon incomplete myelination in the developing brain. Dose reduction likely contributes to the consistent reports of diminished survival

Table 13.7. Outcome in localized pineal region tumors and biopsy proven intracranial germinoma[a]

Histology	No.	RT	5-year DFS	Spinal failures
Germinoma	50	Local	77%	4
	35	CSI	90%	2
Pineal region tumors	78	Local	79%	6
	19	CSI	99%	0

RT, radiation therapy; CSI, craniospinal irradiation; DFS, disease-free survival

[a] Data from series of ABAY et al. (1981), RICH et al. (1985), SHIBAMOTO et al. (1988), GLANZMANN and SEELENTAG (1989), LINSTADT et al. (1988), DEARNALEY et al. (1990), JENKIN et al. (1990b); $n = 12$–30; 1950–78 to 1962–87

Table 13.8. Medulloblastoma and ependymoma: age-related outcome[a] (y.o., years old)

Series	5-year outcome			
Medulloblastoma				
Hughes et al. (1988)	< 2 y.o.	48%	2–12 y.o.	71%
Tait ct al. (1990)	< 2 y.o.	*39%*	2 9 y.o.	*50%*
Evans et al. (1990)	< 4 y.o.	*32%*	≥ 4 y.o.	*64%*
Jenkin et al. (1990a)	≤ 2 y.o.	60%	> 2 y.o.	65%
Ependymoma				
Sutton et al. (1990–91)	< 4 y.o.	*26%*	≥ 4 y.o.	*51%*

[a] Numbers in italics show statistically significant difference

measured overall and in specific tumor types (e.g., medulloblastoma, ependymoma) for children < 2–5 years old (Bloom et al. 1990; Duffner et al. 1986; Evans et al. 1990; Tait et al. 1990; Nazar et al. 1990; Sutton et al. 1990–91; Deutsch 1982). Those surviving still experience greater somatic alterations and cognitive deficits (Kun et al. 1983; Mulhern et al. 1992; Jooma et al. 1984; Packer et al. 1989).

In the context of contemporary trials of initial chemotherapy for malignant tumors in very young children, it is important to recognize baseline data reflecting traditional surgery and irradiation. Jooma et al. (1984) noted overall 5-year survival of 40% in infants less than 1 year old treated conventionally with postoperative irradiation for all tumor types; 80% of long-term survivors had received radiation therapy. Similar results in children < 5 years old had been described by Deutsch (1982). Both series noted intellectual deficits felt to be "acceptable" and, potentially, dose related. Several institutional and cooperative group studies in medulloblastoma and ependymoma indicate survival rates of 20%–35% for young children following surgery and irradiation with or without chemotherapy; although such levels indicate curative potential, they are significantly below those noted in children over 2–4 years old (Table 13.8) (Duffner et al. 1986; Evans et al. 1990; Tait et al.1990; Bloom et al. 1990; Nazar et al. 1990; Sutton et al. 1990–91; Tomita et al. 1988a).

Recent studies substantiate more significant neuropsychological deficits in children treated for brain tumors before age 4–8 years old (Mulhern et al. 1992; Jannoun and Bloom 1990). Multifactorial causes identified in clinical studies include the effect of the primary tumor, possible extension toward the brain stem or subarachnoid seeding, surgery in this age group, frequently associated major sensory deficits (e.g., vision, hearing), and possibly hydrocephalus (Mulhern et al. 1991). Common to most series is a negative correlation between neuropsychological dysfunction and age at the time of cranial irradiation (Kun et al. 1983; Mulhern et al. 1992; Packer et al. 1989; Jannoun and Bloom 1990; Ellenberg et al. 1987)

The tumor type and frequency of neuraxis dissemination in this age group frequently indicate a requirement for CSI. Somatic changes related to bone and soft tissue development, potential visceral changes, and linear growth deficits are greatest among the very young.

The combination of inferior outcome and more pronounced late effects indicates a risk-benefit ratio in younger children with malignant brain tumors supportive of investigational approaches that delay or, less commonly, eliminate radiation therapy. van Eys et al. (1985) initially reported treatment with MOPP chemotherapy postoperatively in young children with a variety of tumors. Follow-up of the medulloblastoma group so treated indicated relapse-free survival beyond 3.5 years in 5 of 12 youngsters; an additional three children survived 3–5 years following subsequent cisplatin (one) or irradiation (two) (Baram et al. 1987). Other reports of initial chemotherapy (MOPP, combinations of cisplatin ± etoposide, cyclophosphamide, vincristine) with delayed irradiation (6 months to 2 years post-surgery) suggest a likelihood of disease control at least as high as is noted following immediate postoperative irradiation (Horowitz et al. 1988; Loeffler et al. 1988).

The recently reported POG trial in children <3 years old utilized postoperative cyclophosphamide/ vincristine and cisplatin/etoposide for 1–2 years, followed by conventional irradiation (with imaging or cytologic evidence of residual disease or with initial neuraxis dissemination) or reduced-dose irradiation (with apparent "complete response" upon initiation of radiation therapy) (Duffner et al. 1993). The 2-year overall progression-free survival of 37% is at least comparable to previous results with postoperative irradiation (Duffner et al. 1993; Evans et al. 1990; Tait et al. 1990; Nazar et al. 1990). Results in specific histologic groups and subset analyses are shown in Table 13.9. Noteworthy are (a) excellent outcome in M_0 cases following initial total resection, (b) apparently comparable outcome in children who achieved and maintained complete tumor response following chemotherapy, and (c) apparent disease control in a small, highly selected subset who refused irradiation while in "complete response" upon completing chemotherapy (Duffner et al. 1993). Results in ependymoma and malignant gliomas are comparable to those in older children treated with

Table 13.9. Infants and young children with malignant brain tumors – results of initial postoperative chemotherapy (POG study). (From DUFFNER et al. 1993)

Subject	No.	2-yr PFS
All patients	198	0.37
0–23 mos. old	132	0.39
24–36 mos. old	66	0.33
Medulloblastoma	62	0.34
Ependymoma	48	0.42
Embryonal tumors	*36*	*0.19*
Malignant gliomas	18	0.54
Brain stem glioma	14	0.28
M_0, resected[a][b]	*29*[b]	*0.75*
< resected, CR to chemotherapy	12	0.68

PFS, progression-free survival; CR, complete response
[a] Italics indicates a statistically less favorable outcome (embryonal tumor group) or more favorable outcome (M_0, resected group)
[b] subset with totally resected M_0 medulloblastoma and ependymoma

standard surgery and irradiation (NAZAR et al. 1990; TOMITA et al. 1988a; SPOSTO et al. 1989). The 60% rate of progressive disease in medulloblastoma is a cause for concern, yet difficult to fault in comparison to radiation results in this age group. Young children with embryonal tumors (primarily pineoblastoma in the POG study) have had a notably poor outcome (DUFFNER et al. 1993; JAKACKI et al. 1993).

A preliminary report by the CCG of "8-in-1" chemotherapy without systematic irradiation indicates a progression-free survival rate of 25% at 2 years in infants <18 months old with medulloblastoma, PNET, or ependymoma. The same therapy is associated with similar outcome in 35% of infants with malignant gliomas (PENDERGRASS et al. 1987; GEYER et al. 1992). The low rate of disease control is not supportive at this treatment regimen.

Limited data detailing functional status following chemotherapy suggest relatively little early neuropsychological impact (DUFFNER et al. 1993). Further follow-up is necessary to assess cognitive outcome. Preexistent deficits apparent in young children with CNS tumors and potential ototoxicity due to cisplatin are likely to affect learning capabilities (MULHERN et al. 1991). Early reports note inconsistent changes in weight gain and linear growth during prolonged chemotherapy; late changes will need to be measured against those associated with radiation therapy.

Data regarding long-term outcome with postoperative chemotherapy alone in malignant brain tumors are limited to those summarized above and anecdotal cases following cisplatin- and MOPP-based chemotherapy (KRETSCHMAR et al. 1989). To measure the overall impact of such an approach requires attention to salvage irradiation for young children who progress during and after planned chemotherapy. A high proportion of medulloblastoma failures include neuraxis dissemination (DUFFNER et al. 1993; KUN et al. 1989; HOROWITZ et al. 1988). Limited data suggest that conventional dose CSI will provide durable disease control in a significant proportion of children more than 18 months old aggressively treated following chemotherapy failure (GAJJAR et al. 1993a). Information regarding functional capacities in long-term survivors of "salvage therapy" awaits further maturation of the POG study quoted above.

Current protocols address intensification of chemotherapy to improve disease control following complete resection and to increase both response and control in the majority of patients with residual or metastatic disease after initial surgery. Obviating mandatory radiation therapy for those with no measurable disease upon completion of drug therapy in an attractive but highly investigational approach now being tested in the cooperative groups.

References

Abay EO, Laws ER, Grado GL, Bruckman JE, Forbes GS, Gomez MR, Scott M (1981) Pineal tumors in children and adolescents. Treatment by CSF shunting and radiotherapy. J Neurosurg 55: 889–895

Albright AL (1986) Surgical aspects of medulloblastoma. In: Zeltzer PM, Pochedly C (eds) Medulloblastomas in children: New concepts in tumor biology, diagnosis and treatment. Praeger, New York, pp 155–163

Albright AL, Wisoff JH, Zeltzer PM, Deutsch M, Finlay J, Hammond D (1989) Current neurosurgical treatment of medulloblastomas in children. Paediatr Neurosurg 15: 276–282

Allen JC, Helson L, Jereb B (1983) Preradiation chemotherapy for newly diagnosed childhood brain tumors: a modified phase II trial. Cancer 52: 2001–2006

Allen JC, Kim JH, Packer RJ (1987) Neoadjuvant chemotherapy for newly diagnosed germ-cell tumors of the central nervous system. J Neurosurg 67: 65–70

Allen JC, Nirenberg A, Donahue B (1992) Hyperfractionated radiotherapy and adjuvant chemotherapy for high risk PNET. J Neurooncol 12: 262

Ashwal S, Hinshaw DB, Bedros A (1984) CNS primitive neuroectodermal tumors of childhood. Med Pediatr Oncol 12: 180–188

Bailey P, Cushing H (1925) Medulloblastoma cerebelli, common type of midcerebellar glioma of childhood. Arch Neurol Psychiatry 14: 192–224

Baram TZ, van Eys J, Dowell RE, Cangir A, Pack B, Bruner JM (1987) Survival and neurologic outcome of infants with medulloblastoma treated with surgery and

MOPP chemotherapy A preliminary report. Cancer 60: 173–177

Bennett JP, Rubinstein LJ (1984) The biological behavior of primary cerebral neuroblastoma: a reappraisal of the clinical course in a series of 70 cases. Ann Neurol 16: 21–27

Berger MS, Edwards MSB, Wara WM, Levin VA, Wilson CB (1983) Primary cerebral neuroblastoma: long-term follow-up and therapeutic guidelines. J Neurosurg 59: 418–423

Bjornsson J, Scheithauer BW, Okazaki H, Leech RW (1985) Intracranial germ cell tumors: pathobiological and immunohistochemical aspects of 70 cases. J Neuropathol Exp Neurol 44: 32–46

Bloom HJG, Wallace ENK, Henk JM (1969) The treatment and prognosis of medulloblastoma in children. AJR 105: 43–62

Bloom HJG, Glees J, Bell J (1990) The treatment and long-term prognosis of children with intracranial tumors: a study of 610 cases, 1950–1981. Int J Radiat Oncol Biol Phys 18: 723–745

Borit A, Blackwood W, Mair WGP (1980) The separation of pineocytoma from pineoblastoma. Cancer 45: 1408–1418

Bouffet E, Bernard JL, Frappaz D et al. (1992) M4 protocol for cerebellar medulloblastoma: supratentorial radiotherapy may not be avoided. Int J Radiat Oncol Biol Phys 24: 79–85

Buetow PC, Smirniotopoulos JG, Done S (1990) Congenital brain tumors, a review of 45 cases. AJNR 155: 587–593

Burger PC, Fuller GN (1991) Pathology—-trends and pitfalls in histologic diagnosis, immunopathology, and applications of oncogene research. Neurol Clin 9: 249–271

Burger PC, Grahmann FC, Bliestle A, Kleihues P (1987) Differentiation in the medulloblastoma. A histological and immunohistochemical study. Acta Neuropathol (Berl) 73: 115–123

Chang CH, Housepian EM, Herbert C Jr (1969) An operative staging system and a megavoltage radiotherapeutic technic for cerebellar medulloblastomas. Radiology 93: 1351–1359

Childhood Brain Tumor Consortium (1988) A study of childhood brain tumors based on surgical biopsies from ten North American institutions: sample description. J Neurooncol 6: 9–23

Cruz-Sanchez FF, Rossi ML, Hughes JT, Moss TH (1991) Differentiation in embryonal neuroepithelial tumors of the central nervous system. Cancer 67: 965–976

Cutler EC, Sosman MC, Vaughan WW (1936) Place of radiation in treatment of cerebellar medulloblastoma: report of 20 cases. Am J Roentgenol Radiat Ther 35: 429–453

Dattoli MJ, Newall J (1990) Radiation therapy for intracranial germinoma: the case for limited volume treatment. Int J Radiat Oncol Biol Phys 19: 429–433

Dearnaley DP, A'Hern RP, Whittaker S, Bloom HJG (1990) Pineal and CNS germ cell tumors: Royal Marsden Hospital experience 1962–1987. Int J Radiat Oncol Biol Phys 18: 773–781

De Pooter CMJ, Scalliet PG, Elst HJ et al. (1991) Resistance patterns between cis-diamminedichloroplatinum (II) and ionizing radiation. Cancer Res 51: 4523–4527

Deutsch M (1982) Radiotherapy for primary brain tumors in very young children. Cancer 50: 2785–2789

Deutsch M (1988) Medulloblastoma: staging and treatment outcome. Int J Radiat Oncol Biol Phys 14: 1103–1107

Deutsch M, Thomas PP, Krischer J et al. (1991) Low stage medulloblastoma: A Children's Cancer Study Group (CCSG) and Pediatric Oncology Group (POG) randomized study of standard vs reduced neuraxis irradiation. Proc ASCO 10: 124

DiSclafani A, Hudgins RJ, Edwards MSB, Wara W, Wilson CB, Levin VA (1989) Pineocytomas. Cancer 63: 302–304

Duffner PK, Cohen ME, Myers MH, Heise HW (1986) Survival of children with brain tumors: SEER Program, 1973–1980. Neurology 36: 597–601

Duffner PK, Horowitz ME, Krischer JP et al. (1993) Postoperative chemotherapy and delayed radiation in children less than 3 years of age with malignant brain tumors: New Eng J Med 328: 1725–1731

Edwards MSB, Hudgins RJ, Wilson CB, Levin VA, Wara WM (1988) Pineal region tumors in children. J Neurosurg 68: 689–697

Ellenberg L, McComb JG, Siegel SE, Stowe S (1987) Factors affecting intellectual outcome in pediatric brain tumor patients. Neurosurgery 21: 638–644

Erlich SS, Apuzzo MLJ (1985) The pineal gland: anatomy, physiology, and clinical significance. J Neurosurg 63: 321–341

Evans AE, Jenkin RDT, Sposto R et al. (1990) The treatment of medulloblastoma. Results of a prospective randomized trial of radiation therapy with and without CCNU, vincristine, and prednisone. J Neurosurg 72: 572–582

Felix I, Becker LE (1990–91) Intracranial germ cell tumors in children: an immunohistochemical and electron microscopic study. Pediatr Neurosurg 16: 156–162

Fertil B, Malaise EP (1985) Intrinsic radiosensitivity of human cell lines is correlated with radioresponsiveness of human tumors: analysis of 101 published survival curves. Int J Radiat Oncol Biol Phys 11: 1699–1707

Finlay J, Walker R, Balmaceda C, Zapater S, Villablanca J, Diez B (1992) Chemotherapy without irradiation (XRT) for primary central nervous system (CNS) germ cell tumors (GCT): report of an international study. Proc ASCO 11: 150

Flannery AM, Tomita T, Radkowski M, McLone DG (1990) Medulloblastomas in childhood: postsurgical evaluation with myelography and cerebrospinal fluid cytology. J Neurooncol 8: 149–151

Friedman HS, Oakes WJ (1987) The chemotherapy of posterior fossa tumors in childhood. J Neuro-Oncol 5: 217–229

Gaffney CC, Sloane JP, Bradley NJ, Bloom HJG (1985) Primitive neuroectodermal tumours of the cerebrum: pathology and treatment. J Neurooncol 3: 23–33

Gajjar AJ, Heideman RL, Douglass EC et al. (1993) Relation of tumor l-cell ploidy to survival in children with medulloblastoma. JCO 11: 2211–2217

Gajjar AJ, Mulhern R, Sanford R et al. (1994) Medulloblastoma in very young children: Outcome of definitive craniospinal irradiation following incomplete response to chemotherapy. JCO 12: 1212–1216

Geyer R, Zeltzer P, Finlay J et al. (1992) Chemotherapy for infants with malignant brain tumors: report of the Children's Cancer Study Group trials CCG-921 and CCG 945. Proc ASCO 11: 365

Glanzmann C, Seelentag W (1989) Radiotherapy for tumours of the pineal region and suprasellar germinomas. Radiother Oncol 16: 31–40

Graziano SL, Paolozzi FP, Rudolph AR, Stewart WA, Elbadawi A, Comis RL (1987) Mixed germ-cell tumor of the pineal region. J Neurosurg 66: 300–304

Gururangan S, Heideman RL, Kovnar EH et al. (1994) Peritoneal metastases in two patients with pineoblastom and ventriculo-peritoneal shunts. Med Pediatr Oncol 22: 417–420

Halberg FE, Wara WW, Fippin LF et al. (1991) Low-dose craniospinal radiation therapy for medulloblastoma. Int J Radiat Oncol Biol Phys 20: 651–654

Hart MN, Earle KM (1973) Primitive neuroectodermal tumors of the brain in children. Cancer 32: 890–897

Herrick MK (1984) Pathology of pineal tumors. In: Neuwelt EA (ed) Diagnosis and treatment of pineal Region Tumors. Williams & Wilkins, Baltimore, pp 31–60

Herrick MK, Rubinstein LJ (1979) The cytological differentiating potential of pineal parenchymal neoplasms (true pinealomas). A clinicopathological study of 28 tumours. Brain 102: 280–320

Ho DM, Liu H-C (1992) Primary intracranial germ cell tumor. Pathologic study of 51 patients. Cancer 70: 1577–1584

Horowitz ME, Mulhern RK, Kun LE et al. (1988) Brain tumors in the very young child. Postoperative chemotherapy in combined-modality treatment. Cancer 61: 428–434

Horten BC, Rubinstein LJ (1976) Primary cerebral neuroblastoma: a clinicopathological study of 35 cases. Brain 99: 735–736

Hughes EN, Shillito J, Sallan SE, Loeffler JS, Cassady JR, Tarbell NJ (1988) Medulloblastoma at the Joint Center for Radiation Therapy between 1968–1984. The influence of radiation dose on the patterns of failure and survival. Cancer 61: 1992–1998

Jakacki R, Zeltzer P, Boyett J et al. (1993) Treatment and survival of pineoblastoma (PBL) in childhood: Report of the Children's Cancer Group Trial CCG-921. Proc ASCO 12: 415

Jannoun L, Bloom HJG (1990) Long-term psychological effects in children treated for intracranial tumors. Int J Radiat Oncol Biol Phys 18: 747–753

Jenkin D, Goddard K, Armstrong D et al. (1990a) Posterior fossa medulloblastoma in childhood: treatment results and a proposal for a new staging system. Int J Radiat Oncol Biol Phys 19: 265–274

Jenkin D, Berry M, Chan H et al. (1990b) Pineal region germinomas in childhood: treatment considerations. Int J Radiat Oncol Biol Phys 18: 541–545

Jennings MT, Gelman R, Hochberg F (1985) Intracranial germ-cell tumors: natural history and pathogenesis. J Neurosurg 63. 155–167

Jereb B, Reid A, Ahuja RK (1982) Patterns of failure in patients with medulloblastoma. Cancer 50: 2941–2947

Jooma R, Kendall BE (1983) Diagnosis and management of pineal tumors. J Neurosurg 58: 654–655

Jooma R, Hayward RD, Grant DN (1984) Intracranial neoplasms during the first year of life: analysis of one hundred consecutive cases. Neurosurgery 14: 31–41

Kersh CR, Constable WC, Eisert DR, Spaulding CA, Hahn SS, Jenrette JM, Marks RD (1988) Primary central nervous system germ cell tumors. Effect of histologic confirmation on radiotherapy. Cancer 61: 2148–2152

Kleihues P (1993) Neuroepithelial tumours. In: Kleihues P, Burger PC, Scheithauer BW (eds) Histological typing of tumours of the central nervous system. Springer-Verlag, New York

Kobayashi T, Yoshida J, Ishyama J, Noda S, Kito A, Kida Y (1989) Combination chemotherapy with cisplatin and etoposide for malignant intracranial germ-cell tumors. An experimental and clinical study. J Neurosurg 70: 676–681

Kollias SS, Barkovich AJ, Edwards MSB (1991–92) Magnetic resonance analysis of suprasellar tumors of childhood. Pediatr Neurosurg 17: 284–303

Kosnik EJ, Boesel CP, Bay J, Sayers MP (1978) Primitive neuroectodermal tumors of the central nervous system in children. J Neurosurg 48: 741–746

Kovnar EH, Kellie SJ, Horowitz ME et al. (1990) Preirradiation cisplatin and etoposide in the treatment of high-risk medulloblastoma and other malignant embryonal tumors of the central nervous system: a phase II study. J Clin Oncol 8: 330–336

Kovnar E, Heideman R, Kellie S et al. (1993) Carboplatin and VP-16 in the treatment of high stage medulloblastoma, pineoblastoma and supratentorial PNET. Proc ASCO 12: 425

Kretschmar CS, Tarbell NJ, Kupsky W et al. (1989) Preirradiation chemotherapy for infants and children with medulloblastoma: a preliminary report. J Neurosurg 71: 820–825

Krischer JP, Ragab AH, Kun L et al. (1991) Nitrogen mustard, vincristine, procarbazine, and prednisone as adjuvant chemotherapy in the treatment of medulloblastoma. A Pediatric Oncology Group study. J Neurosurg 74: 905–909

Kun LE, Constine LS (1991) Medulloblastoma – caution regarding new treatment approaches. Int J Radiat Oncol Biol Phys 20: 897–899

Kun LE, Mulhern RK, Crisco JJ (1983) Quality of life in children treated for brain tumors. Intellectual, emotional, and academic function. J Neurosurg 58: 1–6

Kun LE, Horowitz M, Douglass E et al. (1989) Medulloblastoma in young children: radiation therapy results following failure of primary chemotherapy. Pediatr Neurosci 15: 148

Kun LE, Fontanesi J, Kovnar EH, Greenwald C, Douglass EC, Langston J, Coffey D (1990–91) Hyperfractionated craniospinal irradiation – a phase I trial in children with malignant central nervous system tumors. Pediatr Neurosurg 16: 112

Landberg TC, Lindgren ML, Cavallin-Stahl EK et al. (1980) Improvements in the radiotherapy of medulloblastoma, 1946–1975. Cancer 45: 670–678

Lefkowitz IB, Packer RJ, Ryan SG et al. (1988) Late recurrence of primitive neuroectodermal tumor/medulloblastoma. Cancer 62: 826–830

Legido A, Packer RJ, Sutton LN, D'Angio G, Rorke LB, Bruce DA, Schut L (1989) Suprasellar germinomas in childhood. A reappraisal. Cancer 63: 340–344

Leibel SA, Sheline GE (1987) Radiation therapy for neoplasms of the brain. J Neurosurg 66: 1–22

Linggood RM, Chapman PH (1992) Pineal tumors. J Neurooncol 12: 85–91

Linstadt D, Wara WM, Edwards MSB, Hudgins RJ, Sheline GE (1988) Radiotherapy of primary intracranial germinomas: the case against routine craniospinal irradiation. Int J Radiat Oncol Biol Phys 15: 291–297

Loeffler JS, Kretschmar CS, Sallan SE, LaVally BL, Winston KR, Fischer EG, Tarbell NJ (1988) Pre-radiation chemotherapy for infants and poor prognosis children with meduloblastoma. Int J Radiat Oncol Biol Phys 15: 177–181

Mosijczuk AD, Nigro MA, Thomas PRM et al. (1993) Pre-radiation chemotherapy in advanced medulloblastoma: a Pediatric Oncology Group pilot study. Cancer 72: 2755–2762

Mulhern RK, Ochs J, Kun LE (1991) Changes in intellect associated with cranial radiation therapy. In: Gutin PH, Leibel SA, Sheline GE (eds) Radiation injury to the nervous system. Raven, New York, pp 325–340

Mulhern RK, Hancock J, Fairclough D, Kun L (1992) Neuropsychological status of children treated for brain tumors: a critical review and integrative analysis. Med Pediatr Oncol 20: 181–191

Nazar GB, Hoffman HJ, Becker LE, Jenkin D, Humphreys RP, Hendrick EB (1990) Infratentorial ependymomas in childhood: prognostic factors and treatment. J Neurosurg 72: 408–417

Neuwelt EA (1989) Radiotherapy for tumours of the pineal region and suprasellar germinomas (by Glanzmann and Sellentag), Letter to the Editor. Radiother Oncol 16: 79–80

Neuwelt EA, Frenkel EP (1984) Germinomas and other pineal tumors: chemotherapeutic responses. In: Neuwelt EA (ed) Diagnosis and treatment of pineal region tumors. Williams & Wilkins, Baltimore, pp 332–343

Packer RJ (1990) Chemotherapy for medulloblastoma/primitive neuroectodermal tumors of the posterior fossa. Ann Neurol 28: 823–828

Packer RJ, Sutton LN, Rosenstock JG et al. (1984a) Pineal region tumors of childhood. Pediatrics 74: 97–102

Packer RJ, Sutton LN, Rorke LB et al. (1984b) Intracranial embryonal cell carcinoma. Cancer 54: 520–524

Packer RJ, Sutton LN, Atkins TE et al. (1989) A prospective study of cognitive function in children receiving whole-brain radiotherapy and chemotherapy: 2-year results. J Neurosurg 70: 707–713

Park TS, Hoffman HJ, Hendrick EB, Humphreys RP, Becker LE (1983) Medulloblastoma: clinical presentation and management. Experience at the Hospital for Sick Children, Toronto, 1950–1980, J Neurosurg 58: 543–552

Pendergrass TW, Milstein JM, Geyer JR et al. (1987) Eight drugs in one day chemotherapy for brain tumors: experience in 107 children and rationale for preradiation chemotherapy. J Clin Oncol 5: 1221–1231

Pigott TJ, Punt JAG, Lowe JS, Henderson MJ, Beck A, Gray T (1990) The clinical, radiological and histopathological features of cerebral primitive neuroectodermal tumours. Br J Neurosurg 4: 287–298

Prados M, Wara WM, Edwards MSB et al. (1993) Hyperfractionated craniospinal radiation therapy for primitive neuroectodermal tumors: Early results of a pilot study. Int J Radiat Oncol Biol Phys 28: 431–438

Raffel C, Gilles FE, Weinberg KI (1990) Reduction to homozygosity and gene amplification in central nervous system primitive neuroectodermal tumors in childhood. Cancer Res 50: 587–591

Rich TA, Cassady JR, Strand RD, Winston KR (1985) Radiation therapy for pineal and suprasellar germ cell tumors. Cancer 55: 932–940

Rorke LB (1983) The cerebellar medulloblastoma and its relationship to primitive neuroectodermal tumors (presidential address). J Neuropathol Exp Neurol 42: 1–15

Rorke LB, Gilles FH, Davis RL, Becker LE, (Committee on Pathology, Pediatric Brain Tumor Workshop) (1985) Revision of the World Health Organization classification of brain tumors for childhood brain tumors. Cancer 56: 1869–1886

Rubinstein LJ (1985) Embryonal central neuroepithelial tumors and their differentiating potential. A cytogenetic view of a complex neuro-oncologic problem. J Neurosurg 62: 795–805

Rubinstein LJ (1989) Medulloblastomas (including cerebellar neuroblastoma), 5th edn. In: Russell DS, Rubinstein LJ (eds) Pathology of tumours of the nervous system. Williams & Wilkins, Baltimore, pp 251–279

Sano K, Matsutani M, Seto T (1989) So-called intracranial germ cell tumours: personal experiences and theory of their pathogenesis. Neurol Res 11: 118–126

Schofield DE, Yunis EJ, Geyer JR, Albright AL, Berger MS, Taylor SR (1992) DNA content and other prognostic features in childhood medulloblastoma. Proposal of a scoring system. Cancer 69: 1307–1314

Senan S, Rampling R, Kaye SB (1991) Malignant pineal teratomas: a report on three patients and the case for craniospinal irradiation following chemotherapy. Radiother Oncol 22: 209–213

Shibamoto Y, Abe M, Yamashita J, Takahashi M, Hiraoka M, Ono K, Tsutsui K (1988) Treatment results of intracranial germinoma as a function of the irradiated volume. Int J Radiat Oncol Biol Phys 15: 285–290

Silverman CL, Simpson JR (1982) Cerebellar medulloblastoma: the importance of posterior fossa dose to survival and patterns of failure. Int J Radiat Oncol Biol Phys 8: 1869–1876

Sposto R, Ertel IJ, Jenkin RDT et al. (1989) The effectiveness of chemotherapy for treatment of high grade astrocytoma in children: results of a randomized trial. A report from the Children's Cancer Study Group. J Neurooncol 7: 165–177

Stein BM (1984) Surgical therapy of benign pineal tumors. In: Neuwelt EA (ed) Diagnosis and Treatment of pineal region tumors. Williams & Wilkins, Baltimore, pp 254–272

Sung D, Harisiadis L, Chang CH (1978) Midline pineal tumors and suprasellar germinomas: highly curable by irradiation. Radiology 128: 745–751

Sutton LN, Goldwein J, Perilongo G, Lang B, Schut L, Rorke L, Packer R (1990–91) Prognostic factors in childhood ependymomas. Pediatr Neurosurg 16: 57–65

Tait DM, Thornton-Jones H, Bloom HJG, Lemerle J, Morris-Jones P (1990) Adjuvant chemotherapy for medulloblastoma: the first multi-centre control trial of the International Society of Paediatric Oncology (SIOP I). Eur J Cancer 26: 464–469

Takakura K (1984) Nonsurgical pineal tumor therapy – the Japanese experience. In: Neuwelt EA (ed) Diagnosis and treatment of pineal region tumors. Williams & Wilkins, Baltimore, pp 309–322

Tomita T, McLone DG (1985) Brain tumors during the first twenty-four months of life. Neurosurgery 17: 913–919

Tomita T, McLone DG (1986) Medulloblastoma in childhood: results of radical resection and low-dose neuraxis radiation therapy. J Neurosurg 64: 238–242

Tomita T, McLone DG, Das L, Brand WN (1988a) Benign ependymomas of the posterior fossa in childhood. Pediatr Neurosci 14: 277–285

Tomita T, Yasue M, Engelhard HH, McLone DG, Gonzalez-Crussi F, Bauer KD (1988b) Flow cytometric DNA analysis of medulloblastoma. Prognostic implication of aneuploidy. Cancer 61: 744–749

van Eys J, Cangir A, Coody D, Smith B (1985) MOPP regimen as primary chemotherapy for brain tumors in infants. J Neurooncol 3: 237–243

Walker AE, Robins M, Weinfeld FD (1985) Epidemiology of brain tumors: the national survey of intracranial neoplasms. Neurology 35: 219–226

Wara WM, Jenkin RDT, Evans A et al. (1979) Tumors of the pineal and suprasellar region: Children's Cancer Study Group treatment results 1960–1975. A report from Children's Cancer Study Group. Cancer 43: 698–701

Wisoff JH, Epstein FJ (1984) Pseudobulbar palsy after posterior fossa operation in children. Neurosurgery 15: 707–709

Withers HR, Taylor JMG, Maciejewski B (1988) The hazard of accelerated tumor clonogen repopulation during radiotherapy. Acta Oncol 27: 131–146

Zeltzer PM (1992) Toward a cure for infants with brain tumours: the challenge for the 1990's. Br J Cancer 66(18): S41–S49

Zerbini C, Gelber RD, Weinberg D et al. (1993) Prognostic factors in medulloblastoma including DNA ploidy. J Clin Oncol 11: 616–622

14 Brain Stem Gliomas in Children

PATRICK S. SWIFT

CONTENTS

14.1   Epidemiology 215
14.2   Clinical Presentation.................. 215
14.3   Prognostic Factors................... 215
14.4   Evaluation 217
14.5   Pathology......................... 217
14.6   Therapy.......................... 217
14.6.1 Surgery 217
14.6.2 Radiation Therapy................... 217
14.7   Future Directions.................... 219
        References........................ 219

14.1 Epidemiology

Brain tumors are the most common solid tumors and second most common malignancies in children after the leukemias. Approximately 1100–1200 new cases of brain and central nervous system tumors are seen yearly in children under the age of 14 in the United States. Brain stem tumors account for 10%–20% of all brain tumors in children (ABRAMSON et al. 1974; LITTMAN et al. 1980; BLOOM et al. 1990). For the purposes of this chapter, brain stem will be defined as the medulla oblangata and the pons and will exclude the thalamus and midbrain. No sex or racial predominance is noted in brain stem gliomas. The mean age at diagnosis varies from 6.5 to 8.9 years (HALPERIN 1985; FREEMAN and SUISSA 1986; EIFEL et al. 1987; FREEMAN et al. 1987; STROINK et al. 1987; HALPERIN et al. 1989b; SHRIEVE et al. 1992).

14.2 Clinical presentation

The duration of symptoms prior to diagnosis is highly variable. More than 50% will have a relatively brief duration of symptoms (less than 1 month) before diagnoses, whereas 17% will have symptoms

---

PATRICK S. SWIFT, M.D., Assistant Professor, Department of Radiation Oncology, University of California San Francisco, Long Hospital, Room L-75, Parnassus Avenue, San Francisco, CA 94143-0226, USA

for at least 6 months before diagnosis (HALPERIN 1985; GRIGSBY et al. 1987, 1989; HALPERIN et al. 1989b). Symptoms arise as a result of either obstruction of cerebrospinal flow or local destruction or compression of structure in the region of the brain stem or nerves coursing through the brain stem. The most common presenting symptoms are ataxia (62%–63%), motor disturbances (37%), headaches (42%–61%), and nausea and vomiting (24%–43%). Less common symptoms include dysarthria, personality changes, seizures, and failures to thrive in infants (HALPERIN 1985; EIFEL et al. 1987; GRIGSBY et al. 1987, 1989; HALPERIN et al. 1989b). Cranial nerve deficits, most commonly involving nerves III–VII, occur in 65% of patients, and abnormal cerebellar testing occurs in 63%. Other less common signs include papilledema, head tilt, and long tract signs.

14.3 Prognostic Factors

A wide array of clinical, pathologic, and radiologic characteristics have been reported to be of prognostic significance. Location of the lesion is the most frequently discussed and has been incorporated into the eligibility criteria of three major cooperative group trials in brain stem gliomas (LEE 1975; GREENBERGER et al. 1977; ALBRIGHT et al. 1986; EDWARDS et al. 1987, 1989; EIFEL et al. 1987; FREEMAN et al. 1987, 1988; HALPERIN et al. 1989 a,b). Retrospective reports from Duke and the Joint Center for Radiation Therapy (GREENBERGER et al. 1977; HALPERIN 1985; EIFEL et al. 1987) found that patients with tumors located in the midbrain or thalamus had a superior survival when compared to those with lesions of the pons and medulla after treatment with conventional radiotherapeutic techniques (57%–72% vs 28%–38% 5-year survival). Two special subgroups of brain stem gliomas have been identified that have an improved overall survival and that are often amenable to surgical resection. The first is an exophytic tumor which arises from the dorsum of the brain stem, fills or partially fills the fourth ventricle, and is isodense or hypodense on CT scan. These tumors are generally associated with a prolonged duration for symptoms prior to diagnosis and accounted for 8% of all brain stem lesions in the Toronto series of 121 patients (HOFFMAN et al. 1980; STROINK et al. 1987; SANFORD et al. 1988). Of 16 of these tumors that were approached with a subtotal resection, 13 were pathologically identified as grade I or II astrocytomas, two as gangliogliomas, and only one as an anaplastic glioma. Fifteen of the 16 patients were alive 8 months to 23 years after therapy. EPSTEIN and WISOFF (1988) described a second subgroup of patients with tumors of the cervicomedullary junction. In his series of 24 resected patients, 16 were found to have benign astrocytomas, four gangliogliomas, and four anaplastic astrocytomas or glioblastoma multiforme after gross total resection, and required no postoperative therapy.

The impact of histologic grade on survival is unclear at present. In most series, only a minority of cases have tissue available for histological diagnosis (17%–64%) (HALPERIN 1985; ALBRIGHT et al. 1986; FREEMAN and SUISSA 1986; EIFEL et al. 1987; GRIGSBY et al. 1987, 1989; PACKER et al. 1985, 1990b). Such biopsies often reveal low-grade astrocytomas, and their significance has been called into doubt on the basis of sampling error. Most studies fail to show a major impact of grade on survival; however, there are some notable exceptions. One is the review of prognostic factors in the combined series of cases from the Children's Hospitals of Pittsburg and Philadelphia (ALBRIGHT et al. 1986). The presence of mitoses in histological specimens had a dramatic inverse effect on survival (15 of 18 with mitoses were dead within 6 months and the longest period of survival was only 2.4 years, whereas 18 of 6 without mitoses were alive at 4 years). In this study, the presence of Rosenthal fibers or calcification was associated with improved survival. The recent evaluation of hyperfractionation for brain stem gliomas in children from the CCG (Children's Cancer Group) (EDWARDS et al. 1987, 1989) also suggests that there is a correlation between high-grade malignancy and poor survival. Most studies, however, fail to show a significant correlation between biopsy results and survival (LITTMAN et al. 1980; BERGER et al. 1983; STROINK et al. 1986).

Computed tomographic characteristics of the lesion have been analyzed with respect to survival. Pediatric tumor that appear clearly focal on CT scan or MR scan have a significantly better prognosis than those that are diffusely infiltrative (90% vs 46% 1-year survival in the CCG study) (EPSTEIN 1985; STROINK et al. 1986; EDWARDS et al. 1987, 1989; STROINK et al. 1987; SHRIEVE et al. 1992). Likewise, tumors that display an exophytic pattern tend to fare better than intrinsically expansile lesions. EPSTEIN and WISOFF (1989) reported on 27 cases of diffuse lesions approached surgically, all of which were found to be either anaplastic astrocytomas or glioblastoma multiforme, whereas of six focal lesions, all less than 2.5 cm on MR scan, half were found to be low-grade astrocytomas. The presence of a hypodense lesion prior to enhancement with contrast has been suggested as a poor prognostic factor, as well, and most likely associated with diffuse involvement of the brain stem (ALBRIGHT et al. 1986).

Clinical characteristics associated with a poor prognosis include rapid progression of symptoms over a 2-month course (EDWARDS and PRADOS 1987; EDWARDS et al. 1987, 1989; GRIGSBY et al. 1989; SHRIEVE et al. 1992), the presence of multiple cranial nerve deficits (ALBRIGHT et al. 1986; EDWARDS and PRADOS 1987; EDWARDS et al. 1987, 1989; SHRIEVE et al. 1992), or the presence of long tract signs (ALBRIGHT et al. 1986; FREEMAN and SUSSA et al. 1986). The CCG studies of hyperfractionation have found a highly significant reduction in time to progression and survival for patients whose symptoms began ≤2 months prior to diagnosis (EDWARDS et al. 1989; SHRIEVE et al. 1992). ALBRIGHT et al.'s study (1986) also found a significant decrease in overall survival in patients whose signs had been present for less than 6 months prior to diagnosis. Patients with duration of symptoms ≥ 6 months have been excluded from the Pediatric Oncoloy Group (POG) Study unless they have other evidence suggestive of high-grade malignancy (biopsy positive for anaplastic astrocytoma or glioblastoma or multiple cranial nerve signs) (FREEMAN et al. 1988, 1991). In one series, the 2-year actuarial survival was 71.3% for those without cranial nerve deficits, versus 20.3% for those with cranial nerve deficits (ALBRIGHT et al. 1986).

Aside from the previously mentioned favorable subtypes (cervicomedullary, exophytic dorsal lesions), the impact of surgery on overall survival has been negligible. A retrospective analysis from the Mallinckrodt Institute of 70 pediatric thalamic and brain stem lesion did not find a benefit of subtotal resection over no surgery (GRIGSBY et al. 1987), but the majority of studies have not shown any impact with radical surgery for the most brain stem lesions (GREENBERGER et al. 1977; EPSTEIN 1985; HALPERIN

1985; EDWARDS et al. 1987, 1989; EPSTEIN and WISOFF 1988; HALPERIN et al. 1989 a,b).

14.4 Evaluation

Unquestionably, the cornerstone of the diagnostic evaluation is the MR scan (PACKER et al. 1985, 1990a; EDWARDS et al. 1989). Multiple reports have demonstrated that the extent of disease as seen on MR scan is greater than that revealed on CT scan alone. The characteristic findings on MR are a lesion with decreased signal intensity in T1-weighted images and an increased signal intensity on T2-weighted images.

The incidence of the disseminated disease at presentation is extremely low (GREENBERGER et al. 1977; HALPERIN 1985; EIFEL et al. 1987; GRIGSBY et al. 1987, 1988, 1989; HALPERIN et al. 1989 a,b). MR of the spine is warranted only if the evaluation of the brain shows evidence if diffuse intracerebral disease or if there is clinical symptomatology suggestive of cord involvement. Likewise, spinal taps for CSF cytology are not routinely obtained unless the MR is suggestive of medulloblastoma, primitive neuroelectrodermal tumor, or pineal tumors.

Biopsies of brain lesions have become progressively safer through the use of stereotactic guidance, but are not performed routinely on all brain stem lesions outside of study settings (EDWARDS et al. 1987; EPSTEIN and WISOFF 1989). Indications for biopsy include situations in which the diagnosis is in doubt, or there is serious consideration begin given to maximal debulking procedures, as for cervicomedullary lesions, focal cystic lesions, or dorsally exophytic lesions. The information to be gained from the procedure must be weighed against the potential for adverse effects of such a maneuver.

14.5 Pathology

The number of patients with tissue available for histologic evaluation prior to treatment varies considerably from one report to the next (HALPERIN 1985; PACKER et al. 1985; ALBRIGHT et al. 1986; FREEMAN and SUISSA 1986; EIFEL et al. 1987; GRIGSBY et al. 1987, 1989; PACKER et al. 1990b). In the series of EPSTEIN and WISOFF (1988), in which 66 children underwent attempts at subtotal resection, 24 were found to have low-grade astrocytomas, 38 had either anaplastic astrocytomas to glioblastoma multiforme, and four had gangliogliomas. Studies in which biopsy alone was performed prior to therapy showed low-grade astrocytomas in 0%–72% of cases, anaplastic astrocytomas in 7%–71%, glioblastoma multiforme in 9%–20%, and other or nondiagnostic tissue in 0%–42% (HALPERIN 1985; PACKER et al. 1985, ALBRIGHT et al. 1986; FREEMAN and SUISSA 1986; STROINK et al. 1986; GRIGSBY et al. 1987; EPSTEIN and WISOFF 1988; SANFORD et al. 1988; EDWARDS et al. 1989). Such a disparity lends credence to the belief that biopsies are subject to considerable sampling error. Autopsy studies tend to reveal a very high proportion of malignant astrocytomas and glioblastoma multiforme, suggesting either initial sampling error or else malignant deterioration of the disease over time. Up to 50% of cases will be found at autopsy to have evidence of leptomeningeal spread (HALPERIN 1985; FREEMAN and SUISSA 1986; EIFEL et al. 1987; GRIGSBY et al. 1989; PACKER et al. 1990b).

The differential diagnosis for brain stem lesion includes arteriovenous malformations, abscesses, demyelinating disorders, neurofibromatoses, and encephalitis. MR scanning allows proper delineation of the lesion in the majority of cases (EDWARDS et al. 1987; HEIDEMAN et al. 1989; PACKER et al. 1990a; SMITH et al. 1990).

14.6 Therapy

14.6.1 Surgery

Improvements in neurosurgical instrumentation, notably the introduction of the Cavitron ultrasonic aspirator and the surgical CO_2 or Nd: YAG laser, have reduced the morbidity of such an approach in trained hands. The conditions where an attempted resection by a skilled neurosurgeon are warranted, however, remain quite limited (PACKER et al. 1985; STROINK et al. 1986; EDWARDS et al. 1987; EPSTEIN and WISOFF 1988, 1989; PACKER et al. 1990a). These include lesions in which the diagnosis remains in doubt despite radiologic evaluation, certain lesions in the cervicomedullary junction with minimal involvement of the brain stem, dorsally exophytic lesions, and focal cystic lesions measuring less than 2.5 cm on MR scan. For the majority of brain stem tumors, however, surgery other than biopsy is not recommended.

14.6.2 Radiation Therapy

Radiation therapy remains the cornerstone of treatment despite the poor overall results. Transient symptomatic improvements or stabilization can be expected in up to 85% of patients after irradiation (GREENBERGER et al. 1977; KIM et al. 1980; LITTMAN et al. 1980; FREEMAN and SUISSA 1986; EIFEL et al. 1987). Conventional doses of radiation, using single daily fractions of 1.6–1.8 Gy to a total dose of between 50 and 60 Gy, have resulted in a 5-year survival rate ranging from 0% to 45% (GREENBERGER et al. 1977; KIM et al. 1980; LITTMAN et al. 1980; DUFFNER and COHEN 1985–1986; ALBRIGHT et al. 1986; FREEMAN et al. 1987, 1988, 1991; HALPERIN et al. 1989a,b). The majority of these retrospective reports, however, dealt with small numbers. This broad range of results reflected the fact that certain subsets of patients fared better than others (e.g., those with thalamic lesion fared considerably better than those with pontine or medullary lesions).

In 1977, the CCSG (Children's Cancer Study Group) initiated a study (CCG-944) comparing 50–60 Gy radiation to the brain stem versus the same radiation plus concomitant intravenous vincristine followed by maintenance CCNU, vincristine, and prednisone (PCV) for 1 year (JENKIN et al. 1987). These drugs were considered at that time to be the most efficacious agents available for brain lesions. Focal fields of irradiation were used to deliver dose to the tumor plus 3-cm margins around the tumor. No significant difference was seen in terms of overall survival with the addition of chemotherapy. Median survival time for the overall group was 48 weeks, with a 5-year survival rate of 20%. This trial was followed by a second CCSG trial using preradiation CCNU and flurouracil followed by concomitant misonidazole, hydroxyurea, and radiation (LEVIN et al. 1984). Results of this trial were identical to those seen in the first CCSG trial.

WALKER et al. (1979) demonstrated a dose-response relationship in supratentorial gliomas, improved survival time being correlated with increasing doses of radiation until the threshold of normal tissue toxicity was reached. Hyperfractionated radiotherapy has been evaluated as a means of improving the survival rates by increasing the total dose delivered to the brain stem lesion (EDWARDS and PRADOS 1987; EDWARDS et al. 1987, 1989; FREEMAN et al. 1987, 1988, 1991; PACKER et al. 1987, 1988, 1990a; FREEMAN and LEHNERT 1991). Hyperfractionation, the use of multiple small doses of radiation therapy during a 24-h period instead of the conventional single daily dose, is an attempt to increase the total dose by capitalizing on the different growth rates of the normal tissues of the central nervous system and those of the abnormally proliferating malignant tissues. Increasing the number of fractions increases the likelihood of irradiation of tumor cells during sensitive portions of the cell cycle, diminishing tumor repopulation, and allowing redistribution of rapidly proliferating cell lines thorough the cell cycle into more radiosensitive phases of the cycle (ELLIS 1969; WITHERS 1975; EDWARDS et al. 1987, 1989; FREEMAN et al. 1987, 1988, 1991; PACKER et al. 1990a,b). Spacing the doses at appropriate intervals, no less than 4 h apart and preferably not greater than 8 h, theoretically allows normal repair to take place in healthy, supportive glial and vascular tissues surrounding the tumor to a greater extent than is possible in the abnormal tissue. It is theorized that hyperfractionation will result in overall sparing of normal late-reacting tissues.

Several pilot studies of hyperfractionation were initiated in the 1980s. EDWARDS et al. (1987) at UCSF utilized 1 Gy individual fractions administered twice a day with a 4- to 8-h interval to a total dose of 72 Gy over a 7-week period. The fields were focal, attempting to cover the tumor and edema as seen on CT scan, with a 2- to 3-cm margin around the lesion. The pituitary gland and optic chiasm were shielded when possible at 40 Gy, and the cervical spine was blocked if possible at 60 Gy. Of 41 pediatrics patients treated, the median time to progression was 44 weeks. Median survival time was 72 weeks. Patients with focal tumors in this trial have not yet achieved their median survival, whereas diffuse tumor patients had a median survival of only 51 weeks ($P = 0.0069$) (SHRIEVE et al. 1992). A single patient with a diffuse tumor has survived beyond two years. Patients with duration of symptoms prior to diagnosis of ≤ 2 months had a significantly shorter median survival than those patients with symptoms for ≥ 2 months ($P = 0.001$) (SHRIEVE et al. 1992). Biopsy evidence of glioblastoma multiforme also boded poorly for patients in this trail.

During the same period, a second trial which selected poor prognosis patients was mounted at the Children's Hospital of Philadelphia (CHOP) using 1.2-Gy fractions b.i.d. to a total dose of 64.8 Gy (PACKER et al. 1987). No improvement in overall survival was seen when compared to standard doses, with median survival being 45 weeks. It is of note, however, that no increase in toxicity was observed. A third trial carried out by the POG (FREEMAN et al. 1987) also attempted to select those patients with unfavorable characteristics (clinical course ≤ 6 months prior to diagnosis, presence of cranial nerves findings, long tract signs, and CT characteristics suggestive of high grade). These patients receive 1.1 Gy b.i.d. to a total dose of 66 Gy. Once again, a median survival of approximately 11 months was seen, with a median time to progression of 26 weeks and a 1-year survival of 48%. No significant toxicity increase was noted in either of these trials.

These last two trials were then amended to use higher overall doses (FREEMAN et al. 1988, 1991; PACKER et al. 1990a). The CHOP study was expanded to include other instructions and began treatment with 1-Gy fractions b.i.d. to 72 Gy. This study found a modest but statistically significant increase in progression-free survival rates for the higher dose group and a 20 month progression-free survival of 32%. The recently updated Pediatric Oncology Study of 1.17 Gy fractions b.i.d. to 70.2 Gy found no difference in median survival or median time to progression when compared to the previous trial of 66 Gy. It did, however, find a modest but significant increase in 2-year survival (23% vs 6% for the lower dose trial). In this last trial, the presence of cranial nerve deficits was the single most important factor predicting for poor outcome on multivariate analysis.

The long-term effect of these treatments will require further follow-up. Toxicity at the 70–72-Gy level was slightly greater than that seen at the lower doses, with 50% of patients in the POG study requiring steroid use for more than 3 months after radiation therapy, and reintroduction of steroids in a small portion of patients in the CHOP/NYU study. In the CHOP/NYU higher dose study, six patients out of 35 had transient neurologic deterioration or cystic intralesional changes on MR within 6 weeks of therapy. Similar changes were noted in three of the POG study patients. These trials showed clinical improvement in approximately 70%–77% of patients treated (FREEMAN et al. 1988, 1991; EDWARDS et al. 1989; PACKER et al. 1990a; SHRIEVE et al. 1992). The site of failure in those patients with progressive disease was local in approximately 88% of patients, suggesting no benefits to be derived form treating larger fields.

Chemotherapeutic trials to date have been disappointing in this group of patients. The CCG has recently mounted a trial using b.i.d. radiation to 72 Gy with concomitant interferon-β for patients with high-risk brain stem gliomas.

In summary, it would appear that there is a "standard risk" group of brain stem patients who have biopsy-proven low-grade tumors without early cranial nerve or long tract findings, and with a gradual onset of symptoms over a period of 6 or more months, who have a 6-year survival after standard therapy of 60%. Similarly, patients with midbrain/thalamic lesions are found to have a 67%–73% 5-year survival rate after conventional therapy using focal fields and single daily doses of 1.6–1.8 Gy to a total dose of 54 Gy.

For the poor-risk patients, with biopsy proof of malignancy or without biopsy proof of anaplastic tumor or disease mainly confined to the pons medulla, the outcome after standard therapy is much worse. Use of twice daily radiation in this group improves the median survival in time to progression, but this benefit appears to be limited to patients with focal lesions on MR scan and a duration of symptoms of more than 2 months prior to diagnosis. Those patients with diffuse lesions or rapid onset of symptoms continue to have a rapidly fatal course, with few survivors beyond 2 years.

14.7 Future Directions

Further escalations of dose is unlikely to yield improvements in results due to limitations of normal tissue toxicity (SHRIEVE et al. 1992). Modification of effect is currently being investigated in ongoing trials with biological response modifiers (interferons-β), radiations sensitizers (SR-2508), and chemotherapy dose escalation studies (cisplatin, carboplatin), in conjunction with hyperfractionated radiation.

References

Abramson N, Raben M, Cavanaugh PJ (1974) Brain tumors in children: analysis of 136 cases. Radiology 112: 669–672

Albright AL, Guthkelch AN, Packer RJ, Price RA, Rourke LB (1986) Prognostic factors in pediatric brain-stem gliomas. J Neurosurg 65: 751–755

Berger MS, Edwards MSB, LaMasters D, Davis RL, Wilson CB (1983) Pediatric brain stem tumors: Radiographic, pathological, and clinical correlations. Neurosurgery 12: 298–301

Bloom HJG, Glees J, Bell J (1990) The treatment and long-term prognosis of children with intracranial tumors: a study of 610 cases, 1950–1981. Int J Radiat Oncol Biol Phys 18: 723–745

Duffner PK, Cohen ME (1985–1986) Treatment of brain tumors in babies and very young infants. Pediatr Neurosci 12: 304–310

Edwards MSB, Prados M (1987) Current management of brain stem gliomas Pediatr Neurosci 13: 309–315

Edwards MSB, Levin V, Wara W (1987) Hyperfractionated radiation therapy for brainstem glioma in children. J Neurooncol 5: 170

Edwards MSB, Wara WM, Urtasun RC (1989) Hyperfractionated radiation therapy for brain-stem glioma: a phase I–II trial. J Neurosurg 70: 691–700

Eifel PJ, Cassady JR, Belli JA (1987) Radiation therapy of tumors of the brainstem and midbrain in children: experience of the Joint Center for Radiation Therapy and

Children's Hospital Medical Center (1971–1981). Int J Radiat Oncol Biol Phys 13: 847–852

Ellis F (1969) Dose, time and fractionation: a clinical hypothesis Clin Radiol 20: 1–7

Epstein F (1985) A staging system for brain stem gliomas. Cancer 56: 1804–1806

Epstein F, Wisoff JH (1988) Intrinsic brainstem tumors in childhood: surgical indications. J Neurooncol 6: 309–317

Epstein FJ, Wisoff JH (1989) Brainstem tumors in childhood: surgical indications. In: McLaurin RL (ed) Pediatric Neurosurgery: surgery of the developing nervous system. W.B. Saunders, Philadelphia, pp 357–365

Freeman CR, Lehnert S (1991) Radiotherapy dose-fractionation schedules: hyperfractionation and accelerated treatment regimens. Neurol Clin 9: 351–362

Freeman CR, Suissa S (1986) Brain stem tumors in children: results of a survey of 62 patients treated with radiotherapy. Int J Radiat Oncol Biol Phys 12: 1823–1828

Freeman C, Krischer J, Cohen M, Sanford RA, Burger P (1987) A phase I/II study of hyperfractionated radiotherapy in pediatrics patients with brain stem gliomas. Proceedings of the 29th Annual ASTRO Meeting. Int J Radiat Oncol Biol Phys 13: [Suppl 1]: 105–106

Freeman CR, Krischer J, Sanford RA, Burger PC, Cohen M, Norris D (1988) Hyperfractionated radiotherapy in brain stem tumors: results of a pediatric oncology group study. Int J Radiat Oncol Biol Phys 15: 311–318

Freeman CR, Krischer J, Sanford RA et al. (1991) Hyperfractionated radiation therapy in brain stem tumors. Cancer 68: 474–481

Greenberger JS, Cassady JR, Levene MB (1977) Radiation therapy of thalamic, midbrain and brain stem gliomas. Radiology 122: 463–468

Grisby PW, Thomas PRM, Schwartz HG, Fineberg B (1987) Irradiation of primary thalamic and brainstem tumors in a pediatric population: a 33 year experience. Cancer 60: 2901–2906

Grisby PW, Thomas PR, Simpson JR, Fineberg BB (1988) Long-term results of radiotherapy in the treatment of pituitary adenomas in children and adolescents. Am J Clin Oncol 11: 607–611

Grisby PW, Thomas PR, Schwartz HG, Fineberg BB (1989) Multivarate analysis of prognostic factors in pediatric and adult thalamic brainstem tumors. Int J Radiat Oncol Biol Phys. 16: 649–655

Halperin EC (1985) Pediatric brain stem tumors: patterns of treatment failure and their implications for radiotherapy. Int J Radiat Oncol Biol Phys 11: 1293–1298

Halperin EC, Kun LE, Constine LS, Tarbell NJ (1989a) Pediatric radiation oncology: Raven, New York

Halperin EC, Wehn SM, Scott JW, Djang W, Oakes WJ, Friedmann HS (1989b) Selection of a management strategy for pediatric brianstem tumors. Med Pediatr Oncol 17: 116–125

Heideman RL, Packer RJ, Albright LA, Freeman CR, Rorke LB (1989b) Tumors of the CNS. In: Pizzo PA, Poplack DV (eds) Principles and practice of pediatric oncology. J.B. Lippincott, Philadephia, pp 505–553

Hoffman HJ, Becker L, Craven MA (1980) A clinically and pathologically distinct group of benign brain stem gliomas. Neurosurgery 7: 243–248

Jenkin RDT, Boesel C, Ertel J (1987) Brain-stem tumors in childhood: a prospective randomized trial of irradiation with or without adjuvant CCNU, VCR, and prednisone. A report of the Children's Cancer Study Group. J Neurosurg 66: 227–233

Kim TH, Chin HW, Pollan S (1980) Radiotherapy of primary brain stem tumors. Int J Radiat Oncol Biol Phys 6: 51–57

Lee F (1975) Radiation of infratentorial and supratentorial brain-stem tumors. J Neurosurg 43: 65–68

Levin VA, Edwards MSB, Wara WM (1984) 5FU and CCNU followed by hydroxyurea, misonidazole and irradiation for brainstem gliomas: a pilot study for the BTRC and CCG. Neurosurgery 14: 67–681

Littman P, Jarrett P, Bilanivk L (1980) Pediatric brainstem gliomas. Cancer 45: 2787–2792

Packer RJ, Zimmerman RA, Luerssen TG, Sutton LN, Bilaniuk LT, Bruce DA, Schut L (1985) Brainstem gliomas of childhood: magnetic resonance imaging. Neurology 35: 397–401

Packer RJ, Littman PA, Sposto RM (1987) Results of a pilot study of hyperfractionated radiation therapy for children with brain stem gliomas. Int J Radiat Oncol Biol Phys 13: 1647–1651

Packer R, Wara WM, Albright A (1988) Children's Cancer Study Group Protocol CCG-9882 – hyperfractionated radiation therapy in pediatric brainstem gliomas – a Phase I/II groupwide pilot study. Children's Cancer Study Group

Packer RJ, Allen JC, Goldwein JL (1990a) Hyperfractionated radiotherapy for children with brainstem gliomas: a pilot study using 7,200 cGy. Ann Neurol 27: 167–173

Packer RJ, Schut L, Sutton LN, Bruce D (1990b) Brain tumors of the posterial cranial fossa in infants and children. In: Youmans (ed) Neurological surgery, 3rd edn. W.B. Saunders, Philadelphia, pp 3017–3039

Sanford RA, Freeman CR, Burger P, Cohen ME (1988) Prognostic criteria for experimental protocols in pediatrics brainstem gliomas. Surg Neurol 30: 276–280

Shrieve DC, Wara WM, Edwards MSB (1992) Hyperfractionated radiation therapy for Gliomas of the brainstem and thalamus in children and adults. Int J Radiat Oncol Biol Phys (in press)

Smith RR, Zimmerman RA, Packer RJ (1990) Pediatric brainstem glioma. Post-radiation clinical and MR follow-up. Neuroradiology 32: 265–271

Stroink AR, Hoffman HJ, Hendrick EB, Humphreys RD (1986) Diagnosis and management of pediatric brain-stem gliomas. J Neurosurg 65: 745–750

Stroink AR, Hoffman HJ, Hendrik EB, Humphreys RP, Davidson G (1987) Transependymal benign dorsally exophytic brain stem gliomas in childhood: diagnosis and treatment recommendations. Neurosurgery 20: 439–444

Walker MD, Strike TA, Sheline GE (979) An analysis of dose-effect relationship in the radiotherapy of malignant gliomas. Int J Radiat Oncol Biol Phys 5: 1725–1731

Withers HR (1975) Cell cycle redistribution as a factor in multifractionation radiation. Radiology 114: 199–202

15 Gliomas of the Supratentorium, Ventricular System, and Visual Pathways, and Tumors of the Sellar Region

PATRICK S. SWIFT

CONTENTS

15.1   Supratentorial Gliomas 221
15.1.1 Epidemiology and Etiology 221
15.1.2 Pathology......................... 221
15.1.3 Presentation 222
15.1.4 Evaluation 222
15.1.5 Prognostic Factors................... 222
15.1.6 Management....................... 223
15.2   Oligodendrogliomas 224
15.3   Supratentorial Ependymomas............ 225
15.4   Visual Pathway Gliomas 226
15.4.1 Epidemiology 226
15.4.2 Presenting Symptoms and Signs 227
15.4.3 Pathology......................... 227
15.4.4 Evaluation 227
15.4.5 Management 227
15.4.6 Radiation Technique 229
15.4.7 Complications...................... 229
15.5   Choroid Plexus Tumors 230
15.6   Craniopharyngiomas.................. 230
15.7   Pituitary Adenomas.................. 232
15.8   Future Directions 233
       References 233

15.1 Supratentorial Gliomas

15.1.1 Epidemiology and Etiology

Supratentorial astrocytomas accounted for 36% of all pediatric brain tumors in the SEER registry review of 1973–1980 (25% low-grade astrocytomas and 11% high-grade astrocytomas) (DUFFNER et al. 1986). No predilection for either sex has been noted. Age at time of presentation ranges from infancy to 20 years, with the median at 12.7 years.

Causes are not well defined for the majority of these tumors. In a review of the Connecticut Tumor Registry data on families of children with brain tumors, a relative risk of 8 was found for the subsequent development of a CNS tumor in the siblings of

children with gliomas or medulloblastoma, suggesting a heritable component (FARWELL and FLANNERY 1984). Certain phakomatoses are clearly associated with the development of gliomas, most notably neurofibromatosis (astrocytoma) (LEWIS et al. 1984; HURST et al. 1988) and tuberous sclerosis (giant cell astrocytoma) (PRADOS and LEVIN 1987). Although 40%–50% of adult gliomas have been reported to be associated with oncogene amplification, the exact role of oncogenes in the development of pediatric gliomas has yet to be elucidated (WASSON et al. 1990; BURGER and FULLER 1991). Expression of the c-*erb*B-2 gene product as well as epidermal growth factor receptors has been detected in a variety of pediatric brain tumors, including astrocytoma (KUROIWA et al. 1991). However, in a report of 12 pediatric glial tumors evaluated for 11 different oncogenes, only one was found to have amplification of c-*erb*B-2 (WASSON et al. 1990).

Prior exposure to radiation has been implicated in the development of cerebral gliomas. At least 33 cases of late anaplastic gliomas have been described in children who underwent cranial radiation with or without intrathecal methotrexate for acute lymphoblastic leukemia (ALL) (SHAPIRO and MEALEY 1989). The exact contribution of the radiation to the development of the glioma is unclear, as cases of malignant gliomas have also been reported in the absence of cranial radiation for ALL (REGELSON et al. 1965). In a separate group of more than 10 000 children treated for tinea capitis with low-dose scalp irradiation in Israel, a slightly increased incidence of cerebral gliomas was noted compared to the general population (RON et al. 1988).

15.1.2 Pathology

The differential between low-grade and anaplastic gliomas has prognostic significance in most studies in terms of response to therapy and overall survival (LEIBEL et al. 1975; SHELINE 1975, 1976; DUFFNER and COHEN 1985–1986; LEIBEL and SHELINE 1987;

PATRICK S. SWIFT, M.D., Assistant Professor, Department of Radiation Oncology, University of California San Francisco, Long Hospital, Room L–75, Parnassus Avenue, San Francisco, CA 94143–0226, USA

HALPERIN et al. 1989; BLOOM et al. 1990; BRUCE et al. 1990). Several different schemes are available for the artificial breakdown of these tumors into prognostic subgroups (KERNOHAN et al. 1949; RINGERTZ 1950; RUBINSTEIN 1972a,b; ZULCH 1979; NELSON et al. 1983; DAUMAS-DUPORT et al. 1988; GERMANO et al. 1989), which has resulted in some confusion. These schemes each utilize a different combination of criteria to separate tumors into subgroups with similar outcomes, usually resulting in either three- or four-tiered classifications. The criteria include cellular density, mitotic activity, proliferation potential, nuclear pleomorphism, necrosis, and vascular proliferation. The controversies surrounding the various grading systems for the gliomas are beyond the scope of this chapter and are dealt with in an excellent review by BURGER (1990).

"Low-grade gliomas" generally include fibrillary, protoplasmic, and pilocytic astrocytomas, oligodendrogliomas, and mixed gliomas (RORKE et al. 1985; BURGER 1990), as well as the rarer forms of subependymal giant cell astrocytomas seen in tuberous sclerosis (SHAW et al. 1991). Pilocytic astrocytomas [the classic juvenile pilocytic astrocytoma with an excellent long-term prognosis (PALMA and GUIDETTI 1985)] commonly involve the infratentorial region, but may be found in the supratentorium, the anterior visual pathways, or the diencephalon.

"High-grade gliomas" include glioblastoma multiforme, highly anaplastic astrocytoma, moderately anaplastic astrocytoma (anaplastic gliomas), and malignant gliomas not otherwise specified (RORKE et al. 1985; BURGER 1990). Recent reviews suggest that gemistocytic astrocytomas should also be considered as high-grade lesions (KROUWER et al. 1991), although there is argument on this point (HALPERIN et al. 1989).

15.1.3 Presentation

Symptoms at presentation include headache (60%), focal weakness (34%), personality changes (12%), and a wide variety of less common symptoms referable to tumor location, including nausea, vomiting, aphasia, and developmental regression (MERCURI et al. 1981; PALMA and GUIDETTI 1985; DROPCHO et al. 1987; HEIDEMAN et al. 1989; BRUCE et al. 1990). Seizures have been reported to occur in up to 36%–72% of cases at presentation and are the main presenting symptom for gangliogliomas (BACKUS and MILLICHAP 1962; SUTTON et al. 1983; WALKER et al. 1989). Given the fact that signs are due to local pro-

gression of disease, a host of neurologic deficits can be found, depending on the tumor location.

15.1.4 Evaluation

Magnetic resonance scanning with and without gadolinium enhancement has emerged as the radiologic procedure of choice, although contrast-enhanced CT scanning can provide much of the necessary information (SUTTON et al. 1983; HEIDEMAN et al. 1989; BRUCE et al. 1990; SHAW et al. 1991). MR imaging, particularly the T2-weighted images, can allow detection of small low-grade lesions which might not enhance well on CT scan. MR can also help differentiate between vascular lesions and gliomas, and provides three-dimensional imaging with smooth sagittal and coronal cuts, which is helpful in treatment planning for radiation therapy (BRUCE et al. 1990; Kaiser and KRALENDONK 1991). Tumor cells can, however, be found to extend beyond the limits of contrast enhancement on both CT and MR (KELLY et al. 1987).

Histologic confirmation is obtained in the majority of cases as resection remains the cornerstone of therapy. Routine evaluation of the spine by CSF cytology and MR scans is not warranted since, at presentation, only a 4.5% incidence of leptomeningeal spread is noted (PACKER et al. 1985).

15.1.5 Prognostic Factors

Grade of the glioma is the single most significant prognosticator (SHELINE 1975, 1976; BLOOM 1981a; HEIDEMAN et al. 1989; SHAW et al. 1989b, 1991; Bloom et al. 1990; BRUCE et al. 1990). In the SEER registry, 5-year overall survival for low-grade versus high-grade supratentorial astrocytoma was 71% versus 35% (DUFFNER et al. 1986). Five-year overall survival rates of 71%–95% and greater than 50% 15-year overall survival rates are reported for low-grade lesions. For high-grade lesions, survival at 5 years ranges from 0% to 45% with median survival times of 18–42 months (SHELINE 1975, 1976; BLOOM 1981b; HEIDEMAN et al. 1989; SHAW et al. 1989, 1991; BLOOM et al. 1990; BRUCE et al. 1990). Unlike the situation in adults, a significant 5-year survival rate may be seen in pediatric high-grade astrocytomas (45% 5-year actuarial survival in the UCSF report) (PHUPHANICH et al. 1984).

Other prognostic indicators include age, functional status at the time of surgery, location,

Table 15.1. Pediatric supratentorial astrocytomas: prognostic factors

Factor	References
Histologic grade	LAWS et al. 1984
	DUFFNER et al. 1986
	WOO et al. 1988
	SHAW et al. 1989a
	SPOSTO et al. 1989
	BLOOM et al. 1990
Age	LAWS et al. 1984
	PHUPHANICH et al. 1984
	DUFFNER et al. 1986
	DROPCHO et al. 1987
	SHAW et al. 1989a
	SPOSTO et al. 1989
Functional status prior to surgery	LAWS et al. 1984
Extent of resection	LAWS et al. 1984
	SHAW et al. 1989a
	SPOSTO et al. 1989
	BLOOM et al. 1990
Tumor location	WOO et al. 1988
	SPOSTO et al. 1989
	BLOOM et al. 1990
Radiation dose	LAWS et al. 1984
	SHAW et al. 1989b
	BLOOM et al. 1990
Duration of symptoms	LAWS et al. 1984
Presence of cyst	MERCURI et al. 1981
	LAWS et al. 1984
Necrosis	SPOSTO et al. 1989
BuDR labeling	HOSHINO et al. 1989
Seizures	LAWS et al. 1984
Sex	LAWS et al. 1984

duration of symptoms, 5-bromodeoxyuridine (BUdR) labeling, presence of a cystic component, and extent of resection (Table 15.1) (LAWS et al. 1984; PHUPHANICH et al. 1984; COHADON et al. 1985; PALMA and GUIDETTI 1985; DUFFNER and COHEN 1985–1986; DROPCHO et al. 1987; WOO et al. 1988; HOSHINO et al. 1989; BRUCE et al. 1990). There is no consensus as to the relative importance of these variables.

15.1.6 Management

Low-grade astrocytomas which are surgically accessible should undergo attempts at gross total resection, unless such attempts would result in unacceptable neurologic morbidity. Cystic lesions, most of which will represent benign pilocytic lesions (MERCURI et al. 1981), require aspiration of the cyst, removal of mural nodule, and cyst wall resection. In a series of 42 low-grade gliomas in children followed for a median of 4 years, 40 underwent gross total resection, and only three have failed, for an 8% local failure rate (HIRSCH et al. 1989). In a separate study (MERCURI et al. 1981), 11 of 13 children who underwent a gross total resection with no post-operative radiotherapy are alive, with a median follow-up of 13 years. Of the subtotally resected cases in this report, 11 of 16 remain alive (11 of these 16 received radiation, doses not discussed). Cerebral pilocytic astrocytomas have an excellent outcome after complete resection alone, as do gangliogliomas (SUTTON et al. 1983; SHAW et al. 1989b, 1991). It is unlikely that postoperative radiation will contribute significantly to overall outcome in patients who have undergone gross total excision of low-grade gliomas using today's neurosurgical techniques.

The question of whether or nor to administer adjuvant radiotherapy after subtotal resection has not been definitively answered (SUTTON et al. 1983; LAWS et al. 1984; SHAW et al. 1989b, 1991). Trials by the EORTC and the Brain Tumor Cooperative Group are randomizing adults to observation or immediate treatment after subtotal resection of low-grade gliomas (SHAW et al. 1991). In addition, a current intergroup study (MAYO, NCCTG, ECOG, RTOG, SWOG), as well as a separate EORTC protocol, is randomizing adult patients to different doses of post-operative radiotherapy immediately following incomplete resection (SHAW et al. 1991). In retrospective studies, the use of adjuvant radiation therapy after subtotal resection has been shown to improve the duration of local control in adults with low-grade astrocytoma (LEIBEL et al. 1975; SHELINE 1975; LAWS et al. 1984; LEIBEL and SHELINE 1987; SHAW et al. 1989b, 1991). Given the improved overall prognosis for children with supratentorial astrocytoma (BLOOM 1981a; PHUPHANICH et al. 1984; DROPCHO et al. 1987; BLOOM et al. 1990), however, and the deleterious effects of high doses of radiation on the developing brain (DUFFNER et al. 1985), routine postoperative radiation therapy cannot be recommended in every case. In the young child, close follow-up after subtotal resection with possible reexploration at time of progression may be preferred over immediate radiation. In cases where biopsy only was performed, however, or where further progression of disease would rapidly lead to neurologic deterioration, local-field radiation therapy to the tumor and edema (as seen on the T2-weighted image of the MR) plus a 2-cm margin is recommended. Daily fractions of 180 cGy a day are used to deliver a total dose of 54 Gy. A concerted attempt should be made to limit the dose to the optic chiasm to less than 45 Gy to reduce the risk of visual impairment. (For children less than 5 years of age, some authors suggest that the total dose may be reduced by 10% to 45–60 Gy.)

For patients with high-grade gliomas, the overall prognosis is poor (BLOOM 1981a; DROPCHO et al. 1987; PRADOS and LEVIN 1987; BLOOM et al. 1990). Gross total resection is not usually possible due to the infiltrative nature of the disease (DROPCHO et al. 1987; BRUCE et al. 1990). Radiation therapy is routinely recommended in all patients ≥ 3 years of age, delivering 1.8-Gy fractions to a total dose of 60 Gy to focal fields. Although leptomeningeal spread may occur at some point in the disease process in as many as 30% of cases (DROPCHO et al. 1987), local recurrence is a component in 95% of cases that fail. Little benefit would therefore be derived from craniospinal radiation therapy in light of the inability to control the disease locally at current doses (PRADOS and LEVIN 1987; BLOOM et al. 1990; BRUCE et al. 1990). There are some long-term survivors after surgery and radiation, unlike the more dismal picture in adults (a 26% 10-year survival for 45 children with high-grade supratentorial astrocytomas) (BLOOM et al. 1990).

Chemotherapy may prove to play an important role in pediatric cases. In a prospective randomized CCSG study using CCNU, vincristine, and prednisone in conjunction with radiation therapy and surgery, a 42% 5-year survival was seen, compared to 10% for patients treated without chemotherapy (PRADOS et al. 1988). In a separate UCSF pilot study of 6-thioguanine, procarbazine, dibromodocitol, methyl-CCNU, and vincristine, in addition to surgery and radiation therapy, for 35 high-grade supratentorial pediatric gliomas, only seven failures were seen at a median follow-up of approximately 2 years (PHUPHANICH et al. 1984). A recent report of high-dose multi-agent chemotherapy (thiotepa, VP-16 ± BCNU) followed by autologous bone marrow rescue has shown promising early results in a small group of patients (FINLAY et al. 1990).

15.2 Oligodendrogliomas

Oligodendrogliomas account for only 1% of pediatric CNS tumors (DOHRMANN et al. 1978; BLOOM et al. 1990). Twelve percent of oligodendrogliomas occur in children under the age of 18. The most common location for these infiltrative tumors is the supratentorial region. The slow growth pattern of these tumors is an explanation for the delay in diagnosis, with a mean duration of symptoms prior to diagnosis of 40–42 months. Seizures are a common manifestation of this lesion, being seen in more than 50% of patients in most large series (LUDWIG et al. 1986; BULLARD et al. 1987). Other symptoms are referable to the location of the lesions. On initial evaluation, 40–70% will have radiologic evidence of calcifications, and on pathologic review, more than 90% will have microcalcifications (SHELINE 1975; MORK et al. 1985; LUDWIG et al. 1986; WALKER et al. 1989; BURGER and SCHEITHAUER 1991). The incidence of dissemination in this disease is less than 5% (WALLNER et al. 1988). Grading systems have been proposed and have been shown in at least one major review to be of prognostic significance (SMITH et al. 1983; LUDWIG et al. 1986). The oligodendroglial component is often seen in conjunction with astrocytic elements, and clinical course relates more to the astrocytic grade than the oligodendroglial component (WALLNER et al. 1988). Progression of oligodendrogliomas to more malignant glial histologies at time of recurrence has been reported (WALLNER et al. 1988).

Oligodendrogliomas tend to be sharply demarcated from the white matter of the brain, but insinuate themselves into the surrounding gray matter of the cerebral cortex, making gross total excision exceedingly difficult (BURGER and FULLER 1991). The percentage of patients who have undergone complete resection is very low, 10% in the UCSF series (WALLNER et al. 1988). There is a high incidence of regrowth of incompletely resected lesions, with 5- and 10-year survival rates of only 30% and 15% following surgery alone (LINDEGAARD et al. 1987; SUN et al. 1988). Intracranial tumor recurrence is the main form of failure (WALLNER et al. 1988). The role of radiation therapy after incomplete resection is debated. Reports that failed to show an advantage to postoperative radiation tended to cover long periods of time due to the relative rarity of the tumor (DOHRMANN et al. 1978; REEDY et al. 1983; BULLARD et al. 1987). The use of orthovoltage and wide range of doses employed in these series makes it difficult to draw solid conclusions regarding the delivery of radiation in the megavoltage era. The initial report by SHELINE et al. (1969) showed a significant prolongation in survival with postoperative radiation in 13 subtotally resected lesions. Although this result was difficult to substantiate in later studies, a number suggest improved duration of survival with the addition of radiation after subtotal resection (LINDEGAARD et al. 1987; SUN et al. 1988; WALLNER et al. 1988). At 10 years follow-up, the approach of postoperative radiation for incompletely resected pure oligodendrogliomas has yielded a 56% survival rate compared with 18% for those who received no radiation in the UCSF follow-up study (WALLNER et al. 1988).

The current recommendation is to attempt a complete resection, followed by postoperative radiotherapy for incompletely resected lesions (Wallner et al. 1988). Daily fractions of 1.8–2 Gy are delivered to a total dose of 54 Gy, encompassing a target volume defined by the tumor on MRI with a 2-cm margin. In the young child less than 3 years of age, close follow-up with serial scans may be used to delay the onset of radiation for as long as possible to allow further brain development.

15.3 Supratentorial Ependymomas

Representing 5%–10% of pediatric CNS malignancies (Dohrmann et al. 1976; Bloom 1981a; Duffner and Cohen 1985–1986, 1986; Kun et al. 1988; Heideman et al. 1989; Bloom et al. 1990), ependymomas arise in supratentorial locations in approximately 40% of cases in children, with a predilection for the frontal and temporal lobes (Kun et al. 1988). Most appear to grow adjacent to rather than within the ventricles, arising from rests of subependymal glial cells deposited intracerebrally during embryologic development. Lesions from the supratentorium tend to be more cystic than in other locations, and calcification is commonly seen.

Grading of ependymomas is a controversial topic (Dohrmann et al. 1976; Pierre et al. 1983; West et al. 1985; Kun et al. 1988; Heideman et al. 1989; Ross and Rubinstein 1989). The revised World Health Organization system recognizes four entities which include the common ependymoma ("benign"), the myxopapillary ependymoma (with rare exception confined to the cauda and filum terminale region), the anaplastic ependymoma (characterized by increasing frequency of mitoses, nuclear atypia, endovascular proliferation, and necrosis), and the ependymoblastoma (a primitive neuroectodermal tumor with ependymal elements) (Rorke et al. 1985). Further subdivision of benign ependymomas has been proposed using a 1–4 division, but is of uncertain prognostic significance (Fokes and Earle 1969; Ross and Rubinstein 1989).

In major reviews of the incidence of spinal seeding, benign supratentorial ependymomas are associated with a 0%–2% risk of CSF dissemination (Bloom 1981a; Pierre et al. 1983; Halperin et al. 1989; Bloom et al. 1990), much less than is seen in infratentorial lesions. The risk of seeding in high-grade supratentorial lesions is not well documented, but is estimated to be in the 0%–15% range (Bloom 1981a; West et al. 1985; Kun et al. 1988; Heideman

et al. 1989; Bloom et al. 1990). The current evaluation of an ependymoma necessarily includes a thorough spinal and cranial investigation in the case of all high-grade lesions and symptomatic low-grade lesions. As in astrocytomas, MRI with enhancement is proving superior to the use of CT in cranial studies, and is less invasive than CT myelography for the spine. CSF cytology is routinely sent for cytopathologic review.

Although surgical management is the initial approach to patients with ependymomas, it is not adequate by itself (Fokes and Earle 1969; Salazar et al. 1975, 1983; Salazar 1983; West et al. 1985; Kun et al. 1988). Overall 5-year survival rates following surgery only are less than 20% (Fokes and Earle 1969; Mork and Loken 1977). The extent of resection, however, has been correlated with survival in a number of studies, supporting the approach of radical resection when feasible (Marks and Adler 1982; Jenkin et al. 1987; Kun et al. 1988). Following the use of postoperative radiation after maximal resection, overall survival rates of 35%–70% have been recorded (Table 15.2) (Fokes and Earle 1969; Dohrmann et al. 1976; Mork and Loken 1977; Walker et al. 1989; Bloom et al. 1990). Retrospective analyses suggest a benefit to doses in excess of 45 Gy (Salazar et al. 1975; Kim and Fayos 1977; Marks and Adler 1982; Salazar 1983; Salazar et al. 1983; Read 1984). Local failure remains a major problem, however, even when doses in excess of 50 Gy are used (Read 1984; Shaw et al. 1987; Goldwein et al. 1990a, b). In the treatment of supratentorial ependymomas (low grade), fields encompassing the primary tumor and the ventricular system (essentially whole brain fields) are sufficient, given the low risk of spinal dissemination. The entire ventricular system is treated at 1.6- to 1.8-Gy fractions per day to a dose of 45 Gy, followed by a boost

Table 15. 2. Pediatric supratentorial ependymomas: survival rates with or without radiation

Author	No.	5-yr OS	10-yr OS
Surgery			
Mork and Loken 1977	12	17%	
Dohrmann et al. 1976	19	25%	
Surgery + RT			
Shaw et al. 1989b	18	73%	60%
Wallner et al. 1986	10	50%	
Bloom et al. 1990	51	51%	40%
Salazar et al. 1983	30	48%	
Goldwein et al. 1990a	51	46%	

OS, overall survival

of the primary as defined on MRI to 54–56 Gy. Local control is achieved in up to 78% of low-grade cranial lesions, with 10-year survival rates of 47%–70% achieved after aggressive surgical approaches followed by radiation therapy (SALAZAR 1983; SALAZAR et al. 1983; SHAW et al. 1987; BLOOM et al. 1990). Several institutions are looking at the use of hyperfractionation in an attempt to boost the primary tumor dose to > 60 Gy via twice daily treatment with 1-Gy fractions (UCSF, personal communication).

Controversy exists in the treatment of high-grade supratentorial ependymomas with no radiologic or cytologic evidence of dissemination. Most authors would recommend craniospinal irradiation (24–30 Gy for spine, 36–45 Gy whole brain with boost of the primary to 55 Gy) (SALAZAR et al. 1975, 1983; SALAZAR 1983; SHAW et al. 1987; HALPERIN et al. 1989; HEIDEMAN et al. 1989). Others, however, argue that when ependymoblastomas are excluded, there is no benefit seen with the use of CSI, and treatment of the primary and ventricular system is adequate (WALLNER et al. 1986; ROSS and RUBINSTEIN 1989). In the presence of documented drop metastases or ependymoblastoma in any location, however, craniospinal irradiation is the standard treatment with boost of involved regions to cord tolerance levels. Local control is accomplished using the techniques recommended by SALAZAR et al. (1983) in up to 50% of high-grade lesions, with 10-year survival rates ranging from 10% to 67% reported (SALAZAR 1983; SALAZAR et al. 1983; SHAW et al. 1987; BLOOM et al. 1990). Of note, Goldwein and West have seen no significant difference in 5-year survival rates based on grade (WEST et al. 1985; GOLDWEIN et al. 1990b, 1991). Given significant local failure rates, especially for anaplastic lesions, novel approaches such as hyperfractionation or neoadjuvant chemotherapy or the introduction of new radiosensitizers may be justified.

Chemotherapeutic agents such as vincristine, the nitrosoureas, and cyclophosphamide and combinations such as MOPP (EYS et al. 1985), the "eight in one" regimen (BLEYER et al. 1983), and a combination of 6-thioguanine, procarbazine, dibromodulcitol, CCNU, and vincristine (PETRONIO et al. 1991) have been used in the young child ≤ 3 years of age after surgery in an attempt to delay the use of radiation until the CNS has had further time to mature. Early reports are encouraging but further follow-up is required before such treatment can be considered standard of care. Additional studies have analyzed the use of adjuvant chemotherapy during and/or following radiotherapy, most notably with vincristine and CCNU, but have failed to show a survival advantage (BLOOM et al. 1990).

15.4 Visual Pathway Gliomas

15.4.1 Epidemiology

Gliomas of the visual pathways (VPGs), or optic gliomas, represent 1%–5% of all childhood CNS tumors (DANOFF et al. 1980; WONG et al. 1987; HEIDEMAN et al. 1989; HOUSEPIAN et al. 1990; PIERCE et al. 1990; DUTTON 1991). The mean age at presentation for these tumors is 8.5 years (DUTTON 1991); 71% occur within the first decade and 90% have occurred by the conclusion of the second decade of life. The sex distribution overall is 1:1 male to female. These tumors may involve the orbit and optic disk (intraorbital gliomas), the optic nerve (one or both), the chiasm, the optic tracts, the optic radiations, the visual cortex of the occipital lobes, or combinations of the above, and may extend into locally adjacent structures such as the hypothalamus. Twenty-five percent of tumors are confined to the orbit and/or optic nerve, while the remaining 75% have extension to the chiasm (ALVORD and LOFTON 1988; COHEN and FUFFNER 1991; DUTTON 1991). Forty percent of chiasmal lesions extend into adjacent structures such as the hypothalamus (RUSH et al. 1982; HORWICH and BLOOM 1985; ALVORD and LOFTON 1988; DUTTON 1991).

Visual Pathway Gliomas are often found in association with neurofibromatosis (NF) (STERN et al. 1979; DANOFF et al. 1980; PACKER et al. 1983; LEWIS et al. 1984; HORWICH and BLOOM 1985; IMES and HOYT 1986; ALVORD and LOFTON 1988; HURST et al. 1988; RUBINSTEIN 1988; SPITZER and GOODRICH 1988; LISTERNICK et al. 1989; BATAINI et al. 1991; DUTTON 1991). Between 9% and 50% of patients with VPGs will have clinical evidence of NF (PACKER et al. 1983). Prior to the routine use of MRI for CNS screening of patients with NF, it had been estimated that from 3% to 5% of patients with NF would develop VPGs (PACKER et al. 1983; LISTERNICK et al. 1989). Screening MR scanning in NF patients is revealing a greater number of anomalies of the visual pathways (PACKER et al. 1983; IMES and HOYT 1986; POMERANZ et al. 1987; LISTERNICK et al. 1989), but the significance of these asymptomatic abnormalities in the setting of a disease associated with brain hamartomas is not presently known. Longer follow-up is required to determine what percentage of these anomalies will progress.

Visual pathway gliomas in the setting of NF tend to be more extensive than those found in the absence of NF (PACKER et al. 1983). In a review of cases of VPG from the Children's Hospital of Philadelphia, approximately half of the 29 lesions in patients without NF were confined to the optic chiasm, whereas 0 of 24 were limited to the chiasm in the setting of NF.

15.4.2 Presenting Symptoms and Signs

Lesions confined to the orbit present with painless proptosis (95%), deterioration of vision (50%–85%), and interference with ocular motility (30%) (HOYT and BAGHDASSARIAN 1969; RUSH et al. 1982; HORWICH and BLOOM 1985; WONG et al. 1987; WRIGHT et al. 1989; DUTTON 1991). Findings on evaluable patients reveal optic atrophy (60%), disk edema (20%), visual field defects (46%–61%), and strabismus (30%) (DANOFF et al. 1980; HORWICH and BLOOM 1985; WONG et al. 1987; DUTTON 1991). Tumors involving the intracranial optic nerve and chiasm have bilateral visual acuity decreases, as well as field cuts in up to 90% of cases. The incidence of proptosis and extraocular muscle abnormalities drops to about 20% for chiasmal lesions (HOUSPIAN 1969; McCULLOUGH and JOHNSON 1989; HOUSEPIAN et al. 1990; DUTTON 1991). Pain, headache, papilledema, and nystagmus may also be seen (ALBRIGHT et al. 1986; COHEN and DUFFNER 1991). Extension of disease posteriorly into the hypothalamus may result in precocious puberty, endocrine disturbances, isolated growth delay, and a diencephalic syndrome of Russel (emesis, failure to thrive, and euphoria) (DANOFF et al. 1980; HORWICH and BLOOM 1985; HEIDEMAN et al. 1989; KOVALIC et al. 1990; DUTTON 1991). In infants and children less than 3 years of age, gradual visual loss is often difficult to detect. It is common for this age group to present with nystagmus, strabismus, and developmental abnormalities.

15.4.3 Pathology

HOYT and BAGHDASSARIAN (1969) postulated that optic gliomas represented benign hemartomas with limited growth potential, but this theory is currently opposed by most authors (TAVERAS et al. 1956; DANOFF et al. 1980; RUSH et al. 1982; HORWICH and BLOOM 1985; IMES and HOYT 1986; WONG et al. 1987; FLICKINGER et al. 1988; BLOOM et al. 1990; PIERCE et al. 1990; BATAINI et al. 1991). The review by Alvord and LOFTON (1988) of 623 cases in the literature showed that failure and mortality increased gradually up to 20 years after diagnosis. In a review of 171

biopsied cases in the literature by PIERCE et al. (1990), 89% were found to be low-grade astrocytomas (pilocytic or fibrillary), with a small percentage representing more anaplastic lesions (5%). In the UCSF series of 19 pediatric cases, histologic diagnosis was available in 12: seven had pilocytic astrocytomas, two had moderately anaplastic astrocytomas, two had highly anaplastic astrocytomas, and one had a subependymal giant cell astrocytoma in the setting of tuberous sclerosis (PETRONIO et al. 1991).

15.4.4 Evaluation

The differential diagnosis includes neurofibromas (usually eccentric in location), optic nerve meningiomas (which generally appear on CT or MR as diffuse tubular enlargement with residual optic nerve visible, surrounded by a thickened abnormal sheath), intraorbital rhabdomyosarcoma, orbital angioma, craniopharyngioma, and metastasis from other solid tumors such as neuroblastoma. In the majority of cases, radiologic evaluation clarifies the etiology. MR scanning and CT with contrast are excellent studies for the evaluation of VPGs, although MR scan often reveals a larger extension of tumor than is evident on CT (HAIK et al. 1987; HEIDEMAN et al. 1989; HOUSEPIAN et al. 1990; IMES and HOYT 1991; PETRONIO et al. 1991). The classic MR appearance is that of a fusiform enlargement of the optic nerve or extension of the tumor from the chiasm posteriorly along the optic tracts. On T1-weighted images, the gliomas have an isointense to slightly hypointense image compared to normal optic nerve (DUTTON 1991). On T2-weighted images, the tumor is hyperintense in relation to the nerve. Contrast enhancement with gadopentatate may also yield additional information in selected cases.

Careful neuro-ophthalmologic evaluation with close follow-up, including visual acuity checks, formal visual field testing, and color appreciation, is mandatory. After diagnosis, endocrinologic evaluation and semiannual follow-up are strongly recommended. A neuropsychiatric developmental assessment is also urged. Biopsy is not routinely recommended in this disease, as this procedure may result in further visual deterioration in up to 75% of cases (GLASER et al. 1972; HEIDEMAN et al. 1989). Biopsy is reserved for those cases in which the diagnosis is in doubt.

15.4.5 Management

The approach to patients with VPGs is highly controversial because of the fact that there is a great disparity in growth rates for these lesions (PACKER et al. 1983; ALVORD and LOFTON 1988; HEIDEMAN et al. 1989; DUTTON 1991). Some cases will show no evidence of progression for prolonged periods of time without any intervention (HOYT and BAGHDASSARIAN 1969). Others will progress rapidly, with visual deterioration and extension into the hypothalamus noted. With the advent of MR evaluation of NF patients, asymptomatic lesions of unknown growth potential are being found more commonly (POMERANZ et al. 1987; PACKER et al. 1988b; LISTERNICK et al. 1989; DUTTON 1991; IMES and HOYT 1991). In patients with incidental findings of VPG in the setting of NF, or in the case of asymptomatic lesions with minimal visual loss in a reliable and evaluable patient, close observation with frequent neuro-ophthalmologic and radiographic evaluation is the regimen of choice (PACKER et al. 1988a; HALPERIN et al. 1989).

When lesions limited to the optic nerve are associated with visual deterioration or other evidence of progression, a surgical approach is warranted (HOUSPIAN 1969; RUSH et al. 1982; WONG et al. 1987; ALVORD and LOFTON 1988; FLICKINGER et al. 1988; HALPERIN et al. 1989; HOUSEPIAN et al. 1990). Surgical management has resulted in control rates of 80%–90% when the lesion was confined to the orbit and optic nerve, and the entire nerve to the chiasm was removed (Table 15.3) (TENNY et al. 1982; ALVORD and LOFTON 1988; PIERCE et al. 1990; DUTTON 1991). Unilateral vision was obviously lost in all these patients. Of 81 patients under the age of 20, approached with complete resection in the review by ALVORD and LOFTON (1988), only 15% later failed. The surgical approach used is a frontal craniotomy with initial evaluation of the chiasm prior to unroofing the optic canal and resection of the tumor from orbit to chiasm (HOUSEPIAN et al. 1990). There is no benefit to be gained from leaving any residual optic nerve. Postoperative radiation therapy is not recommended routinely after complete resection (WONG et al. 1987; HALPERIN et al. 1989; PIERCE et al. 1990; DUTTON 1991).

Once disease has progressed to the chiasm or beyond, there is little benefit to be achieved from attempted resection, except perhaps in very young patients with large cystic lesions where debulking may relieve obstructive symptoms prior to definitive therapy (COHEN and DUFFNER 1991; DUTTON 1991). For disease that extends behind the optic nerves with evidence of visual deterioration or progression of disease, radiation therapy is the treatment of choice for all except perhaps very young children (DANOFF et al. 1980; DOSORETZ et al. 1980; FLICKINGER et al 1988; HALPERIN et al. 1989; PIERCE et al. 1990; COHEN and DUFFNER 1991). For this subgroup, chemotherapy may play an important role and will be discussed later.

Radiation therapy has been reported to provide improvement in vision in from 8% to 43% of cases (DANOFF et al. 1980; HORWICH and BLOOM 1985; WONG et al. 1987), and stabilization of disease has been reported in up to 91% of cases (TAVERAS et al. 1956; HOYT and BAGHDASSARIAN 1969; HORWICH and BLOOM 1985; WEISS et al. 1987; FLICKINGER et al. 1988; KOVALIC et al. 1990; PIERCE et al. 1990). Given the fact that there is only a relatively small chance of improvement of vision with therapy, it is essential that intervention occur before deterioration begins in earnest. Mortality rates in untreated patients with hydrocephalus (77% at 10 years), chiasmal involvement (47% at 10 years), and hypothalamic involvement (91% at 10 years) show that observation only is a poor choice in this disease once progression has been documented (ALVORD and LOFTON 1988). Radiation doses in excess of 45 Gy have resulted in long-term survival rates of 60%–100% and 10-year freedom from progression rates of 55%–88% (Table 15.4) (DANOFF et al. 1980; HORWICH et al. 1985; WONG et al. 1987; FLICKINGER et al. 1988; BLOOM et al. 1990; KOVALIC et al. 1990; PIERCE et al. 1990). Doses less than 45 Gy have been associated with a greater percentage of failures (MONTGOMERY et al. 1977;

Table 15.3. Visual pathway gliomas limited to the optic nerve: results after surgery alone

Author	No.	Follow-up (yrs)	Local failures
HOUSPIAN 1969	31	2–21	1/31
ALVORD and LOFTON 1988	89	1–20	12/89
North American Study Group for Optic Gliomas (NASGOG) 1989	44	1–19	2/44

Table 15.4. Visual pathway gliomas: progression-free survival (PFS) after radiotherapy

	No.	5-yr PFS	10 yr	15 yr
FLICKINGER et al. 1988	25	87%	87%	87%
ALVORD and LOFTON 1988	194	80%	60%	50%
PIERCE et al. 1990	24	88%	–	–
HORWICH and BLOOM 1985	29	100%	85%	–
WONG et al. 1987	24	70%	60%	38%
KOVALIC et al. 1990	33	85%	75%	75%
BATAINI et al. 1991	53	82%	82%	–

DOSORETZ et al. 1980). These reports have been small and retrospective, however, and a valid dose-response curve has not yet been established. Even with "adequate" doses of radiation, eventual progression of disease has been seen in approximately 40% of 79 pediatric patients 10 years after diagnosis, with no evidence of a plateau, in the large review by ALVORD and LOFTON (1988). It appears that radiation has the ability to stabilize disease for most patients and may lead to improvement in a small proportion. Eventually, however, a significant proportion of cases will progress beyond 10 years.

In infants and very young children, concern over the deleterious effects of radiation on developing CNS has prompted several groups to examine the use of chemotherapy to delay the need for intervention with radiation therapy. Packer reported on the use of actinomycin D and vincristine in 24 children less than 10 years of age with chiasmal or hypothalamic gliomas (ROSENSTOCK et al. 1985; PACKER et al. 1988b). At a mean follow-up of 4.3 years, all children are alive: 37.5% have progressed at a median of 3 years after initiation of chemotherapy and have gone on to receive radiation therapy, while the remaining 62.5% are progression free at a median follow-up of 3.1 years from diagnosis. MOP was used at the Joint Center for Radiation Therapy for failures after radiotherapy, with stabilization of disease noted in two of three patients treated at 2 years follow-up. A report from UCSF discusses 18 patients with a median age of 2.3 years who were treated at the time of progression of symptoms with a combination of 6-thioguanine, procarbazine, dibromodulcitol, CCNU, and vincristine (PETRONIO et al. 1991). Radiation was delayed until the time of further progression. Fifteen of the 18 patients had initial stabilization of disease, with no complete responders. Only four patients had failed at a median follow-up of 79 weeks, two during chemotherapy and two at 1 and 3 years after initiation of chemotherapy. Carboplatin, as a single agent, is currently being evaluated in a trial by the Pediatric Oncology Group (COHEN and DUFFNER 1991). Although the follow-up is short on all these studies, the results are interesting and suggest a possible alternative to immediate radiation at the time of progression in the young child.

15.4.6 Radiation Technique

Patients should be well immobilized to assure exact set-up on a daily basis. In the very young child, anesthesia or sedation may be necessary. Megavoltage machines, at least 4 MeV and preferably higher energy, should be used to spare as much tissue laterally as possible. Radiation fields for optic nerve gliomas must encompass the posterior retina to include the optic disk. If opposed lateral fields are used, care must be taken to avoid radiation of the opposite lens by divergent beams. This can be accomplished by using a beam split set-up for the anterior portion of the field. Alternatively, rotational therapy or multiple fields with CT planning or conformal therapy can be used to isolate the high-dose portion of the field as effectively as possible. Posteriorly, the field must extend to cover the entire tumor as visualized on MR scan, plus a 2-cm margin. For larger tumors, especially those with involvement of the optic tracts, occipital lobe, and hypothalamus, the fields may be quite extensive. Custom-designed blocks are necessary to limit the dose to uninvolved adjacent tissues. Daily fractions of 1.8 Gy are delivered five times a week to a total dose of 50–54 Gy. Fraction sizes greater than 2 Gy to these overall total doses have been associated with a significant incidence of visual impairment (ARISTIZABEL et al. 1977; WARA et al. 1979).

15.4.7 Complications

Acute complications of radiation therapy for VPGs include hair loss at the beam entrance and exit sites, and occasional irritation of the pinna and external auditory canal in those whose fields must necessarily extend posteriorly to encompass large tumors. Long-term complications include endocrinopathies in 20%–80% of patients (DANOFF et al. 1980; HORWICH et al. 1985; BRAUNER et al. 1990; PIERCE et al. 1990), most commonly growth hormone deficiencies. However, up to half of these patients may present with endocrine abnormalities. Cognitive deficits and learning disabilities have also been reported in a significant proportion of patients (DANOFF et al. 1980; WEISS et al. 1987; KOVALIC et al. 1990; PIERCE et al. 1990). NF is a cofactor for the development of neurologic abnormalities in many, but not all patients with NF are afflicted after therapy. Moyamoya syndrome ("puff of smoke"), the progressive occlusion or narrowing of one or both of the internal carotid arteries resulting in brief repetitive ischemic attacks, scizures, or hemorrhagic episodes, has also been reported in children treated with radiation for VPGs (OKUNO et al. 1985; BEYER et al. 1986; KOVALIC et al. 1990; PIERCE et al. 1990). The potential also exists for the development of second malignancies as a late effect of therapy, especially in the setting of NF (PACKER et al. 1988).

15.5 Choroid Plexus Tumors

Choroid plexus tumors make up 0.4%–0.6% of all intracranial tumors (BLOOM 1981a; DUFFNER and COHEN 1985–1986; ELLENBOGEN et al. 1989; BLOOM et al. 1990), 3%–4% of all pediatric intracranial tumors (COHEN and DUFFNER 1984), and 10%–20% of all intracranial tumors in the first year of life (BOYD and STEINBOK 1987; SCHIJMAN et al. 1990). There is a definite predisposition for location in the lateral ventricles in children, unlike the adult situation, where most occur in the third ventricle (ELLENBOGEN et al. 1989; JOHNSON 1989).

These tumors are composed of epithelial cells and stroma which look strikingly similar to the normal tissues of the choroid plexus (HEIDEMAN et al. 1989; BURGER and SCHEITHAUER 1990). A spectrum of cytologic features are seen, ranging from the benign characteristics of the pure papilloma to the pleomorphic invasive carcinoma with mitotic figures. Most reports break these tumors down into choroid plexus papillomas (PPCs) and choroid plexus carcinomas (CPCs) (PASCUAL et al. 1983; RORKE et al. 1985; BOYD and STEINBOK 1987; ELLENBOGEN et al. 1989; HEIDEMAN et al. 1989; BURGER et al. 1991). The differentiation between the two is occasionally somewhat difficult, however, as they represent ends of a spectrum. The differential diagnosis includes papillary ependymoma. Bilateral papillomas may be seen and are referred to as villous hypertrophy (DAVIS 1924; WELCH et al. 1983; ELLENBOGEN et al. 1989). Dissemination is uncommon in papillomas, although cells may be identified in the CSF at the time of surgery (ELLENBOGEN et al. 1989; JOHNSON 1989). In the case of CPCs, however, seeding has been reported in as many as 44% of cases (ELLENBOGEN et al. 1989; HALPERIN et al. 1989).

A common finding at presentation in the infant is macrocranium and hydrocephalus (ELLENBOGEN et al. 1989). Hydrocephalus is theorized to be a result of a combination of excessive CSF formation by the tumor combined with obstruction of the normal CSF flow (EISENBERG et al. 1974; WELCH et al. 1983; ELLENBOGEN et al. 1989; JOHNSON 1989; BURGER 1990). Intracranial hypertension is always relieved by resection of tumor due to interference with the normal pathways by debris or surgical intervention (ELLENBOGEN et al. 1989; HEIDEMAN et al. 1989).

Proper evaluation of the tumor involves the use of contrast-enhanced CT scan or MR scan (COATES et al. 1989). Angiography may occasionally be helpful in delineating the blood supply of this highly vascular tumor prior to surgery. Calcifications are frequent findings in CPPs.

Surgical resection remains the mainstay of therapy for choroid plexus tumors. In the report of 40 cases operated on at the Children's Hospital and Brigham and Women's Hospital in Boston, 96% of 26 papillomas were amenable to a complete resection (ELLENBOGEN et al. 1989). The 5-year survival rate overall in this group was 84%. In the case of incompletely resected papillomas there remains a low risk of local failure, but most such cases are amenable to re-resection. Radiation therapy is not recommended as routine treatment for benign papillomas (ELLENBOGEN et al. 1989; HALPERIN et al. 1989; HEIDEMAN et al. 1989).

Choroid plexus carcinomas, on the other hand, are more difficult to resect (ELLENBOGEN et al. 1989; JOHNSON 1989). In the Boston series, only 64% of CPCs were amenable to total resection, and the 5-year survival rate dropped to 50% (ELLENBOGEN et al. 1989). A limited series of patients have been reported who have received postoperative radiotherapy after incomplete resection of CPCs (BOHM and STRANG 1961; NASSAR and MOUNT 1968; HAWKINS et al. 1980; PALAZZI et al. 1989). These reports discuss small numbers of patients who were treated with a variety of techniques, including focal radiation and craniospinal irradiation. In cases where craniospinal irradiation was delivered, local failure remained a major problem (HALPERIN et al. 1989). In the infant presenting with a CPC, gross total resection should be attempted. In the event of an incomplete resection, consideration should be given to the use of chemotherapy in an attempt to delay the necessity of local radiation. If progressive or recurrent disease is noted, however, initiation of focal irradiation is a rational approach if there is no evidence on MR or cytologic examination of spinal dissemination. The primary site should be taken to at least 54 Gy, using 1.6 to 1.8 Gy daily fractions with a dose of 25–35 Gy to the entire neural axis if seeding has occurred. Focal areas of seeding should be taken to cord tolerance doses.

15.6 Craniopharyngiomas

Craniopharyngiomas are benign tumors of the suprasellar region composed of embryonic rests of squamous cell epithelium from an incompletely involuted hypophyseal/pharyngeal duct (Rathke's pouch) (CARMEL et al. 1982; BURGER and SCHEITHAUER 1991). These tumors make up 6%–9% of all pediatric CNS tumors (MATSON 1969; RUBINSTEIN 1972b; FARWELL et al. 1977; HEIDEMAN et al. 1989) and occur in a bimodal age distribution, with two-thirds occurring in the first two decades of life (SUNG et al. 1981; CARMEL et al. 1982; SUNG 1982). The second peak incidence is in the fifth and sixth decades of life. No predominance by sex is noted CARMEL et al. 1982; HEIDEMAN et al. 1989).

These tumors may appear as cystic, solid, or a combination thereof, with the cystic component comprising columnar or stratified squamous cell epithelium surrounding a dense viscous greenish-yellow fluid ("crankcase oil") which glitters with cholesterol crystals and cellular debris (CARMEL et al. 1982; BASKIN and WILSON 1986; HEIDEMAN et al. 1989; BURGER and SCHEITHAUER 1991). The solid component often undergoes calcification of the keratinized matrix (BURGER and SCHEITHAUER 1991). These tumors are most frequently found in the suprasellar region, but may infiltrate the sella, hypothalamus, and down along the anterior surface of the brain stem. They are frequently densely adherent to local blood vessels (CARMEL et al. 1982; BASKIN et al. 1986).

The location of the tumor is responsible for the majority of symptoms seen at presentation. Hoffman and RAFFEL (1989) described three growth patterns; small sellar tumors with no impingement of the optic chiasm or vessels, prechiasmatic tumors which tend to present with visual disorders, and postchiasmatic lesions which grow posteriorly and superiorly, filling the third ventricle and leading to obstructive hydrocephalus. Infiltration of or compression of the optic chiasm results in visual field deficits (most notably bitemporal or homonymous hemianopsia) in 50%–90% of patients (LICHTER et al. 1977; CALVO 1983; COHEN and DUFFNER 1985; BASKIN and WILSON 1986; HALPERIN et al. 1989). Visual acuity reduction is noted in 60%–70%. Less commonly, optic atrophy and papilledema may be seen (LICHTER et al. 1977; CALVO 1983; DANOFF et al. 1983; BASKIN and WILSON 1986). Infiltration of the hypothalamus and pituitary regions results in interference with the normal hormonal axis in more than 50% of patients (BASKIN and WILSON 1986). In the UCSF series of 74 patients (BASKIN and WILSON 1986), at initial diagnosis 42% were hypothyroid, 24% were hypoadrenal, and 12% had diabetes insipidus. Growth failure was the most common presenting symptom in children, seen in 26

of 28 patients under the age of 18 (CARMEL et al. 1982; BASKIN and WILSON 1986). Decreased sexual function or impotance was manifested in 88% of men older than 18, and primary or secondary amenorrhea in 18 of 22 women over the age of 18 (BASKIN and WILSON 1986). Growth of tumor into the third ventricle, with resulting obstruction of the foramen of Monro and hydrocephalus, results in severe headaches, nausea, and vomiting in more than 50% of patients (COHEN and DUFFNER 1985; FISCHER et al. 1985, 1990; BASKIN and WILSON 1986).

Preoperative evaluation of these tumors includes an ophthalmologic evaluation with formal visual field and visual acuity testing. A full neuroendocrinologic evaluation should be carried out, including tests for diabetes insipidus as well as complete checks of integrity of the hypothalamic pituitary axis, thyroid, adrenal, and gonadal function. Radiologic evaluation may include plain films which well show calcification in 50%–80% of cases and sellar enlargement in up to 80% (SUNG et al. 1981; SUNG 1982; COHEN and DUFFNER 1984; HEIDEMAN et al. 1989; HOFFMAN and RAFFEL 1989). CT and MR evaluation will delineate the solid and cystic components of disease, and when used with enhancement can highlight the relationship of tumor to nearby vessels (BASKIN and WILSON 1986). Angiography may provide helpful information for the surgeon prior to resection, although MR has reduced the need for this invasive procedure.

Controversy over treatment revolves around the extent of resection necessary. Some authors argue that as complete a resection as possible should be attempted (CARMEL et al. 1982; HOFFMAN and RAFFEL 1989), stating that with improved neurosurgical instrumentation, morbidity should be markedly reduced from earlier reports [down to a surgical mortality of 5% or less (MATSON 1969; SUNG et al. 1981; SUNG 1982; YASARGIL et al. 1990)]. No routine adjuvant therapy is offered in the face of complete resection as evidenced on neurodiagnostic imaging, reserving re-resection for recurrent disease and radiation for unresectable components of disease (HOFFMAN and RAFFEL 1989). Following this path, HOFFMAN and RAFFEL have reported excellent results using modern neurosurgical techniques in 24 totally resected children, with no significant damage to the optic chiasm or hypothalamus. Recurrence rates of 0%–50% are reported after complete resection, with 5-year survival rates of 73%–100% (LICHTER et al. 1977; SHAPIRO et al. 1979; RICHMOND et al. 1980; SUNG et al. 1981; FISCHER et al. 1985, 1990; HALPERIN et al. 1989; HOFFMAN and RAFFEL 1989;

WEISS et al. 1989). Endocrine dysfunction will occur in a large majority of patients treated, regardless of the treatment or modality used.

Other investigators contend that the danger of unacceptable chiasmatic, hypothalamic, or vascular damage makes heroic attempts at resection unwarranted (RICHMOND et al. 1980; DANOFF et al. 1983; BASKIN and WILSON 1986). Functional status of the patient must be taken into account when assessing the successfulness of a given procedure. Recurrence rates after subtotal resection range from 45% to 100% (HALPERIN et al. 1989; HOFFMAN and RAFFEL 1989), and radiation therapy is routinely recommended after anything less than a complete resection (CARMEL et al. 1982; COHEN and DUFFNER 1984; HALPERIN et al. 1989; HEIDEMAN et al. 1989; HOFFMAN and RAFFEL 1989; CARMEL 1990). Some authors argue that the use of less than radical surgery followed by radiation is as effective and less morbid than aggressive attempts at total resection. Reports on the use of radiation after surgery reveal a failure rate of 0%–28%, with 5- and 10-year survival rates of 69%–100% and 66%–86%, respectively (KRAMER et al. 1961; BLOOM and HARMER 1972; LICHTER et al. 1977; RICHMOND et al. 1980; SUNG et al. 1981; SUNG 1982; CALVO 1983; DANOFF et al. 1983; FISCHER et al. 1985, 1990; LEVINE et al. 1988; HALPERIN et al. 1989).

A rational approach to the problem is to attempt surgical resection, which may often be complete in small sellar lesions, but to limit the resection to cyst decompression and removal of easily debulked tissue in larger lesions, avoiding damage to the hypothalamus, chiasm, or cavernous sinus structures (BASKIN and WILSON 1986; HALPERIN et al. 1989; HEIDEMAN et al. 1989). If a complete resection has been accomplished, close follow-up with serial MR scans and frequent neurologic examinations may be appropriate. However, if there is residual disease, focal radiotherapy is indicated to improve the duration of local control (BASKIN and WILSON 1986; HALPERIN et al. 1989; HEIDEMAN et al. 1989).

Radiation doses of 1.8 Gy per day, administered by megavoltage machines of 4 MeV or greater, are delivered daily to a total dose of 54 Gy. Depending on the tumor size, a number of techniques can be used to deliver treatment. For small suprasellar lesions, bilateral moving coronal arc fields with reversible wedge filters are recommended (HALBERG and SHELINE 1987; HALPERIN et al. 1989). The patient is treated on a tilt board, with the chin tucked in. The fields are checked to make sure the plane of rotation is posterior to the orbits. Bilateral 110° arc rotations, with a reversible 30° wedge, are used. Care is taken to

ensure that the beams do not exit through the thyroid. This plan can accurately cover a 5 cm diameter target volume (tumor plus a 1- to 2-cm margin on MR scan), with rapid drop-off of dose to the surrounding temporal lobes. The isocenter is established taking into account the eccentricity of the tumor. For larger lesions with more extensive suprasellar, cavernous sinus, or pontine extension, multiple field plans may be devised using CT treatment planning (HALBERG and SHELINE 1987). Opposed lateral fields are only used in cases which are too massive to be adequately encompassed by one of the more refined plans, due to the fact that such an opposed plan necessarily results in a significant portion of the temporal lobes receiving the full dose of radiation and the chance of permanent alopecia in the treatment sites. During treatment, attention must be paid to the patient's symptoms, as worsening may be an indication of reaccumulation of cyst fluid, requiring drainage (HALBERG and SHELINE 1987; HALPERIN et al. 1989).

After resection and radiation, some degree of pituitary dysfunction can be expected to develop in the majority of patients (45% adrenal dysfunction, 40% hypothyroidism, 23% diabetes insipidus in the UCSF series, post-therapy) (BASKIN and WILSON 1986). Visual improvement, however, can be expected in up to 93% of symptomatic patients. Psychological and social sequelae of the tumor and therapy are indistinguishable for the most part, and may frequently be appreciated with prolonged follow-up.

15.7 Pituitary Adenomas

Tumors of the pituitary gland are exceptionally rare in childhood [0.7%–1.5% of all pediatric CNS tumors (AMADOR 1983)] and will be discussed only briefly here. For a full discussion of radiotherapeutic and surgical management, see HALBERG and SHELINE (1987). The majority of these adenomas are associated with endocrine disorders due to hypersecretion of hormones in the pediatric population: prolactin (prolactinomas – precocious puberty), growth hormone (somatotropinomas – acromegaly), adrenocorticotropic hormone (corticotropinoma – Cushing's disease), follicle-stimulating hormone and luteinizing hormone (gonadotropinoma – hypogonadism, precocious puberty), and thyroid-stimulating hormone (thyrotropinomas – hyperthyroidism). Nonsecretory chromophobe adenomas are less common in the young.

Somatotropinomas, corticotropinomas, and chromophobe adenomas may be seen as part of Werner's syndrome [multiple endocrine neoplasia type I (CHROUSOS 1989) pituitary, parathyroid, and adrenal tumors]. In the McCune-Albright syndrome of polyostotic fibrous dysplasia, café au lait spots, and endocrine dysfunction, prolactinomas and somatotropinomas may occur (CHROUSOS 1989).

The mainstay of therapy for pituitary adenomas in children, as in adults, is surgical treatment. The majority of these tumors are confined to the sella and are amenable to transsphenoidal resection (AMADOR 1983). In cases where complete resection is not possible, radiation therapy may be delivered using arc rotational therapy (45 Gy in 1.8-Gy fractions) with an excellent response rate. Alternatively, bromocriptine can be used to lower prolactin, growth hormone, or ACTH levels in functional adenomas if surgery is unsuccessful in lowering hormone production (HALBERG and SHELINE 1987).

15.8 Future Directions

Gliomas in children are the object of intense scrutiny in a wide array of studies analyzing the usefulness of chemotherapy as an adjuvant to radiation and as a means of delaying the initiation of radiation as long as possible to allow time for the sensitive nervous tissues to develop. These studies are evaluating neoadjuvant therapy with single agents such as carboplatin, etoposide, and thiotepa, combinations including MMOPP (methotrexate plus standard MOPP), and high-dose regimens of cyclophosphamide and L-PAM or etoposide and carboplatin with autologous bone marrow rescue in an attempt to improve duration of survival in patients with high-grade lesions. In subtotally resected low-grade lesions, studies in adult patients are attempting to answer the questions about appropriate dose and whether or not radiation can safely be delayed until the time of progression, information which will undoubtedly be helpful in managing children with such lesions.

References

Albright AL, Guthkelch AN, Packer RJ, Price RA, Rourke LB (1986) Prognostic factors in pediatric brain-stem gliomas. J Neurosurg 65: 751–755

Alvord ECJ, Lofton S (1988) Gliomas of the optic nerve or chiasm. Outcome by patients' age, tumor site, and treatment. Neurosurg 68: 85–98

Amador LV (1983) Brain Tumors in the Young. CC Thomas, Springfield, III

Aristizabel S, Caldwell WL, Avila L (1977) The relationship of time-dose fractionation factors to complications in the treatment of pituitary tumors by irradiation. Int J Radiat Oncol Bio Phys 2: 667–673

Backus RF, Millichap JG (1962) The seizure as a manifestation of intracranial tumors of childhood. Pediatrics 29: 978–984

Baskin DS, Wilson CB (1986) Surgical management of craniopharyngiomas. A review of 74 cases. J Neurosurg 65: 22–27

Bataini JP, Delanian S, Ponvert D (1991) Chiasmal gliomas: results of irradiation management in 57 patients and review of literature. Int J Radiat Oncol Biol Phys 21: 615–623

Beyer RA, Paden P, Sobel DF, Flynn FG (1986) Moyamoya pattern of vascular occlusion after radiotherapy for glioma of the optic chiasm. Neurology 36: 1173–1178

Bleyer W, Milstein J, Balais F et al. (1983) Eight drugs in one day chemotherapy for brain tumors. A new approach and rationale for pre-irradiation chemotherapy. Med Pediatr Oncol 11: 213.

Bloom HJG (1981a) Brain gliomas in children: treatment policy and prognosis. Front Radiat Ther Oncol 16: 90–104

Bloom HJG (1981b) Intracranial tumors: response and resistance to therapeutic endeavors, 1970–1980. Int J Radiat Oncol Biol Phys 8: 1083–1113

Bloom HJG, Harmer CL (1972) Craniopharyngiomas. Br Med J 2: 286–287

Bloom HJG, Glees J, Bell J (1990) The treatment and long-term prognosis of children with intracranial tumors: a study of 610 cases, 1950–1981. Int J Radiat Oncol Biol Phys 18: 723–745

Bohm E, Strang R (1961) Choroid plexus papillomas. J Neurosurg 18: 493–500

Boyd MC, Steinbok P (1987) Choroid plexus tumors: problems in diagnosis and management. J Neurosurg 66: 800–805

Brauner R, Malandry F, Rappaport R, Zucker JM, Kalifa C, Pierre KA, Bataini P et al. (1990) Growth and endocrine disorders in optic glioma. Eur J Pediatr 149: 825–828

Bruce DA, Schut L, Sutlon LN (1990) Supratentorial brain tumors in children. In: Youmans JR (ed) Neurological Surgery, 3rd edn. WB Saynders, Philadelphia, pp 3000–3019

Bullard DE, Rawlings CEI, Phillips B, Cox EB, Schold SC, Burger P, Halperin EC (1987) Oligodendroglioma: an analysis of the value of radiation therapy. Cancer 60: 2179–2188

Burger PC (1990) Classification and biology of brain tumors. In: Youmans JR (ed) Neurological Surgery, 3rd edn. WB Saunders, Philadelphia, pp 2967–2999

Burger PC, Fuller GN (1991) Pathology – trends and pitfalls in histologic diagnosis, immunopathology, and applications of oncogene research. Neurol Clin 9: 249–272

Burger PC, Scheithauer BW, Vogel FS (1991) Brain: tumors. In: Burger PC, Scheithauer BW, Vogel FS (eds) Surgical pathology of the nervous system and its coverings. Churchill Livingstone, New York, pp 193–438

Calvo F (1983) Radiation therapy in craniopharyngiomas. Int J Radiat Oncol Bio Phys 9: 493–496

Carmel PW (1990) Brain tumors of disordered dysembryogenesis. In: Youmans JR (ed) Neurological surgery, 3rd edn. WB Saunders, Philadelphia, pp 3223–3249

Carmel PW, Antunes JL, Chang CH (1982) Craniopharyngiomas in children. Neurosurgery 11: 382–389

Chrousos GP (1989) Endocrine tumors. In: Pizzo PA, Poplack DG (eds) Principles and practice of pediatric oncology. JB Lippincott, Philadelphia, pp 733–758

Coates TL, Hinshaw Jr DB, Peckman N, Thompson JR, Hasso AN, Holshouser BA, Knierim DS (1989) Pediatric choroid plexus neoplasms: MR, CT, and pathologic correlation. Radiology 173: 81–88

Cohadon F, Aouad N, Rougier A (1985) Histologic and nonhistologic factors correlated with survival time in supratentorial astrocytic tumors. J Neurooncol 3: 105–111

Cohen ME, Duffner PK (1984) Brain tumors in children Raven, New York

Cohen ME, Duffner PK (1985) Current therapy in childhood brain tumors. Neurol Clin North Am 3: 147–164

Cohen ME, Duffner PK (1991) Optic pathway tumors. Neurol Clin 9: 467–477

Danoff BF, Kramer S, Thompson N (1980) The radiotherapeutic management of optic nerve gliomas in children. Int J Radiat Oncol Biol Phys 6: 45–50

Danoff BF, Cowchock FS, Kramer S (1983) Childhood craniopharyngioma: survival, local control, endocrine and neurologic function following radiotherapy. Int J Radiat Oncol Biol Phys 9: 171–175

Daumas-Duport C, Scheithauer B (1988) Grading of astrocytomas: a simple and reproducible method. Cancer 62: 2152–2165

Davis LE (1924) A physiopathologic study of the choroid plexus and the report of a case of villous hypertrophy. Med Res 44: 521–534

Dohrmann GJ, Farwell JR, Flannery JT (1976) Ependymomas and ependymoblastomas in children. J Neurosurg 45: 273–283

Dohrmann GJ, Farwell JR, Flannery JT (1978) Oligodendrogliomas in children. Surg Neurol 10: 21–26

Dosoretz DE, Blitzer PH, Wang CC, Lingood RM (1980) Management of gliomas of the optic nerve and/or chiasm. Cancer 45: 1467–1471

Dropcho EJ, Wisoff JH, Walker RW, Allen JC (1987) Supratentorial malignant gliomas in childhood: a review of fifty cases. Ann Neurol 22: 355–364

Duffner PK, Cohen ME (1985–1986) Treatment of brain tumors in babies and very young infants. Pediatr Neurosci 12: 304–310

Duffner PK, Cohen ME, Thomas PRM, Lansky SB (1985) The long-term effects of cranial irradiation in the central nervous system. Cancer 56: 1841–1847

Duffner PK, Cohen ME, Myers MH, Heise HW (1986) Survival of children with brain tumors: SEER program 1973–1980. Neurology 36: 597–601

Dutton JJ (1991) Optic nerve gliomas and meningiomas. Neurol Clin 9: 163–177

Eisenberg HM, McComb JG, Lorenzo AV (1974) CSF overproduction and hydrocephalus associated with choroid plexus papillomas. J Neurosurg 40: 381–385

Ellenbogen RG, Winston KR, Kupsky WJ (1989) Tumors of the choroid plexus in children. Neurosurgery 25: 327–335

Eys VJ, Cangir A, Coody D, Smith B (1985) MOPP regimen as primary chemotherapy for brain tumors in infants. J Neurooncol 3: 237–243

Farwell J, Flannery JT (1984) Cancer in relatives of children with CNS neoplasms. N Engl J Med 311: 749–753

Farwell JR, Dohrmann GJ, Flannery JT (1977) CNS tumors in children Cancer 40: 3123–3132

Finlay JL, August C, Packer R (1990) High-dose multi-agent chemotherapy followed by bone marrow rescue for malignant astrocytomas of childhood and adolescence. J Neurooncol 9: 239–248

Fischer EG, Welch K, Belli JA, Wallman J, Shillito JJJ, Winston KR, Cassady R (1985) Treatment of craniopharyngiomas in children: 1972–1981. J Neurosurg 62: 496–501

Fischer EG, Welch K, Shillito JJ, Winston KR, Tarbell NJ (1990) Craniopharyngiomas in children. Long-term effects of conservative surgical procedures combined with radiation therapy. J Neurosurg 73: 535–540

Flickinger JC, Torres C, Deutsch M (1988) Management of low-grade gliomas of the optic nerve and chiasm. Cancer 61: 635–642

Fokes EC, Earle KM (1969) Ependymomas: clinical and pathological aspects. J Neurosurg 30: 585–594

Germano IM, Ito M, Cho KG, Hoshino T, Davis RL, Wilson CB (1989) Correlation of histopathological features and proliferative potential of gliomas. J Neurosurg 70: 701–706

Glaser JS, Hoyt WF, Carbett J (1972) Visual morbidity and chiasmatic glioma. Arch Opthalmol 85: 3–12

Gliomas NASGfO (1989) Tumor spread in unilateral optic glioma: study report #2. Neurofibromatosis, 2: 195–203

Goldwein JW, Glauser TA, Packer RJ, Finlay JL, Sutton LN, Curran WJ, Laehy JM et al. (1990a) Recurrent intracranial ependymomas in children. Survival, patterns of failure, and prognostic factors. Cancer 66: 557–563

Goldwein JW, Leahy JM, Packer RJ, Sutton LN, Curran WJ, Rorke LB, Schut L et al. (1990b) Intracranial ependymomas in children. Int J Radiat Oncol Biol Phys 19: 1497–1502

Goldwein JW, Corn BW, Finlay JL, Packer RJ, Rorke LB, Schut L (1991) Is craniospinal irradiation required to cure children with malignant (anaplastic) intracranial ependymomas? Cancer 67: 2766–2771

Haik BG, Saint LL, Bierly J, Smith ME, Abramson DA, Ellsworth RM, Wall M (1987) Magnetic resonance imaging in the evaluation of optic nerve gliomas. Ophthalmology 94: 709–717

Halberg FE, Sheline GE (1987) Radiation therapy for pituitary tumors. Endocrinol Metab Clin North Am 16: 667–684

Halperin EC, Kun LE, Constine LS, Tarbell NJ (1989) Pediatric radiation oncology. Raven, New York

Hawkins J (1980) Treatment of choroid plexus papillomas in children: a brief analysis of twenty years' experience. Neurosurgery 6: 380–384

Heideman RL, Packer RJ, Albright LA, Freeman CR, Rorke LB (1989) Tumors of the CNS. In: Pizzo PA, Poplack DV (eds) Principles and practice of pediatric oncology. JB Lippincott, Philadelphia, pp 505–553

Hirsch JF, Rose CS, Pierre-Kahn A, Pfister A (1989) Benign astrocytic and oligodendrocytic tumors of the cerebral hemispheres in children. J Neurosurg 70: 560–572

Hoffman HJ, Raffel C (1989) Craniopharyngiomas. In: McLaurin RL, Schut L, Venes JL, Epstein F (eds) Pediatric neurosurgery, 2nd edn. WB Saunders, Philadelphia, pp 399–408

Horwich A, Bloom HG (1985) Optic gliomas: radiation therapy and prognosis. Int J Radiat Oncol Biol Phys 11: 1067–1079

Hoshino T, Prados M, Wilson CB, Cho KG, Lee KS, Davis RL (1989) Prognostic implications of the bromodeoxyuridine labeling index of human gliomas. J Neurosurg 71: 335–341

Housepian EM (1969) Surgical treatment of unilateral optic nerve gliomas. J Neurosurg 31: 604–607

Housepian EM, Trokel SL, Jakobiec FA, Hilal SK (1990) Tumors of the orbit. In: Youmans JR (ed) Neurological surgery, 3rd edn. WB Saunders, Philadelphia, pp. 3371–3411

Hoyt WG, Baghdassarian SA (1969) Optic glioma of childhood. Natural history and rationale for conservative management. Br J Ophthalmol 53: 793–798

Hurst RW, Newman SA, Cail WS (1988) Multifocal intracranial MR abnormalities in neurofibromatosis. Ajnr 9: 293–296

Imes RK, Hoyt WF (1986) Childhood chiasmal gliomas: update on the fate of patients in the 1969 San Francisco study. Br J Ophthalmol 70: 179–182

Imes RK, Hoyt WF (1991) Magnetic resonance imaging signs of optic nerve gliomas in neurofibromatosis 1. Am J Ophthalmol 111: 729–734

Jenkin RDT, Boesel C, Ertel I, Evans A, Hittle R, Ortega J, Sposto R et al. (1987) Brain-stem tumors in childhood: a prospective randomized trial of irradiation with and without adjuvant CCNU, VCR, and prednisone. A report of the Children's Cancer Study Group. J Neurosurg 66: 227–233

Johnson DL (1989) Management of choroid plexus tumors in children. Pediatr Neurosci 15: 195–206

Kaiser MC, Kralendonk JH (1991) Modern imaging for cerebral gliomas: breakthroughs and limitations. In: Karim ABMF, Laws ER (eds) Glioma, Principles and practice of neuro-oncology. Springer, Berlin Heidelberg New York, pp 37–56

Kelly PJ, Daumas-Duport C, Scheithauer BW (1987) Stereotactic histologic correlations of CT and MRI defined abnormalities in patients with glial neoplasms. Mayo Clin Proc 62: 450–459

Kernohan JW, Mabon RF (1949) A simplified classification of gliomas. Proc Staff Meet Mayo Clin 24: 71–75

Kim YH, Fayos JV (1977) Intracranial ependymomas. Radiology 124: 805–808

Kovalic JJ, Grigsby PW, Shepard MJ, Fineberg BB, Thomas PR (1990) Radiation therapy for gliomas of the optic nerve and chiasm. Int J Radiat Oncol Biol Phys 18: 927–832

Kramer S, McKissock W, Concannon JD (1961) Craniopharyngiomas: treatment by combined surgery and radiation. J Neurosurgery 18: 217–226

Krouwer HG, Davis RL, Silver P, Prados M (1991) Gemistocytic astrocytomas: a reappraisal. J Neurosurg 74: 399–406

Kun LE, Kovnar EH, Sanford RA (1988) Ependymomas in children. Pediatr Neurosci 14: 57–63

Kuroiwa T, Tanabe H, Fujii S, Yamamoto H (1991) Immunohistochemical study of the C-erbB-2 gene product and epidermal: growth factor receptor in pediatric brain tumors. 4th International Symposium on Pediatric Neuro-Oncology, Tokyo, Japan

Laws ERJ, Taylor WJ, Clifton HB, Okazaki H (1984) Neurosurgical management of low-grade astrocytoma of the cerebral hemispheres. J Neurosurg 61: 665–673

Leibel SA, Sheline GE (1987) Radiation therapy for neoplasms of the brain. Neurosurgery 66: 1–22

Leibel SA, Sheline GE, Wara WM (1975) The role of radiation therapy in the treatment of astrocytomas. Cancer 35: 1551–1557

Levine RA, Wara WM, Sheline GE (1988) Radiation therapy for craniopharyngiomas. Int J Radiat Oncol Biol Phys 15 [Suppl 1]: 196

Lewis RA, Gerson LP, Axelson RA, Riccardi VM, Whitford RP (1984) Von Recklinghausen neurofibromatosis II. Incidence of optic gliomata. Ophthalmology 91: 929–935

Lichter A, Wara WM, Sheline GE (1977) The treatment of craniopharyngiomas. Int J Radiat Oncol Biol Phys 2: 675–683

Lindegaard KF, Mork SJ, Eide GE (1987) Statistical analysis of clinicopathologic features, radiation therapy and survival in 170 cases of oligodendroglioma. J Neurosurg 67: 224–230

Listernick R, Charrow J, Greenworld MJ, Esterly NB (1989) Optic gliomas in children with neurofibromatosis type 1. J Pediatr 114: 788–792

Ludwig CL, Smith MT, Godfrey AD, Armbrustmacher VW (1986) A clinicopathologic study of 323 patients with oligodendrogliomas. Ann Neurol 19: 15–21

Marks JE, Adler SJ (1982) A comparative study of ependymomas by site of origin. Int J Radiat Oncol Biol Phys 8: 37–43

Matson DD (1969) Neurosurgery of infancy and childhood. Charles C. Thomas, Springfield, Ill.

McCullough DC, Johnson DL (1989) Optic nerve gliomas and other tumors involving the optic nerve and chiasm. In: Mclaurin RL, Schut L, Venes JL, Epstein F (eds) Pediatric Neurosurgery: surgery of the developing nervous system. WB Saunders, Philadelphia, pp 391–398

Mercuri S, Russo A, Palma L (1981) Hemispheric supratentorial astrocytomas in childhood: long term results in 29 children. J Neurosurg 55: 170–173

Montgomery AB, Griffin T et al. (1977) Optic nerve glioma: the role of radiation therapy. Cancer 40: 2079–2080

Mork SJ, Loken AC (1977) Ependymoma: a follow-up study of 101 cases. Cancer 40: 907–915

Mork SJ, Lindegaard KF, Halvorsen TB, Lehmann EH (1985) Oligodendroglioma: incidence and biologic behavior in a defined population. J Neurosurg 63: 881–889

Nassar SI, Mount LA (1968) Papillomas of the choroid plexus. J Neurosurg 29: 73–77

Nelson JS, Tsukada Y (1983) Necrosis as a prognostic criteria in malignant supratentorial astrocytic gliomas. Cancer 152: 550–554

North American Study Group for Optic Gliomas (1989) Tumor spread in unilateral optic glioma: study report #2. Neurofibromatosis 2: 195–203

Okuno T, Prensky AL, Godo M (1985) The moyamoya syndrome associated with irradiation of an optic glioma in children: report of two cases and review of the literature. Pediatr Neurol 1: 311–316

Packer RJ, Savino PJ, Bilanivk LT (1983) Chiasmatic gliomas of childhood: a reappraisal of natural history and effectiveness of cranial irradiation Childs Brain 10: 393–403

Packer RJ, Seigel KR, Sutton LN, Littman P, Bruce DA, Schut L (1985) Leptomeningeal dissemination of primary central nervous system tumors of childhood. Ann Neurol 18: 217–221

Packer RJ, Bilaniuk LT, Cohen BH, Braffman BH, Obringer AC, Zimmerman RA, Siegel KR (1988a) Intracranial visual pathway gliomas in children with neurofibromatosis. Neurofibromatosis 1: 212–222

Packer RS, Sutton LN, Bilaniuk LT, Radcliffe J, Rosenstock JG, Siegel KR, Bunim GR (1988b) Treatment of chiasmatic/hypothalamic gliomas of childhood with chemotherapy: an update. Ann Neurol 23: 79–85

Palazzi M, DiMarco A, Campostrini F, Grandinetti A (1989) The role of radiation therapy in the management of choroid plexus neoplasms. Tumori 75: 463–469

Palma L, Guidetti B (1985) Cystic pilocytic astrocytomas of the cerebral hemispheres. surgical experience with 51 cases and long-term results. J Neurosurg 62: 811–815

Pascual CI, Villarejo F, Perez HA, Morales C, Pascual PSI (1983) Childhood choroid plexus neoplasms. A study of 14 cases less than 2 years old. Eur J Pediatr 140: 51–56

Petronio J, Edwards MS, Prados M, Freyberger S, Rabbitt J, Silver P, Levin VA (1991) Management of chiasmal and hypothalamic gliomas of infancy and childhood with chemotherapy. J Neurosurg 74: 701–708

Phuphanich S, Edwards MS, Levin VA, Vestnys PS, Wara WM, Davis RL, Wilson CB (1984) Supratentorial malignant gliomas of childhood. Results of treatment with radiation therapy and chemotherapy. J Neurosurg 60: 495–499

Pierce SM, Barnes PD, Loeffler JS, McGinn C, Tarbell NJ (1990) Definitive radiation therapy in the management of symptomatic patients with optic glioma. Survival and long-term effects. Cancer 65: 45–52

Pierre KA, Hirsch JF, Roux FX, Renier D, Sainte RC (1983) Intracranial ependymomas in childhood. Survival and functional results of 47 cases. Childs Brain 10: 145–156

Pomeranz SJ, Shelton JJ, Tobias J, Solia K, Altman D, Viamonte M (1987) MR of visual pathways in patients with neurofibromatosis. AJNR 8: 831–836

Prados M, Levin V (1987) Malignant supratentorial gliomas in childhood. Pediatr Neurosci 13: 144–151

Prados MD, Wara WM, Edwards MSB, Silver P (1988) BTRC Protocol 8725 – a phase II study of hyperfractionated radiotherapy for the treatment of primary brainstem tumors (78 Gy protocol). Brain Tumor Research Center, University of California, San Francisco, CA; Childrens Cancer Group, Los Angeles, CA

Read G (1984) The treatment of ependymoma of the brain or spinal canal by radiotherapy: a report of 79 cases. Clin Radiol 35: 163–166

Reedy DP, Bay JW, Hahn JF (1983) Role of radiotherapy in the treatment of oligodendrogliomas: an analysis of 57 cases. Neurosurgery. 13: 499–503

Regelson W, Bross I, Hananian J (1965) Incidence of second primary tumors in children with cancer and leukemia: a seven year survey of 150 consecutive autopsied cases. Cancer 18: 58–72

Richmond IL, Wara WM, Wilson CB (1980) Role of radiation therapy in the management of craniopharyngiomas in children. Neurosurgery 6: 513–517

Ringertz J (1950) Grading of gliomas. Acta Pathol Microbiol Scand 27: 51–54

Ron E, Modan B, Boice JD, Alfandary E (1988) Tumors of the brain and nervous system after radiotherapy in childhood. N Engl J Med 319: 1033–1039

Rorke LB, Gilles FM, Davis RL, Becker LE (1985) Revision of the World Health Organization classification of brain tumors for childhood brain tumors. Cancer 56: 1869–1886

Rosenstock JG, Packer RJ, Bilaniuk L, Bruce DA, Radcliffe JL, Savino P (1985) Chiasmatic optic glioma treated with chemotherapy. A preliminary report. J Neurosurg 63: 862–866

Ross GW, Rubinstein LJ (1989) Lack of histopatholgic correlation of malignant ependymomas with post-operative survival. J Neurosurg 70: 31–36.

Rubinstein LJ (1972) Tumors of the central nervous system. AFIP, Fascicle 6. Washington, D.C.

Rubinstein LJ (1988) Pathological features of optic nerve and chiasmatic gliomas. Neurofibromatosis 1: 152–158

Rus JA, Younge BR, Campbell RJ, MacCarty CS (1982) Optic glioma. Long-term follow-up of 85 histopathologically verified cases. Ophthalmology 89: 1213–1219

Salazar OM (1983) A better understanding of CNS seeding and a brighter outlook for postoperatively irradiated patients with ependymomas. Int J Radiat Oncol Biol Phys 9: 1231–1234

Salazar OM, Rubin P, Bassano D (1975) Improved survival of patients with intracranial ependymomas by irradiation: dose selection and field extension. Cancer 35: 1563–1573

Salazar OM, Castro VH, VanHoutte P, Rubin P, Aygun C (1983) Improved survival in cases of intracranial ependymomas after radiation therapy. Late report and recommendations. J Neurosurg 59: 652–659

Schijman E, Monges J, Raimondi AJ, Tomita T (1990) Choroid plexus papillomas of the III ventricle in childhood. Their diagnosis and surgical management. Childs Nerv Syst 6: 331–334

Shapiro K, Till K, Grfant DN (1979) Craniopharyngiomas in childhood: a rational approach to treatment. J Neurosurg 50: 617–623

Shapiro S, Mealey J (1989) Late anaplastic gliomas in children previously treated for acute lymphoblastic leukemia. Pediatr Neurosci 15: 176–180

Shaw EG, Evans RG, Scheithauer BW, Ilstryp DM, Earle JD (1987) Post-operative radiotherapy of intracranial ependymoma in pediatric and adult patients. Int J Radiat Oncol Biol Phys 13: 1457–1462

Shaw EG, Daumas-Duport C, Scheithauer BW (1989a) Radiation therapy in the management of low-grade supratentorial astrocytomas. J Neurosurg 70: 853–861

Shaw EG, Scheithauer BW, Gilbertson DT et al. (1989b) Post-operative radiotherapy of supratentorial low-grade gliomas. Int J Radiat Oncol Biol Phys 16: 663–668

Shaw EG, Scheithauer BW, O'Fallon JR (1991) Management of supratentorial low-grade gliomas. Semin Radiat Oncol 1: 23–31

Sheline GE (1975) Radiation therapy of tumors of the CNS of childhood. Cancer 35: 957–964

Sheline GE (1976) The importance of distinguishing tumor grade in malignant gliomas: treatment and prognosis. Int J Radiat Oncol Biol Phys 1: 781–786

Sheline GE, Boldrey E, Karlsberg P (1969) Therapeutic consideration in tumors affecting the CNS: oligodendrogliomas. Radiology 82: 84–89

Smith MT, Ludwig CL, Godfrey AD (1983) Grading of oligodendrogliomas of the brain. Cancer 52: 2017–2114

Spitzer DE, Goodrich JT (1988) Optic gliomas and neurofibromatosis: neurosurgical management. Neurofibromatosis 1: 223–232

Sposto R, Ertel IJ, Jenkin RDT, Boesel CP, Venes JL, Ortega JA, Evans AE et al. (1989) The effectiveness of chemotherapy for treatment of high grade astrocytoma in children: results of a randomized trial. A report from the Childrens Cancer Study Group. J Neurooncology 7: 165–177

Stern J, Digiacinto GV, Housepian EM (1979) Neurofibromatosis and optic glioma: clinical and morphological correlations. Neurosurgery 4: 524–528

Sun ZM, Genka S, Shitara N, Akanuma A (1988) Factors possibly influencing the prognosis of oligodendroglioma. Neurosurgery 22: 886–891

Sung DI (1982) Suprasellar tumors in children: a review of clinical manifestations and managements. Cancer 50: 1420–1425

Sung DL, Chang CH, Harisiadis L, Carnel PW (1981) Treatment results of craniopharyngiomas. Cancer 47: 847–852

Sutton LN, Packer RJ, Rorke LB (1983) Cerebral gangliogliomas during childhood. Neurosurgery 13: 129

Taveras JM, Mount LA, Wood EH (1956) Value of radiation therapy in the management of glioma of the optic nerves and chiasm. Radiology 66: 518–528

Tenny RT, Laws ERJ, Younge BR, Rush JA (1982) The neurosurgical management of optic glioma. Results in 104 patients. J Neurosurg 57: 452–458

Walker ML, Fried A, Pattisapu J (1989) Tumors of the cerebral hemispheres in children. In: McLaurin RL, Schut L, Venes JL, Epstein F (eds) Pediatric neurosurgery: surgery of the developing nervous system. WB Saunders, Philadelphia, pp 372–382

Wallner KE, Wara WM, Sheline GE, Davis RL (1986) Intracranial ependymomas: results of treatment with partial or whole brain irradiation without spinal irradiation. Int J Radiat Oncol Biol Phys 12: 1937–1941

Wallner KE, Gonzales M, Sheline GE (1988) Treatment of oligodendrogliomas with or without post-operative irradiation. J Neurosurg 68: 684–688

Wara WM, Irvine AR, Neger RE, Howes EL, Phillips TL (1990) Radiation retinopathy. Int J Radiat Oncol Biol Phys 5: 81–83

Wasson JC, Saylors RL III, Zeltzer P, Friedman HS, Bigner SH, Burger PC, Bigner DD (1990) Oncogene amplification in pediatric brain tumors. Cancer Res 50: 2987–2990

Weiss L, Sagerman RH, King GA, Chung CT, Dubowy RL et al. (1987) Controversy in the management of optic nerve glioma. Cancer 59: 1000–1004

Weiss M, Sutton L, Marcial V, Fowble B, Packer R, Zimmerman R, Schut L et al. (1989) The role of radiation therapy in the management of childhood craniopharyngioma. Int J Radiat Oncol Biol Phys, 17: 1313–1321

Welch K, Strand R, Bresnan Mea (1983) Cogenital hydrocephalus due to villous hypertrophy of the telencephalic choroid plexuses. Journal of Neurosurgery, 59: 172–175

West CR, Bruce DA, Duffner PK (1985) Ependymomas: factors in clinical and diagnostic staging. Cancer, 56: 1812–1816

Wong JY, Uhl V, Wara WM, Sheline GE (1987) Optic gliomas: A reanalysis of the University of California, San Francisco experience. Cancer 60: 1847–1855

Woo SY, Donaldson SS, Cox RS (1988) Astrocytomas in children: 14 years experience at Stanford UMC. Journal of Clinical Oncology, 6: 1001–1007

Wright JE, McNab AA, McDonald WI (1989) Optic nerve glioma and the management of optic nerve tumors in the young. Br J Ophthalmol, 73: 967–974

Yasargil MG, Curcic M, Kis M, Siegenthaler G, Teddy PJ, Roth P (1990) Total removal of craniopharyngiomas. Approaches and long-term results in 144 patients. J Neurosurg, 73: 3–11

Zulch KL (1979) Histologic subtyping of tumors of the central nervous system. International Histologic Classification of Tumers. World Health Organization, Geneva (No. 21)

16 Tumors of the Spinal Cord in Children

PATRICK S. SWIFT

CONTENTS

16.1   Epidemiology 239
16.2   Pathology......................... 240
16.3   Clinical Presentation................. 241
16.4   Evaluation......................... 241
16.5   Intramedullary Tumors.............. 242
16.5.1 Astrocytomas 242
16.5.2 Ependymomas.................... 244
16.5.3 Vascular Lesions.................. 244
16.5.4 Lipomas 245
16.6   Intradural Extramedullary Tumors........ 245
16.6.1 Nerve Sheath Tumors 245
16.6.2 Epidermoids, Teratomas............. 245
16.6.3 Meningiomas..................... 245
16.6.4 Metastatic Deposits 245
16.7   Extradural Tumors.................. 246
16.8   Complications of Therapy............. 246
16.8.1 Bone Growth.................... 246
16.8.2 Spinal Cord Injury 247
16.9   Future Directions.................. 248
      References....................... 248

16.1 Epidemiology

Involvement of the pediatric spine by malignant or benign tumors is thankfully an uncommon finding. When present, however, the consequences of both the tumor and the treatment chosen to eradicate it can be devastating to the normal course of development of the growing spinal column and paraspinous musculature of the infant or child.

Between 4% and 6% of all pediatric CNS tumors are located in the spinal cord (HALPERIN et al. 1989; HEIDEMAN et al. 1989). When compared to the adult, the ratio of spinal to intracranial tumors in children is much lower, ranging from 1:5.5 to 1:20 (ANDERSON and CARSON 1953; DILORENZO et al. 1982; RAFFEL and EDWARDS 1990). Primary tumors of the spine are divided into extradural, intradural extramedullary, and intramedullary locations (Figs. 16.1–16.3). In a

major view of the literature carried out by DILORENZO, 1234 published cases of pediatric spinal tumors were analyzed. Of all cases, tumor location was extradural in 43%, intradural extramedullary in 24.4%, intramedullary in 31.4%, and transdural in 1% (HAMBY 1935, 1944; DILORENZO et al. 1982).

There appears to be no predilection for a specific spinal segment when these tumors are considered as a group. However, when considering different histological subtypes, certain preferences are noted (DILORENZO et al. 1982). Astrocytomas favor the cervicothoracic spine (79%) and are rarely found in the lumbosacral region (1.4%), whereas ependymomas are uncommon in the cervical region (6%) and frequent in the conus and cauda regions (68%) (DESOUSA et al. 1979; DILORENZO et al. 1982; RIMER and ONOFRIO 1985). Neuroblastomas occur in the thoracolumbar segments in 70%–88% of cases (TRAGGIS et al. 1977; DILORENZO et al. 1982). Dermoids are extremely uncommon in the cervicothoracic segments whereas teratomas are evenly distributed throughout the cord (DESOUSA et al. 1979, DILORENZO et al. 1982; LUNARDI et al. 1989).

There is an increased incidence of primary spinal tumors in the first year of life (12% of all such tumors) (DILORENZO et al. 1982), but no significant

PATRICK S. SWIFT, M.D., Assistant Professor, Department of Radiation Oncology, University of California San Francisco, Long Hospital, Room L-75, Parnassus Avenue, San Francisco, CA 94143-0226, USA

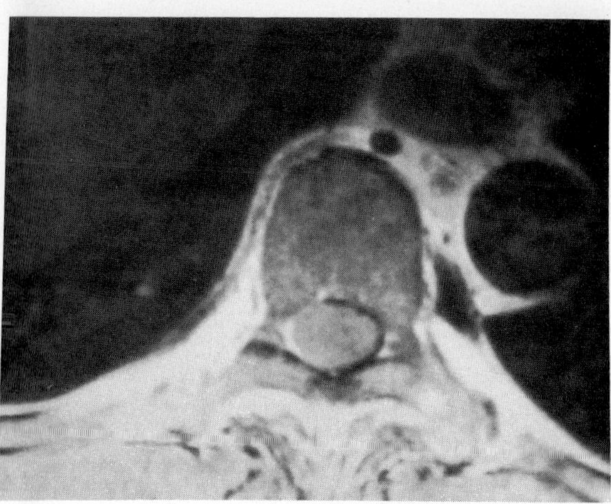

Fig. 16.1. Intramedullary location – astrocytoma

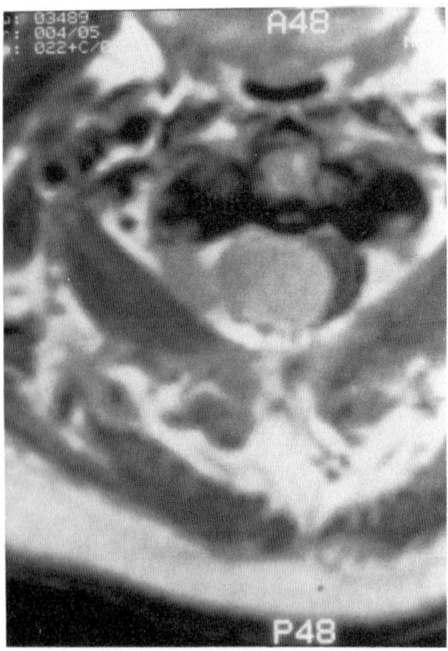

Fig. 16.2. Intramedullary intradural location – cervical meningioma

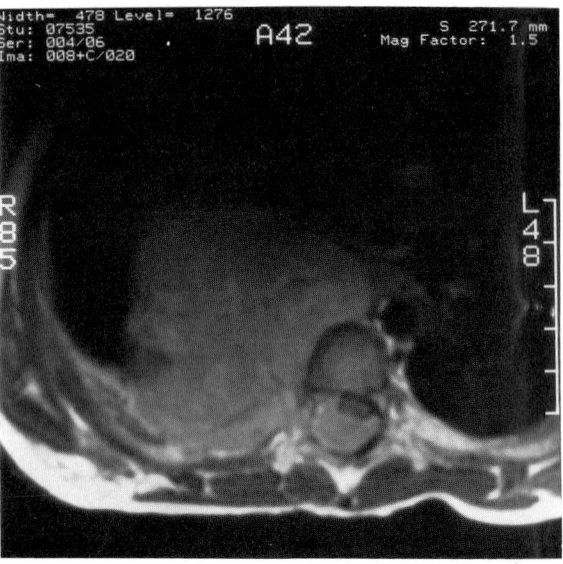

Fig. 16.3. Epidural location – neuroblastoma

predilection for any other childhood age is seen in the overall group. Certain histologic subtypes, however, do vary with age of the child. For instance, 42% of neuroblastomas and 37% of lipomas with spinal involvement will occur in the first year of lie, 46% of dermoids will be found in the first 3 years, and 84% of all teratomas occur under the age of 5 years. No significant sexual predominance has been noted either in the group as a whole or for any specific histologic subtype in most series (HAMBY 1935, 1944; DiLORENZO et al. 1982), but some series suggest a slight predominance in males (RAFFEL et al. 1990).

16.2 Pathology

Breakdown of spinal tumors by pathology is given in Table 16.1. Gliomas, comprising astrocytomas and ependymomas, are the most common tumors in the pediatric population (30%) (DeSOUSA et al. 1979; DiLORENZO et al. 1982; RAFFEL and EDWARDS 1990). The ratio of intracranial to intraspinal occurrence is 10:1 for pediatric astrocytomas and from 3:1 to 20:1 for ependymomas in various series (REIMER and ONOFRIO 1985). Sarcomas, including a variety of cell types such as Ewing's sarcoma, fibrosarcoma, osteogenic sarcoma, and rhabdomyosarcoma, as well as nonclassified sarcomas from the older literature, constitute the next largest group at 19%, followed by embryonal neoplasms (dermoids, epidermoids, and terotomas) at 14% and neuroblastomas at 13%. Neuromas and neurofibromas account for 10.6% of spinal tumors. Various other lesions, including meningiomas, hemangioblastomas, and lipomas, are rare entities.

A variety of congenital malformations coexist with spinal tumors in children. Intramedullary glioblastoma is frequently associated with cord cavitation such as intratumoral necrosis, vascular necrobiosis, syringomyelia, and hydromyelia (DiLORENZO et al. 1982). Glioblastoma may also be seen in association with diastematomyelia [the spinal cord is cleft into two longitudinal portions for a variable length by a bony spur or fibrocartilage, often associated with a lipoma (BRADFORD and HENSINGER 1985)] and spina bifida (EPSTEIN and WISOFF 1989). Teratomas can be associated with a number of malformations including spina bifida, dermal sinus, hypertrichosis, atresia ani, and diplomyelia (DiLORENZO et al. 1982,1986; DiROCCO et al. 1989). Lipomas are relatively commonly found in patients with rachischisis (communication of the neural groove with the exterior) (DiROCCO et al. 1989) and have been associated with other abnormalities, including hydrocephalus, dermal sinus, cutaneous angioma, and subcutaneous

Table 16.1. Pathology of spinal tumors (DiLORENZO et al. 1982; RAFFEL and EDWARDS 1990)

Tumor	%
Astrocytoma	19–34
Neuroblastoma	11–15
Sarcoma	11–18
Nerve sheath tumor	4–11
Ependymoma	8–9
Epidermoid/dermoid	8–14
Meningioma	4–5
Lipoma	1–2

lipoma (DiLorenzo et al. 1982). In the setting of neurofibromatosis, multiple discrete spinal fibromas can be found (Halliday et al. 1991).

16.3 Clinical Presentation

Tumors of the spinal cord manifest themselves by the local destructive action of their growth on adjacent spinal cord, nerve roots, and vertebral bodies. Interference with the longitudinally running nerve tracts results in interruption in or impairment of the functions below the level of the lesion. In most patients, the appearance of symptoms antedates the diagnosis by months to years (DeSousa et al. 1979; Hahn and McLone 1984). The most common initial symptoms of spinal cord tumors in children are weakness (50%–85%: Epstein and Wisoff 1989; Heideman et al. 1989; Raffel and Edwards 1990) and back pain (36%–78%: DeSousa et al. 1979; Hahn and McLone 1984). The weakness can be either spastic (upper motor neuron lesions) or flaccid (conus or cauda equina lesions) (Raffel and Edwards 1990). Gait disturbances are a common finding in the child and adolescent (40%–57%). The pain experienced by the patients may be either back or extremity pain, and may be worse at night due to venous congestion in the supine position or may increase with coughing, the Valsalva maneuver, or sneezing (DiRocco et al. 1989; Epstein and Wisoff 1989). Other symptoms include incontinence (10%–27%), sensory disturbances (5%–10%), hydrocephalus (4%–14%), and spinal curvature (2%–25%). Lesions located in the cervical cord may result in torticollis and monoparesis in one upper extremity, while thoracic lesions may result in mild scoliosis and lower extremity weakness.

The young age of the infant may mask the development of symptoms; for instance, weakness in an infant may only be manifested as an asymmetric kick or preferential use of one arm, or regression of previous developmental milestones (such as rolling over or loss of previously acquired toilet training). Pain may be expressed only as increased irritability. Signs of spinal cord involvement are not always easy to elicit in infants due to lack of cooperation, but weakness and changes in reflex are most commonly seen. Deep tendon reflex examination can be carried out without the full cooperation of the infant (Raffel and Edwards 1990). Sensory abnormalities exist in 30%–54% of cases, and a sensory level is accurately assessed by observing the level of sweat in young children by close inspection or by painting with phe-

nolphthalein (Raffel and Edwards 1990). Scoliosis and spinal rigidity, the presence of a paraspinous mass, torticollis, and muscular atrophy are additional important signs.

16.4 Evaluation

The complete physical examination must include a careful skin evaluation looking for evidence of phakomatoses and developmental defects (café au lait spots, skin dimples), palpation of the nodal regions, fundoscopic examination, skeletal examination for deformities or masses, abdominal examination for associated abdominal masses, genital examination, and full neurologic assessment.

Laboratory examinations, including complete blood count, differential count, platelet count, and renal and hepatic function tests, may help in the evaluation of systemic disease but are often unrevealing in respect to the primary spinal tumor. Serum markers such as ferritin, α-fetoprotein, and β-HCG may be useful in follow-up. In cases where neuroblastoma is suspected, urine should be sent for analysis for homovanillic acid and vanillylmandelic acid.

Plain films of the spine will be abnormal in more than 50% of pediatric spinal tumors (Banna and Gryspeerdt 1971; Naidich et al. 1985). Pathological findings include (DiRocco et al. 1989): (1) destructive vertebral lesions; (2) enlargement of the spinal canal with increased interpedunculate distance; (3) paraspinous soft tissue masses, most easily detected in the thoracic region due to air in the lungs; (4) calcifications; (5) dysraphism; and (6) postural abnormalities. In cases of Langerhans cell hystiocytosis, a skeletal survey should also be performed.

In the infant up to 6 months of age due to the lack of posterior fusion, ultrasonography is useful in the evaluation of spinal malformations. It is also routinely used during neurosurgical spinal procedures as a guide to the removal of intramedullary tumors. Ultrasonography is excellent for differentiating solid nodules from the cystic areas that often accompany intramedullary gliomas (Raghavendra et al. 1984; Raffel and Edwards 1990).

Overall, the most reliable method of evaluation of the spinal cord is magnetic resonance imaging (MRI), which is rapidly replacing CT-myelography as the study of choice (Heideman et al. 1989; Enzmann et al. 1990; Raffel and Edwards 1990). In addition to the obvious benefits of multiplane imaging provided by MRI and the fact that it is less invasive than CT-myelography, the ability to vary the mode of imaging by altering the parameters of repetition time (TR) and echo time (TE) allows for superior soft-tissue contrast and resolution. Different parameters are used for detection of abnormalities in the various compartments of the spinal column (SZE 1991). Vertebral body lesions are well delineated by using short TR spin-echo sequences which reveals the tumors as low-intensity signals against the high signal intensity of the normal marrow. These scans should be performed first without the use of gadopentatate dimeglumine (gadolinium-DTPA), as the tumors may enhance and become isointense with the marrow. In the young child or patient with the anemia of chronic disease, however, the absence of a great deal of fat may cause marrow to be of low signal intensity, necessitating long TR spin-echo sequences for better delineation of tumors (SZE 1991). Epidural tumors with dural impingement are well visualised using a short TR spin-echo approach with enhancement (SZE et al. 1988). In the intradural extramedullary space, CSF has a low signal intensity on T1-weighted images, and a high intensity on T2-weighted images, so compact tumors such as meningiomas and neurofibromas stand out with opposite intensity. Leptomeningeal tumors, such as diffuse drop metastases in this space, may be difficult to visualize, since the high CSF protein content often present and the high water content of these delicate metastases may diminish the difference between the signal intensities. The use of gadolinium in this case will usually show a dramatic change. Therefore short TR scans before and after gadolinium are routinely recommended. In the intramedullary space, short TR sequences deliver excellent characterization of morphologic detail, including the presence of cysts. Gadolinium helps further to highlight focal lesions, and unlike in the brain, where only 50%–60% of gliomas will enhance, the large majority of cord gliomas do enhance (DILLION et al. 1989).

Difficulties do exist with MRI – the high cost of machinery with limited availability in some areas and the need for heavy sedation of the young child to assure immobility for the duration of the scan (30–60 min) (DIROCCO et al. 1989). As mentioned previously, MRI may miss subtle diffuse lesions in which the intradural extramedullary space. Under circumstances in which the degree of suspicion is high and MRI is negative, equivocal, or fails to adequately demonstrate the extent of leptomeningeal disease, CT-myelography with metrizamide enhancement may help clarify the extent of disease (RAFFEL and EDWARDS 1990). Angiography may also be indicated in cases where a high degree of vascularity is suspected prior to surgery, such as an arteriovenous malformation (DIROCCO et al. 1989).

Technetium 99m bone scans are indicated in the evaluation of patients with diffuse bony metastatic disease from a systemic malignancy (DIROCCO et al. 1989). The use of radiolabeled meta-iodobenzyl-guanidine (MIBG), which is structurally similar to norepinephrine and guanethidine and is taken up avidly by chromaffin cells, has shown a high degree of sensitivity for the localization of neuroblastoma. The MIBG scan is superior to a technetium bone scan in the evaluation of metastatic neuroblastoma (JACOBS et al. 1990).

Cerebrospinal fluid evaluation is often performed as part of the routine initial staging and follow-up evaluations of patients with leukemia, lymphoma, medulloblastoma, neuroblastoma, primitive neuroectodermal tumor, and pineal tumors. The CSF examination will show an elevated protein content in 83% of cases, and xanthochromia in 52% (RAFFEL and EDWARDS 1990; EDWARDS et al. 1985). A positive cytology may be the only evidence of spinal involvement in medulloblastoma or leukemia, and necessitate an alternate treatment approach. Tumor markers such as α-fetoprotein and β-HCG for germ cell neoplasms and the polyamines putrescine and spermine for medulloblastoma aid in patient follow-up (ORTEGA and SIEGEL 1989).

16.5 Intramedullary Tumors

16.5.1 Astrocytomas

Surgical resection is the mainstay of treatment for the majority of these tumors. In the past, the ability of the surgeon to perform a complete resection was questioned. These tumors invade local tissue with no clean plane of cleavage, and there was concern over the risk of increasing the already-present neurological deficit (GREENWOOD 1963; GUIDETTI et al. 1981). Given the fact that the majority of these lesions were low grade and the picture was one of a gradually progressive disease (EPSTEIN 1986), there was hesitancy on the part of the surgeon to attempt a complete resection. Prior to the last decade, surgical therapy for intramedullary astrocytomas yielded unsatisfactory results. In a series of 129 intramedullary gliomas approached surgically, only 2 of 53 were able to be completely resected. The remaining 51 underwent subtotal resection or decompression and biopsy. Twenty-two of the 53 received postoperative radiotherapy (techniques and doses not described).

Progression of disease was noted within 3–5 years in more than half of these patients (Guidetti et al. 1981). In a separate series of 32 spinal astrocytomas in children, only two were amenable to a radical resection. All but one of the patients were treated with postoperative radiation (average dose 41 Gy), with 5- and 10-year survival rates of 80% and 55% in those with low-grade tumors (Reimer and Onofrio 1985).

With improvements of neurosurgical instrumentation through the 1980s, the morbidity of the radical surgical approach has decreased dramatically as the ability to completely resect some lesions has increased. In an excellent article by Epstein (1986) which discusses the results of 120 consecutive radical resections in low-grade astrocytomas of the cord, these innovations are described in detail. Sixty percent of these tumors were classified as "holocord" astrocytomas, with spinal widening extending along the entire length of the cord from the cervicomedullary junction to the conus. This widening is due to a combination of solid tumor and extensive non-neoplastic cystic cavities. A limited laminectomy is performed over the solid portion of the tumor. There is no need to resect the cystic non neoplastic portions as draining is sufficient. Transdural ultrasound is used intraoperatively to locate the true extent of tumor and achieve adequate exposure by extending the laminectomy as far as needed before placing the myelotomy (Epstein et al. 1991). The CO_2 laser is then used at low wattage to place the myelotomy over the appropriate level of the cord. Using the Cavitron ultrasonic surgical aspirator (CUSA, Cavitron Lasersonics, Division of Cavitron Corp., Stamford, CT) and the operating microscope, the tumor is then removed from the inside out, with no attempt made to locate a clear surgical cleavage plane between normal cord and tumor. The cavitron tip vibrates and causes tissue fragmentation within 1mm of the tip, irrigates the area, and provide suction for removal of tumor fragments. Intraoperative real-time sensory-evoked potential monitoring is carried out continuously throughout the procedure. Using these techniques, only 5% of patients suffered an increase in their neurological deficit, and a 75% disease-free survival was noted at 3 years in patients who received no post-operative radiation (Epstein et al. 1989).

The role of postoperative radiation is controversial for children with low-grade spinal astrocytomas. It is generally agreed that no further therapy is warranted after a gross total resection until time of recurrence (Wood et al. 1954; Reimer and Onofrio 1985; Halperin et al. 1989; Raffel and Edwards 1990;

Wara and Sheline 1990). In the case of incompletely resected lesions or those which underwent biopsy only, radiation has been advocated to retard tumor regrowth and possibly produce cure (Wood et al. 1954; Schwade et al. 1978; Kopelson et al. 1980; Garcia 1985; Halperin et al. 1989; Linstadt et al. 1989; Chun et al. 1990). The value of this approach has not been conclusively proven (Epstein 1986). The numbers in the reported series are small. In a group compiled from three series of a total of 35 patients with low-grade astrocytomas treated with similar doses of local radiation (45–50 Gy) after subtotal resection, the 5-year survival ranged from 60% to 91%, with a local failure rate of 13/35 (37%) (Linstadt et al. 1989). Reimer and Onofrio reported an 80% 5-year survival for children after subtotal resection and postoperative radiation, but failed to comment on the local status of disease at the end of follow-up (Reimer and Onofrio 1985). Radiation treatment after subtotal resection is justified in the pediatric situation to delay and possibly prevent recurrence with its devastating consequences (Halperin et al. 1989; Raffel and Edwards 1990; Wara and Sheline 1990). The radiation field should be designed to cover the tumor identified on the MR scan with a margin of two vertebral bodies above and below the tumor. No attempts should be made to cover the entire cystic cavity which may be associated with the tumor. Doses of 45–50 Gy at 1.8 Gy per day are within the tolerance of the cord. It remains to be shown in a trial setting whether or not hyperfractionated radiation, 1–1.1 Gy b.i.d. to a total dose of 54 Gy or possibly higher, remains within the tolerance of the spinal cord and whether this modest increase in dose would improve local control rates.

In infants and children less than 2–3 years of age with central nervous system tumors, there is great concern over the long-term damage which could result from radiation therapy delivered to very young nervous tissue. An alternative approach after initial resection is close and frequent observation, delaying the use of radiation until there is evidence of regrowth or progression. A second surgical intervention may be justified at the time of progression. This approach allows further time for development of the cord and spine prior to the insult of radiation. Chemotherapy has also been proposed as a means of delaying or replacing the need for neuraxis radiation (Bleyer 1991). Although chemotherapy (BCNU, PCV) has been shown to have some value in the treatment of intracranial astrocytomas in children (Finlay et al. 1991), its role in the therapy of spinal astrocytomas has yet to be proven.

Anaplastic astrocytomas or glioblastoma multiforme account for only 11% of pediatric spinal astrocytomas (HEIDEMAN et al. 1989). Complete surgical resection is rarely possible due to the diffusely infiltrative nature of the lesion. In 19 patients who were treated with attempts at gross total resections, median survival was a mere 6 months, with only two survivors beyond 1 year, one with a Brown-Séquard syndrome, the other paraplegic (COHEN et al. 1989). No patient improved neurologically following surgery. Eleven of the 19 developed hydrocephalus, and 58% developed disseminated disease. Radical resection is not recommended in these rare lesions. Surgery is utilized instead to obtain tissue for diagnosis, to evacuate the cysts, and to allow cord decompression prior to radiation (HALPERIN et al. 1989). The results of radiation in malignant astrocytomas are disappointing, with a local failure rate of 100% at current doses of 45–54 Gy with standard fractionation (LINSTADT et al. 1989). Some authors recommend craniospinal axis irradiation given the high risk of neuraxis dissemination (EPSTEIN and WISOFF 1989), but most authors recommend only focal radiation for these lesions to provide temporary palliation of symptoms and slow local disease progression (SCHWADE et al. 1978; KOPELSON et al. 1980; GARCIA 1985). Given the poor overall prognosis of these patients, focal palliative radiation to 50 Gy is justified. Craniospinal radiation should be reserved for those cases with documented evidence of multifocal disease.

16.5.2 Ependymomas

Due to the growth pattern of ependymoma which displaces rather than infiltrates normal tissue (RAFFEL and EDWARDS 1990), complete surgical resection is more often accomplished than in astrocytomas (FISCHER and MANSUY 1980; RAFFEL and EDWARDS 1990). This is particularly true in ependymomas of the cauda equina region, where complete excision was accomplished in 43%–80% of cases (GARCIA 1985). In a report on the management of 58 patients with spinal ependymomas of all ages from the Royal Marsden, WHITAKER et al. (1991) found that 66% involved the conus or cauda equina and 25% of these were completely resectable. In the review of 377 cases of spinal ependymoma in the literature, complete surgical resection produced 5- and 10-year survival rates of 86%–100% and 74%–92% respectively, suggesting little benefit to be derived from postoperative radiation after complete surgical resection.

Due to the fact that most patients who undergo less than a gross total excision are treated with postoperative radiation, little can be said about the time to recurrence after subtotal resection alone. In studies of postoperative radiation for focal spinal ependymomas after subtotal resection or biopsy, 5- and 10-year survival rates of 60%–100% have been reported (LINSTADT et al. 1989; WHITAKER et al. 1991). An overall progression-free survival at 10 years of 58%–59% was reported in two large series in which doses of 45–54 Gy were administered to focal fields (LINSTADT et al. 1989; WHITAKER et al. 1991). Grade of the tumor and extent of surgery were found to be important prognosticators. Of patients who failed local radiation, 75% of relapses occurred at the primary site of disease. Intracranial relapse occurs in only 6% of cases, suggesting that little benefit would be derived from craniospinal irradiation over local radiation alone. The addition of postoperative radiation was associated with an improvement in symptoms in a significant percentage of patients. Doses in excess of 40 Gy were associated with a higher local control rate than doses less than 40 Gy (GARCIA 1985). Local radiation to the lesion as seen on preoperative MRI and a margin of two vertebral bodies to a dose of 45 Gy in 5 weeks is standard treatment for incompletely resected ependymomas (HALPERIN et al. 1989). In children under the age of 2–3, this approach must be weighed against the potential for severe structural deformity as a result of interference with normal bone growth. In this situation, as for astrocytomas, close observation with routine neurologic examinations and frequent MR scans may allow delay in institution of radiation therapy until further developmental time has elapsed. In the case of malignant ependymoma of the spinal cord or those cases with positive CSF cytology, the decision whether or not to deliver craniospinal radiation must be addressed. The entire craniospinal axis is taken to 36 Gy at doses of 1.5–2 Gy per day, with the original tumor volume boosted to 50 Gy (HALPERIN et al. 1989).

16.5.3 Vascular Lesions

Rarely, arteriovenous malformations and hemangioblastomas (seen in association with von Hippel-Lindau syndrome) can involve the pediatric spine. Only 15% of 85 hemangioblastomas of the spine reported in the literature were found in children under the age of 18 (BROWNE et al. 1976). Surgical extirpation is the treatment of choice. Low-dose radiation has been described in single cases of spinal hemangioblastomas in the literature with no clear documentation of efficacy (HELLE et al. 1980; NEUMANN et al. 1989); however, radiation has proven to be effective in cerebellar lesions treated at doses of 45–50 Gy (SUNG et al. 1982). Postoperative radiation for incompletely resected spinal hemangioblastomas to a dose of 45–50 Gy is warranted in the older child. The role of radiation in the treatment of arteriovenous malformations of the spine not responsive to embolization is unknown (KORNBLITH et al. 1987).

16.5.4 Lipomas

This group of tumors is associated with congenital developmental defects in 33%–90% of cases reported in the literature. Lipomas fall into two general categories depending on whether or not there is communication between the subdural space and subcutaneous tissues (KLEIN 1989; LUNARDI et al. 1990). They are most commonly located in the thoracic region, but can be found in the sacral region as well. The therapeutic approach is to remove enough tissue to allow decompression of the cord. No attempt should be made to perform a complete excision (EPSTEIN and WISOFF 1989). No postoperative therapy is necessary.

16.6 Intradural Extramedullary Tumors

16.6.1 Nerve Sheath Tumors

These benign tumors, referred to in the literature as neurinomas, neurofibromas, neurilemmomas, and schwannomas, are slightly more common than meningiomas and are also seen in conjunction with neurofibromatosis. As in childhood meningiomas, there is a predilection for males and a uniform distribution of tumors throughout the spine. Forty-eight percent will be extradural or have an extradural component (FORTUNA et al. 1981). Surgical resection is adequate therapy, although malignant degeneration has been reported in a small number of these tumors (KLEIN 1989) Neurofibromatosis type 1 (peripheral neurofibromatosis – NF) is an autosomal dominant disorder associated with a gene near the centromere of the long arm of chromosome 17 (HALLIDAY et al. 1991). It is characterized by café au lait spots, neurofibromas, and iris hamartomas. Spinal nerve sheath tumors in this setting are uniformly neurofi-

bromas. In NF type 2, with its locus on the long arm of chromosome 22, multiple intracranial and spinal tumors including bilateral acoustic neurinomas and spinal schwannomas, are found.

16.6.2 Epidermoids, Teratomas

These congenital tumors are due to implantation of ectodermal rests during the period of closure of the neural tube during early embryonic development. Although they constitute only 1% of all spinal tumors, they make up 17% of all spinal tumors seen in the first year of life (LUNARDI et al. 1989). These tumors may be seen in conjunction with spina bifida, dermal sinus tracts, myelomeningocele, diastematomyelia, hemivertebra, and syringomyelia. Sacral teratomas may present as large masses in the newborn. The recurrence rate after surgical resection alone is less than 10% (LUNARDI et al. 1989). No adjuvant therapy is warranted.

16.6.3 Meningiomas

Meningiomas are rare benign tumors that account for only 2% of intraspinal lesions in children. Unlike the picture in adults, where the great majority are found in women and there is a predilection for the thoracic spine, these rare tumors in children occur more commonly in males and are uniformly distributed through the spine (FORTUNA et al. 1981). They may be found in the setting of neurofibromatosis. Results following surgical extirpation alone have been excellent, with 150/156 cases undergoing gross total resection and a local recurrence rate of only 7% at 5-year minimum follow-up (KLEIN 1989; SOLERO et al. 1989).

16.6.4 Metastatic Deposits

Drop matastases from intracranial malignancies are seen in patients with medulloblastoma, pineoblastoma, pineal germ cell tumors, ependymomas, primitive neuroectodermal tumors, retinoblastoma, cranial astrocytomas, glioblastoma multiforme, and choroid plexus carcinomas (KLEIN 1989). The finding of metastatic deposits in the asymptomatic spine dramatically alters the therapeutic approach for these children. Surgery is indicated only if the tissue diagnosis is in doubt or if there is rapid deterioration in the setting of disease unlikely to respond to chemotherapy or radiation therapy. The role and technique of craniospinal radiation are described elsewhere in the text. Local radiation may be utilized effectively for palliative purposes in end-stage disease (STANLEY et al. 1985).

16.7 Extradural Tumors

Tumors which may present with epidural compression of the cord may be primary or metastatic in nature. Primary lesions include tumors of the sympathetic ganglia (neuroblastoma, ganglioneuroma), sarcomas (Ewing's, paraspinal rhabdomyosarcoma), lymphomas, and rarer lesions like chordomas. In addition to metastatic epidural involvement of the cord by the above-mentioned histologies, compression may also be seen in cases of osteosarcoma, leukemia, and primitive neuroectodermal tumors. These lesions are discussed in other chapters in the text and will not be dealt with here.

16.8 Complications of Therapy

16.8.1 Bone Growth

Growth of the vertebral bodies continues throughout childhood and adolescence via growth plates located at the upper and lower surfaces of the bodies (BRADFORD and HENSINGER 1985). In addition, the spinous processes undergo secondary ossification and are formed during the first year of life by amalgamation of the neural arches. This process is not complete in the cervical region until the second year and in the sacrum as late as the seventh to tenth year. Ossification of the vertebral bodies is not complete until the 18th year (FREEMAN 1991) in some children. Spinal deformity is a common result of laminectomy for spinal tumors in children (RISEBOROUGH et al. 1976; LONSTEIN 1977; RISEBOROUGH 1977). At laminectomy, there is removal of the structures necessary for counterbalance of the flexion force of gravity (the spinous process, inter- and supraspinous ligaments, the laminae, ligamenta flava, and partial or complete removal of the facet joints) (LONSTEIN 1977). Kyphosis is the most common deformity seen following laminectomy, and has been reported in from 33% to 100% of children after laminectomy for spinal tumors without radiation (LONSTEIN 1977). The lower estimates are probably incorrect due to the fact that many children died of their diseases before adequate time had passed to develop the structural

abnormality. The deformity is gradually progressive and becomes most severe during the adolescent growth spurt. Avoidance of the facet joints at the time of surgery can reduce the incidence and severity of the disorder (FREEMAN 1991). Patients who undergo laminectomy between the ages of 15 and 18 have a much less severe degree of kyphosis compared to younger patients (YASUOKA et al. 1981). Laminectomies of the cervical region have the highest incidence of deformity, followed by those in the thoracic region and least commonly those in the lumbar region. In a review from Mayo Clinic, 8/9 cervical, 8/15 thoracic, and 2/11 lumbar procedures resulted in spinal deformities (YASUOKA et al. 1981).

Spinal deformity is a well-known consequence of radiation of the developing spine as well (NEUHAUSER et al. 1952; RISEBOROUGH et al.1976; LONSTEIN 1977; RISEBOROUGH 1977; MAYFIELD 1979; MAYFIELD et al. 1981; YASUOKA et al. 1981; BRADFORD and HENSINGER 1985; FREEMAN 1991). The epiphyseal plates of the vertebral bodies are susceptible to radiation damage. The deformity most commonly described is scoliosis, but kyphosis, lordosis, or a combination may be seen (RISEBROUGH 1977). Deformity is believed to be due to a combination of asymmetric dose distribution in the vertebral body and paraspinous soft tissue fibrosis (MAYFIELD 1979; MAYFIELD et al. 1981). Although the inclusion of the entire spinal body may reduce the serverity of the curvature, it will not completely prevent it, perhaps due to the fact that dose falloff is noted along one side of the vertebral body closest to the field edge.

In animal studies, doses as low as 6 Gy caused some growth disturbance, and growth arrest was noted after 20 Gy (MAYFIELD 1979; MAYFIELD et al. 1981). Most early clinical reports dealing with radiation-induced spinal deformity dealt with orthovoltage treatment, which has a higher degree of absorption in bone than does megavoltage at comparable soft tissue doses. In general, dose, patient age, and length of irradiated spine are the most relevant factors in predicting damage. Doses less than 20 Gy failed to produce significant degrees of curvature in a series of 74 children (mean age at treatment of 17 months) treated for neuroblastoma (median follow-up of 12.9 years) (MAYFIELD et al. 1981) and in a series of 59 children (mean age at treatment of 3 years) treated for Wilms' tumor (median follow-up of 11.9 years) (RISEBOROUGH et al. 1976). In both of these studies, doses between 20 and 30 Gy were associated with mild to moderate scoliotic changes, while doses in excess of 30 Gy tended to produce severe deformities. As with surgery, these deformities became most severe during the adolescent growth spurt. It is recommended that any child who has undergone a laminectomy and/or received radiation doses in excess of 20 Gy to the spinal column during childhood undergo thorough orthopedic evaluation as soon as possible after therapy and continue under close observation at least until the end of adolescence (FREEMAN 1991). If significant degrees of curvature are noted, the use of a Milwaukee brace may prevent aggravation of the deformity during the growing years. Approximately 50% of these children will be helped with the use of orthotics alone, but the remaining 50% will require eventual surgical intervention with a spinal fusion (either anterior or combined anterior/posterior) to correct a worsening deformity (BRADFORD and HENSINGER 1985; FREEMAN 1991).

16.8.2 Spinal Cord Injury

Radiation injury to the cord occurs predominantly in the white matter. Two general modes of damage have been described – a direct effect on the oligodendroglial cells which results in eventual white matter necrosis, and a delayed effect on the capillary endothelial cells which may proceed to the development of vasogenic edema, hemorrhagic necrosis, and cord infarction (SCHULTHEISS et al. 1988; LEIBEL and SHELINE 1991). A transient manifestation consisting of very brief shock-like sensations that originate in the neck and radiate down the extremities associated with flexion of the cervical vertebrae, known as Lhermitte's sign, is due to temporary demyelination of the posterior and lateral spinothalamic tracts of the irradiated cord (JONES 1964; GOLDWEIN 1987; LEIBEL and SHELINE 1991). This may occur at approximately 1–4 months after the radiation, is self-limiting, and requires no intervention. The devastating syndrome of progressive delayed radiation myelopathy occurs after a latency period of several months to years. There is a bimodal distribution of latency periods noted in adults that reflects the dual nature of radiation injury (SCHULTHEISS et al. 1984; LEIBEL and SHELINE 1991). The first peak occurs 12–14 months after radiation, the second at 24–28 months. In the pediatric population, however, the latent period is consistently shorter than in the adult (SCHULTHEISS et al. 1984). The number of reported cases of pediatric mayelitis associated with radiation is exceedingly low (SUNDARESEN et al. 1978).

Delayed radiation myelitis may occur in a rapid and dramatic fashion due to sudden cord infarction, progressing over a matter of hours to days. More commonly, however, it tends to progress as a gradual deterioration of sensory and motor functions distal to the level of the cord lesion. A combination of paresthesias, motor deficits, sphincter disturbances, and eventually paralysis may occur. A Brown-Séquard syndrome, with impairment of superficial pain sensation on one side and contralateral motor deficits due to hemisection of the cord, can also occur (GOLDWEIN 1987). Lower motor neuron disease in the absence of sensory disturbance has been reported as well. These deficits are irreversible and lead to death in approximately half of cases (LAMBERT 1978; LEIBEL and SHELINE 1991).

The development of myelitis is related to the extent of cord irradiated, the individual daily fraction size, the overall dose, and the concomitant use of certain forms of chemotherapy such as actinomycin D (WARA et al. 1975; LITTMANN et al. 1978; SCHWADE et al. 1978; LEIBEL and SHELINE 1991). Dogmatic statements have been made that certain portions of the cord are more susceptible to damage than others (i.e., the thoracic region was felt to be more sensitive than the cervical region due to a supposed "watershed" effect of blood supply (KRAMER et al. 1989), but this belief has been disputed by some authors (SCHULTHEISS 1990). Reviews of cases of radiation myelitis have, however, documented that there is an increased risk if longer segments are treated to full doses.

The threshold for damage has not been clearly defined despite numerous attempts in the literature to create isoeffect curves for the development of radiation myelitis (BODEN 1948; PALLIS et al. 1961; PHILLIPS and BUSCHKE 1969; WARA et al. 1975; COHEN et al. 1981). BODEN, in 1948, drew on his institutions's experience of six cases of progressive and four cases of transient radiation myelopathy from a group of 164 cases treated with radiation to the cervical cord, and concluded that 3500 R in 17 days was the limit of tolerance (BODEN 1948). Pallis later expanded recommendations to the thoracic cord, stating that the limits for fields less than or more than 10 cm in length were 4300 or 3300 rads, respectively, delivered over 42 days (PALLIS et al. 1961). Wara used an ED (estimated dose) formula (total dose $= ED \times N^{0.377} \times T^{0.058}$) and concluded that the 1% incidence level was 1015 rets (WARA et al. 1975). The 50% incidence level was determined to be 1746 rets. According to these observations, 50 Gy in 25 fractions was felt to be safe in cases of thoracic radiation. In a report of three cases of pediatric radiation myelitis, however, all were found to occur at between 1100 and 1200 rets

(SUNDARESEN et al. 1978). A review of 1112 patients followed for more than 12 months after radiation to the cervical cord for primary head and neck malignancies using modern equipment and techniques revealed only two cases of radiation myelitis (0.18% overall) (MARCUS and MILLION 1990). No cases were reported for doses less than 45 Gy, both cases having been seen in the 45–50 Gy range; none of the 75 patients treated with more than 50 Gy developed myelopathy. Such reviews of the literature reveal that sporadic cases occur in patients treated with what are considered to be the "safe" regimens described above. These levels are quite conservative, and higher doses may well be tolerated in the adult.

Recent work has been performed in experimental animal models, testing tolerance of the cord to reduced individual fraction sizes taken to higher doses. The doses chosen were derived from predictions of the linear-quadratic (LQ) model of radiation repair. The work of Van der Scheuren and Ang revealed that there is no additional spinal tissue repair seen with a reduction of dose fraction from 2 to 1.3 Gy, as had been predicted by the LQ model (ANG et al. 1985), but that there may be a modest 12% benefit as a result of reduction of fraction size from 2 to 1 Gy (VAN DER SCHUEREN et al. 1988). In the pediatric brain stem glioma population, doses of 1 Gy given twice daily at an interval of 4–6 h to a total of 72 Gy have been well tolerated (SHRIEVE et al. 1992). Caution must be used, however, in the use of the LQ formula for predicting new and safe dosing regimens for the spinal cord. In designing the CHART protocol (continuous hyperfractionated accelerated radiation therapy – 1.5 Gy tid at 6-h intervals with total cord dose limited to less than 50 Gy), a TD5 of 68 Gy was predicted by the LQ model to be a safe dose for the cord (DISCHE 1991). Four cases of radiation myelitis have now occurred unexpectedly at doses of 45–48 Gy.

Given the clinical information available, a total dose of 45–50 Gy in 1.8-Gy fractions is certainly well tolerated by the cord. The tolerance of the cord to higher cumulative doses delivered in multiple daily fractions of 1–1.2 Gy has yet to be tested in a prospective fashion and should be attempted cautiously.

16.9 Future Directions

Advances in imaging techniques for more complete delineation of the spinal lesion as well as further improvements in the tools available to the surgeon are critical, since the completeness of resection remains the main determinant of long-term control in spinal lesions. Alternative fractionation schemes for the delivery of higher doses of radiation for incompletely resected lesions are being examined in protocol settings as well. Extrapolating from the experience of the use of chemotherapy for intracranial malignancies in children, protocols have been established for the use of intensive chemotherapeutic regimens with or without bone marrow rescue of the infant and young child with spinal tumors in an attempt to delay the need for radiotherapy to the developing spine. The long-term efficacy of these approaches remains to be determined.

References

Anderson FM, Carson MJ (1953) Spinal cord tumors in children: a review of the subject and presentation of 21 cases. J Pediatr 43: 190–207

Ang KK, van der Kogel AJ, van der Schueren (1985) Lack of evidence for increased tolerance of rat spinal cord with decreasing fraction doses below 2 Gy. Int J Radiat Oncol Biol Phys 11: 105–110

Banna M, Gryspeerdt GL (1971) Intraspinal tumors in children (excluding dysraphism). Clin Radiol 22: 17–32

Bleyer WA (1991) Pediatric neuro-oncology: ten predictions for the future of therapy. 4th International Symposium on Pediatric Neuro-Oncology. Tokyo, Japan

Boden G (1948) Radiation myelitis of the cervical spinal cord. Br J Radiol 21: 64–469

Bradford DS, Hensinger RN (1985) The pediatric spine. Thieme, New York

Browne TR, Adams RD et al. (1976) Hemangioblastoma of the spinal cord: review and report of five cases. Arch Neurol 33: 435–441

Chun HC, Schmidt-Ullrich RK et al. (1990) External beam radiotherapy for primary spinal cord tumors. J Neurooncol 9: 211–217

Cohen AR, Wisoff JH, Allen JC, Epstein F (1989) Malignant astrocytomas of the spinal cord. J Neurosurg 70: 50–54

Cohen L, Creditor M (1981) An isoeffect table for radiation tolerance of the human spinal cord. Int J Radiat Oncol Biol Phys 7: 961–966

DeSousa AL, Kalsbeck JE, Mealey J (1979) Intraspinal tumors in children: a review of 81 patients. J Neurosurg 51: 437–445

Dillon WP, Norman D, Newton TH, Bolla K, Mark A (1989) Intradural spinal cord lesions: Gd-DTPA-enhanced MR image. Radiology 170: 229–237

DiLorenzo N, Giuffre R, Fortuna A (1982) Primary spinal neoplasms in childhood: analysis of 1234 published cases (including 56 personal cases) by pathology, sex, age and site. Differences from the situation in adults. Neurochirurgia (stuttg) 24: 153–164

DiLorenzo N, Nardi P, Ciappetta P, Fortuna A (1986) Benign tumors and tumorlike conditions of the spine. Surg Neurol 25: 449–456

DiRocco C, Iannelli A, Colosirno C (1989) Intraspinal tumors. In: Raimondi AJ, Choux M, DiRocco C (eds) The pediatric spine. Springer, New York Berlin Heidelberg, pp 45–120

Dische S (1991) Accelerated treatment and radiation myelitis (editorial). Radiat Oncol 20: 1–2

Edwards MSB, Davis RL, Laurent JP (1985) Tumor markers and cytologic features of cerebrospinal fluid. Cancer 1773–1777

Enzmann DR, DeLaPat RL, Rubin JB (1990) Magnetic resonance of the spine. C.V. Mosby, St. Louis

Epstein F (1986) Spinal cord astrocytomas of childhood. Adv Tech Stand Neurosurg 13: 135–169

Epstein FJ, Wisoff JH (1989) Intramedullary tumors of the spinal cord. In: McLaurin RL, Schut L, Venes JL, Epstein F Pediactric neurosurgery: surgery of the developing nervous system. W.B. Saunders, Philadelphia, pp 428–442

Epstein FJ, Farmer JP, Schneider SJ (1991) Intraoperative ultrasonography: an important surgical adjunct for intramedullary tumors. J Neurosurg 74: 729–733

Finlay J, Boyett J (1991) A randomized phase III trial in childhood high-grade astrocytoma, comparing VCR, CCNU and prednisone chemotherapy with the "eight-drugs-in-one-day" regimen: a report of the CCSG, CCG-945 trial. 4th International Symposium on Pediatric Neuro-oncology. Tokyo, Japan

Fischer G, Mansuy L (1980) Total removal of intramedullary ependymomas: follow-up study of 16 cases. Surg Neurol 14: 243–249

Fortuna A, Noletti A, Nardi P (1981) Spinal neurinomas and meningiomas in children. Acta Neurochir (Wien) 55: 329–341

Freeman BL (1991) The pediatric spine. In: Canale SJ, Beaty JH (eds) Operative pediatric orthopedics. Mosby Year Book, St. Louis, pp 451–610

Garcia DM (1985) Primary spinal cord tumors treated with surgery and postoperative irradiation. Int J Radiat Oncol Biol Phys 11: 1933–1939

Goldwein JW (1987) Radiation myelopathy: a review. Med Pediatr Oncol 15: 89–95

Greenwood J (1963) Intramedullary tumors of the spinal cord. A follow-up study after total surgical removal. J Neurosurg 20: 665–668

Guidetti B, Mercuri S, Vagnozzi R (1981) Longterm results of surgical treatment of 129 intramedullary spinal gliomas. J Neurosurg 54: 323–330

Hahn YS, McLone DG (1984) Pain in children with spinal cord tumors. Childs Brain 11: 36–46

Halliday AL, Sobel RA, Martuza (1991) Benign spinal nerve sheath tumors: their occurrence sporadically and in neurofibromatosis types 1 and 2. J Neurosurg 74: 248–253

Halperin EC, Kun LE, Constine LS, Tarbell NJ (1989) Tumors of the posterior fossa of the brain and the spinal canal. Pediatric radiation oncology. Raven, New York, pp 76–107

Hamby WB (1935) Tumor in the spinal canal in childhood. J Nerv Ment Dis 81: 24–42

Hamby WB (1944) Tumors in the spinal canal in childhood. II. Analysis of the literature of a subsequent decade (1933–1942). J Neuropathol Exp Neurol 3: 397–412

Heideman RL, Packer RJ, Albright LA, Freeman CR, Rorke LB (1989) Tumors of the central nervous system. In: Pizzo PA, Poplack DG (eds) Pediatric oncology. J.B. Lippincott, Philadelphia, pp 505–553.

Helle TL, Conley FK, Britt RH (1980) Effect of radiation therapy on hemangioblastoma: a case report and review of the literature. Neurosurgery 6: 82–86

Jacobs A, Delree M, Desprechins B, Otten J, Ferster A, Jonchkmer MH, Mertens J et al. (1990) Consolidating the role of *I MIBG-scintigraphy in childhood neuroblastoma: five years of clinical experience. Pediatr Radiol 20: 157–159

Jones A (1964) Transient radiation myelopathy (with reference to Lhermitte's sign of electrical parasthesias). Br J Radiol 37: 727–744

Klein DM (1989) Extramedullary spinal tumors. In McLaurin RL, Schut L, Venes JL, Epstein F (eds) Pediatric neurosurgery: surgery of the developing spine, W.B. Saunders, Philadelphia, pp 443–452

Kopelson G, Linggood RM et al. (1980) Management of intramedullary spinal cord tumors. Radiology 135: 473–479

Kornblith PL, Walker MD, et al. (1987) Neurologic oncology. JB Lippincott, Philadelphia

Kramer ED, Lewis D et al. (1989) Neurologic complications in children with soft tissue and osseous sarcomas. Cancer 64: 2600–2603

Lambert PM (1978) Radiation myelopathy of the thoracic cord in long term survivors treated with radical radiotherapy using conventional fractionation. Cancer 41: 1751–1760

Leibel SA, Sheline GE (1991) Tolerance of the brain and spinal cord to conventional radiation. In: Gutin PH, Leibel SA, Sheline GE (eds) Radiation injury to the nervous system. Raven, New York, pp 257–270

Linstadt DE, Wara WM, Leibel SA, Gutin PH, Wilson CB, Sheline GE (1989) Postoperative radiotherapy of primary spinal cord tumors. Int J Radiat Oncol Biol Phys 16: 1397–1403

Littmann P, Rosenstock JG, Bailey C (1978) Radiation myelitis following craniospinal irradiation with concurrent actinomycin-D therapy. Med Pediatr Oncol 5: 145–151

Lonstein JE (1977) Post-laminectomy kyphosis. Clin Orthop 128: 93–100

Lunardi P, Missori P, Gogliardi FM, Fortuna A (1989) Long term results of the surgical treatment of spinal dermoid and epidermoid tumors. Neurosurgery 25: 860–864

Lunardi P, Missori P, Ferrante L, Fortuna A (1990) Long-term results of surgical treatment of spinal lipomas. Report of 18 cases. Acta Neurochir (Wien) 104: 64–68

Marcus RB, Million RR (1990) The incidence of myelitis after irradiation of the cervical spinal cord. Int J Radiat Oncol Biol Phys 19: 3–8

Mayfield JK (1979) Postradiation spinal deformity. Orthop Clin North Am 10: 829–844

Mayfield JK, Riseborough EJ, Jaffe N, Nehme AME (1981) Spinal deformity in children treated for neuroblastoma. J Bone Joint Surg [Am] 63: 183–193

Naidich TP, Doundoulakis SH, Poznaski AK (1985) Intraspinal masses: efficacy of plain spine radiography. Pediatr Neurosci 12: 10–17

Neuhauser EBD, Wittenborg MH, Berman CZ, Cohen J (1952) Irradiation effects of roentgen therapy on the growing spine. Radiology 59: 637–650

Neumann HP, Eggert HR, Weigel K, Friedburg H, Wiestler OD, Schollmeyet P (1989) Hemangioblastomas of the central nervous system. A 10-year study with special reference to von Hippel-Lindau syndrome. J Neurosurg 70: 24–30

Ortega JA, Siegel SE (1989) Biological markers in pediatric cancer. In: Pizzo PA, Poplack DG (eds) Principles and practice of pediatric oncology. JB Lippincott, Philadelphia, pp 149–162

Pallis CA, Louis S, Morgan RL (1961) Radiation myelopathy. Brain 84: 460–479

Phillips TL, Buschke F (1969) Radiation tolerance of the thoracic spinal cord. AJR 105: 659–664

Raffel C, Edwards MSB (1990) Intraspinal tumors in children

3rd edn. In: Youmans JR (ed) Neurological surgery. W.B. Saunders, Philadelphia, pp 3574–3588

Raghavendra BN, Epstein FJ, McCleary L (1984) Intramedullary spinal cord tumors in children: localization by intraoperative sonography. Am J Neuroradiol 5: 395–397

Reimer R, Onofrio BM (1985) Astrocytomas of the spinal cord in children and adolescents. J Neurosurg 63: 669–675

Riseborough EJ (1977) Irradiation induced kyphosis. Clin Orthop 128: 101–106

Riseborough EJ, Grabias SL, Burton RI, Joffe N (1976) Skeletal alterations following irradiation for Wilms' tumor. J Bone Joint Surg [Am] 58: 526–536

Schultheiss TE (1990) Spinal cord radiation "tolerance": doctrine versus data. Int J Radiat Oncol Biol Phys 19: 219–221

Schultheiss TE, Higgins EM, El-Mahdi AM (1984) The latent period in clinical radiation myelopathy. Int J Radiat Oncol Bio Phys 10: 1109–1115

Schultheiss TE, Stephens LC, Maor MH (1988) Analysis of the histopathology of radiation myelopathy. Int J Radiat Oncol Biol Phys 14: 27–32

Schwade JG, Wara WM, Sheline GE, Sorgen S, Wilson CB (1978) Management of primary spinal cord tumors. Int J Radiat Oncol Biol Phys 4: 389–393

Shrieve D, Wara WM Edward MCB, Prados MD, Cogan PH, Levin VA, Sneed PK et al. (1992) Hyperfractionated radiation therapy for brain stem gliomas in children and adults. Int J Radiat Oncol Biol Phys (in press)

Solero CL, Fornari M, Giombini S, Lasir G, Oliveri G, Limino C, Pluchino F (1989) Spinal meningiomas: review of 174 operated cases. Neurosurgery 25: 153–160

Stanley P, Senac MO, Segall HD (1985) Intraspinal seeding from intracranial tumors in children. Am J Radiol 144: 157–161

Sundaresen N, Gutierrez FA, Larson MB (1978) Radiation myelopathy in children. Ann Neurol 4: 47–50

Sung DI, Chang CH, Harisiadis L (1982) Cerebellar hemangioblastoma. Cancer 49: 553

Sze G (1991) Magnetic resonance imaging in the evaluation of spinal tumors. Cancer 67: 1229–1241

Sze G, Krol G, Zimmermann RD, Deck MDF (1988) Gadolinium-DTPA: malignant extradural spinal tumors. Radiology 167: 217–233

Traggis DG, Filler RM, Druckman H, Jaffe N, Cassady JR (1977) Prognosis for children with neuroblastoma presenting with paralysis. J Pediatr Surg 12: 419–425

Van der Schueren E, Landuyt W, Ang KK, Van der Kogel AJ (1988) From 2 Gy to 1 Gy per fraction: sparing effect in rat spinal cord? Int J Radiat Oncol Biol Phys 14: 297–300

Wara WM, Sheline GE (1990) Radiation therapy of tumors of the spinal cord. In: Youmans JR (ed) Neurological surgery, 3rd edn. W.B. Saunders, Philadelphia, pp 3589–3593

Wara WM, Phillips TL, Sheline GE, Schwade JG (1975) Radiation tolerance of the spinal cord. Cancer 35: 1558–1562

Whitaker SJ, Bessell EM, Ashley SE, Bloom HJ, Bell BA, Broda M (1991) Postoperative radiotherapy in the management of spinal cord ependymoma. J Neurosurg 74: 720–728

Wood EH, Berne AS, Taveras JH (1954) The value of radiation therapy in the management of intrinsic tumors of the spinal cord. Radiology 63: 11–24

Yasuoka S, Peterson HA, Laws ER, Maclarty CS (1981) Pathogenesis and prophylaxis of post-laminectomy deformity of the spine after multiple level laminectomy: difference between children and adults. Neurosurgery 9: 145–152

17 Wilms Tumor

MOODY D. WHARAM, JR.

CONTENTS

17.1 Introduction. 251
17.2 Patterns of Spread and Clinical Presentation. . . . 252
17.3 Diagnostic Evaluation 252
17.4 Surgery. 254
17.5 Staging System 254
17.6 Pathology 254
17.7 Population Characteristics 255
17.8 Treatment 255
17.9 Treatment of Bilateral Wilms Tumor. 256
17.10 Radiation Therapy. 257
17.11 Treatment Outcome: Stage and Histology 258
17.12 Treatment Outcome: Influence of
       Other Factors 259
17.13 Treatment Outcome: Bilateral
       Wilms Tumor. 260
17.14 Treatment Outcome: Patients with Relapse. 260
17.15 Late Effects 260
       References. 262

17.1 Introduction

Carefully designed, controlled clinical trials conducted by the National Wilms Tumor Study (NWTS) committee have refined the indications for adjuvant chemotherapy and radiotherapy in the management of Wilms tumor (WT) patients. Fewer patients now require radiotherapy and those that do, need a smaller dose than was historically given. At the same time, treatment outcome has improved. Reduction in therapy duration, intensity, and dose holds the promise of fewer late effects of decreased severity. Despite the reduced requirement for radiotherapy, the radiation oncologist remains an essential member of the management team. The purpose of this chapter is to review the clinical science that the radiation oncologist will require in the current management of patients with WT.

MOODY D. WHARAM, JR., M.D., Professor, Division of Radiation Oncology, Johns Hopkins Oncology Center, 600 N. Wolfe Street, Baltimore, MD 21287, USA

Wilms tumor arises in the kidney. It has a peak incidence in the third year of life, with a median age for males of 36 months, and for females of 43 months. The male/female ratio is 1:1. After central nervous system tumors and neuroblastoma, WT is the third most common childhood solid tumor in the United States for children under the age of 15 (CRIST and KUN 1991b). The annual incidence is 7.7 cases per million children.

The cause of WT is unknown; however, certain paternal occupations may be associated with the disease. A case control study of 200 children registered on the NWTS protocols from 1984 through 1986 found an elevated odds ratio which predicted a significantly increased risk for WT in the children of welders, vehicle mechanics, and autobody repairmen (OLSHAN et al. 1990). This apparent association and any other postulated environmental factors, however, do not imply an elevated risk of WT in siblings, as might be expected. Only 15 instances of WT in siblings were ascertained in 3442 NWTS patients (D'ANGIO et al. 1989b). In this same survey, only 1% of patients had a positive family history. A comparable figure (0.5%) was found in the International Society of Pediatric Oncology (SIOP) trial (PASTORE et al. 1988), whereas it was 2.4% in the French WT study (BONAITI-PELLIE et al. 1991). It has been estimated that up to one-fifth of WT cases are hereditary. This was not supported, however, by a survey of 36 surviving patients who were parents of 59 children, none of whom had WT (GREEN et al. 1982).

Associated malformation syndromes of childhood include neurofibromatosis and Beckwith-Wiedemann (BECKWITH 1969), Drash (DRASH et al. 1970), and Perlman (PERLMAN et al. 1973) syndromes. The most commonly associated congenital anomalies are aniridia, hemihypertrophy, cryptorchidism, hypospadias, and cardiac or pericardial anomalies (BONAITI-PELLIE et al. 1991).

Cytogenetic and molecular biologic studies of WT are evolving. Between 30% and 50% of patients may have a deletion (loss of heterozygosity favoring the maternal allele) of the 11p-13-15 region. The constitutional deletion associated with the WAGR syndrome (WT, aniridia, genitourinary anomalies, and mental retardation) usually maps to 11p-13 and the Beckwith-Wiedemann syndrome to 11p-15 (NWTS Committee 1991; CRIST and KUN 1991a; PING et al. 1989). Different transcripts which map to the 11p-13 region appear to correlate with different histopathologic patterns of WT (YEGER et al. 1991). The failure to map a genetic defect to chromosome 11p in two studies of familial WT supports the concept of a complex etiology and implicates other, undetermined chromosomal loci (GRUNDY et al. 1988; HUFF et al. 1988; MOUTOU et al. 1991).

17.2 Patterns of Spread and Clinical Presentation

Wilms tumor may extend both locally and distantly. It has a capsule which may be either infiltrated or penetrated by tumor. If penetrated, the tumor is upstaged. This is the most frequent reason for elevation from stage I to stage II. Beyond the tumor capsule, tumor will infiltrate into perirenal fat and if more extensive, may involve by extension, adjacent intestine, spleen, pancreas, stomach, diaphragm, psoas, or peritoneal surfaces. Preoperative rupture of the tumor capsule into the peritoneal cavity will contaminate the entire peritoneal surface. Gross tumor nodules may be found at the time of surgery. The tumor may protrude or infiltrate into the structures of the renal sinus. It may traverse the renal vein and extend into the inferior vena cava as distantly as the right atrium (Fig. 17.1). Other means of peritoneal contamination include intraoperative disruption of the tumor capsule with spillage of contents either locally in the flank or diffusely throughout the peritoneal cavity. Preoperative biopsy (posterior flank approach) is considered to produce a "local" or flank spillage, whereas biopsy from the anterior route is considered to predict for diffuse contamination of the peritoneal cavity.

In addition to direct and regional patterns of spread, WT may metastasize to lymph nodes in the renal hilus or the ipsilateral and contralateral, or more distant, lymph node groups. In patients who present with metastatic disease, 85% have only pulmonary metastases. The remaining 15% have lung and hepatic metastases. Patients with clear cell sarcoma of the kidney may also have bone metastases.

Wilms tumor will typically produce few symptoms. The first clinical sign may be the discovery of an asymptomatic, large abdominal mass. Associated symptoms include abdominal pain and fever, which occur in up to 30% of patients. Associated signs include hematuria, again occurring in up to about 30%, and hypertension, present in up to 63%.

17.3 Diagnostic Evaluation

The laboratory and imaging studies recommended in the protocol for NWTS-4 are listed in Table 17.1. They are required to establish the extent of the primary, extension beyond the renal sinus and the renal vein, the presence of adenopathy, and distant metastases. In addition, the location and function of the opposite kidney and its architecture are studied. It is important to distinguish between patients with a normal chest x-ray who have apparent pulmonary metastases diagnosed on computerized axial tomography (CT) of the chest and patients whose pulmonary lesions are apparent on routine chest x-ray. Therefore, all patients should have chest CT. Preoperative sonography and CT scanning of the tumor may allow distinction between malignant rhabdoid tumor and WT (SISLER and SIEGEL 1989). This appears not to be true for clear cell sarcoma of the kidney (GLASS et al. 1991). Both radiography and radionuclide bone scanning are essential to maximize detection of bone metastases from clear cell sarcoma of the kidney (FEUSNER et al. 1990).

For the occasional patient with a massive, unresectable primary tumor, treatment may be initiated without biopsy. It is estimated that the error rate in diagnosis from tissue subsequently at the time of nephrectomy may be as high as 10%. Without biopsy, less than sufficiently aggressive therapy may be administered for the least common but more malignant histologies. An adequate pretreatment specimen may be obtained by percutaneous needle biopsy from the posterior approach, which will not increase the risk of peritoneal dissemination (SAARINEN et al. 1991).

Table 17.1. Laboratory and imaging evaluation

Complete blood count
Blood chemistry
Urinalysis
Chest radiograph and CT scan
Abdominal CT scan and ultrasonography
(CCSK: cranial CT or MRI and skeletal survey and isotope scan)

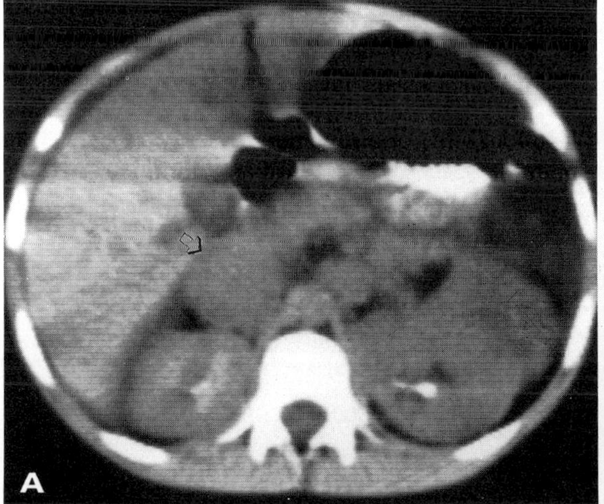

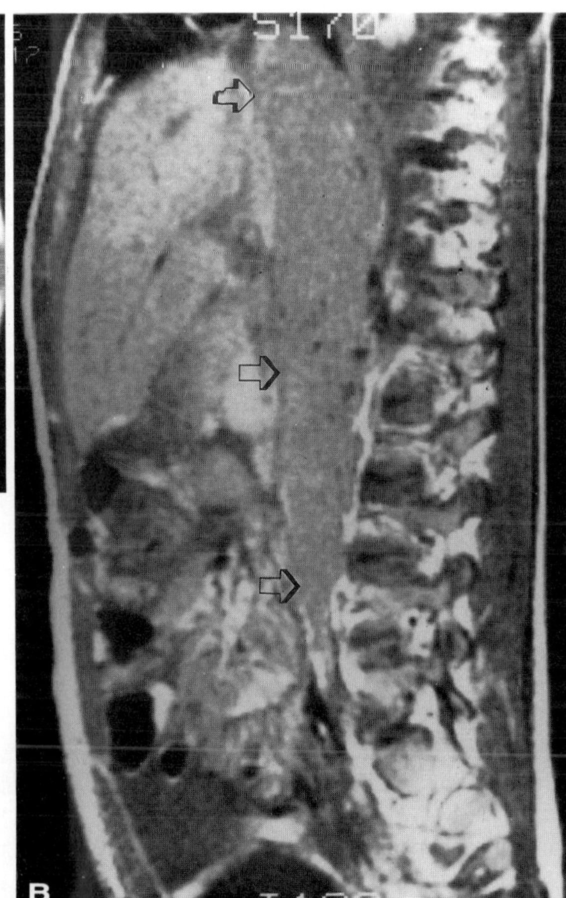

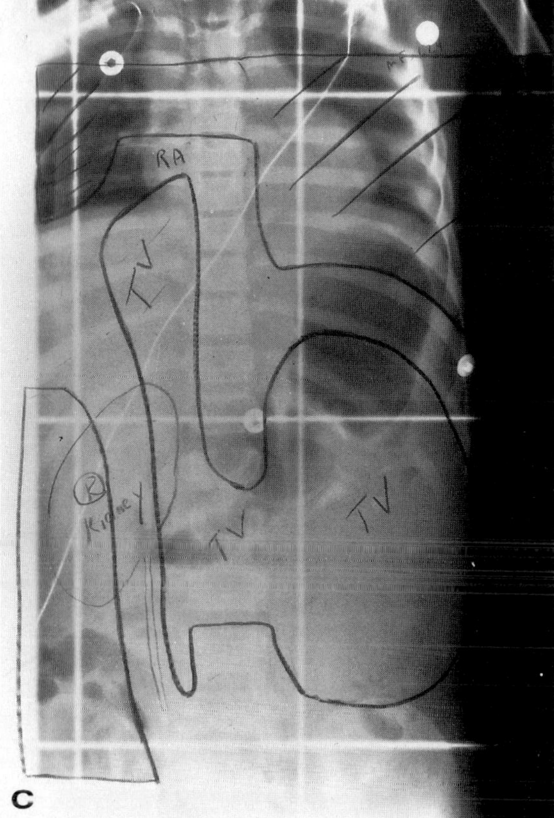

Fig. 17.1 A–C. A 9-year-old white female presented with abdominal and left shoulder pain. Open biopsy: favorable histology WT. **A** CT scan demonstrating WT of the left kidney with tumor thrombus filling the inferior vena cava (*arrow*). **B** Sagittal MRI scan demonstrating that the tumor thrombus in the vena cava extends above the diaphragm (*arrows*). **C** Simulation film for preoperative radiotherapy. A total dose of 11.2 Gy was given (1.60 Gy/day). The subsequent surgical specimen contained no viable tumor in the vena cava

17.4 Surgery

With few exceptions, patients with even the largest tumors may successfully undergo transabdominal, transperitoneal nephrectomy. The goal of surgery is to remove the primary tumor, to sample regional lymph nodes, to inspect by vision and palpation the opposite kidney, and to similarly inspect the peritoneum and liver for evidence of dissemination. Care is taken to avoid rupture of cysts that typically comprise the tumor substance. Tumor infiltrating the renal vein and vena cava should be removed and notation made of whether or not it is attached to the vessel intima or penetrates through the vessel wall. Should the tumor capsule be violated with spillage of cyst contents, the surgeon must know whether the spillage is confined to the ipsilateral flank (flank radiotherapy not indicated) or whether the entire peritoneum is "contaminated" (abdominal radiotherapy indicated).

Table 17.2. Staging system (adapted from National Wilms' Tumor Study-4, c/o National Wilms' Tumor Study Statistical Center, Fred Hutchinson Cancer Research Center, 1124 Columbia Street, Seattle, WA 98104)

Stage I – The tumor is limited to the kidney and was completely excised. The surface of the renal capsule is intact. The tumor was not ruptured before or during removal. There is no residual tumor apparent beyond the margins of resection.

Stage II – The tumor extends beyond the kidney, but was completely excised. There is regional extension of tumor (i.e., penetration of tumor through the outer surface of the renal capsule) into the perirenal soft tissues. Blood vessels outside the kidney substance are infiltrated by or contain tumor thrombus. The tumor may have been biopsied or there has been local spillage of tumor, but the spillage was confined to the ipsilateral flank. No residual tumor is apparent at or beyond the margins of excision.

Stage III – Residual nonhematogenous tumor is present, and confined to the abdomen. Any one or more of the following may occur:

> Lymph nodes (renal hilar, para-aortic, or beyond) are found on biopsy to be involved by tumor.
> There has been diffuse peritoneal contamination by tumor, such as by spillage of tumor beyond the ipsilateral flank before or during surgery, or the tumor has penetrated through the peritoneal surface.
> Tumor implants are found on the peritoneal surface.
> Gross or microscopic tumor remains postoperatively (e.g., tumor cells are found at the margin of surgical resection on microscopic examination).
> Preoperative chemotherapy or radiotherapy was given.

Stage IV – Hematogenous metastases are present.

Stage V – Bilateral renal involvement is present at diagnosis. An attempt should be made to stage each side according to the above criteria on the basis of the extent of disease prior to biopsy.

17.5 Staging System

Staging for WT in accordance with NWTS-4 consists of imaging, surgical, and pathologic criteria. The diagnosis of stage IV is usually made on the basis of pulmonary metastases detected on chest x-ray. A small subset of patients with lung lesions found only on chest tomography are given less aggressive treatment. The criteria which determine the stage assignment (Table 17.2) for non-metastatic patients are also applicable for stage IV patients. This "local" stage has been designated in a retrospective review as the "C" (for computer determined) stage (BRESLOW et al. 1986). Similarly, for the patient with bilateral WT, which is designated as stage V, each kidney is given a local stage as if it were the sole primary. For the occasional patient with an inoperable primary who receives preoperative therapy, the "local" stage is always considered to be stage III.

The NWTS staging system is described in Table 17.2. The extent of involvement of the renal sinus affects staging. A distinction is drawn based upon the "hilar plane," an imaginary line which extends from the upper to the lower medial borders of the intact kidney. That portion of the renal sinus lateral to the hilar plane is considered to be intrarenal. Tumor that protrudes beyond the hilar plane remains as stage I. *Invasion* beyond the hilar plane constitutes stage II. A positive surgical margin at any point without regard to the hilar plane constitutes stage III.

17.6 Pathology

The WT rubric includes three neoplasms and several variants. The majority of patients have classical, "favorable histology" (FH), WT, which is to be contrasted with the less common and more aggressive tumor types called clear cell sarcoma of the kidney (CCSK) (BECKWITH and PALMER 1978) and malignant rhabdoid tumor of the kidney (RTK) (WEEKS et al. 1989), both of which are included under the appellation "unfavorable histology Wilms tumor." The classic form of WT also exists in infrequent, unfavorable subtypes identified as "anaplastic." At one time the CCSK and the RTK were lumped together with anaplastic WT to constitute the "unfavorable histology" types. Together they accounted for about 12% of patients entered on NWTS-3. Presently, RTK patients are not eligible for randomization on NWTS-4; however, they may be registered and managed in accordance with that protocol. The differential diagnosis of patients with renal masses presenting in infancy includes congenital mesoblastic nephroma. Although the latter tumor may extend into perinephric tissues, it may have a benign natural history and not require adjuvant chemotherapy or radiotherapy when radical surgical resection is accomplished. Occasionally, local recurrence and metastases occur (STEINFELD et al. 1984).

In a review of 1,156 NWTS patients, 7.3% had anaplastic histology (BONADIO et al. 1985). The anaplastic patients had a mean age at diagnosis of 63 months compared to 41 months for the non anaplastic patients. Presentation before the age of 2 years was rare and more of the anaplastic tumor group were nonwhite (31% compared to 11%). They were more likely to have lymph node metastases (30% vs 16%). There was no significant effect of focal versus diffuse anaplasia; however, the presence of anaplasia in extrarenal tumor sites and a predominantly blastemal tumor pattern were both associated with poor outcome (ZUPPAN et al. 1988). The anaplastic subtype is more likely to feature hyperdiploid DNA content and to have chromosomal rearrangement (DOUGLASS et al. 1986).

In its mode of presentation and age distribution at diagnosis, CCSK is similar to classic WT; however, it is more likely to be associated with both bone and brain metastases (MARSDEN et al. 1978). RTK is an infrequent but aggressive lesion that typically presents at a younger age than classic WT. In a review from the NWTS, the median age at diagnosis was 11 months. The patients are more likely to present as stages III or IV and there is an association with hypercalcemia and neuroectodermal brain tumors (WEEKS et al. 1989). A variant of FH WT has been described which occurs rarely and in patients of median age 12 months. The cystic partially differentiated nephroblastoma (papillonodular variant) may have an excellent prognosis with nephrectomy alone (JOSHI and BECKWITH 1990).

17.7 Population Characteristics

The age range at diagnosis for WT extends into adulthood; however, the peak is between ages 2 and 3. The median age for males with unilateral disease is 36 months and for females 43 months. The annual incidence is 460 patients (CRIST and KUN 1991b), of whom approximately 76% are registered on the NTWS protocols. The stage distribution for FH patients randomized on NWTS-3 was: I, 47.7%; II, 21.5%; III, 21.5%; IV, 9.3%. Patients with unfavorable histology (UH) (all stages) accounted for 11.1%

Table 17.3. NWTS-4 patients requiring radiotherapy: stage, histology, age, and gender ratio (adapted from BRESLOW NE, personal communication, 1991)

Stage/histology	Percent	Median age (months)	Female:male ratio
III/FH	50	45	1.3
IV/FH	29	50	1.9
II-IV/ANA	11	53	1.1
I-IV/CCSK	10	27	0.5

ANA, anaplastic

Table 17.4. Proportion of randomized NWTS-4 patients receiving radiotherapy (RT) by age group (adapted from BRESLOW NE, personal communication, 1991)

Age group (months)	Percentage of patients	Percentage receiving RT
0–23	31	19
24–47	33	42
≥48	36	48
All	100	37

of the total randomized patients (D'ANGIO et al. 1989a). The histological types and patient number were: FH, 1248; anaplastic, 61; CCSK, 56; RTK, 32. In NWTS-4 at a point when 1101 patients had been randomized and analyzed, 37% were in a category requiring radiotherapy. The characteristics of this population subset are shown in Table 17.3. The median ages cited (except in the case of CCSK) exceed the median ages for patients not requiring radiotherapy: I/FH, 23 months; II/FH, 41 months. Of all patients who require RT, the proportion aged 48 months or more is 47%. For randomized NWTS-4 patients, the children under the age 24 months were least likely to require RT (Table 17.4).

The incidence of synchronous bilateral WT is approximately 5% (BLUTE et al. 1987; COPES et al. 1989). It is 3% for metachronous tumors (BISHOP et al. 1977; COPPES et al. 1989), with a time interval between diagnoses of 11–21 months in one series (MALCOLM et al. 1980). For patients on NWTS-2 and -3, the incidence of unfavorable histology in patients with synchronous bilateral WT was 10% (BLUTE et al. 1987).

17.8 Treatment

For unilateral WT, initial nephrectomy can be accomplished in 94% of patients (ZUPPAN et al. 1991). The determination of surgical/pathologic staging and the histologic subtype provides the prognostic information upon which a decision for treatment is based. Since 1969, the majority of patients in the United States have been enrolled in one of the NWTS protocols. The current study (4) began in 1986 and remains open in 1992. The protocols have led to gradual improvements in disease-free survival and simplification of therapy by reduction of treatment duration, elimination of certain chemotherapeutic agents, reduced requirement for radiotherapy, and reduced duration of chemotherapy. Important findings from the NWTS trial include the observation that postoperative radiotherapy is unnecessary for patients with stages I and II, FH and those with stage I anaplastic histology. For these same stages, actinomycin D and vincristine in combination are more efficacious than each drug alone. For patients who are staged III or IV, FH, the addition of adriamycin to actinomycin D and vincristine improves outcome. When the same three drugs are given for stage III, FH patients, the administration of 10 Gy (fractionated) to the flank or abdomen is as efficacious as 20 Gy. During NWTS-2, the duration of actinomycin D and vincristine therapy was restricted to 10 weeks for stage I patients and was equivalent to the 6-month regimen. For patients with stage IV, FH, the addition of the alkylating agent cyclophosphamide did not improve survival when added to adriamycin, actinomycin D, and vincristine.

The current NTWS-4 protocol has evolved from predecessor studies and is predicated upon the opportunity to reduce the cost (in terms of time and money) of treatment. All randomized patients are placed in one of four risk groups that are defined by stage and histology:

Stage I, favorable histology or anaplastic histology

Stage II, favorable histology

Stage III or IV, favorable histology or CCSK all stages

Stage II–IV, anaplastic histology

Patients are randomized to a standard regimen of conventional intensity or to a regimen employing the same drug in a pulsed, intensive regimen which requires fewer hospital visits. For the second and third risk groups, there is a second randomization after 18–26 weeks (depending on regimen) to either stop or continue therapy so that the efficacy of shorter versus standard duration may be assessed in a factorial design. Postoperative radiation therapy is utilized for all patients in the third and fourth risk groups.

Carefully selected stage I, FH patients may not require postnephrectomy adjuvant chemotherapy.

A study of stage I, FH patients from NWTS-3 was done of all 24 patients who relapsed. They were compared retrospectively with 48 matched controls on the same study. Four histopathologic features were assessed, any one of which raised the likelihood of relapse. They were: invasion of the tumor capsule, presence of an inflammatory pseudocapsule, renal sinus invasion, and tumor in intrarenal vessels. The absence of all four features was associated with a zero relapse risk (WEEKS et al. 1987). A different set of criteria were described in a two institution report of eight patients who were stage I by the Cassady criteria. The criteria are: unilateral and favorable histology, no metastases, specimen weight less than 550 g, and age less than 24 months (CASSADY et al. 1973).

Some patients will not be amenable to initial nephrectomy. In NWTS-3, 140 of 2489 patients (5.6%) with unilateral disease had preoperative therapy (ZUPPAN et al. 1991). For the inoperable patient, actinomycin D, vincristine, and adriamycin chemotherapy is initiated and continued as long as tumor shrinkage continues. Nephrectomy is recommended within 6 weeks of diagnosis. In the absence of prompt response to the chemotherapy, preoperative, fractionated radiotherapy is utilized to a dose of 12 Gy. These patients are considered to be stage III regardless of subsequent, operative findings. Preoperative chemotherapy is considered to be the standard approach for WT in the studies conducted by the SIOP (LEMERLE et al. 1983) and by The Hospital for Sick Children, Toronto (GREENBERG et al. 1990).

17.9 Treatment of Bilateral Wilms Tumor

The guiding principle in the treatment of bilateral WT is one of conservatism and the preservation of as much renal parenchyma as possible. In the NWTS review, 64% of patients were stage I (most advanced side) and 90% had favorable histology (BLUTE et al. 1987). Current recommendations for management are predicated upon the good results that these numbers would suggest and the favorable response to chemotherapy that permits renal parenchymal preservation.

The diagnosis of bilateral WT can be predicted by CT scanning in about 80% of synchronous cases. Laparotomy is recommended to establish the diagnosis and accomplish the staging procedures noted earlier. Where both kidneys are extensively involved, each should be biopsied to confirm the diagnosis and the histologic subtype. The tumors on each side should be resected in their entirety, leaving sufficient parenchyma for renal function. Where the tumor cannot be completely excised, it should be left in situ. Thereafter, post-operative chemotherapy is initiated with actinomycin D and vincristine. After a standard 13-week course, a CT scan is repeated and the patient subjected to a second-look operation. If no tumor is found, the patient continues to receive actinomycin D/vincristine chemotherapy for a total of 65 weeks. If any tumor is found, and regardless of the resection accomplished by surgery, adriamycin should be added to the postoperative course as utilized in regimen DD of the NWTS-4 protocol. At second-look surgery, the most involved side may be subjected to nephrectomy with the contralateral side having complete tumor excision only, and with sufficient renal parenchyma to support renal function. If only tumor excision is done for the most involved side, marking or clips should be employed to indicate disease extent for subsequent radiotherapy. After an additional 13 weeks of triple-drug chemotherapy, repeat evaluation is done to assess response. Further surgery or radiotherapy alone or a combination of both may then be required, depending upon the radiographic and/or surgical evaluation. If radio-therapy is required for favorable histology, the portal should, whenever possible, spare some renal parenchyma. After 10.5 Gy, the portal can be reduced to the actual tumor nodule and an additional 10.5 Gy administered.

17.10 Radiation Therapy

The recommendation in the NWTS-4 protocol is that radiotherapy be initiated within 9 days of surgery. To delay to day 10 or beyond was associated with an increased relapse risk in NWTS-2 (THOMAS et al. 1984), and this was confirmed in the NWST-3 study (THOMAS et al. 1991a). Treatment of the intact kidney is rarely required. It will occasionally be necessary for bilateral WT (see above) for the patients with an initially unresectable tumor that does not respond to a brief course of vincristine and actinomycin D. With concurrent vincristine, the daily radiotherapy dose is 1.5–1.8 Gy to a total of 12.6 Gy.

The indications for postoperative infradiaphragmatic radiation therapy are based upon pathologic stage and histology. For stage I and II patients with FH, postoperative radiation is not given. It is administered for patients who are stage III and those patients who are stage IV whose "local, abdominal" stage is equivalent to stage III. The indications for treating the entire abdomen include preoperative tumor rupture, diffuse intraoperative spillage, and peritoneal seeding. Rarely, there will be gross residual abdominal tumor. A more conservative portal restricted to the tumor bed but extending to include the contralateral para-aortic node chain is designed for the patient with positive nodes, or if there is gross or microscopic tumor confined to the operative bed.

The whole abdominal portal extends from above the dome of each diaphragm down to the level of the lower aspect of the obturator foraminae. Laterally it extends beyond the edge of the flank. The more restricted flank portal is based upon the preoperative imaging studies. It is tightly drawn with its medial border extending to the contralateral side of the vertebral column to include potentially involved nodes but to exclude the remaining kidney. The lateral border "falls off" at the margin of the flank. The superior and inferior margins are determined by the initial tumor site. When one pole is spared, as is usually the case, the margin is just beyond that uninvolved pole. A margin of at least 1 cm delimited with a focused block technique is recommended. For the remaining portal border that approximates the pole of the kidney containing tumor, the margin recommended by the NWTS protocol is again 1 cm. The author employs 2–2.5 cm with the margin defined by a focused block technique. The ipsilateral iliac crest is protected to the extent possible, and for the whole abdominal portal, the femoral heads are similarly protected. For the occasional patient with gross residual disease, a supplemental portal is designed according to that tumor distribution, again with tight margins.

Stage IV patients usually have dissemination only to the lung. In this case, the radiotherapy portal includes the entire lung with an extension to cover the tumor bed as described above. This large portal is generally well tolerated. For the patient who requires lung and whole abdominal radiotherapy, this large portal should be employed initially; if hematologic tolerance is exceeded, the portal is restricted to the pulmonary component until radiotherapy to the lungs is complete, at which time the abdominal component is resumed. The whole lung portal includes all of the lung parenchyma with no shielding of the cardiac and mediastinal structures. The shoulder girdle is excluded by shielding. The lower border of the whole lung portal (when flank or abdominal radiation therapy is not indicated) extends to the bottom of L1. Following the dose recommendations of NWTS (see below), treatment of the flank or abdominal portal is concluded 1 day prior to the lung

Table 17.5. NWTS-4 recommended radiotherapy total dose (Gy) (adapted from National Wilms' Tumor Study-4 c/o National Wilms' Tumor Study Statistical Center, Fred Hutchinson Cancer Research Center, 1124 Columbia Street, Seattle, WA 98104)

Favorable histology		Anaplastic Histology	
Stage III	10.8		
		Age in	
Stage IV		months	
Lungs	12	0–12	12.6–18
Lung boost		13–18	21.6
(additional)	7.5	19–30	27
Abdomen if		31–40	32.4
local stage III	10.8	≥41	37.8
Liver metastases			
(unresected)	19.8		
		Clear cell sarcoma	
Stage III bulk			
residual boost	10.8	Stages I, II, and III	10.8
Preoperative	12–12.6		
		Stage III bulk	10.8
		residual boost	
		Stage IV (same as FH)	
		except unresected	
		liver metastases	30.6

radiotherapy, thus requiring design of the lung portal for the last treatment. The need for supplemental radiation to pulmonary metastases is determined 2 weeks after whole lung radiation therapy. Thoractomy with resection is an option.

Portal design is not influenced by favorable versus unfavorable histology, whereas dose is. Table 17.5 indicates the total doses recommended for the radiotherapy portals described above. When large volumes are included within the portal, the daily dose is 1.5 Gy. For smaller volumes such as flank treatment and boosts to intra-abdominal disease, the daily dose is 1.8 Gy. These same dose fractions are employed for patients with unfavorable histology and the total dose is escalated in accordance with age at diagnosis, as indicated in Table 17.5. This scale derives from the early experience in treating all patients with WT and is meant to reflect a concept of "tolerance" based on age. Patients with unfavorable histology are treated with portals as described above; however, patients with clear cell sarcoma receive flank radiotherapy even if they are stage I or II. Similarly, patients with stage II anaplastic histology receive flank radiotherapy. The portals are designed according to the same principles as described above for FH, stage III.

17.11 Treatment Outcome: Stage and Histology

A subset of children with stage I FH WT may not require adjuvant therapy after nephrectomy. Eight consecutive stage I (CASSADY et al. 1973) patients were disease-free after a mean follow-up of 5 years, none having received postoperative adjuvant therapy. One patient had a metachronous second primary (LARSEN et al. 1990).

The outcome of therapy for WT patients in the United States is accurately represented by the results of the NWTS cooperative clinical trials. The NWTS-4 study in 1991 enrolled approximately 76% of the estimated 1991 United States incidence of 460 cases (BRESLOW NE, personal communication, 1991; CRIST and KUN 1991b).

The results of the first three NWTS protocols have been published (D'ANGIO et al. 1976,1981,1989a). The conclusions pertaining to radiotherapy are that postoperative radiotherapy is not indicated in three circumstances: (a) stage I FH, (b) stage I anaplastic histology, and (c) stage II FH if chemotherapy consists of both actinomycin D and vincristine. In addition, the NWTS-3 stage III FH randomization between either 10 Gy or 20 Gy postoperatively demonstrated no significant difference. NWTS-4 uses 10 Gy along with three drug chemotherapy regimens that contain adriamycin, actinomycin D, and vincristine. The 4-year survival rates for NWTS-3 are listed in Table 17.6. The subset of patients aged 12 months or less at diagnosis were recommended to receive chemotherapy at one-half dose levels. The 4-year survival results did not differ from those of older patients with FH, stages I–III (CORN et al. 1991). A single institution report noted 5-year survival in seven of eight children with anaplastic histology, stages II–IV (COREY et al. 1991). The comparable NWTS-3 data are 40 patients, 54% survival (NWTS Committee 1991).

Results of the SIOP trials of preoperative radiotherapy, chemotherapy, or both approximate those published by the NWTS committee (LEMERLE et al. 1983; TOURNADE et al. 1991). A comparison of the trial results is precluded by the different eligibility cri-

Table 17.6. Survival at 4 years, NWTS-3 (adapted from D'ANGIO et al. 1989a and NWTS Committee 1991)

Stage/histology	Percent alive
I/FH	97
II/FH	94
III/FH	88
IV/FH	82
I/ANA	89
II–IV/ANA	54
All/CCSK	75
All/RTK	25

teria and the use within SIOP of staging determined after preoperative treatment. The advantage of the SIOP approach is an apparent reduction in the proportion of stage III patients and in the incidence of intraoperative rupture/spillage (BURGERS et al. 1986) with a consequent reduction in the requirement for whole abdominal radiotherapy or any radiotherapy. Contrary to the SIOP policy of not requiring initial biopsy, the group at the Hospital for Sick Children, Toronto successfully obtained histologic diagnosis in each of 32 patients who had percutaneous retroperitoneal biopsy (GREENBERG et al. 1990)

17.12 Treatment Outcome: Influence of Other Factors

The NWTS committee has reported the prognostic factor affecting outcome in studies 1,2, and 3. For NWST-1, the most important predictors of relapse (not treatment related) for patients with non-metastatic disease were unfavorable histology, specimen weight of more than 250 g, positive regional lymph nodes, and age exceeding 2 years (BRESLOW et al. 1978). Unfavorable histology or positive regional adenopathy remained the major prognostic factors in the equivalent population in NWTS-2 (BRESLOW et al. 1985). Other factors of importance depending on endpoint were: operative spillage, tumor thrombosis in the renal vein or inferior vena cava, and intrarenal vascular invasion. The effect of prognostic factors in the population with FH only were ascertained using the method of recursive partitioning analysis. Patients with FH and positive nodes were four times as likely as FH node-negative patients to experience distant metastasis, relapse at any site, or death.

The comparable study for NWTS-3 excluded patients with UH and analyzed patients by stage corrected after review of surgery and pathology reports ("calculated" or "C" stage). Positive adenopathy remained a major factor, raising the percentage of patients having lung relapse from 7% (negative nodes) to 15% (positive hilar nodes) and 22% (positive aortic nodes). Specimen weight reemerged as the major factor in "C" stage I patients. For example, there were similar numbers of patients with a specimen weight of less than 250 g and 500 999 g. The percentage with any relapse was 2.8% versus 9.7% respectively. Age at diagnosis of more than 24 months predicted poorer outcome in "C" stage II and III patients. The percentage of "C" stage II patients with abdominal relapse was, for example,

0% when diagnosis was achieved at 0–23 months of age, but 4.4% when age at diagnosis exceeded 48 months. Using death from tumor as the endpoint, the comparable percentage for "C" stage III patients were 14.1% and 15.9% respectively. (BRESLOW et al. 1991).

Intra-abdominal relapse (IAR) is an infrequent event in patients who receive postoperative radiotherapy. The 1984 report of NWTS-2 noted only ten such patients out of 259 (3.8%) with stage II or III FH or UH disease. Factors associated with this pattern of failure were UH, inadequate radiotherapy portal size, and delay of radiotherapy beyond postoperative day 10 (THOMAS et al. 1984). A similar analysis of NWTS-3 restricted to stage III, FH patients reported an IAR rate of 5.4%. IAR was more likely to occur in patients who started radiotherapy more than 10 days after surgery. A higher IAR rate was seen in patients who received dactinomycin/vincristine/10 Gy than those who also received doxorubicin (7 of 61 vs 3 of 70 patients) (THOMAS et al. 1991a).

Patients with stage II WT are not upstaged by virtue of specimen adhesion to the liver or tumor invasion of the liver, provided the surgical margin is negative. There is no apparent adverse effect for FH patients when these occur. The same is true for stage III FH patients, whose radiotherapy portal must include a positive hepatic margin but not the entire liver. Three-year survival of NWTS-3 FH patients was *not* reduced for 13 patients with liver metastasis only (92% survival) or 20 patients with liver and lung metstasis (80% survival) compared to 169 stage IV patients without liver metastasis (82% survival) (THOMAS et al. 1991b).

Survival rates are adversely affected by involvement of the vena cava or by intracardiac extension. Surgical management is of greater complexity and operative complications are increased (NAKAYAMA et al. 1986; RITCHEY et al. 1988). Preoperative chemotherapy in this circumstance will reduce or eliminate the intra vascular tumor, thereby simplifying subsequent surgery and reducing its risk (KOGAN et al. 1986; OBERHOLZER et al. 1992).

The 4-year survival for stage IV FH patients has improved with successive NWTS protocols: 1, 62%; 2, 73%; and 3, 84%. (BRESLOW et al. 1986). Similar patients receiving treatment at the Boston Children's Hospital had a 10-year survival of 77% (MACKLIS et al. 1991). In this series and the NWTS protocols, patients received whole lung radiotherapy. In contrast, patients treated in accordance with a SIOP study received pulmonary radiotherapy only if they did not achieve lung complete remission by chemotherapy or thoracotomy. With this approach, 26 of 36 patients survived without pulmonary radiotherapy. Five-year survival for the entire group was 83% (DE KRAKER et al. 1990). As noted above, patients with lung metastases at diagnosis (FH) do not fare worse if liver metastases are also present. There is no apparent survival advantage for FH patients with lung metastases that are apparently solitary, or confined to one lung, compared to patients with bilateral metastases (BRESLOW et al. 1986). As small cohort of NWTS-3 patients were considered stage IV on the basis of pulmonary metastases detected only on CT and not on routine chest x-ray. The 4-year survival of 94% for the patients treated according to the stage IV protocol did not differ significantly from the 88% survival for patients whose management was less intense and did not include whole lung radiotherapy (GREEN et al. 1991a).

Stage IV patients may be divided according to the stage of their primary tumor, i.e., their "local" stage as corrected by NWTS investigators, "C stage" I and II versus III. This division affects prognosis for FH patients. The 4-year survival rate for 77 patients with local C stage I and II was approximately 83% compared to 68% for C stage III patients (NWTS 1–3). The difference was statistically significant for FH patients, whereas no difference was observed for UH patients (approximately 20% survival) (BRESLOW et al. 1986).

17.13 Treatment Outcome: Bilateral Wilms Tumor

In a review of synchronous (stage V) bilateral WT in NWTS-2 and -3, patients were staged according to the most advanced side. The 3-year survival figure by that stage for FH patients: I, 92%; II, 69%; III, 75%; and IV, 72%. The 3-year survival for all FH patients was 84% compared to 16% for UH patients. Patients were compared by initial surgical attempt, i.e., either biopsy only (followed by chemotherapy and a subsequent operation) or attempted tumor removal. Three-year survival was lower in the initial biopsy group (57% vs 82%), but the result was not statistically significant. Also lacking statistical significance for effect on survival was the administration (or withholding) of tumor bed radiotherapy in those patients with postsurgical tumor residual (BLUTE et al. 1987).

17.14 Treatment Outcome: Patients with Relapse

Long-term survival is possible for WT patients who relapse. For FH patients on NWTS-1,-2, and -3

with relapse confined to lung, 4-year survival is 53% (BRESLOW et al. 1986). The 10-year result in the Boston Children's Hospital report was 52% (MACKLIS et al. 1991). The addition of liver metastases in the NWTS report reduced the survival probability to 20%. Liver metastasis, however, accompanied lung relapse in only 12% of patients. In the small cohort of NWTS-1, -2, and -3 patients (initially FH, stage I, II, or III) with a solitary pulmonary relapse, the influence of surgical resection (followed by lung radiotherapy and chemotherapy) was compared to that of radiotherapy and chemotherapy without surgery. The 4-year survival rates were each approximately 75%. FH patients with multiple lung lesions at relapse who received radiotherapy and chemotherapy had a 44% 4-year survival rate. Radiation doses ranged from 10.5 Gy (whole lung) to 20 Gy (hemithorax). "Boost" radiotherapy to visible lesions was infrequently administered. Five FH patients with resection of solitary metastasis did not receive radiotherapy. Four relapsed in the ipsilateral lung (GREEN et al. 1991b).

Patients on NWTS-2 and -3 who were stage I–IV (UH or FH) and achieved complete remission and subsequently relapsed were studied for prognostic factors. The overall 3-year survival was 30%. It was 42% for FH and 16% for UH (NWTS-3). Other factors influencing 3-year, postrelapse survival for FH patients were: (a) abdominal relapse on NWTS-3, no prior radiotherapy, 77%; (b) original stage I, 57%; (c) recurrence more than 12 months after original diagnosis, 47%; (d) original chemotherapy only actinomycin D and vincristine (stages II and III), 41%; and (e) lung relapse only, 44%. This last figure differs from the more favorable data recorded above by the inclusion of initial stage IV patients (GRUNDY et al. 1989). These results were achieved mainly with standard treatment. Response rates to second-line chemotherapy have been reported in patients who relapsed on the first WT study of the United Kingdom Children's Cancer Study (PINKERTON et al. 1991).

17.15 Late Effects

An extensive literature documents the wide range of late effects that resulted from the early, higher dose era of radiotherapy for WT patients (RISEBOROUGH et al. 1976; GIBSON et al. 1977; OLIVER et al. 1978; JONES et al. 1984). These effects are becoming less likely with current multidisciplinary management for three reasons. First, the doses required for FH patients are lower for abdominal and thoracic portals. Second, the proportion of patients needing radiotherapy is reduced, having been restricted principally to initial stage III, and IV patients. Third, the average age of patients receiving radiotherapy is now higher as the indications for radiotherapy have been restricted to higher stages where the more vulnerable, younger patient is less frequently found. The incidence and severity of late radiotherapy effects that may follow the use of lower doses in the smaller number of older patients is difficult to predict but will certainly not exceed those that have been reported in the Late Effects Study from NWTS-1 and -2 (Evans et al. 1991).

Late radiotherapy effects may be described in five categories: pulmonary/cardiovascular; musculoskeletal/integument; endocrine/fertility; renal; and second malignant neoplasms.

Stage IV WT patients receive whole lung radiotherapy and are at risk for developing radiation pneumonitis. For NWTS-2, the protocol dose was 14 Gy; 3 of 49 patients developed a fatal pneumonitis (Thomas et al. 1988). A lower dose (12 Gy) was utilized for NWTS-3, stage IV FH patients. Diffuse interstitial pneumonitis was reported in 19 patients (13% of the total), of whom three had *Pneumocystis carinii* and survived. Of 15 patients with presumed radiation pneumonitis, 11 died. The median elapsed time from the end of chest radiotherapy to pneumonitis did not differ according to pneumopathy: *P. carinii* 54 days; radiation 58 days. Prophylactic treatment with trimethoprim/sulfamethoxazole is now recommended (Green et al. 1989). Significant late cardiac toxicity has not been seen in NWTS-1 and -2 patients enrolled in the long-term follow-up study; however, a longer observation time is required (Evans et al. 1991).

The musculoskeletal and integumentary system late effects due to radiotherapy include scoliosis, kyphosis, bone growth impairment, muscle atrophy, and breast hypoplasia. Two single institution reports that include patients from the orthovoltage era report an incidence of scoliosis of 54% (Thomas et al. 1983) and 58% (Rate et al. 1991). It was 61% in the NWTS Late Effects Study, where it was also observed in 9% of group I patients not having radiotherapy (Evans et al. 1991). Kyphosis is less common but may be more likely to progress after the adolescent growth spurt. Orthopedic intervention was not required in one series of patients who received megavoltage treatment exceeding 30 Gy (Heaston et al. 1979). Flank and abdominal radiotherapy to doses between 20 and 30 Gy impairs spinal growth, producing a disproportion between standing and sitting height. In one series, the calculated height loss by age at treatment was: age 1 year, 9 cm: age 5, 7 cm; age 10, 5.5 cm (Wallace et al. 1990). These data correspond closely to the prediction for males given 25 Gy utilizing the model developed at the Children's Hospital of Philadelphia. For patients receiving the current recommended dose of 10 Gy, the model predicts an eventual stature loss which declines with age at the time of radiotherapy; age 1 year, 3 cm; age 5, 2 cm; age 10, 1 cm (Silber et al. 1990). The incidence of flank muscle and soft tissue atrophy is difficult to estimate since radiation-related rib and iliac wing hypoplasia may contribute to its perception. It was considered grossly visible in 3 of 26 patients in one report (Thomas et al. 1983); however, the incidence was 30% in irradiated patients in the NWTS long-term follow-up study (Evans et al. 1991). Failure of breast development can follow chest radiotherapy in females. The greater skin-sparing effect of modern accelerators and a reduction in dose to 12 Gy may ameliorate this sequela.

Whole abdomen radiotherapy in prepubertal females with WT will impair ovarian function with a resulting increase in the plasma level of follicle-stimulating hormone. In one series, prepubertal males had a similar effect with a corresponding elevation of luteinizing hormone. No difference was noted between the effect of whole versus "hemiabdomen" portals. The lower extent of the whole abdomen portal was the "symphysis pubis." Details of portal boundaries for the "hemiabdomen" portal were not given (Perrone et al. 1988). Flank irradiation which does not extend beyond one hemipelvis in females is compatible with subsequent normal menses. Three of three such patients older than 12 years reported normal menses (Thomas et al. 1983).

Pregnancy outcome was unaffected in 13 females WT survivors who did not receive radiation and no significant adverse outcome was observed in 64 children of male WT survivors who did receive radiation. In contrast, child-bearing female survivors who received radiation were at excess risk (compared to American white females) for adverse pregnancy outcome (fetal death, neonatal mortality, and low birth weight). Thirty percent of 114 pregnancies had an adverse outcome (Li et al. 1987). Another study compared pregnancy outcome in WT survivors with that in their siblings. Females who survived WT were at risk mainly for early delivery or birth defects in their offspring, the rates for these sequelae being four times higher than in their sisters (Byrne et al. 1988). The mechanism for the aforementioned sequelae is postulated to be a direct effect on the uterus. Experimental confirmation is lacking.

Nephrectomy in childhood is followed by contralateral compensatory renal hypertrophy. This process occurs in all WT survivors (LANDMAN PARKER et al. 1991), but to a significantly diminished extent compared to children who had nephrectomy for hydronephrosis. The difference for WT patients is attributed to both chemotherapy and radiotherapy; however, the relative contribution of each could not be assessed. The contralateral kidney of irradiated patients received total radiation doses of 5–15 Gy (WIKSTAD et al. 1986). Functional reserve of the remaining kidney is not compromised (BHISITKUL et al. 1990), and hypertension in adulthood does not significantly exceed the expected incidence (KANTOR et al. 1989).

The NWTS committee has studied the second malignant neoplasms (excluding metachronous, contralateral WT) detected in survivors treated between 1969 and 1982. There were 15 patients, or about 1% of survivors. The relative risk was greater for children who received radiotherapy than for those who did not, but the difference was not significant. Affected children were more likely to be older or higher stage than the norms for the entire WT population. Second cancers attributable to radiation include those with a low probability of mortality (basal epithelioma and thyroid carcinoma) and types with uniform fatality (hepatocellular carcinoma and mesothelioma) (BRESLOW et al. 1988; KOVALIC et al. 1991; ANTMAN et al. 1984).

References

Antman KH, Ruxer RL, Aisner J, Vawter G (1984) Mesothelioma following Wilms' tumor in childhood. Cancer 54: 367–369

Beckwith JB (1969) Macroglossia, omphalocele, adrenal cytomegaly, gigantism and hyperplastic visceromegaly. In: Bergsma D, McKusick VA, Hall JG, Scott CI (eds) Birth defects. Original article series, vol 5. Stratton Intercontinental, New York, pp 188–196

Beckwith JB, Palmer NF (1978) Histopathology and prognosis of Wilms tumor. Cancer 41: 1937–1948

Bhisitkul DM, Morgan ER, Vozar MA, Langman CB (1990) Renal functional reserve in long term survivors of unilateral Wilms' tumor. J Pediatr 118: 698–702

Bishop HC, Tefft M, Evans AE, D'Angio GJ (1977) Survival in bilateral Wilms' tumor – review of 30 national Wilms' tumor study cases. J Pediatr Surg 12: 631–638

Blute ML, Kelalis PP, Offord KP, Breslow N, Beckwith JB, D'Angio GJ (1987) Bilateral Wilms' tumor. J Urol 138: 968–973

Bonadio JF, Storer B, Norkool P, Farewell VT, Beckwith JB, D'Angio GJ (1985) Anaplastic Wilms' tumor: Clinical and pathologic studies. J Clin Oncol 3: 513–520

Bonaiti-Pellie C, Chompret A, Tournade MF, Zucker JM, Sommelet D, Brunat M (1991) Genetics and epidemiology of Wilms' tumor: the French Wilms' Tumor Study. Med Pediatr Oncol 19: 339

Breslow NE, Palmer NF, Hill LR, Buring J, D'Angio GJ (1978) Wilms' tumor: Prognostic factor for patients without metastases at diagnosis. Cancer 41: 1577–1589

Breslow NE, Churchill G, Beckwith JB, Fernbach DJ, Otherson HB, Tefft M, D'Angio G (1985) Prognosis of Wilms' tumor with nonmetastatic disease disease at diagnosis-results of the second National Wilms' Tumor Study. J Clin Oncol 3: 521–531

Breslow NE, Churchill G, Nesmith B, Thomas PM, Beckwith JB, Othersen HB, D'Angio GJ (1986) Clinicopathologic features and prognosis for Wilms' tumor patients with metastases at diagnosis. Cancer 58: 2501–2511

Breslow NE, Norkool PA, Olshan A, Evans A, D'Angio GJ (1988) Second malignant neoplasms in survivors of Wilms' tumor: a report from the National Wilms' Tumor Study. J Natl Cancer Inst 80: 592–595

Breslow NE, Sharples K, Beckwith JB, Takashima J, Kelalis PP, Green DM, D'Angio GJ (1991) Prognostic factor in nonmetastatic, favorable histology Wilms' tumor. Cancer 68: 2345–2353

Burgers JMV, Tournade MF, Bey P et al. (1986) Abdominal recurrence in Wilms' tumors : a report from the SIOP Wilms' tumors trial and studies. Radiother Oncol 5: 175–182

Byrne J, Mulvihill JJ, Connelly RR et al. (1988) Reproductive problems and birth defects in survivors of Wilms' tumor and their relatives. Med Pediatr Oncol 16: 233–40

Cassady JR, Tefft M, Filler RM, Jaffe N, Hellman S (1973) Consideration in the radiation therapy of Wilms' tumor. Cancer 32: 598–608

Coppes MJ, deKraker J, van Dijken PJ et al. (1989) Bilateral Wilms' tumor: long-term survival and some epidemiological features. J Clin Oncol 7: 310–315

Corey SJ, Anderson JW, Vawter GF, Lack EE, Sallan SE (1991) Improved survival for children with anaplastic Wilms' tumor. Cancer 68: 970–974

Corn B, Goldwein JW, Norkool P, D'Angio GJ (1991) The outcome of babies treated according to the third National Wilms' Tumor Study. Med Pediatr Oncol 19: 412

Crist WM, Kun LE (1991a) Common solid tumors of childhood. N Engl J Med 324: 461–471

Crist WM, Kun LE (1991b) Common solid tumors of childhood. N Engl J Med 324: 1295

D'Angio GJ, Evans AE, Breslow N et al. (1976) The treatment of Wilms' tumor. Cancer 38: 633–646

D'Angio GJ, Evans A, Breslow N et al. (1981) The treatment of Wilms' tumor: results of the second National Wilms' Tumor Study. Cancer 47: 2302–2311

D'Angio GJ, Breslow N, Beckwith JB et al. (1989a) Treatment of Wilms' tumor: results of the third National Wilms' Tumor Study. Cancer 64: 349–360

D'Angio GJ, Bekwith JB, Breslow N, Finklestein J, Green, DM, Kelalis P (1989b) Wilms' tumor (nephroblastoma, renal embryoma). In: Pizzo PA, Poplack DG (eds) Pediatric oncology. JB Lippincott, Philadelphia, 583

de Kraker J, Lemerle J, Voute PA, Zucker JM, Tournade MF, Caril M (1990) Wilms' tumor with pulmonary metastases at diagnosis: the significance of primary chemotherapy. J Clin Oncol 8: 1187–1190

Douglass EC, Look AT, Webber B, Parham D, Wiliams JA, Green AA, Roberson PK (1986) Hyperdiploidy and chromosomal rearrangements define the anaplastic variant of Wilms' tumor. J Clin Oncol 4: 975–981

Drash A, Sherman F, Hartmann WH, Blizzard RM (1970) A syndrome of pseudohermaphorditism, Wilms' tumor, hypertension, and degenerative renal disease. J Pediatr 76: 585–593

Evans AE, Norkool P, Evans I, Breslow N, D'Angio GJ (1991) Late effects of treatment for Wilms' tumor. Cancer 67: 331–336

Feusner JH, Beckwith JB, D'Angio GJ (1990) Clear cell sarcoma of the kidney: accuracy of imaging methods for detecting bone metastases. Reports from the National Wilms' Tumor study. Med Pediatr Oncol 18: 225–227

Gibson AAM, Busuttil AA, Young DG, Flatman GE (1977) Glomerulosclerosis following irradiation and cytoxic therapy for nephroblastoma. Br J Urol 49: 199–201

Glass BJ, Davidson AJ, Fernbach SK (1991) Clear cell sarcoma of the kidney: CT, sonographic, and pathologic correlation. Radiology 180: 715–717

Green DM, Fine WE, Li FP (1982) Offspring of patients treated for unilateral Wilms' tumor in childhood. Cancer 49: 2285–2288

Green DM, Finklestein JZ, Tefft ME, Norkool P (1989) Diffuse interstitial pneumonitis after pulmonary irradiation for metastatic Wilms' tumor. Cancer 63: 450–453

Green DM, Fernbach DJ, Norkool P, Kollia G, D'Angio GJ (1991a) The treatment of Wilms' tumor patients with pulmonary metastases detected only with computed tomography: a report form the National Wilms' Tumor Study. J Clin Oncol 9: 1776–1781

Green DM, Breslow NE, Li Y, Grundy PE, Shochat SJ, Takashima J, D'Angio GJ (1991b) The role of surgical excision in the management of relapsed Wilms' tumor patients with pulmonary metastases. J Pediatr Surg 26: 728–733

Greenberg ML, Thorner P, Weitzman S et al. (1990) Pre-operative biopsy and chemotherapy for Wilm tumor. Proc ASCO 9: 292

Grundy P, Koufos A, Morgan K, Li FP, Meadows AT, Cavenee WK (1988) Familiar predisposition to Wilms' tumor does not map to the short arm of chromosomes 11. Nature 336: 374–376

Grundy P, Breslow N, Green DM, Sharpless K, Evans A, D'Angio GJ (1989) Prognostic factors for children with recurrent Wilms' tumor: results from the second and third National Wilms' Tumor Study. J Clin Oncol 7: 638–647

Heaston DK, Libshitz HI, Chan RC (1979) Skeletal effects of megavoltage irradiation in survivors of Wilms' tumor. AJR 133: 389–395

Huff V, Compton DA, Chao LY, Strong LC, Geiser CF, Saunders GF (1988) Lack of linkage familial Wilms' tumour to chromosomal band 11p13. Nature 336; 377–378

Jones B, Breslow NE, Takashima J (1984) Toxic deaths in the second National Wilms' Tumor Study. J Clin Oncol 2: 1028–1033

Joshi VV, Beckwith JB (1990) Pathologic delineation of the papillionodular type of cystic partially differentiated nephroblastoma. Cancer 66: 1568–1577

Kantor AF, Li FP, Janov AJJ, Tarbell NJ, Sallan SE (1989) Hypertension in long-term survivors of childhood renal cancers. J Clin Oncol 7: 912–915

Kogan SJ, Marans H, Santorineau M, Schneider K, Reda E, Levitt SB (1986) Successful treatment of renal vein and vena caval extension of nephroblastoma by preoperative chemotherapy. J Urol 136; 312–317

Kovalic JJ, Thomas PRM, Beckwith JB, Feusner JH, Norkool PA (1991) Hepatocellular carcinoma as second malignant neoplasms in successfully treated Wilms' tumor patients. Cancer 67: 342–344

Landman Parker J, Tournade MF, Salloum E et al. (1991) Minimal renal sequelate twenty years after unilateral nephrectomy for Wilms' tumor (WT) treatment. Med Pediatr Oncol 19: 430

Larsen E, Perez-Atayde A, Green DM, Retik A, Clavell LA, Sallan SE (1990) Surgery only for the treatment of patients with stage I (Cassady) Wilms' tumor. Cancer 66: 264–266

Lemerle J, Vouted PA, Tournade MF et al. (1983) Effectiveness of preoperative chemotherapy in Wilms' tumor: results of an International Society of Paediatric Oncology (SIOP) Clinical trial. J Clin Oncol 1: 604–609

Li FP, Gimbrere K, Gelber RD et al. (1987) Outcome of pregnancy in survivors of Wilms' tumor. JAMA 257: 216–219

Macklis RM, Oltikar A, Salla SE (1991) Wilms' tumor patients with pulmonary metastases. Int J Radiat Oncol Biol Phys 21: 1187–1193

Malcolm AW, Jaffe N, Folkman J, Cassady RJ (1980) Bilateral Wilms' tumor. Int J Radiat Oncol Biol Phys 6: 167–174

Marsden HB, Lawler W, Kumar PM (1978) Bone metastasizing renal tumor of childhood. Cancer 42: 1922–1928

Moutou C, Chompret A, Hochez J, Tournade MF, Zucker JM, Lemerle J, Bonaiti-Pellie (1991) Mutation theory of carcinogeneses in Wilms' tumor. Med Pediatr Oncol 19: 352

Nakayama K, deLorimier AA, O'Neill JA, Norkool P, D'Angio GJ (1986) Intracardiac extension of Wilms' tumor. Ann Surg 204: 693–697

National Wilms' Tumor Committee (1991) Wilms' tumor: status report, 1990. J Clin Oncol 9: 877–887

Oberholzer HF, Falkson G, DeJager LC (1992) Successful management of inferior vena cava and right atrial nephroblastoma tumor thrombus with preoperative chemotherapy. Med Pediatr Oncol 20: 61–63

Oliver JH, Gluck G, Geldhill RB, Chevalier L (1978) Musculoskeletal deformities following treatment of Wilms' tumour. Can Med Assoc J 119: 459–464

Olshan AF, Breslow NE, Daling JR et al. (1990) Wilms' tumor and paternal occupation. Cancer Res 50: 3212–3217

Pastore G, Carli M, Lemerle J et al. (1988) Epidemiological features of Wilms' tumor: results of studies by the International Society of Pediatric Oncology (SIOP). Med Pediatric Oncol 16: 7–11

Perlman M, Goldberg GM, Bar-Ziv J, Danovitch G (1973) Renal hamartomas and nephroblastomatosis with fetal gigantism: a familial syndrome. J Pediatr 83: 414–418

Perrone L, Sinisi AA, Sicuranza R et al. (1988) Prepubertal endocrine follow-up in subjects with Wilms' tumor. Med Pediatr Oncol 16: 255–258rd

Ping AJ, Reeve AE, Law DJ, Young MR, Boehnke M, Feinberg AP (1989) Genetic linkage of Beckwith Wiedemann syndrome to 11p15. Am J Hum Genet 44: 720–723

Pinkerton CR, Groot-Loonen JJ, Morris-Jones PH, Pritchard J (1991) Response rates in relapsed Wilms' tumor. Cancer 67: 567–571

Rate WR, Butler MS, Robertson WW, D'Angio GJ (1991) Late orthopedic effects in children with Wilms' tumor treated with abdominal irradiation. Med Pediatr Oncol 19: 265–268

Riseborough EJ, Grabias SL, Burton RI, Jaffe N (1976) Skeletal alterations following irradiation for Wilms' tumor. J Bone Joint Surg [AM] 58: 526–536

Ritchey ML, Kelais PP, Breslow N, Offord KP, Shochat SJ, D'Angio GJ (1988) Intracaval and atrial involvement with nephroblastoma: review of National Wilms' Tumor Study-3. J Urol 140: 1113–1118

Saarinen UM, Wikstrom S, Koskimies O, Sariola H (1991) Percutaneous needle biopsy preceding preoperative chemotherapy in the management of massive renal tumors in children. J Clin Oncol 9: 406–415

Silber JH, Littman PS, Meadows AT (1990) Stature loss following skeletal irradiation for childhood cancer. J Clin Oncol 8: 304–312

Sisler CL, Siegel MJ (1989) Malignant rhabdoid tumor of the kidney: radiological features. Radiology 172: 211–212

Steinfeld AD, Crowley CA, O'Shea PA, Tefft M (1984) Recurrent and metastatic mesoblastic nephroma in infancy. J Clin Oncol 2: 956–960

Thomas PRM, Griffith KD, Fineberg BB, Perez CA, Land VJ (1983) Late effects of treatment for Wilms' tumor. Int J Radiat Oncol Biol Phys 9: 651–657

Thomas PRM, Tefft M, Farewell VT, Norkool P, Storer B, D'Angio GJ (1984) Abdominal relapses in irradiated second National Wilms' Tumor Study patients. J Clin Oncol 2: 1098–1101

Thomas PRM, Tefft M, D'Angio GJ, Norkool P (1988) Acute Toxicities associated with radiation in the second National Wilms' Tumor Study. J Clin Oncol 6: 1694–1698

Thomas PRM, Tefft M, Compaan PJ, Norkool P, Breslow NE, D'Angio GJ (1991a) Results of two radiation therapy randomizations in the third National Wilms' Tumor Study. Cancer 68: 1703–1707

Thomas PRM, Schochat SJ, Norkool P, Beckwith JB, Breslow NE, D'Angio GJ (1991b) Prognostic implication of hepatic adhesion, invasion, and metastases at diagnosis of Wilms' tumor. Cancer 68: 2486–2488

Tournade MF, Ludwig R, Voute PA et al. (1991) Preliminary report of the nephroblastoma clinical trial SIOP 9. Med Pediatr Oncol 19: 437

Wallace WHB, Shalet SM, Morris-Jones PH, Swindell R, Gattamaneni HR (1990) Effect of abdominal irradiation on growth in boys treated for a Wilms' tumor. Med Pediatr Oncol 18: 441–446

Weeks DA, Beckwith JB, Luckey DW (1987) Relapse-associated variables in stage I favorable histology Wilms' tumor. Cancer 60: 1204–1212

Weeks DA, Beckwith JB, Mierau GW, Luckey DW (1989) Rhabdoid tumor of kidney: a report of 111 cases from the National Wilms' Tumor Study Pathology Center. Am J Surg Pathol 13: 439–458

Wikstad I, Pettersson BA, Elinder G, Sokucu S, Aperia A (1986) A comparative study of size and function in the remnant kidney in patients nephrectomized in childhood for Wilms' tumor and hydronephrosis. Acta Pediatr Scand 75: 408–414

Yeger H, Huang A, Flenniken A, Bonetta L, Campbell C, Coppes MJ, Williams BRG (1991) Tumor specific expression of two 11p13 transcripts provide a basis for the histopathologic heterogeneity in Wilms' tumor. Med Pediatr Oncol 19: 340

Zuppan CW, Beckwith JB, Luckey DW (1988) Anaplasia in unilateral Wilms' tumor: a report form the National Wilms' Tumor Study Pathology Center. Hum Pathol 19: 1199–1209

Zuppan CW, Beckwith JB, Weeks DA, Luckey DW, Pringle KC (1991) The effect of preoperative therapy on the histologic features of Wilms' tumor. Cancer 68: 385–394

18 Ewing's Sarcoma

ROBERT B. MARCUS, JR.

CONTENTS

18.1　Introduction 265
18.2　Epidemiology and Clinical Features 265
18.3　Diagnosis 266
18.4　Prognostic Features 266
18.5　Treatment of Localized Disease 267
18.5.1 General 267
18.5.2 Systemic Therapy 267
18.5.3 Local Therapy 268
18.5.4 Pulmonary Irradiation 273
18.6　Treatment of Patients with Metastatic
　　　Disease at Diagnosis 273
18.7　Prognosis 273
18.8　Salvage 274
18.9　Follow-up 274
18.10 Complications 275
18.11 New Directions 277
　　　References 278

18.1 Introduction

Ewing's sarcoma is one of a number of small-round-cell sarcomas that occur in childhood, though its exact origin continues to elude investigators. Pathologically, the best definition is that it is a tumor of small, round, blue cells, usually but not always associated with bone, that lacks markers for lymphoma, neuroblastoma, or rhabdomyosarcoma (WOMER 1991). It is not yet clear whether it is a heterogeneous group of tumors that contains subgroups, or a single entity to which several other diagnoses belong. There are two different opinions regarding the origin of Ewing's sarcoma: that it is of neuroectodermal origin, or that it arises from primitive, undifferentiated, mesenchymal cells (WOMER 1991). If the latter is true, the tumor might be better regarded as a blastoma than as a true sarcoma.

Many Ewing's sarcomas have a translocation between chromosomes 11 and 22 [t(11;22)] (TURC-

ROBERT B. MARCUS, JR. M.D. Professor of Radiation Oncology and Pediatrics, Department of Radiation Oncology, University of Florida Health Science Center, PO Box 100385, Gainesville, FL 32610-0385, USA

CAREL et al. 1988). This translocation is present only in tumor cells and not in normal cells taken from the same patients (WOMER 1991). It is present in both osseous and extraosseous variants, as well as primitive neuroectodermal tumors (PNETs) and peripheral neuroectodermal tumors (malignant neuroepitheliomas).

The relationship between classic Ewing's sarcoma of bone and PNET of bone is still controversial: are they variants of the same tumor or are they completely different tumors with some similarities? The former is most likely, and, except where specific reference is made to PNET of bone, they will be considered together as Ewing's sarcoma.

18.2 Epidemiology and Clinical Features

Ewing's sarcoma is primarily a disease of the second decade of life, being less common before age 8 years and after age 25 years (Fig. 18.1a) (KISSANE et al. 1983). Only rare cases have been reported in blacks. Whereas osteosarcomas have been shown to be related to increased stature, Ewing's sarcoma is probably not (PENDERGRASS et al. 1984). Males are more frequently affected than females; 61% of the patients were males and 39% females in the first Intergroup Ewing's Sarcoma Study (IESS-I) (KISSANE et al. 1983).

In IESS-I, two-thirds of the cases of primary Ewing's sarcoma of bone occurred in the lower half of the skeleton, with 22.8% presenting in the pelvis, 20.8% in the femur, and 24.8% below the knee. In the upper half of the body, 10.6% presented in the humerus and 6.9% in the ribs. All other sites are less common, as shown in Fig. 18.1b (KISSANE et al. 1983).

Pain and swelling are the most frequent presenting symptoms. Both tend to be progressive, though pain can appear, then ebb for a few weeks or months. Symptoms of systemic disease occur at times, including low-grade fevers, malaise, and weakness.

Ewing's sarcoma patients exhibit a mean lag time between the onset of symptoms and diagnosis of 146

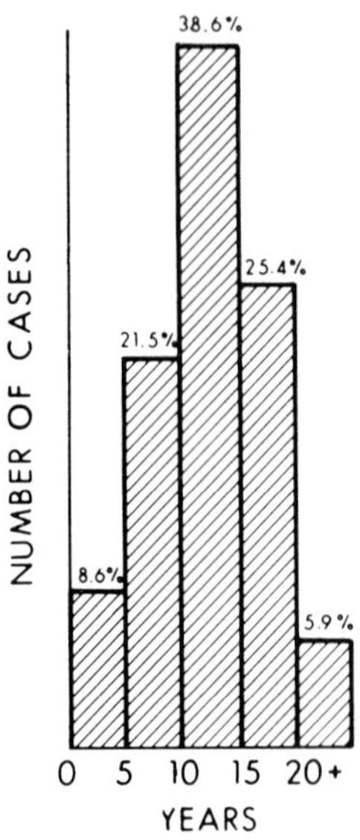

Fig. 18.1a,b. First Intergroup Ewing's Sarcoma Study (IESS-1) – 303 patients. **a** Distribution by age. **b** Distribution by site. (From Kissane et al. 1983)

days, the longest lag time of any pediatric solid tumor (POLLOCK et al. 1991).

18.3 Diagnosis

Even though Ewing's sarcoma may be strongly suspected, it is preferable to thoroughly evaluate the lesion before the biopsy. This evaluation would include plain films, computed tomography (CT), and magnetic resonance imaging (MRI) of the primary lesion. Plain films usually reveal a mottled or moth-eaten lesion involving the bone. Lytic and blastic areas may be present; lytic areas are more commonly seen. Subperiosteal reactive new bone may be present, producing an "onion-skin" appearance. This characteristic is not pathognomonic but may be found in many other bone lesions. At times Ewing's sarcoma, like an osteosarcoma, may produce spicules radiating from the cortex of the involved bone. At other times it may cause expansion of the bone, producing a cystic-appearing tumor. Occasionally the tumor may appear to arise on the surface of the bone, producing a saucerlike indentation of the surface (EDEIKEN and KARASICK 1987).

The radiographic differential diagnosis includes osteosarcoma, osteomyelitis, eosinophilic granuloma, primary lymphoma of the bone, and even an occasional metastatic malignancy.

Both CT and MRI of the primary lesion are valuable in determining the extent of the lesion. An MRI scan will show the extent of bone marrow involvement and soft tissue invasion, while bone destruction is best seen using CT.

The systemic workup should include blood studies (a complete blood cell count, differential count, platelet count, renal function studies, liver function studies, and erythrocyte sedimentation study), a chest roentgenogram, a CT scan of the chest, a bone scan, and a bone marrow biopsy. Approximately 20% of patients present with metastatic disease, most frequently lung metastasis. Cortical bone metastasis is not uncommon, and bone marrow involvement occasionally occurs. Brain metastasis, as well as metastasis to other organs, is extremely rare at diagnosis.

18.4 Prognostic Features

Multiple prognostic features have been suggested in the literature. Metastasis at diagnosis, unfavorable site of the primary tumor, a large primary tumor, the presence of a large soft tissue mass, a high lactic dehy-

Table 18.1. Five-year survival according to tumor size

Institution	Small		Large	
	Survival (%)	Definition	Survival (%)	Definition
University of Florida (MARCUS and MILLION 1984)	72	≤8 cm	22	>8 cm
CESS-81 (SAUER et al. 1987)	72	<100 cm³	32	≥100 cm³
Massachusetts General Hospital (SAILER et al. 1988)	70	<500 cm³	34	≥500 cm³
Instituto Radioterapia, Bologna (BARBIERI et al. 1990)	58	<100 cm³	32	≥100 cm³

drogenase (LDH) level at diagnosis, poor response to induction chemotherapy, failure to use surgery as part of the treatment of the primary lesion, and a filigree histologic pattern have all been proposed as poor prognostic factors (JÜRGENS et al. 1988; MARCUS and MILLION 1984; OBERLIN et al. 1985; SAILER et al. 1988; SAUER et al. 1987). Some of these are interrelated, since tumors in the pelvis, prognostically the worst site, are usually large and have a large soft tissue mass. In general, large tumors have a higher rate of metastatic disease at diagnosis, though small tumors can present with metastases as well.

The two most significant prognostic features known at this time are the size of the primary tumor and the presence of metastatic disease at diagnosis. Most institutions that have reported results by tumor size have divided lesions into two groups, small and large, though, in general, each institution has developed its own criteria for that differentiation. MARCUS and MILLION (1984) and Marcus et al. (1988) at the University of Florida used 8 cm in greatest diameter as the cutoff between large and small tumors, as did ARAI et al. (1991) at St. Jude Children's Research Hospital. SAILER et al. (1988) at Massachusetts General Hospital reported a tumor volume of 500 cm³ as the cutoff, while the German Cooperative Group (JÜRGENS et al. 1988; SAUER et al. 1987) used a tumor volume of 100 cm³ as the cutoff. As shown in Table 18.1, the results for "large" and "small" tumors were very similar at all of these institutions, even though different criteria were used.

The presence of distant metastases reduces the 5-year survival rate to approximately 20%, with essentially all of the survivors coming from the group of patients with lung metastases only. Patients with bone metastases or bone marrow metastases are exceedingly difficult to cure.

18.5 Treatment of Localized Disease

18.5.1 General

Effective local therapy *and* effective systemic therapy are necessary for the cure of Ewing's sarcoma. Alone, neither will produce a cure rate above 5%–10%.

18.5.2 Systemic Therapy

A number of drugs are effective in the treatment of Ewing's sarcoma, including cyclophosphamide, doxorubicin hydrochloride (Adriamycin), vincristine, dactinomycin, ifosfamide, and etoposide. Most regimens are a combination of these (ARAI et al. 1991; BADER et al. 1989; BURGERT et al. 1990; CANGIR et al. 1990; CAPANNA et al. 1990; DUNST et al. 1991; EVANS et al. 1991; HAYES et al. 1989; KINSELLA et al. 1983; NESBIT et al. 1990; OBERLIN et al. 1985; SAILER et al. 1988; WILKINS et al. 1986). In the past, when radiation therapy was the local treatment, the systemic regimen would begin simultaneously with the local therapy. For those patients who had a surgical excision, the systemic therapy was not started until after the resection. Now, many institutions have switched to using induction chemotherapy, whether the local treatment is surgery or irradiation. The advantages of this approach are several: (a) giving the chemotherapy first allows an evaluation of the effectiveness of the regimen for each patient; (b) shrinkage of the soft tissue mass may help the surgeon or radiation oncologist to decrease the volume of the local therapy; and (c) some bone healing takes place during the chemotherapy, which may diminish the risk of pathologic fracture if radiation therapy is used to treat the primary lesion. The response to induction chemotherapy is quite good, with complete response rates of 50% and partial response rates of 40% reported by several groups (Marcus et al. 1991; Hayes et al. 1989; Oberlin et al. 1985). Those patients who do not respond, however, and especially those whose lesions progress during induction chemotherapy, do very poorly, but it is doubtful that they would fare better with any other approach.

18.5.3 Local Therapy

Historically, radiation therapy has been the treatment of choice for the control of disease at the primary tumor site. This philosophy evolved because of the dismal prognosis of the disease before the use of systemic chemotherapy. Almost every patient with the disease died, so there was no advantage to ablative surgery over local radiotherapy, which could preserve limb function for the remainder of the patient's life. If there were a large number of local recurrences (which was usually the case, since local control without chemotherapy was <70%), it hardly mattered because of the high mortality.

However, because of the improved prognosis with present therapy, there is renewed interest in the surgical treatment of the primary disease. The evaluation of both local therapies is continuing, but it is clear that both will play an important role in the management of Ewing's sarcoma for years to come.

18.5.3.1 Surgery

Surgery is necessary for a biopsy, and some lesions are best treated with a surgical approach. The biopsy should be performed in the same institution in which the treatment will be performed. Preferably the bone should not be violated, and since most Ewing's tumors have a soft tissue component, it is usually not necessary to biopsy the bone. An adequate amount of tissue should be obtained for both light and electron microscopy. Usually an open biopsy is preferred, but in experienced hands a large needle biopsy may be sufficient.

The biopsy incision should be directly over the portion of the tumor to be sampled. A limited amount of dissection should be performed, and in general it is better to go through a muscle rather than dissect extensively around it (Pritchard 1989). It is important to maintain hemostasis throughout the procedure. Drains, if needed, should be brought out as near the incision as possible, as the drain site is a potentially contaminated area. If it is necessary to penetrate the cortex of the bone, the tension site of the bone should be avoided to reduce the risk of pathologic fracture. Proximal femur lesions have the highest risk of fracture and should not be approached laterally (O'Connor and Pritchard 1991; Pritchard 1989), but rather anteriorly, medially, or posteriorly. Plugging the biopsy site with methylmethacrylate may also help decrease the risk of subsequent pathologic fracture.

If surgery is chosen for the treatment of the primary lesion, then it is necessary to determine whether limb salvage therapy is possible. Certain sites are more amenable to conservative surgery than others. Lesions of the proximal fibula, ribs, clavicle, and wing of the ilium are easier to resect than those of most other sites. Lesions of the bones of the hands and feet may be resectable with a ray resection. Amputation, however, remains an option for some patients.

Lesions of the fibula, tibia, and foot in younger patients, where the growth deficits caused by radiation therapy result in major deformities, are certainly candidates for primary surgery.

18.5.3.2 Radiation Therapy

Ewing's sarcoma is thought to be a disease originating in the marrow cavity. Because of this, radiation oncologists traditionally included the entire marrow cavity for at least part of the treatment.

This philosophy has been questioned in three recent trials. In 1980, St. Jude Children's Research Hospital began a pilot study where less-than-whole-bone treatment was given (Arai et al. 1991), followed in 1982 by a pilot study at the University of Florida (Marcus et al. 1991). Both studies demonstrated excellent local control rates for small lesions (<8 cm in maximum diameter), but the local control rates for larger lesions have been poor in the St. Jude Children's Research Hospital series, and though local control rates for these lesions have been excellent in the University of Florida series, patients with large lesions usually received total body irradiation of 8 or 12 Gy, thus giving them some treatment to the entire marrow cavity. In 1983 the Pediatric Oncology Group started a randomized trial comparing standard whole-bone irradiation with tailored irradiation consisting of the lesion at diagnosis (including the soft tissue extension) plus a 2-cm margin. The study closed in 1989, and an analysis is ongoing (Donaldson S.S., personal communication, 1992). It is probable that irradiation of the entire

Table 18.2. Local control by method of treatment to primary lesions (localized lesions only)

Treatment, institution	Total dose to tumor (Gy)	Dose per fraction (Gy)	Local control (%)			5-year relapse- free survival (%)
			Small	Large	All	
Radiotherapy alone (q.d. fractionation)						
IESS-1 (Nesbit et al. 1990)	55–65	2.0	ND	ND	85	24–60
IESS-2 (pelvic) (Evans et al. 1991)	55	2.0	ND	ND	85	55
University of Florida (Marcus R.B. Jr, unpublished data, 1991)	50–60	1.8–2.0	94	66	76	45
St. Jude (Arai et al. 1991)	30-60	1.75 median	94	44	57	52
CESS-81 (Jürgens et al. 1988)	45–60	1.8–2.0	65	31	52	43
CESS-81 (Dunst et al. 1991)	60	1.8–2.0 or 1.6 b. i. d.	ND	ND	87	67 (3 yr)
National Cancer Institute (Kinsella et al. 1988)	55–60	2.0	ND	ND	87	50[a]
Instituto Radioterapia, Bologna (Barbieri et al. 1990)	45–60	1.8–2.0	93	57	69	30
Massachusetts General Hospital (Sailer et al. 1988)	40–50	ND	86	57	79	54
Radiotherapy alone (b.i.d. fractionation)						
University of Florida (Marcus R.B. Jr, unpublished date, 1992)	50.4–67.2[b]	1.2 b.i.d.	88	87	88	70
Combined treatment (surgery + radiotherapy)						
CESS-81 (Jürgens et al. 1988)	36	1.8–2.0	94	69	83	68[c]
Instituto Radioterapia, Bologna (Barbieri et al. 1990)	45–55	1.8–2.0	ND	ND	93	48[c]
Memorial Sloan-Kettering (Jereb et al. 1986)	30–45	2.0	ND	ND	89	63
Surgery alone						
CESS-81 (Jürgens et al. 1988)	–	–	94	100	96	65[c]
Instituto Radioterapia (Barbieri et al. 1990)	–	–	ND	ND	94	59[c]

[a] Patient population includes some with other round-cell tumors as well as those with Ewing's sarcoma.
[b] Includes total body irradiation (8 or 12 Gy) to patients with large lesions.
[c] Selection toward using surgery for the smaller lesions occurred in these studies.

marrow cavity is not necessary, but no series has yet reported acceptable local control using less-than-whole-bone treatment for large lesions.

The dose to be used with standard fractionation schemes is well established, even though no dose-response curve has been demonstrated for this disease. Doses of 40–50 Gy at 1.8–2 Gy per day to the entire marrow cavity (if this volume is to be treated) are given, with a boost to the primary tumor site of 10–15 Gy, also at 1.8–2 Gy per day, for a total tumor dose of 50–60 Gy. Local control rates of 50%–88% have been reported with these doses (Table 18.2). Lower doses have not been studied recently except at St. Jude Children's Research Hospital (Arai et al. 1991). In this study, patients received 35 Gy if a complete remission was obtained with induction chemotherapy, and though local control was good for small lesions (<8 cm), it was poor for larger lesions, as noted previously. It is unclear whether the poor local control for large lesions is a result of decreasing the volume treated or decreasing the dose, though the latter seems more likely, as the

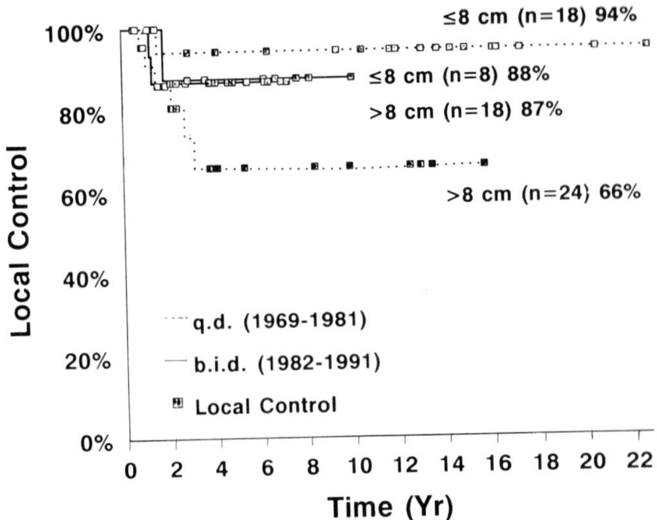

Fig.18.2. Actuarial local control of patients treated with radiation therapy alone at the University of Florida from 1969 through 1990. Patients treated from 1969 through 1981 were treated with standard q.d. regimens. Patients treated from 1982 through 1990 were treated with b.i.d. regimens as described in the text. Small lesions were controlled well with all fractionations, but larger lesions were controlled better with the b.i.d. regimens. The majority of patients with large primary lesions also underwent total body irradiation (8 or 12 Gy) and autologous bone marrow transplantation

majority of local failures appeared to occur in the middle of the treatment field.

The type of chemotherapy used may also influence the local control rate. In IESS-I, the use of doxorubicin was shown to increase local control rates (THOMAS et al. 1984).

Twice-a-day irradiation has been used by the University of Florida and as one arm of the CESS-86 study of the German Cooperative Ewing's Sarcoma Study Group. The fractionation used at the University of Florida since 1982 is 1.2 Gy b.i.d. (with a 6-h interfraction interval) to a total dose of 50.4 Gy, 55.2 Gy, or 60 Gy, depending on the response to induction chemotherapy (Marcus et al. 1991). Whole-bone irradiation was not intended, but for large lesions, particularly those occurring in the pelvis, the entire medullary cavity was included in the majority of patients to encompass the original tumor volume. A reduction to just the residual tumor volume after induction chemotherapy was made after 36 Gy. Patients in the high-risk category (metastases at diagnosis or primary lesions >8 cm in maximum diameter) also received a total body irradiation dose of either 8 or 12 Gy (see Sect. 18.11). Though the total dose and fractionation for this protocol were designed primarily to decrease late effects and not necessarily to increase local control, the local control has been good, as shown in Fig. 18.2 and Table 18.2.

In the CESS-86 study, doses of 1.6 Gy b.i.d. to a total of 60 Gy were used. Results of this study show no difference between the b.i.d. regimen and standard irradiation, though follow-up is short to date (DUNST et al. 1991). However, this fractionation

scheme is not likely to decrease late effects, and may even increase them.

The most important factor in the treatment of Ewing's sarcoma is the treating radiation oncologist, as shown in the CESS-81 study of the German Cooperative Group. In this study, the relapse-free survival in patients treated with radiation therapy alone was improved from 50% to 80% by requiring all treatment volumes to be planned by a central planning agency (SAUER et al. 1987). This eliminated one of the most frequent sources of failure: geographic miss. It is crucial to carefully map out the tumor volume from a good CT scan or MRI scan (or both). Even though less-than-whole-bone irradiation has not definitely been proven to be adequate for large lesions, the standard of care (including the present Intergroup Ewing's Sarcoma Study) is evolving to such "tailored fields." If such an approach is chosen, the initial field should include the prechemotherapy volume with a 4-cm margin, if possible, to a dose of 35–40 Gy. At that point, a reduction to the residual tumor volume should be made and a boost given for another 15–20 Gy (total dose 50–60 Gy) (Fig. 18.3). It may be adequate to use smaller volumes (Arai et al. 1991) for the entire course of treatment, but additional information is required before considering this to be the standard therapy, as large lesions were not well controlled with this approach. If volumes that do not include the entire marrow cavity are employed, then a prechemotherapy MRI scan is necessary. *Any* abnormal signals from the marrow cavity in the same bone as the primary lesion, even if distant from that lesion, should be considered disease and treated.

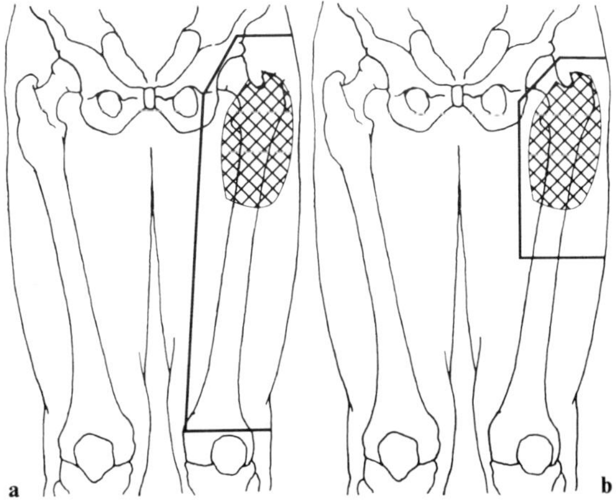

Fig.18.3a,b. A comparison of "whole-bone" fields versus "tailored" field. **a** A standard whole-bone field drawn around the *initial* tumor volume. In this example, the distal femoral epiphysis is spared, though this is not a universally accepted approach. **b** Tailored fields around the same lesion. The margins used for such an approach vary widely. Some institutions plan the radiation therapy based on the initial tumor volume (as shown here), while others treat based on the volume after induction chemotherapy. There is no universally accepted approach; at the University of Florida the former approach is used. The tailored fields are, in fact, similar to the boost fields commonly used after the delivery of whole-bone irradiation (also see text)

During the treatment of extremity lesions, it is necessary to spare at least a 1- to 2-cm strip of tissue to prevent lymphedema. Occasionally, particularly in arm lesions, this can be very difficult. A dose of 20–30 Gy can usually be given to the entire circumference of an arm without significant sequelae, but for further treatment it is necessary to reduce to a field that spares a strip of tissue. The leg is less tolerant. Neoadjuvant chemotherapy, with the significant shrinkage of disease that occurs during this phase of treatment, often allows for tighter margins than would be possible if the course of irradiation was concomitant with the first course of chemotherapy.

In extremity lesions, it is preferable to spare at least one epiphysis. For reference, the amount of growth potential remaining in each epiphysis is discussed in Sect. 18.10. It is usually not possible to choose which epiphysis to spare; in a diaphyseal lesion it is sometimes possible to spare both.

Pelvic lesions can usually be treated with opposed anterior and posterior fields. With present chemotherapy, which includes high doses of cyclophosphamide or ifosfamide, the most important structure to avoid in the pelvis is the bladder. Radiation cystitis can be a significant risk even at doses as small as 20 Gy. Since pelvic lesions rarely infiltrate into the tissues around the bladder, but

instead tend to push aside those structures, neoadjuvant chemotherapy allows additional bladder to be spared if good shrinkage is obtained. A 2-cm medial margin is adequate.

Rib lesions are difficult to irradiate, as damage to the heart, lungs, or liver can be fatal. Irradiating the entire rib with opposed anterior and posterior fields is not worth the risk of complications to these organs, though great care must be taken not to miss any area of involvement. It is usually necessary to use tangential fields or wedged pairs of fields. Surgical resection can be of great value in decreasing morbidity.

The choice of energies is also important. For lesions in areas where the bone is close to the surface of the skin, such as hand, foot, forearm, distal leg, or some rib lesions, it is necessary to use no greater than 6 MV, and sometimes cobalt-60 or 4 MV may be preferable. Lesions in the pelvis or proximal lower extremity are best treated with a higher-energy beam. The biopsy site should be included in the field, but scar recurrences are rare. It is usually not necessary to add a bolus to the scar.

If doxorubicin or dactinomycin is given during the course of radiation therapy, moist desquamation will often occur in areas of tangential irradiation or skin folds, particularly if lower energy beams (6 MV or less) are used. If a course of chemotherapy containing one or both of these drugs is given within a few weeks after finishing irradiation, a "recall" phenomenon can occur, in which dry or moist desquamation appears where none was present before.

18.5.3.3 Postoperative Irradiation

The question of when to add postoperative irradiation is controversial. Patients who undergo a radical resection (usually an amputation) probably do not need postoperative irradiation, but when conservative surgery is used, postoperative irradiation is usually given. Data from JEREB et al. (1986) indicate that the local recurrence rate after conservative surgery is high without irradiation; in the Memorial Sloan-Kettering Cancer Center (MSKCC) protocols involving induction chemotherapy followed by conservative surgery, 6 of 11 patients who did *not* receive postoperative irradiation (including two of five patients with no tumor found at the time of surgery) suffered a local recurrence, while only 5 (11%) of 47 patients who did receive postoperative irradiation developed a local recurrence (Table 18.3). The actuarial absolute survival rate for patients receiving postoperative irradiation was 63% at 5 years

Table 18.3. Local control and survival for patients receiving postoperative radiotherapy versus no postoperative radiotherapy[a]

Surgical pathologic findings[b]	Local failure		5-Year survival	
	RT	No RT	RT	No RT
No tumor	0/23	2/5	21/23	2/5
Residual tumor, margins negative	4/19	2/4	9/19	0/4
Residual tumor, margins positive	1/5	2/2	0/5	0/2

[a] Data from Jereb et al. (1986).
[b] All patients underwent surgery after induction chemotherapy.

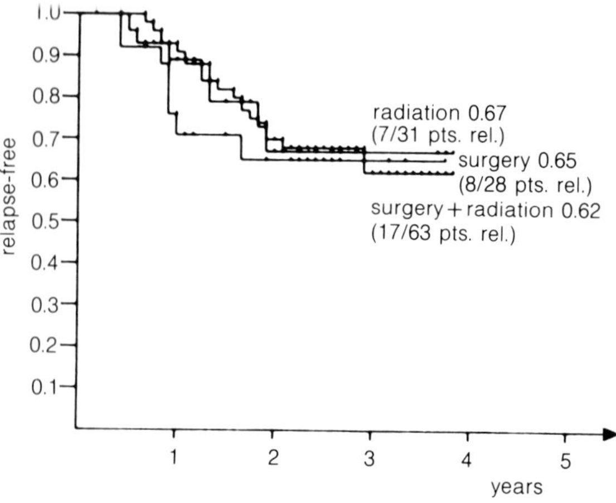

Fig. 18.4. Relapse-free survival in the German Cooperative Ewing's Sarcoma Study CESS-86 according to type of treatment given the primary lesion: radiation alone, surgery alone, or combined surgery and radiation therapy. The difference between the types of local treatment was not significant ($p = 0.74$, long rank test). (From Dunst et al. 1991)

compared with 13% for those who did not receive it. Therefore, it appears that the majority of patients need postoperative radiotherapy if conservative surgery is employed. The poor survival results for patients with residual tumor and positive margins probably reflect a lack of response to the systemic therapy rather than a failure of local therapy.

As shown in Table 18.2, doses in the range of 30–40 Gy are clearly effective in the postoperative treatment of subclinical disease. The fields used should be generous, however, covering the entire surgical bed and residual bone with 3- to 5-cm margins.

18.5.3.4 Choice of Local Therapy

Table 18.2 shows the local control and survival rates for patients treated with radiation alone, surgery alone, and a combination of surgery and irradiation in several recent series.

Before the 1980s, radiation therapy was the accepted local therapy for most primary Ewing's sarcomas of bone. However, several recent reports have stated that patients treated with a component of surgery have a better prognosis than patients treated with radiation therapy alone. Wilkins et al. (1986) reported a 74% 5-year survival rate for patients receiving a surgical resection, while those who received only radiation therapy to the primary lesion had a 34% 5-year survival rate. Sailer et al. (1988), from Massachusetts General Hospital, reported a 91% 5-year survival rate for patients undergoing surgery (with or without radiation therapy), with only a 54% 5-year survival rate for those receiving radiation therapy as the primary treatment. The German Cooperative Group reported similar results

from CESS-81 (Jürgens et al. 1988; Sauer et al. 1987), as did Barbieri et al. (1990). The problem with these studies is the difficulty in determining whether selection of surgery for small, peripherally located tumors, which have a better prognosis, may have influenced the results. Barbieri et al. (1990) clearly show a selection bias toward treating large lesions with radiation therapy alone, using surgery or combined local therapy on smaller lesions.

Other studies show no advantage for patients undergoing surgery. In IESS-II, for the nonpelvic lesions, it was recommended that surgery be used whenever possible to treat the primary lesion; 92 patients underwent surgery (an unknown number had postoperative irradiation), whereas 106 received radiation therapy alone. The 5-year relapse-free survival rates were 65% for the surgery group and 63% for the radiation therapy group. The 5-year relapse-free survival rate for the 25 patients undergoing an amputation was 66%, while it was 63% for a "complete resection" and 64% for an "incomplete resection" (Burgert et al. 1990).

In CESS-86, institutions have a choice between radiotherapy alone, surgery alone, and combined surgery and postoperative radiotherapy. Comparing the results of treatment of 122 patients treated between January 1986 and November 1989, there is no difference to date between the three arms of the study (Fig. 18.4). The longest follow-up reported, however, is less than 4 years; additional follow-up may change the results (Dunst et al. 1991).

Based on these results, it is difficult to strongly conclude that surgery plays a critical role in the treatment of Ewing's sarcoma patients. More than 90% of Ewing's sarcoma patients have either detectable or subclinical metastases at diagnosis, so that local therapy (either surgery, irradiation, or a combination), if delivered correctly, is probably not the critical event in determining survival. If local therapy is delivered poorly, however, or given with inadequate chemotherapy, survival can be greatly compromised.

18.5.4 Pulmonary Irradiation

Because of the success of chemotherapy, prophylactic lung irradiation, popular in the 1970s, has been largely abandoned. However, a long-term update of IESS-I clearly shows that it can be effective (NESBIT et al. 1990). IESS-I was a three-arm study: treatment 1, VAC (vincristine, dactinomycin, and cyclophosphamide) chemotherapy; treatment 2, VAC chemotherapy plus 15-Gy whole-lung irradiation; and treatment 3, VACA (vincristine, dactinomycin, cyclophosphamide, and doxorubicin) chemotherapy. The latter arm clearly showed the best results, but arm 2 was superior to arm 1. The 5-year relapse-free survival rates were 24% for treatment 1, 44% for treatment 2, and 60% for treatment 3 (NESBIT et al. 1990). Thus, prophylactic lung irradiation provided a survival advantage when added to VAC. Whether it would improve survival when added to more aggressive chemotherapy has never been studied.

18.6 Treatment of Patients with Metastatic Disease at Diagnosis

Approximately 20% of patients have overt metastatic disease at diagnosis (SAILER et al. 1988; MARCUS et al. 1988). Although the prognosis of these patients is poor, patients who present with only lung metastases warrant aggressive therapy, as some will be cured. In addition to chemotherapy and treatment to the primary lesion, lung irradiation is probably of value, though not all institutions subscribe to this philosophy (HAYES et al. 1983). A dose of 15–18 Gy in ten fractions is standard, with boosts of 20–25 Gy to any large lesions. Usually, chemotherapy should be given first, with radiation therapy added after two or three cycles. With intensive chemotherapy, complete disappearance of the lung lesions usually occurs before irradiation, and the whole-lung irradiation serves as consolidation. In spite of this, the most common site of failure for patients with lung metastases at diagnosis is the lung, though not always in the same sites within the lung.

The prognosis for patients with bone or bone marrow (often both) metastases is dismal, though five long-term survivors are reported from IESS-I and IESS-II (CANGIR et al. 1990). These patients are labeled as having multifocal bone disease by some authors. The usual strategy is aggressive chemotherapy followed by radiation therapy to all sites of original disease. A dose of 40–50 Gy at 1.8–2 Gy/day is standard, but this author has used courses as short as 30 Gy in ten fractions if the number of fields is large, as it can be in patients with multifocal bone disease.

In reports from IESS-I and IESS-II, patients with rib lesions and a pleural effusion were considered to have metastatic disease at diagnosis. The prognosis for such patients is better than for other patients with metastatic disease (CANGIR et al. 1990).

18.7 Prognosis

Ewing's sarcoma is a disease for which the ultimate cure rate may not be established for 10 years because of late recurrences and deaths from complications. Unfortunately, most reports in the literature are published with a majority of patients having less than 5 years of follow-up. Table 18.4 lists those reports in which the majority of patients treated (all with localized disease at diagnosis) had 10 years of follow-up. The survival rates are very similar. Two-year survival rates range from 66% to 76%, 5-year survival rates from 42% to 60%, and by 10 years the survival rates have dropped to 38%–47%. There are a number of recent reports in the literature with encouraging early survival rates, but more follow-up is needed to determine whether these will hold up (DUNST et al. 1991; HAYES et al. 1987; JEREB et al. 1986; MARCUS et al. 1988).

Table 18.4. Five- and 10-year survival rates for Ewing's sarcoma of bond (localized lesions only) (from MARCUS 1991)

Investigators	Survival		
	2-year	5-year	10-year
KINSELLA et al. (NCI) (1991)	68%	51%	39%
WILKINS et al. (Mayo Clinic) (1986)	70%	42%	38%
SAILER et al. (Mass. General) (1988)	76%	60%	47%
MARCUS (Univ. Florida) (unpublished data, October 1990)	66%	45%	43%
NESBIT et al. (IESS-1) (1990)	75%	52%	40%

Patients with metastases at diagnosis fare much worse, with a 20% 10-year survival rate at best (SAILER et al. 1988), excluding patients with rib lesions and pleural effusion as the only site of metastasis.

At present, the prognosis of primitive neuroectodermal tumor of bone (PNET) versus classic Ewing's sarcoma of bone is controversial. Most authors believe that PNET occurs in older patients on the average (though occasionally it is diagnosed in very young patients) and carries a worse prognosis, but since there is little agreement on the exact criteria to be used to differentiate PNET from classic Ewing's sarcoma, there is no definitive proof to support this hypothesis. Until further information is available, both should probably be treated in a similar fashion.

18.8 Salvage

Treatment of Ewing's sarcoma should be aggressive at the time of diagnosis, as it is difficult to salvage patients who relapse, particularly those who experience failure rapidly after the end of the first treatment. Patients who experience failure with only a local relapse warrant aggressive salvage therapy with whatever combination of surgery and irradiation can be used, along with additional chemotherapy. Some of these can be salvaged (HAYES et al. 1987).

Patients who develop lung metastases can also be salvaged, rarely, with additional chemotherapy and lung irradiation. Patients who develop bone metastases, however, are essentially incurable with standard therapy. Protocols using bone marrow transplantation have been tried, but further follow-up is needed.

18.9 Follow-up

After irradiation of a primary lesion, plain roentgenograms should be taken every 3–4 months for the first 2 years, then every 6 months for the next 3 years. CT and/or MRI scans of the primary site should be done every 6 months for 2 years, along with a CT of the lungs and a bone scan. The usefulness of such procedures after 2 years is debatable. If MRI is used in follow-up, soft tissue changes due to radio-

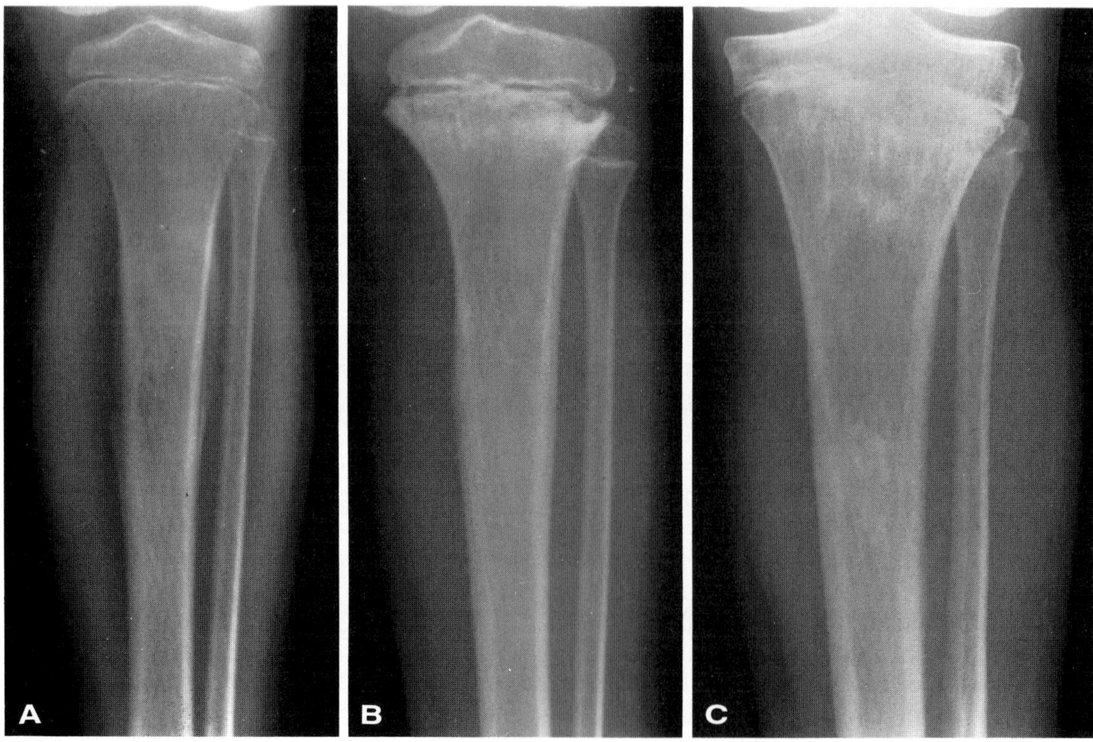

Fig.18.5A–C. An 8-year-old girl with a small lesion of the proximal tibia. **A** Periosteal elevation is present circumferentially around the femur. The patient had VAC (vincristine, dactinomycin, and cyclophosphamide) chemotherapy and 51.87 Gy radiation to the lesion, including 40 Gy to the entire tibia. **B** One year after treatment, the cortex is smooth and the periosteal elevation has disappeared. **c** Eight years after treatment, a residual abnormality is present but the cortex remains uninterrupted. Often, long term follow up films show considerably more sclerosis than in this patient. The patient is now 20 years post-treatment with no evidence of recurrence

therapy are often seen in the irradiated field. These changes, which consist of increased signal intensity on T2-weighted and gadolinium-DTPA-enhanced, T1-weighted images, can occur as early as a few weeks after the completion of irradiation and can persist for several months (FLETCHER et al. 1990). The changes occur more frequently with low-energy (<6 MV) photons and hyperfractionated treatment. Because late failures can occur, it is our policy to continue yearly films as long as the patient returns to our clinic for follow-up. Even after maximum healing, a residual abnormality exists permanently in the treated bone (Fig. 18.5). This makes the evaluation of a possible local recurrence difficult. Maximum ossification should occur by 8–24 months. Until then, cortical changes, particularly new breaks in the cortex, should be viewed with suspicion. After 24 months, *any* change in the treated bone should be evaluated further (Fig. 18.6). Further evaluation should probably include both CT and MRI, since bony changes can be best evaluated by CT, while changes in soft tissue extent and marrow involvement are best seen using MRI.

18.10 Complications

The treatment of Ewing's sarcoma is necessarily aggressive, resulting in considerable risks and complications.

The complications secondary to irradiation are numerous. Since doses of 50 Gy and above are used, the most common complication is abnormal growth and development of the irradiated tissues. For extremities, this can mean both a cosmetic and a functional abnormality. Functionally, the extremity can be shorter, since doses above 20 Gy will prematurely close the irradiated epiphysis. This is usually only a minor cosmetic problem in the upper extremities, but may produce major morbidity in the lower extremities, since a leg length discrepancy will produce a gait abnormality. The degree of discrepancy will depend upon the epiphysis or epiphyses irradiated as well as the age of the patient at the time of treatment. It is important to be able to predict the potential leg-length discrepancy before treatment of a patient with a lower extremity lesion, since this may affect the decision to use surgery versus radiation therapy. The treatment required for the different categories of leg-length discrepancy is shown in Table 18.5.

Obviously, in predicting the degree of leg-length discrepancy that will result from irradiation, one has to take into account which epiphysis or epiphyses are irradiated. Sixty-five percent of future growth comes from the knee, 37% from the distal femoral plate and 28% from the proximal tibial plate. Only 15% occurs at the proximal femoral plate and 20% from the distal tibial plate (MOSELEY 1990).

For practical purposes, rough estimates according to age of the growth remaining for the four major lower extremity epiphyses are shown in Table 18.6. These estimates can be used as a rough guide to predict leg-length discrepancies, but for a more thorough review of the subject, see MOSELEY (1990).

One of the more common side-effects of the tumor and its treatment is permanent weakening of the affected bone. This is obviously more of a problem in long-bone lesions, particularly those in the femur, and can result in a pathologic fracture. The highest risk for such a fracture is within the first 18 months of the completion of radiation therapy, and it should be emphasized to the patient that contact sports and other high-stress activities to the leg should be avoided during that time. The patient should also be informed that the involved bone will never attain normal strength and extremely high-risk activities should be permanently avoided, since such a pathologic fracture will not heal without internal fixation.

Since 1982, the use of induction chemotherapy (which allows some healing to occur before the start of irradiation) and the b.i.d. fractionation regimen as well as a better knowledge of the risk factors has virtually eliminated pathologic fractures at the University of Florida (Table 18.7).

Other functional abnormalities include extremity weakness; decreased range of motion secondary to fibrosis; pain in the extremity, particularly in the early morning; discoloration of the skin; and lymphedema. The latter should be extremely rare with careful planning and sparing of an adequate strip of tissue.

Other risks include damage to organs in the irradiated field; the heart, lungs, kidneys, and bladder are the most frequently affected.

Table 18.5. Recommended treatment for categories of leg-length discrepancies (from MOSELEY 1990)

Leg-length discrepancy (cm)	Treatment
0–2	None required
2–6	Shoe lift, epiphysiodesis
6–15	Leg lengthening
>15	Prosthetic fitting

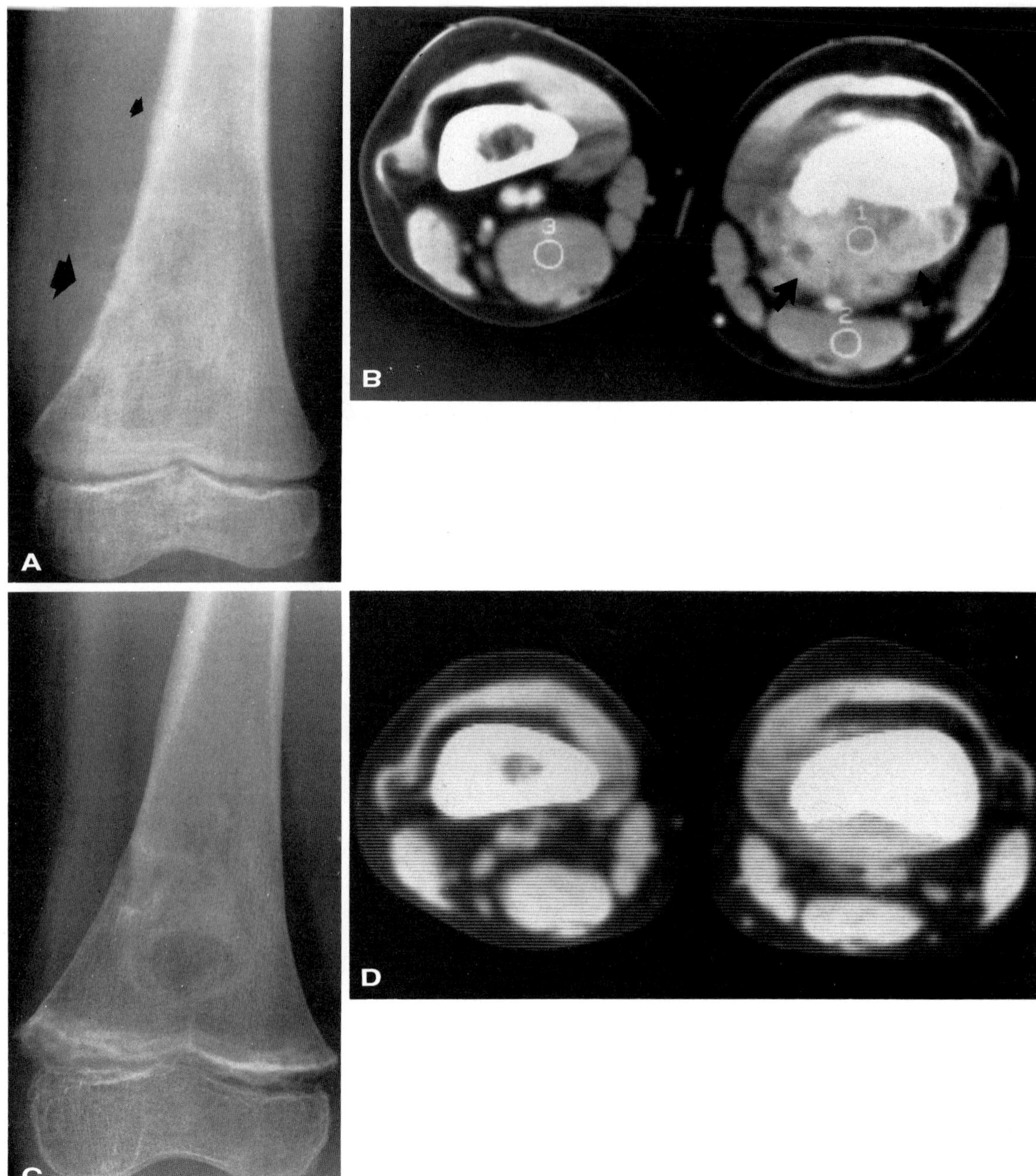

Fig.18.6A–F. An 8-year-old girl with a lesion of the left distal femur. **A** Plain film at diagnosis shows a destructive lesion, a small amount of diffuse new bone formation (*large arrow*), and periosteal elevation (*small arrow*). **B** A CT slice though the femur 2 cm proximal to the epiphysis shows sclerosis of the femur, irregularity of the cortex, and a soft tissue mass (*arrow*). **C** The patient was treated with VACA (vincristine, dactinomycin, cyclophosphamide, and doxorubicin) chemotherapy and 55 Gy radiation to the primary lesion. Plain film at the end of all treatment (1 year after diagnosis) shows that the cortex of the bone has healed. **D** CT at the same time, showing that the soft tissue mass has disappeared. **E** Two years after treatment, plain films of the distal femur show extensive destruction and periosteal elevation. **F** CT confirms this finding, and shows a soft tissue mass anterior, lateral, and posterior to the femur (*arrows*). Biopsy revealed recurrent Ewing's sarcoma

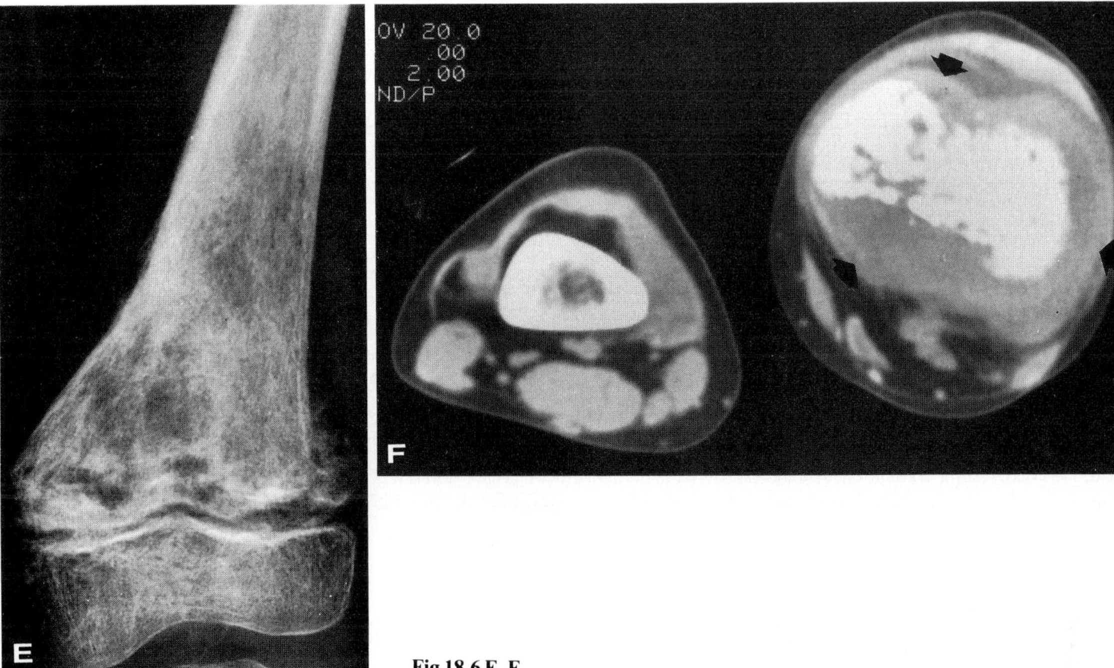

Fig 18.6 E, F

Table 18.6. Average growth (in cm) remaining for each lower extremity epiphysis by age and sex (adapted from ANDERSON et al. 1963)

Epiphysis	Boys – age in yr					Girls – age in yr				
	8	10	12	14	16	8	10	12	14	16
Proximal femur	3.5	3.0	2.0	0.8	<0.5	2.8	1.9	0.8	<0.5	0
Distal femur	8.5	7.5	5.0	2.0	0.5	7.0	4.7	2.0	0.8	0
Proximal tibia	6.0	5.0	3.5	1.0	<0.5	4.5	3.0	1.0	<0.5	0
Distal tibia	4.2	3.7	2.5	1.0	<0.5	3.4	2.3	1.0	<0.5	0

Table 18.7. Pathologic fractures in Ewing's sarcoma patients irradiated for extremity lesions (University of Florida data, 1969–1990, analysis 4/92, 2-year minimum follow-up)

Treatment	No. of patients	No. of fractures
RT q.d. (1969–1976)	9	5
Induction chemotherapy and RT q.d. (1977–1981)	8	2
Induction chemotherapy and RT b.i.d. (1982–1990)	26	0

In addition, there is the risk of secondary neoplasia at the site of the primary lesion. Osteosarcoma is the most common secondary tumor, though others have been reported. For orthovoltage treatment the risk may be quite high, but the exact risk for megavoltage treatment is just now being defined (TUCKER et al. 1987). In the IESS-I experience, the risk to date is 1% (NESBIT et al. 1990). In a joint analysis from St. Jude Children's Research Hospital, the National Cancer Institute, and the University of Florida, the risk of secondary neoplasia was 12 (4%) of 315 patients, with eight (2.5%) cases related to the radiation therapy. Only two of the eight were osteosarcomas (KUTTESCH, unpublished data). The risk appears to increase if the dose is greater than 60 Gy (BORIANI et al. 1988).

18.11 New Directions

Even though patients with small lesions and no metastatic disease at diagnosis do well, it is essential to continue to seek new regimens and methods to improve survival, since, overall (including patients

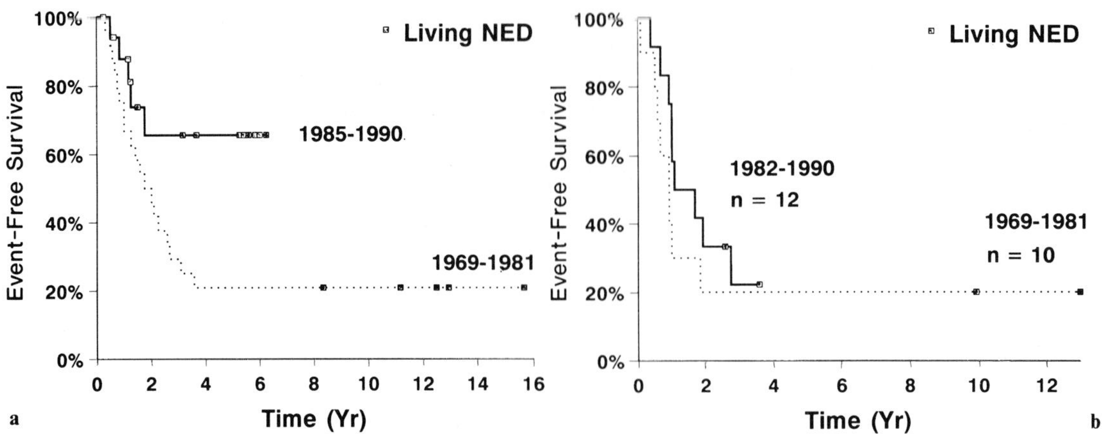

Fig. 18.7a,b. Event-free survival for patients with high-risk Ewing's sarcoma treated at the University of Florida, comparing results from 1969 to 1981 with results from the latest bone marrow transplant protocols (HR-3 and HR-4) from 1985 to 1990, **a** for patients with localized disease and large primary lesions (>8 cm in maximum diameter) and **b** for patients with metastatic disease at diagnosis.

with metastatic disease at diagnosis), less than 50% of all Ewing's sarcoma patients survive. Presently, the addition of an ifosfamide-etoposide combination appears most promising and is being studied by a number of groups, with randomized studies in the United States by both the Pediatric Oncology Group and the Children's Cancer Study Group. It will obviously take years to determine the cure rates obtained from the addition of these drugs.

Total body irradiation (TBI) has also been used as a systemic treatment. Rider used a single 3-Gy treatment (and no chemotherapy), resulting in a 5-year survival rate of 30% (JENKIN et al. 1976). Low-dose TBI, 15 cGy twice a week to a total dose of 1.5 Gy, was employed by the NCI in the S-5 protocol for high-risk patients (KINSELLA et al. 1983). However, the long-term survival rate was still poor. In the 1980s, with the development of autologous bone marrow transplantation (ABMT) technology, the use of TBI in a conditioning regimen was studied at the NCI and the University of Florida, as well as Europe. The NCI protocol treated all high-risk, small-round-cell sarcoma patients with the same protocol, ending with TBI and a combination of vincristine, doxorubicin, and cyclophosphamide as a conditioning regimen before ABMT. The 5-year survival rate on this protocol for patients with localized disease was 50%, and for patients with metastatic disease at diagnosis, 20% (BADER et al. 1989). For patients with high-risk disease (primary lesions >8 cm in maximum diameter or metastatic disease at diagnosis), similar protocols have been used at the University of Florida from 1985 to date, one protocol using 8 Gy TBI (4 Gy q.d. for 2 days) and one using 12 Gy TBI (2 Gy b.i.d. for 3 days) (MARCUS

et al. 1988, 1991). Four-year event-free survival rates for these two protocols combined are 65% for patients with localized disease and 25% for patients with metastatic disease at diagnosis (MARCUS RB Jr, unpublished data). These results appear to be superior to those previously shown for patients with large primary lesions (Fig. 18.7a). Unfortunately, for patients with metastatic disease at diagnosis, there does not seem to be a major improvement (Fig. 18.7b).

One potential source of failure in patients with metastases is the reinfusion of tumor cells from the previously harvested marrow. The limited experience at the University of Florida and in Europe indicates better results for patients receiving allogeneic (three of three patients survived free of relapse) or syngeneic (the sole patient survived free of relapse) marrow, even for those with multifocal bone disease at diagnosis (LADENSTEIN et al. 1992; MARCUS RB Jr, unpublished data). Approaches which eliminate the reinfusion of tumor-contaminated marrow may prove to be particularly useful for patients with metastatic disease at diagnosis.

References

Anderson M, Green WT, Messner MB (1963) Growth and predictions of growth in the lower extremities. J Bone Joint Surg [Am] 45: 1–14

Arai Y, Kun LE, Brooks MT et al. (1991) Ewing's sarcoma: local tumor control and patterns of failure following limited-volume radiation therapy. Int J Radiat Oncol Biol Phys 21: 1501–1508

Bader JL, Horowitz ME, Dewan R et al. (1989) Intensive combined modality therapy of small round cell and undifferentiated sarcomas in children and young adults: local control and patterns of failure. Radiother Oncol 16: 189–201

Barbieri E, Emiliani E, Zini G et al. (1990) Combined therapy of localized Ewing's sarcoma of bone: analysis of results in 100 patients. Int J Radiat Oncol Biol Phys 19: 1165–1170

Boriani S, Picci P, Sudanese A et al. (1988) Radio-induced sarcomas in survivors of Ewing's sarcoma. Tumori 74: 543–551

Burgert EO Jr, Nesbit ME, Garnsey LA et al. (1990) Multimodal therapy for the management of nonpelvic, localized Ewing's sarcoma of bone: Intergroup Study IESS-II. J Clin Oncol 8: 1514–1524

Cangir A, Vietti TJ, Gehan EA et al. (1990) Ewing's sarcoma metastatic at diagnosis: results and comparisons of two Intergroup Ewing's Sarcoma Studies. Cancer 66: 887–893

Capanna R, Toni A, Sudanese A, McDonald D, Bacci G, Campanacci M (1990) Ewing's sarcoma of the pelvis. Int Orthop 14: 57–61

Dunst J, Sauer R, Burgers JMV et al. (1991) Radiation therapy as local treatment in Ewing's sarcoma: results of the Cooperative Ewing's Sarcoma Studies CESS 81 and CESS 86. Cancer 67: 2818–2825

Edeiken J, Karasick D (1987) Imaging in bone cancer. CA 37: 239–245

Evans RG, Nesbit ME, Gehan EA et al. (1991) Multimodal therapy for the management of localized Ewing's sarcoma of pelvic and sacral bones: a report from the Second Intergroup Study. J Clin Oncol 9: 1173–1180

Fletcher BD, Hanna SL, Kun LE (1990) Changes in MR signal intensity and contrast enhancement of therapeutically irradiated soft tissue. Magn Reson Imaging 8: 771–777

Hayes FA, Thompson EI, Hustu HO, Kumar M, Coburn T, Webber B (1983) The response of Ewing's sarcoma to sequential cyclophosphamide and adriamycin induction therapy. J Clin Oncol 1: 45–51

Hayes FA, Thompson EI, Kumar M, Hustu HO (1987) Long-term survival in patients with Ewing's sarcoma relapsing after completing therapy. Med Pediatr Oncol 15: 254–256

Hayes FA, Thompson EI, Meyer WH et al. (1989) Therapy for localized Ewing's sarcoma of bone. J Clin Oncol 7: 208–213

Jenkin RDT, Rider WD, Sonley MJ (1976) Ewing's sarcoma: adjuvant total body irradiation, cyclophosphamide and vincristine. Int J Radiat Oncol Biol Phys 1: 407–413

Jereb B, Ong RL, Mohan M, Caparros B, Exelby P (1986) Redefined role of radiation in combined treatment of Ewing's sarcoma. Pediatr Hematol Oncol 3: 111–118

Jürgens H, Exner U, Gadner H et al. (1988) Multidisciplinary treatment of primary Ewing's sarcoma of bone: a 6-year experience of a European cooperative trial. Cancer 61: 23–32

Kinsella TJ, Glaubiger D, Diesseroth A, Makuch R, Waller B, Pizzo P, Glatstein E (1983) Intensive combined modality therapy including low-dose TBI in high-risk Ewing's sarcoma patients. Int J Radiat Oncol Biol Phys 9: 1955–1960

Kinsella TJ, Miser JS, Triche TJ, Horvath K, Glatstein E (1988) Treatment of high-risk sarcomas in children and young adults: analysis of local control using intensive combined modality therapy. NCI Monogr 6: 291–296

Kinsella TJ, Miser JA, Waller B, Venzon D, Glatstein E, Weaver-McClure L, Horowitz ME (1991) Long-term follow-up of Ewing's sarcoma of bone treated with combined modality therapy. Int J Radiat Oncol Biol Phys 20: 389–395

Kissane JM, Askin FB, Foulkes M, Stratton LB, Shirley SF (1983) Ewing's sarcoma of bone: clinicopathologic aspects of 303 cases from the Intergroup Ewing's Sarcoma Study. Hum Pathol 14: 773–779

Ladenstein R, Lasset C, Biron P et al. (1992) The impact of megatherapy on response and survival in high-risk Ewing's sarcoma. A report of the EBMT Solid Tumor Registry (abstract). High-dose chemotherapy and stem-cell transplant in solid tumors, an international symposium. Berlin, Society for International Oncology

Marcus RB Jr (1991) Ewing's sarcoma – a local or systemic problem? Int J Radiat Oncol Biol Phys 20: 901–902

Marcus RB Jr, Million RR (1984) The effect of primary tumor size on the prognosis of Ewing's sarcoma (abstract 24). Int J Radiat Oncol Biol Phys 10 [Suppl 2]: 88

Marcus RB Jr, Graham-Pole JR, Springfield DS et al. (1988) High-risk Ewing's sarcoma: End-intensification using autologous bone marrow transplantation. Int J Radiat Oncol Biol Phys 15: 53–59

Marcus RB Jr, Cantor A, Heare TC, Graham-Pole J, Mendenhall NP, Million RR (1991) Local control and function after twice-a-day radiotherapy for Ewing's sarcoma of bone. Int J Radiat Oncol Biol Phys 21: 1509–1515

Moseley CF (1990) Leg-length discrepancy. In: Morrissy RT (ed) Lovell and Winter's pediatric orthopaedics, 3rd edn, vol. 2. Lippincott, Philadelphia, pp 767–813

Nesbit ME Jr, Gehan EA, Burgert EO Jr et al. (1990) Multimodal therapy for the management of primary, nonmetastatic Ewing's sarcoma of bone: a long-term follow-up of the First Intergroup Study. J Clin Oncol 8: 1664–1674

Oberlin O, Patte C, Demeocq F et al. (1985) The response to initial chemotherapy as a prognostic factor in localized Ewing's sarcoma. Eur J Cancer Clin Oncol 21: 463–467

O'Connor MI, Pritchard DJ (1991) Ewing's sarcoma: prognostic factors, disease control, and the reemerging role of surgical treatment. Clin Orthop 262: 78–87

Pendergrass TW, Foulkes MA, Robison LL, Nesbit ME (1984) Stature and Ewing's sarcoma in childhood. Am J Pediatr Hematol Oncol 6: 33–39

Pollock BH, Krischer JP, Vietti TJ (1991) Interval between symptom onset and diagnosis of pediatric solid tumors. J Pediatr 119: 725–732

Pritchard DJ (1989) Small round cell tumors. Orthop Clin North Am 20: 367–375

Sailer SL, Harmon DC, Mankin HJ, Truman JT, Suit HD (1988) Ewing's sarcoma: surgical resection as a prognostic factor. Int J Radiat Oncol Biol Phys 15: 43–52

Sauer R, Jürgens H, Burgers JMV, Dunst J, Hawlicek R, Michaelis J (1987) Prognostic factors in the treatment of Ewing's sarcoma: the Ewing's Sarcoma Study Group of the German Society of Paediatric Oncology CESS 81. Radiother Oncol 10: 101–110

Thomas PRM, Perez CA, Neff JR, Nesbit ME, Evans RG (1984) The management of Ewing's sarcoma: role of radiotherapy in local tumor control. Cancer Treat Rep 68: 703–710

Tucker MA, D'Angio GJ, Boice JD Jr et al. (1987) Bone sarcomas linked to radiotherapy and chemotherapy in children. N Engl J Med 317: 588–593

Turc-Carel C, Aurias A, Mugneret F et al. (1988) Chromosomes in Ewing's sarcoma: I. An evaluation of 85 cases and remarkable consistency of t(11;22) (q24;q12). Cancer Genet Cytogenet 32: 229–238

Wilkins RM, Pritchard DJ, Burgert EO Jr, Unni KK (1986) Ewing's sarcoma of bone: experience with 140 patients. Cancer 58: 2551–2555

Womer RB (1991) The cellular biology of bone tumors. Clin Orthop 262: 12–21

19 Rhabdomyosarcoma

J. ROBERT CASSADY

CONTENTS

19.1 Introduction 281
19.2 Epidemiology. 281
19.3 Etiology 282
19.4 Pathology. 283
19.5 Natural History and Evaluation. 283
19.6 Staging. 284
19.7 Treatment. 285
19.7.1 General Principles. 286
19.7.2 Chemotherapy. 286
19.7.3 Radiation Therapy 287
19.8 Individual Primary Sites. 289
19.8.1 Orbit. 289
19.8.2 Nasopharynx. 290
19.8.3 Middle Ear 292
19.8.4 Larynx. 293
19.8.5 Paratesticular. 293
19.8.6 Vagina 293
19.8.7 Bladder and Prostate. 294
19.8.8 Extremity 295
19.8.9 Trunk. 296
19.9 Results. 297
19.10 Complications. 298
19.10.1 Cataract Formation. 299
19.10.2 Bony Effects 299
19.11 Future Prospects. 299
        References. 300

19.1 Introduction

Rhabdomyosarcoma (RMS) represents a heterogeneous group of diseases occurring at widely diverse sites. Collectively they represent the most common soft tissue sarcomas of childhood (YOUNG et al. 1978). Progress made in the treatment of this challenging condition has influenced pediatric oncology for 25 years and existing problems continue to challenge pediatric oncologists in all specialties. Newer molecular genetic information has been revolutionary in changing our concept of the condition.

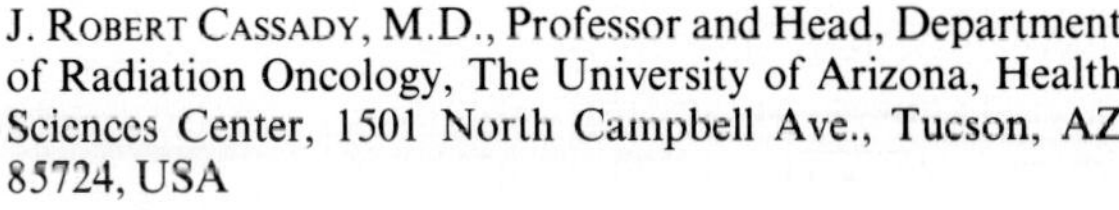

J. ROBERT CASSADY, M.D., Professor and Head, Department of Radiation Oncology, The University of Arizona, Health Sciences Center, 1501 North Campbell Ave., Tucson, AZ 85724, USA

19.2 Epidemiology

Approximately 250–300 children develop RMS in the United States each year. Annual incidence rates approximate 4 cases per million US children less than 15 years of age. Males are seen with an increased frequency of 10%–40% when compared with females (MAURER et al. 1977).

The disease occurs in two age peaks, one with a mean age of approximately 2–2.5 years and one with a mean age of approximately 10–12 years (LI and FRAUMENI 1977). As the younger peak accounts for nearly 70% of all cases, the overall mean age of presentation is 4–5 years (LACEY et al. 1986).

The disease, presumably originating from embryologic precursors of striated muscle, may appear at any body site regardless of whether striated muscle is present or not (STOUT 1946; HORN 1958; GREEN and JAFFE 1978; GREEN 1985). Site is predictive of prognosis (Fig. 19.1) and also varies with age and histology (Table 19.1). The approximate mean age for alveolar histology patients in the series reported by KINGSTON et al. (1983) was 9.0 years, in contrast to a

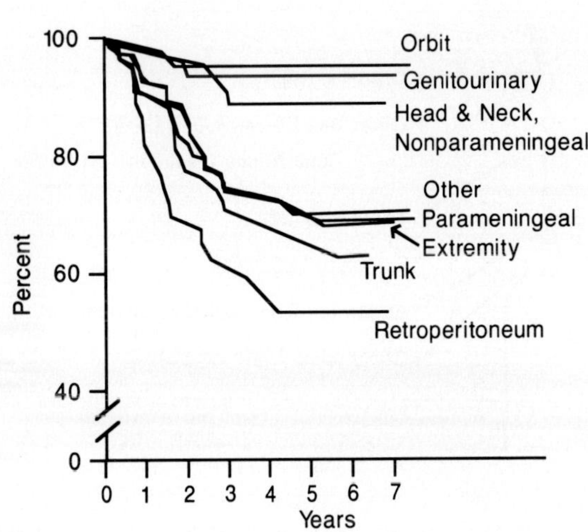

Fig. 19.1. Survival by anatomic site of presentation for 401 non-metastatic cases of RMS registered and treated in IRS II. (adapted from RUYMANN 1987).

Table 19.1. Histologic variation of RMS by site

	Head/neck	Extremities	G/U	Trunk	Retroperitoneum
Embryonal/botryoid	72%	24%	90%	18%	59%
Alveolar	14%	48%	9%	41%	20%
Pleomorphic/other	14%	28%	1%	51%	21%

G/U, genitourinary sites

Table 19.2. Frequency by site for RMS (573 cases)

Head and neck (257 cases), 45%
Orbit	13%
Nasopharynx[a]	11.5%
Middle ear, temporal bone[a]	6%
Parotid, cheek, face[b]	6%
Neck and larynx	5%
Others	3%

Genitourinary sites (164 cases), 28%
Paratesticular	8%
Retroperitoneum	4%
Pelvis	4%
Bladder	3.5%
Prostate	3%
Vagina	2.5%
Uterus, cervix	2%
Others	1%

Trunk and extremity (152 cases), 27%
Lower extremity	10.5%

Trunk (includes buttocks, perineum, and abdominal wall), 10.5%
Upper extremity	5%
Others	< 1%

[a] Parameningeal site
[b] Includes some parameningeal patients

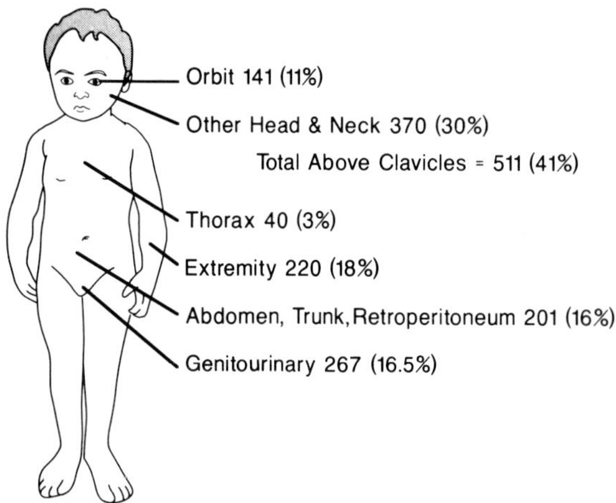

Fig. 19.2. Frequency by site of RMS in 1239 cases (pooled data from Li and Fraumeni 1969; Dritschilo et al. 1978; Kingston et al. 1983; Green 1985; Lacey et al. 1986; Maurer et al. 1988)

mean age of 6.6 years for the embryonal group. Thus children of younger age tend to present with primaries of the genitourinary region and head and neck area with embryonal histology; older children tend to have primaries which occur in the extremities, trunk, and head and neck region, with a substantially higher incidence of alveolar tumors (Pizzo et al. 1989). Tumors occurring above the clavicles, accounting for 35%–40% of all tumors, have been separated into parameningeal and nonparameningeal sites by the Intergroup Rhabdomyosarcoma Study Group (IRS) based on apparent differences in prognosis and natural history (Tefft et al. 1978; Raney et al. 1981). Tumors of the nasopharynx, paranasal sinuses, middle ear, infratemporal fossa, nasal cavity, and pterygopalatine region are included in the parameningeal group (Raney et al. 1981).

Table 19.2 and Fig.19.2 show primary sites by overall frequency. As a single anatomic site, orbital tumors are seen most frequently (Green 1985).

It is notable that congenital anomalies of all types are seen with greater frequency in children with RMS than in "normal" children. In the IRS study, an anomaly was detected in 37 of 115 children (32%). Major anomalies were also seen with eight fold greater frequency (14 major congenital anomalies). As with many childhood tumors, neurofibromatosis is seen with a greater than expected frequency (McKeen et al. 1978).

19.3 Etiology

Like virtually all childhood malignancies, the etiology for RMS is not known. As noted above, children with neurofibromatosis are seen with greater than expected frequency (McKeen et al. 1978). In addition, families with the Li-Fraumeni syndrome may contain members affected by RMS (Li and Fraumeni 1969). The mothers of children with RMS have a significantly higher than expected rate of breast cancer, suggesting a significant genetic aspect to the disease (Li and Fraumeni 1969).

19.4 Pathology

As noted in the introduction, the term RMS covers a diverse collection of neoplasms. Included are "classical" RMS, soft tissue Ewing's tumor (identical in most respects to bony Ewing's tumor but occurring outside bone), and unspecified sarcomas. Askin's tumor, a primitive small cell tumor of neuroectodermal origin which arises has also been included with RMS in some series. Recent molecular genetic studies suggest even greater diversity, with a distinct separation in the "classical" group (PIZZO et al. 1989; SCRABLE et al. 1989).

Grossly, the tumor usually presents as a fleshy, friable mass. When the embryonal subtype arises in a submucosal location and contains a unique band of cells, the "cambium" layer of Nicholson, a peculiar sacculated, grape-like (hence botryoid) appearance may result which has been termed sarcoma botryoides (MCFARLAND 1911; STOBBE and DARGEON 1950; NICKOLSON 1950). These tumors most commonly arise from the bladder, vagina, or oronasal region and usually occur in very young children.

Microscopically, RMS has classically been divided into embryonal, alveolar, pleomorphic/undifferentiated, and soft tissue Ewing groups (HORN and ENTERLINE 1958; MAURER et al. 1977; NEWTON et al. 1988). Only about one-third can be demonstrated to contain cross-striations despite careful search (ENZINGER and SKIRAKI 1969). The embryonal type is present in nearly 60% of all patients and the great majority of these cases are genitourinary and head and neck tumors. They rarely contain cross-striations and are characterized by containing short spindle cells with a syncytial-like appearance, so-called tennis-racquet cells, and a variety of other small round cells (STOBBE and DARGEON 1950).

Alveolar tumors represent nearly 20% of all cases; they are the predominant group appearing in the trunk and extremities and account for some tumors in the head and neck region (RIOPELLE and THERIAULT 1956; ENTERLINE and HORN 1958). They have been called alveolar in view of their low/intermediate power microscopic appearance, which is reminiscent of lung tissue. Finally, about 20% of RMS are considered undifferentiated or pleomorphic types. The latter group is seen mostly in adults and contains frequent cross-striations (STOUT 1946). The undifferentiated group includes the soft tissue Ewing's group and other unclassified tumors (TEFFT et al. 1969; ANGERVALL and ENZINGER 1975; SOULE et al. 1978; GAIGER et al. 1981; NEWTON et al. 1988).

Molecular genetic studies have recently shown that embryonal tumors are associated with a deletion of the 11p (short arm) chromosome which may be homozygous or in which the critical site may demonstrate apparent genome imprinting (SCRABLE et al. 1989). In contrast, the alveolar tumors frequently may be shown to contain a 2/13 translocation similar to small cell osteosarcoma (TURC-CAREL et al. 1986). This new molecular genetic information suggests a biologic separation which may account for the marked diversity in prognosis observed between the embryonal (generally favorable) and alveolar (generally unfavorable) subtypes.

Palmer and co-workers suggested a new histologic classification based on cellular appearance. Three patterns are recognized: anaplastic, monomorphous, and mixed. Although possibly offering better prognostic separation than the previous system, it is probably that characterization of these tumors by their molecular genetic abnormality(ies) will ultimately provide the most benefit (PALMER et al. 1982; PALMER and FOULKES 1983).

19.5 Natural History and Evaluation

Most children present with a mass noted either by themselves, their parents, a physician, or a friend. However, presentation may be insidious, particularly with tumors of the middle ear, antrum, parapharyngeal space, retroperitoneum, or bile ducts, and on occasion a history of facial pain, stuffy nose, or altered hearing may be all that alerts the astute clinician. Children with genitourinary primaries may present with urinary retention or obstruction while those with genitourinary or head and neck disease may present with hematuria or nasal bleeding.

Unlike most sarcomas, especially those occurring in adults, lymph node involvement is relatively common. In repeated series, frequencies of microscopic node involvement average about 20% (range 0%–50%), with overall frequency dependent on primary site and whether first eschelon node dissection/sampling has been routine or frequently performed (MASSON and SOULE 1965; BURRINGTON 1969; LAWRENCE et al. 1977, 1987a; GREEN and JAFFE 1978; RANEY et al. 1978, 1987a; EXELBY et al. 1978; KINGSTON et al. 1983; GREEN 1985; PEDRICK et al. 1986; MANDELL et al. 1990b). Routine lymph node sampling is rarely performed for patients with group III and IV (IRS) disease. Since this group represents >50% of all patients with RMS, the "true" incidence of lymph node involvement in initially diagnosed patients with RMS probably lies at the higher end of the range given.

Certain sites, especially the orbit, appear to have a very low incidence of node involvement (LAWRENCE et al. 1977, 1987a; PEDRICK et al. 1986). However, in other head and neck sites (e.g., nasopharynx), the reportedly low incidence of node involvement appears to be, at least in part, a function of infrequent pathologic sampling combined with the arbitrary decision that clinically palpable abnormal nodes are not sufficient justification for pathologic staging (PEDRICK et al. 1986; MANDELL et al. 1990b) (Table 19.3). Of perhaps greater relevance, Table 19.4 lists frequency of lymph node involvement at death (autopsy data IRS I/II) (SHIMADA et al. 1987).

In addition to wide and insidious local extension and lymph node spread, metastases to distant sites are frequently observed, with pulmonary, hepatic, and bony sites predominating. Parameningeal tumors, by virtue of their location, can extend into the central nervous system and subsequently develop cerebrospinal fluid (CSF) extension and/or local meningeal spread.

Chest wall tumors frequently develop pleural extension and seeding, while retroperitoneal tumors can extend widely along tissue planes.

Evaluation for the child with RMS should thus include a careful physical examination with particular attention paid to primary draining lymph node regions. A careful neurologic examination should also be performed, especially in children with a primary above the clavicles.

Table 19.3. Frequency of pathologically confirmed lymph node involvement in group I–III RMS (LAWRENCE et al. 1977; GREEN 1985)

Site	No.	%
Orbit	0/17	0
Other head and neck	2/62	3
Trunk	3/30	10
Extremities	8/46	17
Genitourinary sites	10/52	19

Table 19.4. Frequency of lymph node involvement at death by primary site (IRS I/II) (SHIMADA et al. 1987)

Primary site	No.	%
Lower extremity	24/48	50
Upper extremity	6/19	32
Parameningeal	8/46	17
Genitourinary	13/32	41

Laboratory studies should include a complete blood count and platelet analysis as well as an SMAC 20 or similar battery of standard serum hepatic and renal function tests. Bone marrow aspiration and biopsy are routine in many clinics and are important for staging in alveolar and far-advanced embryonal tumors. In one series, 50% of positive bone marrow examinations occurred in patients with an alveolar histology, despite their relative rarity (RUYMANN et al. 1984).

Radiographic analysis should include computed tomography (CT) and/or magnetic resonance imaging (MRI) studies of the primary region. Posteroanterior and lateral films of the chest should be obtained and CT of the lungs is strongly recommended. In addition, a radioisotopic bone scan is performed in most clinics and definitely should be performed if there are any suggestive symptoms.

Controversy also exists over the place of routine surgical lymph node sampling for RMS. This procedure will certainly reveal cases with unsuspected nodal extension. If this information were to alter therapy, then the procedure should be routinely performed. However, if reliance is to be placed on systemic therapy for management of microscopic nodal disease, then routine sampling becomes more controversial. Routine sampling for patients with extremity, genitourinary, retroperitoneal, and paratesticular primaries is strongly encouraged as sizable nodes may be present yet remain undetected by routine radiographic studies.

A lumbar puncture and CSF analysis with cytospin study for tumor cells is performed for all patients with parameningeal primaries. For those with spine or paraspinous disease and worrisome symptoms, MRI and possibly myelography with CSF analysis should also be performed.

19.6 Staging

Considerable controversy exists with respect to the most appropriate staging system (DONALDSON 1989). The system most frequently used in the literature is the original grouping devised by the IRS committee for IRS study I. (Table 19.5) (MAURER 1975; MAURER et al. 1977).

Historically, IRS staging has depended on the adequacy of surgical resection (irrespective of primary size) and the presence of nodal or distant metastases. It has been criticized for relying extensively on the postsurgical state, this reliance causing it to be dependent on the facility and aggressiveness

Table 19.5. IRS grouping system (MAURER 1975)

Group I	Localized disease, completely resected A. Confined to organ or muscle of origin B. Infiltration outside organ or muscle of origin: regional nodes not involved
Group II	Total gross resection with evidence of regional spread A. Grossly resected tumors with microscopic residual B. Regional disease with involved nodes, completely resected with no microscopic residual C. Regional disease with involved nodes, grossly resected, but with evidence of microscopic residual and/or histologic involvement of the most distal regional node (from the primary site) in the dissection
Group III	Incomplete resection, or biopsy with presence of gross residual disease
Group IV	Distant metastases present at onset

Table 19.6. Pretreatment clinical staging system proposed by International Union Against Cancer (UICC) (HARMER 1982)

T-1	Tumor confined to organ or tissue of origin 1a. 5 cm or less in size 1b. More than 5 cm in size
T-2	Tumor involves contiguous organs or structures 2a. 5 cm or less in size 2b. More than 5 cm in size
N-0	No clinical or radiographic evidence of involvement of regional lymph nodes (not histologic determination)
M-0	No distant metastases on clinical, radiographic, or bone marrow examination
M-1	Evidence of distant metastasis
H-1	Favorable histology (embryonal, botryoid, mixed, or undifferentiated)
H-2	Unfavorable histology (alveolar, monomorphous, or anaplastic)

TNM staging system

Clinical stage	Invasiveness	Size[a]	Nodal status	Metastasis status
I	T1	A or B	N0	M0
II	T2	A or B	N0	M0
III	T1 or T2	A or B	N1	M0
IV	T1 or T2	A or B	N0 or N1	M0

[a] A, tumor size 5 cm or less; B, tumor size greater than 5 cm

of the surgeon (DONALDSON and BELLI 1984). Comparison of results with patients treated more conservatively with limited surgery or biopsy, chemotherapy, and radiation therapy is difficult as a consequence.

BELLI and DONALDSON have drawn attention to this problem and they and the UICC have proposed an alternative system based on tumor extent, nodal and distant metastases, and histology (HARMER 1982; DONALDSON and BELLI 1984; LAWRENCE et al. 1987b; RODARY et al. 1988b) (Table 19.6). The IRS is currently testing a similar clinical staging system (LAWRENCE et al. 1987b). Nevertheless, a 5-cm tumor in a 23-lb infant is logically more serious than the same size tumor in a 15 year old.

In the United States, 10%–20% of patients will present with nonnodal distant metastases and, using the initial IRS grouping system, at least one-half of all patients will present with group III or IV disease even when aggressive surgery is routinely performed. Thus, in IRS I, 410 of 686 (60%) patients presented with group III (281) or group IV (129) disease. Slightly less than 15% (101) presented with group I disease (MAURER et al. 1988). Table 19.7 illustrates frequency of IRS group by primary site. This separation does not give an accurate portrayal of primary size by site as many orbit and head and neck primaries are not surgically resected and are therefore group III.

At this time it is strongly recommended that presurgical clinical staging be performed in all patients based on available clinical and radiographic studies. Careful pathologic assessment of surgical

Table 19.7. IRS group by primary site (LACEY et al. 1986)

Site	No. of patients	I	II	III	IV
Head and neck	126	17	52	25	6
Orbit	22	64	27	5	4
Thorax	16	31	31	25	13
Abdomen	32	22	50	6	22
G/U and Pelvis	87	46	35	10	9
Extremities	62	43	10	24	23

G/U, gastrourinary sites

specimens continues, of course, to be required, and may have a significant influence on the use of other therapeutic modalities especially radiation.

19.7 Treatment

When the limitless diversity of anatomic sites, histologic types, and possible clinical presentations of RMS are considered, no text can discuss all individual presentations in depth. However, general principles of available treatment modalities can be emphasized and a number of common clinical presentations covered.

19.7.1 General Principles

The great majority of all children who present with RMS will receive surgery, radiation therapy, and systemic chemotherapy in their initial management. Thus all patients must be seen by all participating disciplines prior to initiation of invasive management, including biopsy when possible.

The therapeutic team must weigh considerations of patient age, tumor size, and ease of resectability, as well as the cosmetic and functional effects of various treatment options. The team should choose that combination which ensures optimum function and cosmesis without significant sacrifice in tumor control efficacy. Unlike in the case of certain pediatric tumors (e.g., Hodgkin's disease), it is extremely important to obtain overall tumor control with initial therapy, as "salvage" of relapse is rarely accomplished and death usually results (RANEY et al. 1983).

The surgeon should seek to remove, with clear margins, as much tumor as possible without grave functional or cosmetic consequences. In certain sites such as the orbit, tumor biopsy or local excision suffices as more radical attempts involve orbital exenteration with unnecessary loss of the eye and vision and the probable need for local irradiation (plus systemic therapy) in any case. Certain presentations (e.g., limited, lower extremity RMS of favorable histology in a young child) may profit from more aggressive primary surgery which may eliminate the need for radiation, thus reducing long-term functional risks and eliminating other hazards of irradiation. The most vexing group of children remain those with genitourinary primaries (vide infra), where the local modalities of surgery and irradiation are critically important but uniformly toxic (HAYS et al. 1991a).

19.7.2 Chemotherapy

Essentially all children with RMS should receive multiagent systemic chemotherapy, as either neoadjuvant or adjuvant therapy, or for probable palliation with a remote likelihood of cure when they present with distant visceral metastatic disease. Even the mildly controversial group of patients with extremely limited orbital tumors of favorable histology appear to profit from this routine approach (ABRAMSON et al. 1979).

HEYN et al. (1974) were the first to demonstrate in a randomized controlled fashion the disease-free and overall survival benefits of routine multiagent (vin-

cristine/actinomycin D; VA) chemotherapy even for patients with early disease. Although many confirmatory studies using historical controls exist, this remains the only randomized study demonstrating this point. Tables 19.8 and 19.9 demonstrate response of RMS to several chemotherapeutic agents and combinations and Fig. 19.3 shows representative VAC (VA plus cyclophosphamide) and "T2" regimens. Sites of action of many of the effective agents are shown in Fig. 19.4. Table 19.10 lists a general treatment plan by histology and group utilized by the IRS (LACEY et al. 1986; RANEY et al. 1989).

Despite a sequential increase in the number of agents delivered, which has increased the complexity of regimens and the normal tissue toxicity engendered, it is unclear at this time whether more aggressive chemotherapy regimens have produced substantial additional disease-free and overall survival benefits or whether progressive improvements in survival have occurred for other reasons. Thus the IRS (IRS I) evaluated the efficacy of doxirubicin (adriamycin) added to VAC for patients with group III and IV disease who were also treated uniformly with irradiation. No difference was noted in disease-free survival or length of remission. In a parallel study, VAC was not shown to be superior to VA in patients with group II disease (MAURER et al. 1988). In subsequent studies, pulse VAC was not shown to be superior to VA or VAC plus adriamycin for children with group II or group III and IV disease (RANEY et al. 1979).

Although the recent IRS III study reportedly demonstrates improved survival for patients with group III disease, this benefit could reflect substantial improvements in radiation therapy techniques with more uniform fields and total tumor doses, especially in children with parameningeal head and neck

Table 19.8. Single-agent response of RMS according to GREEN and JAFFE (1978)

Drug	CR	PR	CR + PR	Total responses	
Vincristine	2	17		19/32	(59%)
Actinomycin D	1	7		8/33	(24%)
Cyclophosphamide	5	11	14	35/55	(54%)
Adriamycin	3	6	12	21/67	(31%)
Imidazole carboxamide	0	2		2/18	(11%)
5-Fluorouracil				0/7	(0%)
Mitomycin C	1	3		4/11	(36%)

CR, complete response; PR, partial response

Table 19.9. RMS response rates to single agents and combinations according to various authors[a] (RANEY et al. 19)

Drug(s)	No. of Patients Evaluable	CR	PR	% PR + CR	References
Actinomycin D	14	0	6	43%	PINKEL 1959; TAN et al. 1959, SHAW et al. 1960
Cyclophospha-mide	26	2	11	50%	SUTOW 1967; HADDY et al. 1967
Vincristine	42	3	10	33%	SUTOW et al. 1966; SUTOW 1968; SELAWRY et al. 1968
Doxorubicin	40	1	11	30%	BONADONNA et al. 1970; SUTOW et al 1972; TAN et al. 1973; O'BRYAN et al. 1973
Cisplatin	19	1	3	21%	BAUM et al. 1981
VAC	11	2	7	82%	PRATT 1969; GREEN 1978
VA	6	1	5	100%	JAMES et al. 1966

V, vincristine; A, actinomycin D; C, cyclophosphamide; CR, complete response; PR, partial response
[a] Single-agent CR rate = 5% (7/141); combination CR rate = 18% (3/17)

Table 19.10. Chemotherapy protocols: IRS study (LACEY et al. 1986)

Group I:	(Favorable histology) No radiation is needed Chemotherapy consists of vincristine 2 mg/m^2 i.v. once a week starting in week 3 for 6 doses repeated 5 times in 48 weeks and actinomycin D 0.015 mg/kg daily i.v. for 5 days, 5 times in 48 weeks
Group II:	(Favorable histology) Same as for group I except include radiation; there are two treatment regimens in this group; patients in one regimen receive adriamycin 30 mg/m^2 day for 2 days with first through third course of vincristine; patients in the other regimen receive no adriamycin
Groups I and II:	(Unfavorable histology) Radiation plus "pulse" VAC alternating adriamycin with the actinomycin D every 4 weeks for 1 year. Also cisplatin every 3 weeks for 4 doses, starting at week zero
Groups III and IV:	(Excluding some head primaries with favorable histology) All receive radiation All receive variations of "pulse" VAC There are three randomized arms that are plus or minus the following in a variety of schedules: cisplatin 90 mg/m^2 i.v. infusion, adriamycin 30 mg/m^2 day for 2 days, VP-16 100 mg/m^2 day i.v. infusion for 3 days, DTIC 200 mg/m^2/day i.v. push for 5 days

and genitourinary primaries, rather than improved systemic therapy. Careful analysis of subgroups with improved outcomes will be necessary to resolve this question (RANEY et al. 1987b, 1991; HEYN et al. 1989; CRIST et al. 1990, 1991; HAYS et al. 1991a; ORTEGA et al. 1991).

At this time, no known chemotherapy regimen is able to consistently control gross disease at the primary site, and although responses have been frequent and occasionally dramatic, nonnodal metastatic disease is usually fatal.

19.7.3 Radiation Therapy

Following demonstration of its ability to control both microscopic and gross residual RMS, radiation therapy has been utilized in most children with RMS. IRS I demonstrated no survival benefit from the addition of irradiation to surgery and systemic chemotherapy (VA) when children with group I disease (no microscopic residual and no lymph node disease) were randomly treated (MAURER et al. 1977, 1988). However, subset analysis of IRS II and unirradiated IRS I, group I patients demonstrated an inordinately high rate of locoregional relapse in those with unfavorable histology, and routine radiation of this latter group is now recommended (TEFFT et al. 1985). Thus more than 90% of children with RMS will currently receive local or regional irradiation, usually with curative intent.

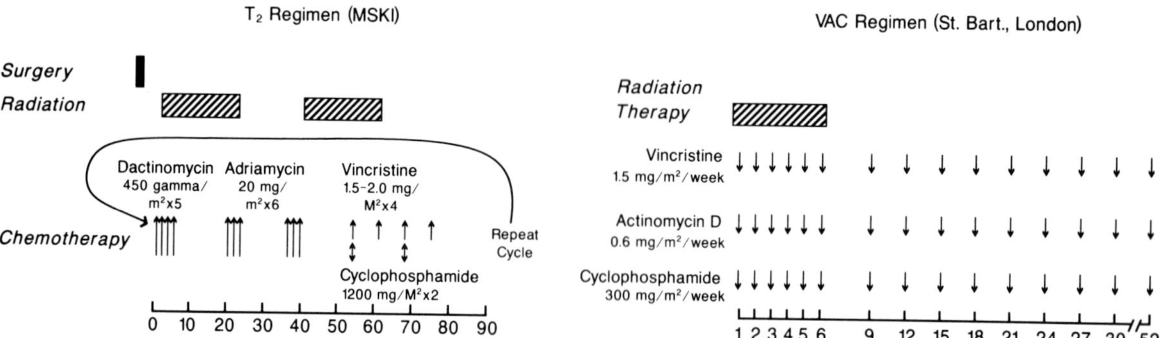

Fig. 19.3. Two representative combination chemotherapy regimens utilized in children with RMS. (T₂ regimen: Ghavimi et al. 1981; VAC regimen: Kingston et al. 1983)

19.7.3.1 Dose

Controversy exists over the dose of radiation necessary to ensure a high rate of local control, especially when gross postsurgical residual disease exists. Numerous uncontrolled single-institution studies have demonstrated improved control when radiation doses of greater than 50 Gy with conventional fractionation have been used for gross residual disease compared to doses of less than 40–45 Gy (CASSADY et al. 1968; DONALDSON et al. 1973; FERNANDEZ et al. 1975; JEREB et al. 1976; DRITSCHILO et al. 1978; CHAN et al. 1979; GHAVIMI et al. 1981; MAURER et al. 1988). A similar trend was noted in IRS I, where doses could vary as a function of the child's age at the time of treatment (MAURER et al. 1988). Local control also varied as a function of tumor bulk, with local failure rates of 30%–40% being reported in patients with tumors greater than 5 cm and/or those with extensive bony invasion (TEFFT et al. 1981; TARBELL et al. 1987; MANDELL et al. 1989).

To date, no series has reported a large group of children with gross residual RMS randomly treated to different total doses of radiation in whom a careful analysis of treatment volume has also been carried out using pretreatment tumor extent (assessed clinically and radiographically), simulation films, and treatment port films to assess adequacy. As "tumor dose" is irrelevant if a portion of the tumor has been significantly underdosed or excluded from the treatment volume, this analysis is critical in combination with appropriate subgroup analysis for tumors of differing size. Generally high local control rates have been published for tumors of the orbit at doses of 45–50 Gy even when gross disease was present (WHARAM et al. 1987a).

Thus the question of "necessary" dose for gross residual disease when irradiation is combined with current chemotherapy regimens is unresolved although clearly 45 Gy (CASSADY et al. 1968; DRITSCHILO et al. 1978; WHARAM et al. 1987b; MAURER et al. 1988) or more should be used as consistent failure rates of

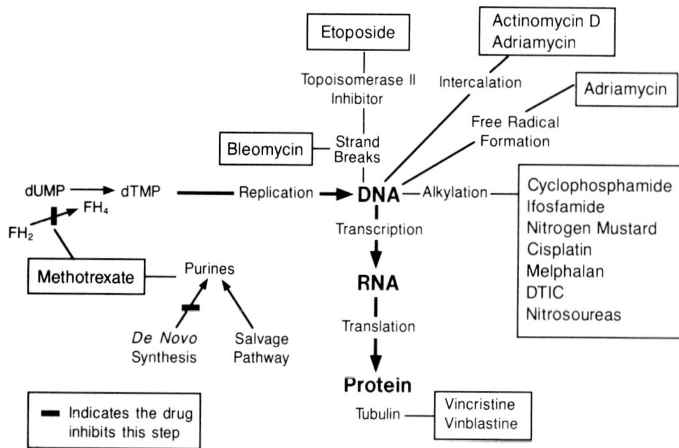

Fig. 19.4. Presumed site(s) of action of many commonly used chemotherapeutic agents or classes of agents. (BERG et al. 1991)

more than 30% have been reported when patients with group III disease (especially >5 cm) have been treated in the IRS. As doses of ≥45 Gy already prevent of eliminate significant further bony growth and soft tissue development, we currently recommend a dose in excess of 50–54 Gy in these adverse settings when conventional fractionation is utilized (MAURER et al. 1988; TEFFT et al. 1988).

Excellent local control rates have been published when patients with presumed microscopic residual disease have been treated to adequate volumes using conventional fractionation and 40–45 Gy in combination with multiagent chemotherapy (JEREB et al. 1976; DRITSCHILO et al. 1978; GHAVIMI et al. 1981; PEDRICK et al. 1986; MAURER et al. 1988; TEFFT et al. 1988). When gross residual disease exists, higher doses must be used to obtain similar levels of efficacy. Using conventional fractionation, a minimum of 55 Gy is suggested for gross residual disease.

Recent attempts to improve tumor control while reducing late normal tissue injury have been initiated using altered fractionation schedules similar to those frequently employed for adult head and neck squamous cell cancer (RANEY et al. 1989; MANDELL et al. 1988, 1990a; CASSADY 1991). Inadequate information currently exists to determine whether this laudable approach will succeed in either or both goals, although follow-up information on one study is encouraging (MANDELL et al. 1988, 1990a).

19.7.3.2 Tumor Volume

General agreement exists among radiation oncologists that the pretreatment volume of tumor should be treated with an adequate margin of 3–5 cm (JEREB et al. 1976; DRITSCHILO et al. 1978; TEFFT et al. 1985, 1988; PEDRICK et al. 1986; RANEY et al. 1987b, 1989; WHARAM et al. 1987b; MANDELL et al. 1988; ORTEGA et al. 1990). Attempts to reduce tumor volumes to postsurgical or postchemotherapy residual disease negate one of the principal advantages of irradiation (control of microscopic disease) and often lead to local failure. However, a shrinking field approach in which graded doses are delivered adjusted to presumed residual tumor cell burden is appropriate.

It is imperative that the therapist appreciate the insidious nature of this tumor and its ability to occultly infiltrate widely. This is of particular importance when tumors of the head and neck or extremity region are being treated. It is also imperative, when considering volume and dose in an individual patient, that the consequences of local failure – both cosmetic/functional and in terms of survival – be kept in mind. Generally, the consequences of a somewhat larger volume or somewhat higher (~5 Gy) dose are modest in relation to the effects of radical surgery and/or reirradiation.

19.7.3.3 Lymph Node Treatment

The role of regional nodal irradiation is controversial. The relative frequency of gross or microscopic nodal disease has been previously noted.

Excellent regional control results have been obtained in series in which routine regional nodal treatment was carried out (DRITSCHILO et al. 1978). However, TEFFT et al. (1980), reporting for the IRS, were unable to demonstrate an advantage for such treatment in their patients with genitourinary primaries who were not randomized for this treatment variable. Although the value of such treatment is unproven and awaits a randomized study, we currently recommend inclusion and treatment of proximal regional lymph nodes in patients who have not undergone node biopsy, especially those who present with head and neck (e.g., nasopharynx) or extremity primaries (MANDELL et al. 1990b).

Should regional node sampling be negative, then no treatment is warranted. Clinically positive and/or pathologically confirmed positive lymph node sites should be treated usually with radiation doses of 45–50 Gy using conventional fractionation dependent on the extent of surgical dissection.

19.8 Individual Primary Sites

In the following section, discussion of specific tumor sites will be undertaken. Complications engendered by treatment will be discussed separately.

19.8.1 Orbit

The orbit is the most common presenting site of RMS (GREEN and JAFFE 1978; GREEN 1985; RANEY 1989). Most patients present with an eyelid mass; however, other symptoms may include proptosis, epistaxis, and ptosis (JONES et al. 1965; ASHTON and MORGAN 1965; WHARAM et al. 1987a).

The orbit is reported to be poorly supplied with lymphatics and the great majority of children have no palpable primary echelon (preauricular and jugulodigastric) lymph nodes or distant metastases (CASSADY et al. 1968). Although not considered "parameningeal tumors" by virtue of their excellent prognosis, orbital tumors are, in fact, proximate to the meninges, especially at the optic canal region, and, when sufficiently advanced, these tumors can extend to the CNS and demonstrate meningeal seeds (FUSNER et al. 1978). Bony orbital erosion is more common but is nevertheless relatively infrequent (JONES et al. 1965; ASHTON and MORGAN 1965; CASSADY et al. 1968).

Most tumors are embryonal and patients are best treated with limited surgery (biopsy or limited excision, not exenteration), combination chemotherapy, and irradiation (WHARAM et al. 1987a). Figure 19.5 demonstrates two possible treatment plans depending on the extent of posterior involvement. It is of importance to recognize that the orbit extends superiorly and medially in its posterior

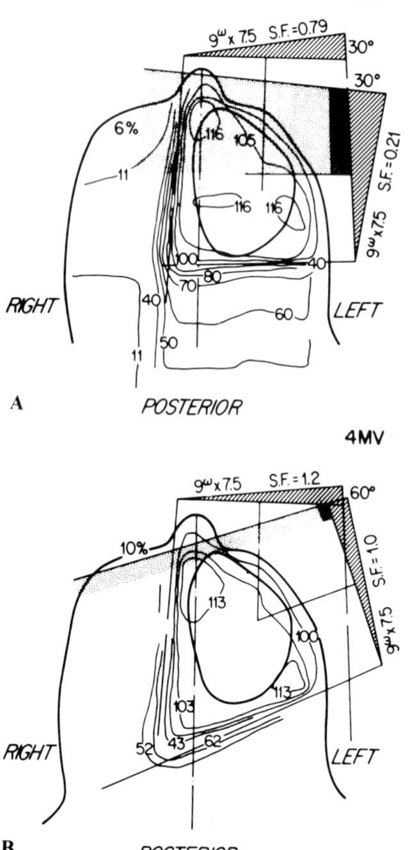

Fig. 19.5A,B. Two representative treatment plans for patients with orbital or antral tumors. Choice of the "best" plan requires a careful assessment of tumor extent which has been demonstrated by optimum imaging techniques or by clinical features. In particular, the posteromedial extent is critical in choice of plan. (DEVITA et al. 1982)

segment and coverage of this region is critical. It is also critical that patients be treated with the eyelids open to avoid a bolus effect on the cornea and conjunctiva of the eye with resultant debilitating keratoconjunctivitis. This sparing of the cornea and conjunctiva is possible as the globe itself is rarely invaded by tumor.

For unexplained reasons, local control at this site is unusually good with radiation doses 5–10 Gy less than those usually needed for equivalent control rates at other sites (WHARAM et al. 1987a; HALPERIN et al. 1989). A tumor dose of approximately 50 Gy is therefore favored in order to balance tumor control with visual function. More than 90% of children with orbital primaries survive following treatment, with equivalent rates of local control (ABRAMSON et al. 1979; WHARAM et al. 1987a).

19.8.2 Nasopharynx

Patients with nasopharyngeal primaries tend to present with a mass, nasal and/or airway obstruction, and/or cranial nerve or visual difficulties (GREEN 1985).

Although nonnodal metastases are overt in less than 10%, radiographic studies frequently show bony erosion at the base of the skull and may show actual invasion into the CNS. Tumors at this site are representative of the parameningeal group discussed earlier (TEFFT et al. 1978; RANEY et al. 1981, 1987b).

Resection is virtually never possible and tumor control relies on locoregional radiation therapy and chemotherapy. Following biopsy confirmation, two to four cycles of multiagent chemotherapy are administered prior to irradiation unless symptoms or signs of tumor progression or lack of response is noted earlier. IN IRS III, radiation therapy was begun on day 14 or 42 following diagnosis, depending on stage (RANEY et al. 1989).

Radiation volumes and treatment plans should resemble those used for nasopharyngeal carcinomas, ensuring that the cranial meninges at the base of the skull are routinely included with an adequate margin (Fig. 19.6). Care should also be taken to include possible nasal extension in this infiltrative tumor and all volumes must include at least the posterior nasal turbinates anteriorly. Cervical lymph nodes should be included, as should the primary parapharyngeal node of Rouviere. In the presence of clinically positive cervical adenopathy, we routinely include the supraclavicular fossae.

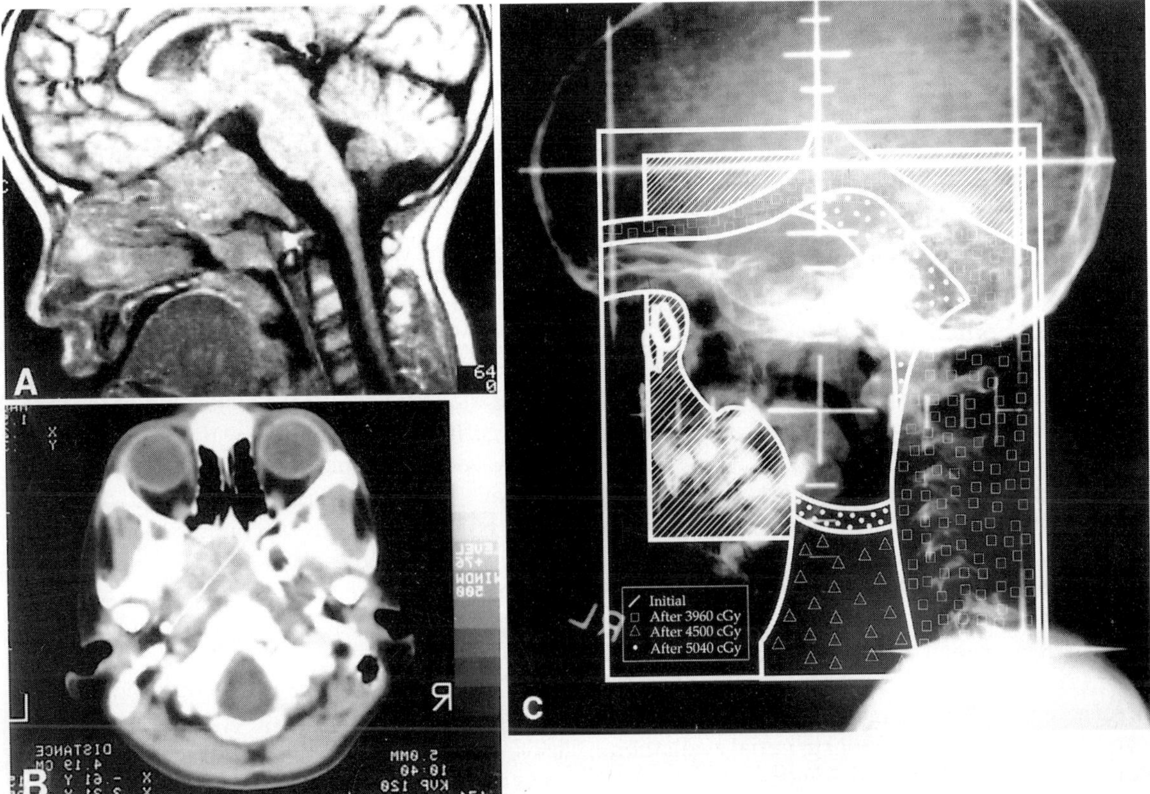

Fig. 19.6A–C. Six-year-old Hispanic female with recent onset of diplopia, a left-sided sixth nerve palsy, headache, and paranasal sinus distress. Imaging studies (**A**, **B**) demonstrate a massive nasopharyngeal lesion involving the clivus and base of skull. The tumor also had significant anterior extension to the posterior antral and pterygoid region. Pulmonary metastases were present initially. Biopsy demonstrated undifferentiated RMS. CSF cytology was negative for tumor cells. After initial modest partial response to combination chemotherapy, radiation therapy was delivered to the head and neck region utilizing a shrinking field approach (**C**). A dose of 57.6 Gy was delivered by photons from a 6-MV linear accelerator to the final cone down field by equally weighted opposing lateral fields utilizing daily 1.8-Gy fractions. Although local control was maintained for 2 years and complete reversal of the sixth nerve palsy occurred following irradiation, relapse of pulmonary metastases (unirradiated) occurred which ultimately led to her demise. Meningeal relapse did not occur

Extensive bony destruction with a large mass may be present. In our experience this finding is more frequent in girls, and others have also noted a female sex predominance (KINGSTON et al. 1983; TARBELL et al. 1987). Local failure rates in this group are significant using conventional 1.5- to 2-Gy fractions and radiation doses of 55–60 Gy. Studies assessing hyperfractionation efficacy are therefore warranted (RANEY et al. 1989; MANDELL et al. 1988, 1990a; CASSADY 1991). Patients with clinically positive nodal disease also fare less well (Fig. 19.6) (RANEY et al. 1989; LAWRENCE et al. 1987a).

Although the IRS observed a high frequency of meningeal relapse in IRS I in patients with parameningeal primaries, lack of primary control was noted in the majority of these patients and both dose and tumor volume were frequently insufficient when analyzed in a retrospective fashion (TEFFT et al. 1978; BERRY and JENKIN 1981; JEREB et al. 1985). When no evidence of gross intracranial disease is present and adequate doses and volumes are utilized with reasonable margins, the incidence of meningeal spread or seeding will be quite low and whole brain or craniospinal treatment volumes are not recommended prophylactically as suggested by some (TEFFT et al. 1978; CHAN et al. 1979; GASPARINI et al. 1983; ORTEGA et al. 1990). Whether intrathecal chemotherapy is warranted with more benefits than risks is unclear. Unusual CNS toxicity (myelopathy) has been reported (RANEY et al. 1990).

When gross intracranial extension is present, the therapist must decide whether the benefits of possibly increased regional control warrant the substantial risks and limitations such wide-field approaches will place on systemic therapy attempts.

At least 50% of cases of nasopharyngeal RMS are locally and systemically controlled with treatment regimens as outlined (DRITSCHILO et al. 1978; CHAN et al. 1979; RANEY et al. 1981; TEFFT et al. 1985; JEREB et al. 1985; ORTEGA et al. 1990).

19.8.3 Middle Ear

Children with RMS of the middle ear usually present because of a mass in the external auditory canal (GREEN 1985). However, the only symptoms may be a facial nerve palsy, diminished hearing, or an apparent chronic otitis media (POTTER 1966). Middle ear tumors occur primarily in young children. Therefore, in addition to infection, a differential diagnosis of histiocytosis or cholesteatoma must be considered and occasionally neuroblastoma is entertained. Lymphoma presenting at this site and age is extraordinarily rare. A pathologic diagnosis of neoplasm is generally not difficult and the absence of Langerhans giant cells, histiocytes, and other cellular characteristics of Langerhans cell histiocytosis usually make the diagnosis easy.

Perhaps more than tumors of any other site, these lesions routinely invade bone and can readily gain direct access to the CNS and CSF. Cytology of CSF (cytospin) is therefore essential in initial evaluation, along with other radiographic studies.

Although radical mastoidectomy can be performed, long-term control and cure of children with tumors at this site require combinations of irradiation and chemotherapy. Very generous margins are needed for radiation portals and inclusion of the entire petrous and temporal bone and structures of the ear is essential. The ipsilateral cervical lymph nodes should be treated and nodal extent may require inclusion of ipsilateral supraclavicular nodes and/or contralateral neck nodes.

At least partial use of a "wedge-pair" approach is highly desirable to avoid severe, permanent xerostomia from irradiation of both parotid glands. Representative treatment plans are shown in Fig. 19.7. Radiation doses at the higher end of the range noted earlier should be used, with attempts to progressively shield normal tissues in a "shrinking field" approach. Such shielding is essential to avoid nerve, brain, bone, and soft tissue complications. When a wedged pair is used, extension of the head is necessary in order to lift the eyes out of the path of the exit radiation beam from the posterior oblique field (KEUS et al. 1991).

Perhaps because of the routine presence of bone involvement and/or prior use of inadequately small fields, control rates for this site have generally been lower than those reported for other head and neck sites (POTTER 1966). Comments regarding parameningeal tumors in the section on nasopharynx are applicable.

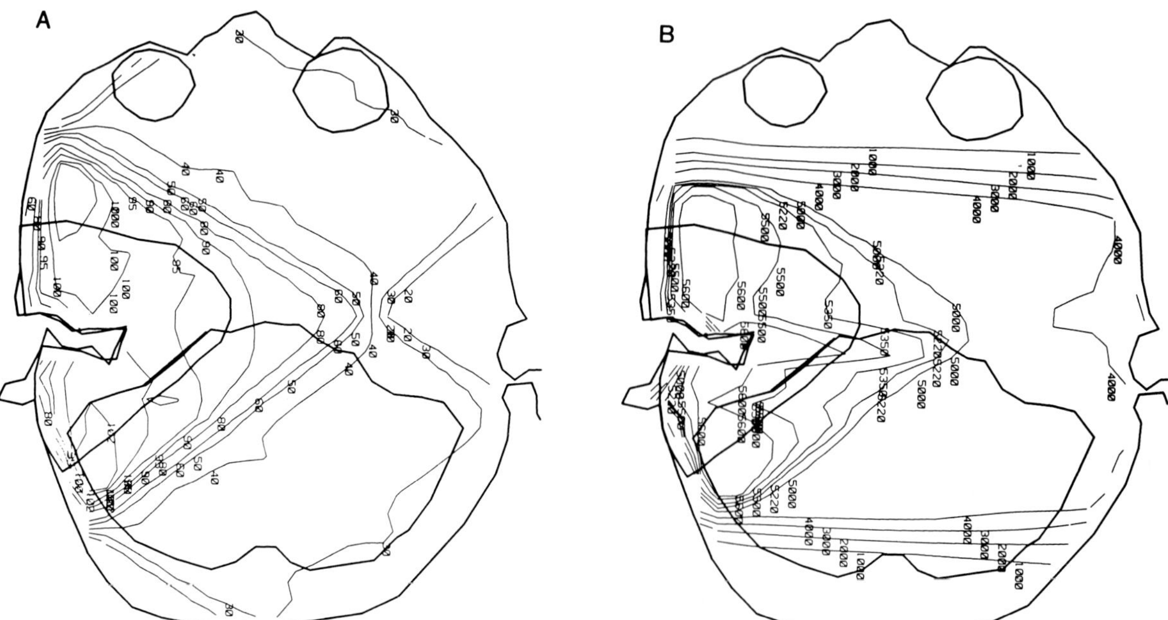

Fig. 19.7A,B. Isodose distributions for a wedge-pair 6 MV photon plan utilized with or without an opposing lateral field component. The plan utilizing lateral fields in addition to the wedge-pair includes 40 Gy from the lateral fields (calculated to midline) and 15 Gy from the wedge-pair

19.8.4 Larynx

Although uncommon, tumors of the larynx are important to consider because of the functional consequences of total laryngectomy. Children with glottic primaries present with hoarseness and signs of airway obstruction. A tracheostomy is frequently necessary at the time of biopsy to avoid acute or subsequent airway compromise during treatment (GREEN 1985).

Although tumor control can often be obtained by total laryngectomy and radiation may thus be avoided if specimen margins and lymph nodes are negative, the functional consequences of this approach are substantial. They can be avoided with excellent outcome by substitution of high-dose irradiation and chemotherapy (WHARAM et al. 1984; KATO et al. 1991). It is possible that a hyperfractionated approach will further benefit functional outcome with equivalent or improved tumor control. Radiation fields and treatment plan should resemble those used for squamous cell tumors in adults with modifications made in accordance with the more infiltrative nature of RMS.

19.8.5 Paratesticular

Rhabdomyosarcoma represents the most common neoplastic cause of a scrotal or "testicular" mass in the young child of 18 months to 7 years. In the first year of life, embryonal carcinoma of the infant occurs with greater frequency, while as adolescence approaches, other testicular carcinomas predominate. However, in the intermediate age period, RMS predominates as a primary tumor with leukemic testicular involvement , lymphomatous involvement and carcinomas providing alternative possibilities. Virtually all carcinomas in this age group are embryonal in type.

Between 20% and 40% of patients with paratesticular RMS will be found to have microscopic or gross nodal involvement when routine retroperitoneal node dissection or sampling is performed (BURRINGTON 1969; LAWRENCE et al. 1977, 1987a; RANEY et al. 1978, 1987a). The success of radiographic studies in predicting node involvement has not been adequate to rely on these studies and not perform nodal dissection or sampling. Lymph nodes at risk parallel those affected by testicular carcinoma. Contralateral "skip" or "cross-over" nodes have not been noted by the IRS and thus unilateral node dissection may be appropriate and hopefully elimi-

nate or reduce the incidence of subsequent retrograde ejaculation (RANEY et al. 1987a). A European study suggests that node sampling or dissection is unnecessary when adjuvant chemotherapy is given in patients with normal lymphangiograms (LAG) and intravenous urograms (15/17 2 yr+ NED) (OLIVE et al. 1984). However, the location of the primary lymph node in left-sided lesions is lateral to nodes routinely opacified by bipedal LAG and microscopic disease may be missed. This observation, combined with our lack of knowledge regarding the ability of combination chemotherapy to control overt nodal disease, makes this author recommend routine sampling (RANEY et al. 1987a). Ninety-seven percent of paratesticular primary patients (vs 53% overall) had embryonal histology in IRS I/II and 60% (vs 13%) were in group I (RANEY et al. 1987a).

If inguinal (radical) orchiectomy and node sampling show no tumor at margins or in nodes (~ 65%–70% of all children), adjuvant treatment with only chemotherapy is indicated. Should nodes (or margins) be positive then irradiation is recommended. Between 40 and 50 Gy to opposed equally weighted AP/PA or mixed AP/PA fields and four-field treatment plans are highly effective. Fields similar to those appropriate in treating testicular seminoma are utilized. Should transscrotal biopsy contamination or tumor involvement occur, placement of the contralateral testis in an untreated site (i.e., the contralateral groin) and electron beam irradiation of the scrotum and, if warranted, ipsilateral inguinal region should be considered. Excellent overall survival of 89% has been reported by the IRS (vs 59% overall) and even children with positive lymph nodes fare better than their counterparts with tumors at other sites (85% vs 65%) (RANEY et al. 1987a; LAWRENCE et al. 1987a).

19.8.6 Vagina

Although not common (2.5%), this site accounts for a significant percentage of the botryoid tumors (McFARLAND 1911). Children usually present with a vaginal mass, bleeding, urinary tract symptoms, or, less commonly, vague abdominal complaints. Most tumors are embryonal or sarcoma botryoides histologically (GREEN 1985).

The "classical" treatment approach has involved an anterior exenteration followed by regional irradiation and/or chemotherapy (WEICHSELBAUM et al. 1977; HAYS et al. 1981; MAURER et al. 1988). Successive attempts by both the IRS and the

International Society of Pediatric Oncology (SIOP) to eliminate or markedly reduce local therapy with surgery and/or irradiation for this site and other genitourinary primaries, relying on chemotherapy for control, have not been successful (RIVARD et al. 1975; HAYS et al. 1982; FLAMANT et al. 1985). Surgery and irradiation have been required to obtain locoregional control. More recent IRS data reveal that conservative surgery frequently delayed until multiagent chemotherapy followed by routine regional, irradiation (≥ 45 Gy) has been given led to substantial improvements (HAYS et al. 1991b). With this approach, about 50% of all patients with genitourinary primaries can avoid functionally destructive exenterative procedures and obtain tumor control. Results with vaginal lesions are similar. More radical surgical approaches have generally been reserved for patients who have developed local relapse after either limited surgery and chemotherapy or, occasionally, limited surgery, chemotherapy, and irradiation.

The French have reported excellent results in a series of children and young women with uterine and vaginal primaries of several histologic subtypes, including RMS, by utilizing brachytherapy in conjunction with more limited external beam therapy (EBRT) (FLAMANT et al. 1979; STOWE et al. 1982; NOVAES 1985; CURRAN et al. 1988). GERBAULET et al. (1985; personal communication, 1990) reported 80% 5-year survival and 72% 5-year relapse-free survival in a series of 37 girls and young women with tumors of the vulva, vagina, and uterus. Eleven had RMS, and at last follow-up, 12 of 17 patients in the entire group were menstruating. The functional advantages of this approach are considerable and should serve as a strong incentive to investigate this approach further.

At this time, initial evaluation should determine whether resection with organ preservation is feasible. If it is, local removal should be accomplished in addition to regional lymph node sampling. If complete excision has been obtained with adequate margins and nodes are negative, adjunct chemotherapy should be delivered and radiation reserved for possible relapse. If resection margins are positive (nodes negative) then brachytherapy or EBRT should be considered in addition to chemotherapy. Should intraoperative radiation capabilities exist, the possible use of this radiation modality should be entertained at the time of surgical resection (with frozen section analysis of surgical margins).

Should tumor removal not be possible without organ sacrifice (bladder, rectum, or uterus and vagina), or should even exenterative surgery not be feasi-

ble, then reliance should be placed on high-dose regional irradiation in conjunction with multiagent chemotherapy in an attempt to control tumor with less functional loss, especially of bladder and/or bowel function. Regional irradiation should also be delivered for patients with pathologically involved lymph nodes.

The radiation therapist must be alert to the likely interaction between cyclophosphamide, which is excreted in active form by the kidneys through the ureters and bladder, and local irradiation (JAYALAKSHMAMMA and PINKEL 1976). In some instances, nitrogen mustard has been substituted for cyclophosphamide in this setting, because of substantial bladder toxicity using cyclophosphamide. Use of iphosphamide with MESNA may also obviate this local problem. Overall, nearly 75% of these patients will be long-term disease-free survivors and, as noted, roughly two-thirds of this group will have preservation of bladder and bowel function.

19.8.7 Bladder and Prostate

Children with primaries of the bladder or prostate tend to present with voiding difficulties including acute urinary retention hematuria and dysuria (Green 1985). A significant male predominance (1.6:1.0) has been noted with bladder primaries, perhaps due to difficulty in distinguishing them from prostate tumors appearing as base of bladder lesions. Virtually all the considerations discussed with regard to vaginal tumors apply, with two exceptions: (1) It is almost always necessary to supplement surgery, including radical cystoprostatectomy, with local and/or regional irradiation for tumors of the prostate because of the invasive nature of tumors at this location, coupled with technical difficulties in achieving wide, tumor-free margins. (2) Tumors of the bladder pose particular difficulties in attempts at organ-preserving treatment. Occasionally, tumors may present at the dome of the bladder and be readily resected, and if clear margins and negative lymph nodes are present no irradiation need be given. However, much more commonly these tumors arise in the trigone or base of bladder region and urethral and/or ureteral obstruction is present. Because of toxicity issues mentioned previously, cytotoxic chemotherapy, especially the use of cyclophosphamide, is compromised and, perhaps in part because of this, responses to initial chemotherapy are usually modest. When radiation is delivered, the likely presence of significant residual tumor often requires an indwelling Foley catheter or, preferably, a suprapubic cystostomy and perhaps ureteral stents with their associated difficulties. Should tumor response to irradiation be slow and a catheter be required for several weeks, both acute and especially chronic complications, including stricture formation, are amplified. Finally, irradiation frequently follows (or is given concurrently with) intensive multiagent chemotherapy and interactions between several of the commonly utilized agents (cyclophosphamide, actinomycin D, and/or adriamycin) and irradiation combined with myelotoxic effects of wide-field irradiation which include the pelvis often cause severe normal tissue side-effects which may be life threatening or lethal.

This group of patients therefore requires the closest possible collaboration between disciplines for successful treatment and, even so, it may not be possible to attain the desired goal of tumor control with organ and function preservation.

Despite these may difficulties, the IRS and others have documented the importance of moderate- to high-dose irradiation in addition to aggressive multiagent chemotherapy in achieving tumor control and bladder preservation in this group (WEICHSELBAUM et al. 1977; HAYS et al. 1982a, 1991b). In IRS I, most children had initial cystectomy or radical cystoprostatectomy and although local control was achieved in many, function was suboptimal (MAURER et al. 1988). In IRS II, attempts were initiated to utilize multiagent chemotherapy in a neoadjuvant fashion and radiation therapy, when used, was not adequate (25 Gy in 5 weeks) (HAYS et al. 1982a). In 1980 radiation doses were increased and in IRS III (1985), moderate- to high-dose radiation therapy was given at 6 weeks to all but children who had tumors at the bladder dome in conjunction with intensified primary chemotherapy. Results have correspondingly improved (HAYS et al. 1991b). In IRS II, about 70% of these patients survived at 3 years and less than 25% had bladder function preserved (HAYS et al. 1982a). In contrast, in IRS III, 90% (73/81) survive and 60% have retained bladders (HAYS et al. 1991b).

19.8.8 Extremity

In most children, a mass is noted although a limp or signs and symptoms of metastatic disease may initially be the reason for presentation (GREEN 1985).

Lymph nodes are often involved (MANDELL et al. 1990b). In the IRS series, 12% of patients with lower extremity primaries were noted to have positive lymph nodes, but only 35% of these children (181/517) were biopsied and no data were provided for children with group III or IV disease (LAWRENCE et al. 1987a). A disproportionate number (~ 30%) of children with extremity lesions present with metastatic disease (HAYS et al. 1982; KINGSTON et al. 1983; GREEN 1985; DONALDSON 1989). The lungs and bones are most commonly affected; however, children may present with only bone or marrow disease and both a bone scan and bone marrow biopsy should be done in this group (RUYMANN et al. 1984).

More than half of the children with extremity primaries have alveolar histology, and other nonembryonal types such as soft tissue Ewing's tumor and the pleomorphic subtype are not uncommon (RANEY et al. 1983). Treatment results are suboptimal for both function and cure (HAYS et al. 1982b; RODARY et al. 1988c).

Initial amputation is not warranted. Five of six children in IRS I subjected to amputation died of tumor (HAYS et al. 1982b). Function-conserving surgical approaches should therefore be attempted. The high rate of local recurrence noted in unirradiated, unfavorable histology group I patients in IRS I and II makes postoperative irradiation of this group necessary, and this fact combined with young age at presentation may reduce functional outcome (TEFFT et al. 1985).

Ideally, the child with an embryonal extremity primary and no nodal disease may be managed with function-preserving resection with clear pathologic margins and subsequently receive only adjuvant chemotherapy. Unfortunately this is an uncommon occurrence and the great majority of these children will require irradiation. Principles developed in the management of adult soft tissue sarcomas should generally be used. Possible differences include the lack of clear evidence requiring treatment from muscle origin to insertion [as opposed to wide (2–5 cm) margins]. In addition, young age and small size may make it difficult to comply with certain principles (e.g., a constant sparing of a 0.75- to 1-cm strip of unirradiated skin and subcutaneous tissue carried out with rigid immobilization). However, these technical aspects are very important and appropriate measures (including general anesthesia) must be pursued to carry them out. KINSELLA et al. (1983) have particularly stressed these factors in the optimal treatment of hand and foot lesions. Radiation doses should not be compromised and total doses of 40–45

Gy should be used for presumed microscopic residual disease and higher doses utilized for gross residual disease in conjunction with multiagent chemotherapy.

Overall, survival in this group is less favorable than for sites such as the orbit or paratesticular region (see Fig. 19.1) (HAYS et al. 1982b; RODARY et al. 1988c). HAYS et al. have reported the results of "PRE" (primary reexcision following initial excision). In this study, a retrospective review of children with trunk and extremity RMS treated by IRS I and II was performed and a group of children subjected to radical re-resection at major centers prior to the administration of adjuvant treatment were found to have significantly improved 3-year survival (91% vs 74%). Of note was the observation that 15/41 (36%) had residual tumor identified which was gross in some patients despite apparent initial complete resection (HAYS et al. 1989). Possible favorable selection factors in the PRE group included tumor size (3.5 cm vs 5.5 cm), location of treatment (major centers vs community hospitals), and exclusion of certain patients (11) who had PRE but, because margins of second excision were still positive, were analyzed with group II rather than PRE. It is also uncertain how many PRE patients had positive lymph nodes found at reexcision and were therefore also excluded (i.e., a "Will Rogers effect") (HAYS et al. 1989). Thus although encouraging in this generally adverse group, routine reresection should be carried out with caution when the quality and extent of initial surgery are known to be appropriate, and optimally these data should be confirmed by a randomized study where possible selection factors will be more rigorously controlled.

Children and young adults with sarcomas of the hands and feet have classically been treated with amputation rather than more conservative surgery and irradiation because of concern about long-term function after moderate- to high-dose irradiation of these structures. Kinsella et al. and several other groups have now demonstrated that functional preservation can be achieved at these sites if reasonable selection is ensured and meticulous attention is paid to technique and immobilization. Use of electron beam therapy of appropriately limited energy, use of entrance dose sparing aspects of high-energy photon beams to restrict dose to certain sites [e.g., treatment of the dorsum of the distal foot with a high ($\geq$ 10 MV) energy photon beam entering from the plantar surface], and use of novel beam directions (e.g., trans-table lateral apparatus) are all potentially important technical aids to ensure optimal results.

19.8.9 Trunk

Children with primary tumors of the trunk, including the perineum, collectively fare less well with current therapy (RANEY et al. 1981, 1989; KINGSTON et al. 1983). Most children will have tumors of alveolar or nonembryonal histology and a disproportionate number will present with detectable distant metastases. Truncal location makes assessment of nodal involvement and likely drainage sites difficult because of the many possible options. The possibility of dissemination by pleural or peritoneal spread often makes adequacy of locoregional therapies difficult or impossible to achieve. Radical surgical resection is recommended where possible (RANEY et al. 1982).

Radiation therapy is frequently necessary either for treatment of microscopically positive surgical margins or because gross resection has not been technically possible. In addition to conventional photon techniques, electron beam treatment may be highly desirable to minimize underlying normal tissue damage.

For children with chest wall disease when probable pleural contamination has occurred and lung tolerance precludes treatment of the entire pleural space to adequate doses with photons, we have been impressed with the efficacy of wide-field photon treatment (18–20 Gy) combined with instillation of the beta emitter 32P. Although dosimetry is uncertain, this approach enables a higher pleural dose to be delivered without substantial lung damage than do conventional photon approaches and it also delivers a substantial radiation dose to hilar and other draining nodal groups. KUTCHER et al. (1987) have described a complex approach for treating the chest wall with combined photons and electrons that may also be used.

Despite these technical options, therapy for this group of children continues to be suboptimal and additional improvements, especially of systemic therapy, are needed.

KINSELLA et al. (1988) and the group at the National Cancer Institute have combined this unfavorable group of patients with other high-risk groups (e.g., patients with pelvic Ewing's tumor) and treated them with very intensive chemoradiation therapy following initial surgery and then attempted to consolidate treatment with ablative doses of chemotherapy, systemic, total body irradiation, and autologous bone marrow transplantation. Although data for patients with initial overt metastatic disease suggest no marked increase in long-term cures, data for nonmetastatic high-risk tumors are very encouraging and support additional clinical studies of this type.

19.9 Results

Remarkable improvements have occurred in cure rates achieved in RMS in the past three decades (CASSADY 1991). Published historical results document that fewer than 10%–15% of all children presenting with RMS were cured prior to 1960 (GREEN 1985). Even children presenting with RMS in an extremely favorable site – the orbit – fared poorly in this period, with only one in three surviving (MASSON and SOULE 1965). Utilization of irradiation has substantially improved locoregional control rates, while the development of effective multiagent chemotherapy has both facilitated local control achieved by surgery and radiation therapy and made possible the control of distant micrometastatic disease in many patients, especially those with embryonal RMS. Today approximately 60%–65% of all children presenting with RMS will be long-term tumor-free survivors (RANEY et al. 1989; CASSADY 1991).

Figures 19.8–19.11 demonstrate survival in recent IRS studies as a function of tumor stage, histology, lymph node involvement (groups I and II), and the presence or absence of metastatic disease. Local control should exceed 90%–95% in patients treated with appropriate chemoradiotherapy for presumed microscopic disease (DRITSCHILO et al. 1978). Figure 19.12 demonstrates local control achieved in 41 patients with gross residual disease (group III) who were seen and treated with high-dose, wide-field regional irradiation and multiagent chemotherapy at Boston's Children Hospital (author's own data).

Prognostic factors in achieving local control include tumor size (> 5–6 cm in adverse), presence of extensive bony involvement (Table 19.11) (TARBELL et al. 1987; MANDELL et al. 1989), and, perhaps, sex

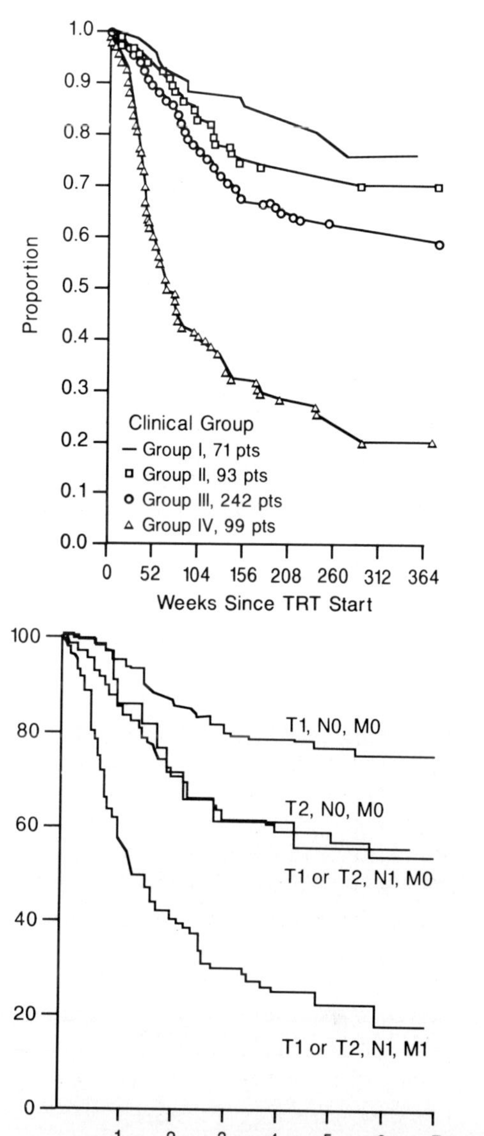

Fig. 19.8. Survival as a function of clinical IRS group (*top*) or UICC TNM stage (*bottom*). The similar prognostic impact of large (> 5 cm) primary size or regional nodal involvement is evident. (RUYMANN 1987; LAWRENCE et al. 1987b)

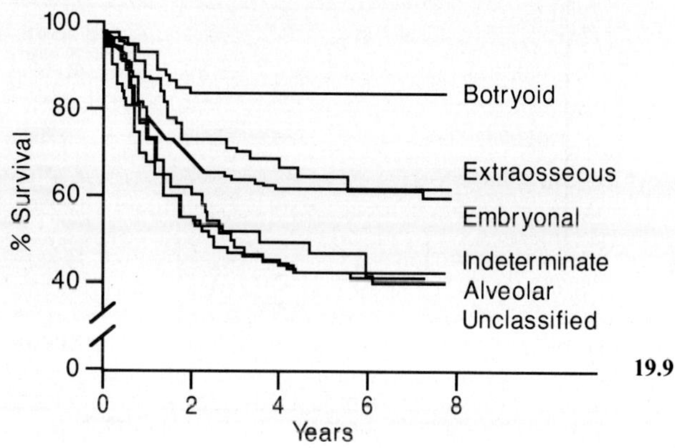

Fig. 19.9. Survival as a function of histologic subtype (including patients with extraosseous Ewing's tumor). The decreased survival in patients with alveolar histology is evident. (adapted from NEWTON et al. 1988)

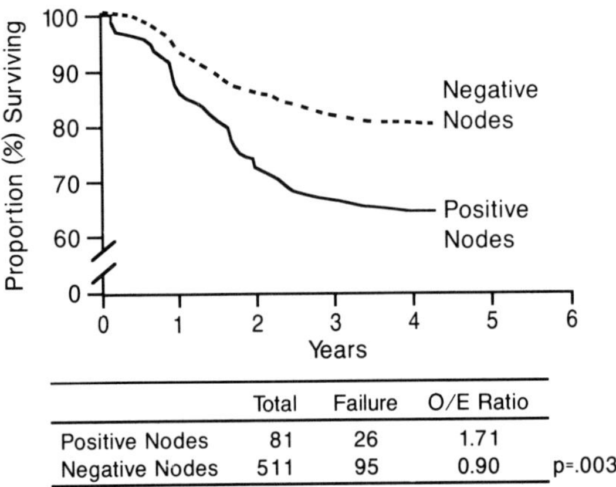

Fig. 19.10. Influence on survival of pathologic nodal involvement in children with group I or II disease in IRS I and II. (adapted from LAWRENCE et al. 1987a)

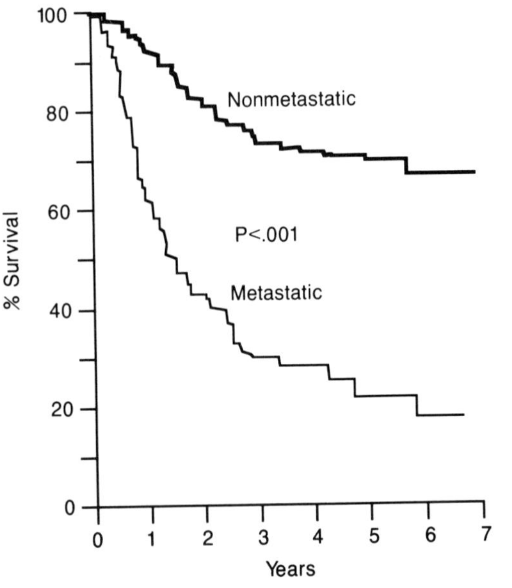

Fig. 19.11. Survival curves for children presenting with and without distant metastatic disease in IRS II. (adapted from LAWRENCE et al. 1987b)

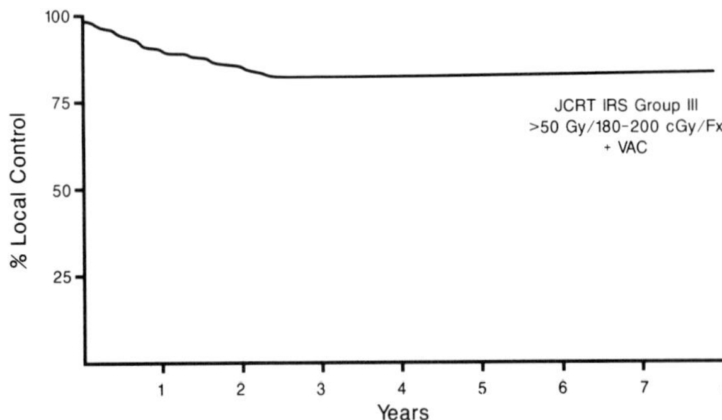

Fig. 19.12. Survival for 41 children with group III RMS following surgical confirmation/treatment with known gross residual disease treated with aggressive chemotherapy (VAC) and irradiation at the Joint Center for Radiation Therapy

Table 19.11. Influence of extensive bone erosion on local and distant relapse in head and neck RMS

Author	No. of patients	Local and distant relapse	Local failure
TARBELL et al. 1987	11	8 (73%)	3 (27%)
MANDELL et al. 1989	22	8 (38%)	8 (38%)
Total	33	16 (49%)	11 (33%)

(KINGSTON et al. 1983; TARBELL et al. 1987) and primary site, with orbital tumors faring well (GREEN 1985; RANEY 1989; RODARY et al. 1988c). However, maintenance of local control continues to represent a significant problem in overall results with RMS. Examination of IRS autopsy results and SIOP pathology data for children who relapse, which include site of first relapse, demonstrates that a significant (15%–20%) number of children fail with evidence of only local relapse and a much larger group (40%–45%) fail with evidence of both local/regional and distant disease (see Table 19.4) (SHIMADA et al. 1987; CAILLAUD et al. 1989).

Treatment programs for children with metastatic disease continue to be relatively ineffective, especially for those with alveolar histology (OKAMURA et al. 1977; RANEY et al. 1989). Finally, salvage attempts for children who relapse after initial management are rarely adequate for long-term control. Only 3 of 60 (5%) children with initial group I–III RMS had long-term salvage after relapse (RANEY et al. 1983).

19.10 Complications

As RMS may occur at virtually any body site and as moderate to high doses of irradiation are usually necessary in conjunction with interactive multiagent chemotherapy and surgery, almost all described radiation complications of bone, soft tissue, and organs are possible. As very young children are often treated, complications of growth and development (Chap. 3) are frequent and second tumor formation is a risk. HEYN et al. (1991) have described 17 second malignant neoplasms in 1820 patients entered on IRS studies I and II. Bone tumors (seven of eight in radiated field) and myeloid leukemia (four) were most frequently seen.

It is beyond the scope of this chapter to list and/or describe all possible complications. However, certain complications occur with relative frequency and uniqueness in RMS and deserve comment.

19.10.1 Cataract Formation

Cataract formation is almost always seen, after an appropriate latent period, following fractionated doses of 8–10 Gy to the lens using conventional (2–3 Gy/min) dose rates (MERRIAM and FOCHT 1957). Although lens opacities formed at these relatively low doses may be visually minimal or modest, cataracts engendered following doses of higher than 40–45 Gy in the treatment of orbital RMS are always dense and ultimately require correction. However, onset of cataract formation rarely occurs until 16–18 months following treatment and no intervention is usually necessary until 20–24 months following irradiation. As RMS of the orbit frequently is primary in the eyelid and tumor may extend throughout the orbit (including posteriorly), attempts at lens shielding are hazardous and may shield tumor and facilitate local failure.

Another frequent complication of treatment of orbital and other head and neck primary sites is orbital, facial, and paranasal sinus cellulitis (HEYN et al. 1986; WHARAM et al. 1987a). This complication is frequently temporally associated with cyclic administration of pulsed chemotherapy with agents, such as actinomycin D and adriamycin, that are known to interact and cause "recall" radiative reactions (D'ANGIO et al. 1959). Prompt antibiotic treatment is necessary and signs and symptoms of erythema, pain, and fever usually subside rapidly when latent drug effects have dissipated somewhat (usually 2–3 weeks after drug administration). These effects are usually most notable after the first three or four cycles of drug administration following irradiation and become progressively less of a problem after that time.

If dose guidelines are exceeded or technical factors such as lid retraction are not adhered to, a number of other orbital and ocular complications are possible, including severe keratoconjunctivitis (PARSONS et al. 1983; HEYN et al. 1986).

19.10.2 Bony Effects

As RMS affects the pelvic region in nearly one-third of all patients, another unusual complication which has been noted is unilateral or bilateral slipped caput femoral epiphysis (WOLFE et al. 1977). Although femoral head irradiation may cause this problem in patients who do not have the usual body habitus of the idiopathic form, the precise mechanism of causation is unclear but may be vascular in nature. If possible, femoral head irradiation doses should be kept to less than 15 Gy in children below 12 years of age in order to minimize this problem.

CARIES and other dental problems associated with head and neck irradiation are frequently seen, and routine fluoride prophylaxis should be initiated early in treatment and continued as needed should head and neck treatment be undertaken (DOLINE et al. 1980; HAZRA and SHIPMAN 1982).

The wide range of complications that may occur or develop over time in these children emphasizes the importance of continued lifetime follow-up (PROBERT et al. 1973; PHILLIPS and FU 1976; TEFFT et al. 1976; HEYN 1985; FROMM et al. 1986). We feel this is best accomplished in a clinic established primarily for this purpose and that this clinic should be restricted to children who have probably been cured of their primary malignancy (i.e., 3–5 years following initiation of treatment). Participants should include all treatment disciplines, and participation of endocrinologists, plastic surgeons, orthopedists, dentists, psychiatrists, and other health care professionals (i.e., nurses and social workers) is critical.

As treated children become teenagers and young adults, there is a natural tendency to put this unpleasant part of their childhood behind them and avoid follow-up appointments, etc. This tendency must be prevented if possible for optimal management.

19.11 Future Prospects

Although much progress has been made, the catalog of improvements needed in the management of RMS is a long one:

1. Better systemic agents and combinations are needed for management of metastatic disease in all groups of patients. This is especially true for children with alveolar and pleomorphic RMS, where available regimens are less effective than with embryonal histology even when given in adjuvant fashion for the control of possible occult microscopic disease.

2. Better irradiation approaches are needed for control of currently unfavorable local settings e.g., children with large tumors or with extensive bone disease. It is possible that current clinical hyperfractionation studies will contribute to the solution to this problem.

3. Optimal sequencing of surgery, chemotherapy, and irradiation needed to be established on a scientific rather than an empirical basis both from the standpoint of tumor control and to minimize acute, subacute, and late normal tissue toxicity.

4. With increasing knowledge of the different molecular makeup of the tumors lumped together in the category RMS, it will be necessary, as has been done in Wilms' tumor, non-Hodgkin's lymphomas, and other tumors, to separate these tumors into their individual types. It is probable that different treatment combinations rather than uniform therapy will be necessary for many of these tumors, and a continued "waste basket" approach will only serve to confuse treatment issues.

5. Current local treatment approaches with radiation therapy and surgery, although necessary for tumor control and cure, are suboptimal. Ultimately, less toxic and less destructive forms of treatment are necessary in these very young children, who, despite considerable functional gains, continue to suffer substantial long-term consequences. Prevention of some of these adverse effects by means of radioprotectors, alternative fractionation patterns, and tumor prevention agents such as retinoids needs to be actively investigated in group studies.

References

Abramson DH, Ellsworth RM, Tretter P, Wolff JA, Kitchen FD (1979) The treatment of orbital rhabdomyosarcoma with irradiation and chemotherapy. Ophthalmology 86: 1330–1335

Angervall L Enzinger FM (1975) Extraskeletal neoplasm resembling Ewing's sarcoma. Cancer 36: 240–251

Ashton N, Morgan G (1965) Embryonal sarcoma and embryonal rhabdomyosarcoma of the orbit. J Clin Pathol 18: 699–714

Baum ES, Gaynon P, Greenberg L, Krivit W, Hammond D (1981) Phase II trial of cisplatin in refractory childhood cancer. Children's Cancer Study Group Report. Cancer Treat Rep 65: 815–822

Berg SL, Grisell DL, DeLaney TF, Balis FM (1991) Principles of treatment of pediatric solid tumors. Pediatr Clin North Am 38: 249–267

Berry MP, Jenkin RDT (1981) Parameningeal rhabdomyosarcoma in the young. Cancer 48: 281–288

Bonadonna G, Monfardini S, Delena M, Fosati-Bellani F, Beretta G (1970) Phase and preliminary phase II evaluation of adriamycin (NSC-12327). Cancer Res 30: 2572–2582

Burrington JD (1969) Rhabdomyosarcoma of the paratesticular tissues in children. Report of eight cases. J Pediatr Surg 4: 503–510

Caillaud JM, Gerard-Marchant R, Marsden HB, Van-Unnik AJ, Rodary C, Rey A, Flamant F (1989) Histopathological classification of childhood rhabdomyosarcoma: a report from the International Society of Pediatric Oncology Pathology Panel. Med Pediatr Oncol 17: 391–400

Cassady JR (1991) Keynote address: contributions of pediatric oncology: examples derived from advances made in the treatment of rhabdomyosarcoma and neuroblastoma. Int J Radiat Oncol Biol Phys 20: 1177–1182

Cassady JR, Sagerman RH, Tretter P, Ellsworth RM (1968) Radiation therapy for rhabdomyosarcoma. Radiology 91: 116–120

Chan RC, Sutow WW, Lindberg RD (1979) Parameningeal rhabdomyosarcoma. Radiology 131: 211–214

Crist WM, Kun LE (1991) Common solid tumors of childhood. N Engl J Med 324: 461–471

Crist WM, Garnsey L, Gehan EA, Maurer HM (1990) Evidence of "stage shift" in IRS studies? J Clin Oncol 8: 1768–1769

Curran WS, Littman P, Raney RB (1988) Interstitial radiation therapy in the treatment of childhood soft tissue sarcomas. Int J Radiat Oncol Biol Phys 14: 169–174

D'Angio GJ, Farber S, Maddock CL (1959) Potentiation of x-ray effects by actinomycin-D. Radiology 73: 175–177

De Vita V, Hellman S, Rosenberg S (1982) Cancer. Principles and Practice of Oncology, 1st ed., J.B. Lippincott, Philadelphia

Doline S, Needleman HL, Petersen R, Cassady JR (1980) The effect of radiotherapy in the treatment of retinoblastoma upon the developing dentition. J Pediatr Ophthalmol 17: 109–113

Donaldson SS (1989) Rhabdomyosarcoma: contemporary status and future directions. Ann Surg 124: 1015–1020

Donaldson SS, Belli JA (1984) A rational clinical staging system for childhood rhabdomyosarcoma. J Clin Oncol 2: 135–139

Donaldson SS, Castro JR, Wilbur JR, Jesse R (1973) Rhabdomyosarcoma of head and neck in children; combination treatment by surgery, irradiation and chemotherapy. Cancer 31: 26–35

Dritschilo A, Weichselbaum RR, Cassady JR, Jaffe N, Green D, Filler RM (1978) The role of radiation therapy in the treatment of soft tissue sarcomas of childhood. Cancer 42: 1192–1203

Egbert PR, Donaldson SS, Moazed K, Rosenthal AR (1978) Visual results and ocular complications following radiotherapy for retinoblastoma. Arch Ophthalmol 96: 1826–1830

Enterline HT, Horn RC Jr (1958) Alveolar rhabdomyosarcoma. Am J Clin Pathol 29: 356–366

Enzinger FM, Skiraki M (1969) Alveolar rhabdomyosarcoma. Cancer 24: 18–31

Exelby RP, Ghavimi F, Jereb B (1978) Genitourinary rhabdomyosarcoma in children. J Pediatr Surg 13: 746–752

Fernandez CH, Sutow WW, Merino OR, George SL (1975) Childhood rhabdomyosarcoma: analysis of coordinated therapy and results. AJR 123: 588–597

Flamant F, Chassagne D, Cosset JM, Gerbaulet A, Lemerle J (1979) Embryonal rhabdomyosarcoma of the vagina in children. Conservative treatment with curietherapy and chemotherapy. Eur J Cancer 15: 527–532

Flamant F, Rodary C, Voute PA, Otten J (1985) Primary chemotherapy in the treatment of rhabdomyosarcoma in children: trial of the International Society of Pediatric Oncology (SIOP), preliminary results. Radiother Oncol 3: 227–236

Fromm M, Littman P, Raney RB, Nelson L, Handler S, Diamond G, Stanley C (1986) Late effects after treatment of twenty children with soft tissue sarcomas of the head and neck: experience at a single institution with a review of the literature. Cancer 57: 2070–2076

Fusner JE, Pizzo PA, Poplack DG, Freeman C (1978) Meningeal relapse of orbital rhabdomyosarcoma. Med Pediatr Oncol 4: 247–251

Gaiger AM, Soule EH, Newton WA Jr (1981) Pathology of rhabdomyosarcoma: experience of the Intergroup Rhabdomyosarcoma Study, 1972–1978, NCI Monogr 56: 19–27

Gasparini M, Lombardi F, Gianni C, Lovati C, Fossati-Bellami F (1983) Childhood rhabdomyosarcoma with meningeal extension: results of combined therapy including central nervous system prophylaxis. Am J Clin Oncol 6: 393–398

Gerbaulet A, Panis X, Flamant F, Chassagne D (1985) Iridium afterloading curietherapy in the treatment of pediatric malignancies. Institute Gustave-Roussy experience. Cancer 56: 1274–1279

Ghavimi F, Exelby PR, D'Angio GJ et al. (1973) Combination therapy of urogenital embryonal rhabdomyosarcoma in children. Cancer 32: 1178–1184

Ghavimi F, Exelby PR, Lieberman PH, Scott BF, Kosloff C (1981) Multidisciplinary treatment of embryonal rhabdomyosarcoma in children: a progress report. NCI Monogr 56: 111–120

Green DM (1978) Evaluation of single-dose vincristine, actinomycin D, and cyclophosphamide in childhood solid tumors. Cancer Treat Rep 62: 1517–1520

Green DM (1985) Rhabdomyosarcoma. In: Green DM (ed) Diagnosis and management of malignant solid tumors in infants and children. Martinus Nijhoff, Boston, pp 15–89

Green DM, Jaffe N (1978) Progress and controversy in the treatment of childhood rhabdomyosarcoma. Cancer Treat Rev 5: 7–27

Grosfeld JL, Weber TR, Weetman RM, Baehneer RL (1983) Rhabdomyosarcoma in childhood: analysis of survival in 98 cases. J Pediatr Surg 18: 141–146

Haddy TB, Nora AHJ, Sutow WW, Vietti TJ (1967) Cyclophosphamide treatment for metastatic soft tissue sarcoma: intermittent large doses in the treatment of children. Am J Dis Child 114: 301–308

Halperin EC, Kun LE, Constine LS, Tarbell NJ (eds) Rhabdomyosarcoma. In: Pediatric Radiation Oncology. Raven, New York, pp 223–246

Harmer MH (1982) TNM classification of pediatric tumors. UICC (Union Internationale Contre le Cancer), Geneva, pp 23–28

Hays DM, Raney RB Jr, Lawrence W Jr, Gehan EA, Soule EH, Tefft M, Maurer HM (1981) Rhabdomyosarcoma of the female urogenital tract. J Pediatr Surg 16: 828–834

Hays DM, Raney RB, Lawrence W Jr et al. (1982a) Primary chemotherapy in the treatment of children with bladder-prostate tumors in the Intergroup Rhabdomyosarcoma Study (IRS-II). J Pediatr Surg 17: 812–820

Hays DM, Soule EH, Lawrence W Jr et al. (1982b) Extremity lesions in the Intergroup Rhabdomyosarcoma Study (IRS-1). A preliminary report. Cancer 48: 1–8

Hays DM, Lawrence W Jr, Wharam M et al. (1989) Primary reexcision for patients with 'microscopic residual' tumor following initial excision of sarcomas of trunk and extremity sites. J Pediatr Surg 24: 5–10

Hays D, Raney RB, Crist W et al. for the IRS Committee of the Childrens Cancer Study Group and Pediatric Oncology Group (1991a) Improved survival and bladder preservation among patients with bladder/prostate primary tumors in Intergroup Rhabdomyosarcoma Study III (IRS) (abstract C-1119). Proc Am Soc Clin Oncol 10: 318

Hays D, Raney RB, Crist W et al. (1991b) Improved survival and bladder preservation among patients with bladder/prostate primary tumors in Intergroup Rhabdomyosarcoma Study II (IRS) (abstract CO-1119). Proc Am Soc Clin Oncol 10: 318

Hazra TA, Shipman B (1982) Dental problems in pediatric patients with head and neck tumors undergoing multiple modality therapy. Med Pediatr Oncol 10: 91–95

Heyn RM (1985) Late effects of therapy in rhabdomyosarcoma. Clin Oncol 4: 287–297

Heyn RM, Holland R, Newton WA Jr, Tefft M, Breslow N, Hartmann JR (1974) The role of combined chemotherapy in the treatment of rhabdomyosarcoma. Cancer 34: 2128–2142

Heyn R, Ragab A, Raney B et al. (1986) Late effects of therapy in orbital rhabdomyosarcoma in children. A report from the Intergroup Rhabdomyosarcoma Study. Cancer 57: 1738–1743

Heyn R, Beltangady M, Hays D et al. (1989) Results of intensive therapy in children with localized alveolar extremity rhabdomyosarcoma: a report from the Intergroup Rhabdomyosarcoma Study. J Clin Oncol 7: 200–207

Heyn R, Haeberlen V, Newton WA, Ragab A, Raney RB, Tefft M, Garnsey L for the IRS Committee of CCSG, POG and UKCCSG (1991) Second malignant neoplasms: inpatients treated on Intergroup Rhabdomyosarcoma Studies I-II (IRS I–II) (abstract C-1090). Proc Am Soc Clin Oncol 10: 311

Horn RC Jr, Enterline HT (1958) Rhabdomyosarcoma: a clinic pathological study and classification of 39 cases. Cancer 11: 181–199

James DH, Hustu O, Wrenn EL, Johnson WW (1966) Childhood malignant tumors: concurrent chemotherapy with dactinomycin and vincristine sulfate. JAMA 197: 1043–1045

Jayalakshmamma B, Pinkel D (1976) Urinary-bladder toxicity following pelvic irradiation and simultaneous cyclophosphamide therapy. Cancer 38: 701–707

Jereb B, Cham W, Lattin P, Exelby P, Ghavimi F, D'Angio GJ, Tefft M (1976) Local control of embryonal rhabdomyosarcoma in children by radiation therapy when combined with concomitant chemotherapy. Int J Radiat Oncol Biol Phys 1: 217–225

Jereb B, Haik BG, Ong R, Ghavimi F (1985) Parameningeal rhabdomyosarcoma (including the orbit): results of orbital irradiation. Int J Radiat Oncol BIol Phys 11: 2057–2065

Jones IS, Reese AB, Krout J (1965) Orbital rhabdomyosarcoma: an analysis of sixty-two cases. Trans Am Opthalmol Soc 63: 223–255

Kato MADP, Flamant F, Terrier-Lacombe MJ et al. (1991) Rhabdomyosarcoma of the larynx in children: a series of five patients treated in the Institute Gustave Roussy (Villejuif, France). Med Pediatr Oncol 19: 110–114

Keus R, Noach P, de Boer R, Lebesque J (1991) The effect of customized beam shaping on normal tissue complications in radiation therapy of parotid gland tumors. Radiother Oncol 21: 211–217

Kingston JE, McElwain TJ, Malpas JS (1983) Childhood rhabdomyosarcoma: experience of the children's solid tumor group. Br J Cancer 48: 198–207

Kinsella TJ, Loeffler JS, Fraass BA, Tepper J (1983) Extremity preservation by combined modality therapy in sarcomas of the hand and foot: an analysis of local control, disease-free survival and functional results. Int J Radiat Oncol Biol Phys 9: 1115–1119

Kinsella TJ, Miser JS, Triche TJ, Horvath K, Glatstein E (1988) Treatment of high-risk sarcomas in children and young adults: analysis of local control using intensive combined modality therapy. NCI Monogr 6: 291–296

Kutcher GJ, Kestler C, Greenblatt D et al. (1987) Technique for external beam treatment for mesothelioma. Int J Radiat Oncol Biol Phys 13: 1747–1752

Lacey SR, Jewett TC, Karp MP, Allen JE, Cooney DR (1986) Advances in the treatment of rhabdomyosarcoma. Semin Surg Oncol 2: 139–146

Lawrence W Jr, Hays DM, Moon TE (1977) Lymphatic metastasis with childhood rhabdomyosarcoma. Cancer 39: 556–559

Lawrence W Jr, Hays DM, Heyn R et al. (1987a) Lymphatic metastases with childhood rhabdomyosarcoma. A report from the Intergroup Rhabdomyosarcoma Study. Cancer 60: 910–915

Lawrence W, Gehan EA, Hays DM, Beltangady M, Maurer HM (1987b) Prognostic significance of staging system in childhood rhabdomyosarcoma: a report from the Intergroup Rhabdomyosarcoma Study (IRS II). J Clin Oncol 5: 46–54

Li FP, Fraumeni JF (1969) Rhabdomyosarcoma in children: epidemiologic study and identification of a familial cancer syndrome. JNCI 43: 1365–1373

Malpas JS, Freeman JE, Paxton A, Smith JW, Stansfeld AG, Wood CBS (1976) Radiotherapy and adjuvant combination chemotherapy for childhood rhabdomyosarcoma. Br Med J I: 247–249

Mandell LR, Ghavimi F, Exelby PR, Fuks Z (1988) Preliminary results of alternating combination chemotherapy (CT) and hyperfractionated radiotherapy (HART) in advanced rhabdomyosarcoma (RMS). Int J Radiat Oncol Biol Phys 15: 197–203

Mandell LR, Massey V, Ghavimi F (1989) The influence of extensive bone erosion on local central in non-orbital rhabdomyosarcoma of the head and neck. Int J Radiat Oncol Biol Phys 17: 649–653

Mandell L, Ghavimi F, La Quaglia M (1990a) Alternating chemotherapy (CT) and hyperfractionated (HF) radiotherapy (RT) in advanced rhabdomyosarcoma (RMS): an update (abstract C-1157). Proc Am Soc Clin Oncol 9: 298

Mandell L, Ghavimi F La Quaglia M, Exelby P (1990b) Prognostic significance of regional lymph node involvement in childhood extremity rhabdomyosarcoma. Med Pediatr Oncol 18: 466–471

Masson JK, Soule EH (1965) Embryonal rhabdomyosarcoma of the head and neck. Report on eighty-eight cases. Am J Surg 110: 585–591

Maurer HM (1975) The Intergroup Rhabdomyosarcoma Study (N.I.H.) objectives and clinical staging classification. J Pediatr Surg 10: 977–978

Maurer HM, Moon T, Donaldson M et al. (1977) The Intergroup Rhabdomyosarcoma Study, a preliminary report. Cancer 40: 2015–2026

Maurer HM, Beltangady M, Gehan EA et al. (1988) The Intergroup Rhabdomyosarcoma Study-I, a final report. Cancer 61: 209–220

McFarland J (1911) Sarcoma of the vagina. Am J Med Sci 141: 570–588

McKeen EA, Bodurtha J, Meadows AT, Douglass EC, Mulvihill SJ (1978) Rhabdomyosarcoma complicating multipe neurofibromatosis. J Pediatr 93: 992–993

Merriam GR, Focht EF (1957) A clinical study of radiation cataracts and the relationship to dose. AJR 77: 759–785

Newton WA, Soule EH, Hamoudi AB et al. (1988) Histopathology of childhood sarcomas. Intergroup Rhabdomyosarcoma Studies I and II: clinical pathological correlation. J Clin Oncol 6: 67–75

Nickolson GW (1950) DeP in studies on tumour formation. C.V. Mosby, St. Louis, p 194

Novaes, PERS (1985) Interstitital therapy in the management of soft tissue sarcoma in childhood. Med Pediatr Oncol 13: 221–224

O'Bryan RM, Luce JK, Talley RW, Gottlieb JA, Baker LH, Bonadonna G (1973) Phase II evaluation of adriamycin in human neoplasia. Cancer 32: 1–8

Okamura J, Sutow WW, Moon TE (1977) Prognosis in children with metastatic rhabdomyosarcoma. Med Pediatr Oncol 3: 243–251

Olive D, Flamant F, Zucker JM et al. (1984) Periaortic lymphadenectomy is not necessary in the treatment of localized paratesticular rhabdomyosarcoma. Cancer 54: 1283–1287

Ortega JA, Fryer C, Gehan E et al. for the IRS Committee of the Children's Cancer Study Group (CCSG), the Pediatric Oncology Group (POG) and United Kingdom CCSG (1990) Efficacy of reducing tissue volume irradiation in children with cranial (CR) parameningeal (PM) rhabdomyosarcoma (RMS). A report for the Intergroup Rhabdomyosarcoma Study (IRS) III (abstract C-1147). Proc Am Soc Clin Oncol 9: 296

Ortega J, Ragab A, Gehan EA, Donaldson SS, Wiener E, Maurer HM for the IRS Committee of the Children's Cancer Study Group (CCSG) and the Pediatric Oncology Group (POG) (1991) Ifosfamide (IF), actinomycin-D, and vincristine (VCR) for the treatment of childhood rhabdomyosarcoma (RMS): a feasibility and toxicity study. A report for the Intergroup Rhabdomyosarcoma Study (IRS) IV (abstract C-1102). Proc Am Soc Clin Oncol 10: 314

Palmer N, Foulkes M (1983) Histopathology and prognosis in the second Intergroup Rhabdomyosarcoma Study (IRS II) (abstract C-899). Proc Am Soc Clin Oncol 2: 229

Palmer N, Sachs N, Foulkes M (1982) Histopathology and prognosis in rhabdomyosarcoma (IRS I) (abstract C-660). Proc Am Soc Clin Oncol 1: 170

Parsons JT, Fitzgerald CR, Hood CI, Ellingwood KE, Bova FJ, Millian RR (1983) The effects of irradiation on the eye and optic nerve. Int J Radiat Oncol Biol Phys 9: 609–622

Pedrick TJ, Donaldson SS, Cox RS (1986) Rhabdomyosarcoma: the Stanford experience using a TNM staging system. J Clin Oncol 4: 370–378

Phillips T, Fu K (1976) Quantification of combined radiation therapy and chemotherapy effects on critical normal tissues. Cancer 37: 1186–1200

Pinkel D (1959) Actinomycin D in childhood cancer: a preliminary report. Padiatrics 23: 342–347

Pizzo PA, Horowitz ME, Poplack DG, Hays DM, Kun LE (1989) Solid tumors of childhood. In: DeVita VT Jr Hellman S, Rosenberg SA (eds) Cancer: principles and practice of oncolgy, 3rd edn. JB Lippincott, Philadelphia, pp 1647–1654

Potter GD (1966) Embryonal rhabdomyosarcoma of the middle ear in children. Cancer 19: 221–226

Pratt CB (1969) Response of childhood rhabdomyosarcoma to combination chemotherapy. J Pediatr 74: 791–794

Probert JC, Parker BR, Kaplan HS (1973) Growth retardation in children after megavoltage irradiation of the spine. Cancer 32: 634–639

Raney RB Jr, Hays DM, Lawrence W Jr, Soule EH, Tefft M, Donaldson MH (1978) Paratesticular rhabdomyosarcoma in childhood. Cancer 42: 729–736

Raney RG Jr, Gehan EA, Maurer HM et al. (1979) Evaluation of intensified chemotherapy in children with advanced rhabdomyosarcoma (clinical group III and IV). Clin Cancer Trials 3: 1928

Raney RB, Donaldson MH, Sutow WW, Lindberg RD, Maurer HM, Tefft M (1981) Special considerations related to primary site in rhabdomyosarcoma: experience of the Intergroup Rhabdomyosarcoma Study 1972–1976. NCI Monogr 56: 69–74

Raney RB Jr, Ragab AH, Ruymann FB, Lindberg RD, Hays DM, Gehan EA, Soule EH (1982) Soft-tissue sarcoma of the trunk in childhood. Results of the Intergroup Rhabdomyosarcoma Study. Cancer 49: 2612–2616

Raney RB Jr, Crist WM, Maurer HM, Foulkes MA for the Intergroup Rhabdomyosarcoma Study Committee (1983) Prognosis of children with soft tissue sarcoma who relapse after achieving a complete response. Cancer 52: 44–50

Raney RB, Tefft M, Lawrence W et al. (1987a) Paratesticular sarcoma in childhood and adolescence: a report from the Intergroup Rhabdomyosarcoma Studies (IRS) I and II (1973–1983). Cancer 60: 2337–2343

Raney RB Jr, Tefft M, Newton WA Jr et al. (1987b) Improved prognosis with cranial soft tissue sarcomas arising in nonorbital parameningeal sites: a report from the Intergroup Rhabdomyosarcoma Study. Cancer 59: 147–155

Raney RB Jr, Hays DM, Tefft M, Triche TJ (1989) Rhabdomyosarcoma and undifferentiated sarcomas. In: Pizzo PA, Poplack O (eds) Principles and practice of pediatric oncology. JB Lippincott, Philadelphia, pp 635–658

Raney RB, Tefft M, Newton WA, Maurer HM, Gehan EA for the IRS Committee of the Children's Cancer Study Group (CCSG), Pediatric Oncology Group (POG) and United Kingdom Children's Cancer Study Group (UKCCSG) (1990) Ascending transverse myelitis in patients with parameningeal sarcoma treated intensively on Intergroup Rhabdomyosarcoma Studies (IRS) (abstract C-1129). Proc Am Soc Clin Oncol 9: 291

Raney RB Jr, Crist WM, Donaldson SS, Gehan EA, Maurer HM (1991) A pilot study of ifosfamide/mesna and doxorubicin (I Fos/Dox) followed by vincristine, actinomycin D, and cyclophosphamide (VAC) and hyperfractionated irradiation (HFRT) for children with metastatic soft tissue sarcoma: a report from the Intergroup Rhabdomyosarcoma Study (IRS) (abstract C 1098). Proc Am Soc Clin Oncol 10: 313

Riopelle JL, Theriault JP (1956) Sur une forme meconnue de sarcome des parties molles; le rhabdomyosarcoma alveolaire Ann Anat Pathol 1: 88–111

Rivard G, Ortega J, Hittle R, Nitschke R, Karon M (1975) Intensive chemotherapy as primary treatment for rhabdomyosarcoma of the pelvis. Cancer 36: 1593–1597

Rodary C, Rey A, Olive D et al. (1988a) Prognostic factors in 281 children with nonmetastatic rhabdomyosarcoma (RMS) at diagnosis. Med Pediatr Oncol 16: 71–77

Rodary C, Rey A, Olive D et al. (1988b) Prognostic factors in 281 children with non-metastatic rhabdomyosarcoma (RMS) at diagnosis. Med Pediatr Oncol 16: 71–77

Rodary C, Rey A, Olive D et al. (1988c) Prognostic factors in 281 children with nonmetastatic rhabdomyosarcoma (RMS) at diagnosis. Med Pediatr Oncol 16: 71–77

Ruymann TB (1987) Rhabdomyosarcoma in children and adolescents: A review Hematol Oncol Clin NA 1: 621–654

Ruymann FB, Newton WA Jr, Ragab AH, Donaldson MD, Foulkes M (1984) for the Intergroup Rhabdomyosarcoma Study Committee. Bone marrow metastases at diagnosis in children and adolescents with rhabdomyosarcoma. A report from the Intergroup Rhabdomyosarcoma Study. Cancer 53: 368–373

Ruymann FB, Maddux HR, Ragab A et al. (1988) Congenital anomalies associated with rhabdomyosarcoma: An autopsy study of 115 cases: a report from the Intergroup Rhabdomyosarcoma Study Committee representing the Children's Cancer Study Group and the Pediatric Intergroup Statistical Center. Med Pediatr Oncol 16: 33–39

Scrable H, Cavenee W, Ghavimi F, Lovell M, Morgan K, Sapienza C (1989) A model for embryonal rhabdomyosarcoma that involves genome imprinting. Proc Natl Acad Sci USA 86: 7480–7484

Selawry OS, Holland JR, Wolman IJ (1968) Effect of vincristine (NSC-67574) on malignant solid tumors in children. Cancer Chemother Rep 52: 497–500

Shaw RK, Moore EW, Mueller PS, Frei E III, Watkin DM (1960) The effect of actinomycin D on childhood neoplasms. Am J Dis Child 99: 628–635

Shimada H, Newton WA Jr, Soule EH et al. (1987) Pathology of fatal rhabdomyosarcoma: reports from Intergroup Rhabdomyosarcoma Studies (IRSI-II). Cancer 59: 459–465

Soule EH, Newton WA Jr, Moon TE, Tefft M (1978) Extraskeletal Ewing's sarcoma. Cancer 42: 259–264

Stobbe GD, Dargeon HW (1950) Embryonal rhabdomyosarcoma of the head and neck in children and adolescents. Cancer 3: 826–836

Stout AP (1946) Rhabdomyosarcoma of the skeletal muscles. Ann Surg 123: 447–472

Stowe SM, Littman P, Wara W, Raney RB, Tefft M (1982) The use of implantation in childhood tumors. The experience of the Children's Cancer Study Group member institutions (abstr 16). Proc Am Soc Clin Oncol 5: 129

Sutow WW (1967) Cyclophosphamide (NSC-2627) in Wilms' tumor and rhabdomyosarcoma. Cancer Chemother Rep 51: 407–409

Sutow WW (1968) Vincristine (NSC-67574) therapy for malignant solid tumors in children (except Wilms' tumor). Cancer Chemother Rep 52: 485–487

Sutow WW, Berry DH, Haddy TB, Sullivan MP, Watkins WL, Windmiller J (1966) Vincristine sulfate therapy in children with metastatic soft tissue sarcoma. Pediatrics 38: 465–472

Sutow WW, Vietti TJ, Lonsdale D, Talley RW (1972) Daunomycin in the treatment of metastatic soft tissue sarcoma in children. Cancer 29: 1293–1297

Tan CTC, Dargeon HW, Burchenal JH (1959) The effect of actinomycin D on cancer in childhood. Pediatrics 24: 544–561

Tan C, Etcubanas E, Wollner N et al. (1973) Adriamycin – an antitumor antibiotic in the treatment of neoplastic disease. Cancer 32: 9–27

Tarbell NJ, Schwenn M, Delorey M, Sheldon T, McGill T, Cassady JR (1987) Extent of bone erosion predicts survival in non-orbital rhabdomyosarcoma of the head and neck in children. Proc Am Soc Clin Oncol 6: 222

Tefft M, Vawter GF, Mitus A (1969) Paravertebral "round cell" tumors in children. Radiology 92: 1501–1509

Tefft M, Lattin PB, Jerb B et al. (1976) Acute and late effects on normal tissues following combined chemotherapy and radiotherapy for childhood rhabdomyosarcoma and Ewing's sarcoma. Cancer 37: 1201–1217

Tefft M, Fernandez C, Donaldson M et al. (1978) Incidence of meningeal involvement by rhabdomyosarcoma of the head and neck in children. Cancer 42: 253–258

Tefft M, Hays D, Raney RB Jr et al. (1980) Radiation to regional nodes for rhabdomyosarcoma of the genitourinary tract in children: Is it necessary? A report from the Intergroup Rhabdomyosarcoma Study #1 (IRS-1). Cancer 45: 3065–3068

Tefft M, Lindberg R, Gehan E (1981) Radiation therapy combined with systemic chemotherapy of rhabdomyosarcoma in children: local control in patients enrolled into the Intergroup Rhabdomyosarcoma Study. NCI Monogr 56: 75

Tefft M, Wharam M, Ruymann F, Foulkes M, Gehan EA (1985) Radiotherapy (RT) for rhabdomyosarcoma in children. A report from the Intergroup Rhabdomyosarcoma

Study #2 (IRS-2) (abstract C-909). Proc Am Soc Clin Oncol 4: 234

Tefft M, Wharam M, Gehan E (1988) Local and regional control of rhabdomyosarcoma by radiation in IRS-II. Int J Radiat Oncol Biol Phys 15# [Suppl 1]: 159

Turc-Carel C, Lizard-Wacol S, Justrabu S et al. (1986) Consistent chromosome translocation in alveolar rhabdomyosarcoma. Cancer Genet Cytogenet 19: 361–362

Weichselbaum RR, Cassady JR, Jaffe N, Filler RM (1977) The evolution of combination therapy of genitourinary rhabdomyosarcoma in children: a preliminary report. Int J Radiat Oncol Biol Phys 2: 267–272

Wharam M, Foulkes M, Lawrence W Jr et al. (1984) Soft tissue sarcoma of the head and neck in childhood: non-orbital and non-parameningeal sites. Cancer 53: 1016–1019

Wharam M, Beltangady M, Hays D et al. (1987a) Localized orbital rhabdomyosarcoma. An interim report of the Intergroup Rhabdomyosarcoma Study Committee. Ophthalmology 94: 251–254

Wharam M, Beltangady MS, Heyn RM et al. (1987b) Pediatric orofacial and laryngopharyngeal rhabdomyosarcoma: an Intergroup Rhabdomyosarcoma Study report. Arch Otolaryngol Head Neck Surg 113: 1225–1227

Wolfe EL, Berdon WE, Cassady JR, Baker DH, Freiberger R, Pavlou H (1977) Slipped femoral capital epiphysis as a sequela to childhood irradiation for malignant tumors. Radiology 125: 781–784

Young JH, Heise HW, Silverberg E, Myers MH (1978) Cancer incidence, survival and mortality for children under 15 years of age. American Cancer Society, New York, pp 8–9

20 Osteosarcoma and the Less Common Sarcomas of Childhood

K. William Harter

CONTENTS

20.1   Osteosarcoma 305
20.1.1 Introduction........................ 305
20.1.2 Historical Experience 306
20.1.3 Adjuvant Treatment: Chemotherapy........ 307
20.1.4 Adjuvant Treatment: Radiation Therapy 308
20.1.5 Osteosarcoma in Unusual Sites: Treatment
        and Results......................... 309
20.1.6 Osteosarcoma and Secondary Oncogenesis.... 310
20.1.7 Palliation 311
20.1.8 Conclusion......................... 311
20.2   The Less Common Pediatric Sarcomas 311
20.2.1 Introduction........................ 311
20.2.2 Clinical Experience and Results 312
20.2.3 Conclusions 314
        References 315

20.1 Osteosarcoma

20.1.1 Introduction

Osteosarcoma is the second most common primary tumor of bone after plasmacytoma (myeloma) (Dahlin and Unni 1986). Within the pediatric age group, it is the most common primary bone tumor (Dahlin and Unni 1986; Lichtenstein 1977; Jaffe 1958). According to Dahlin and Unni, the sine qua non for histopathologic definition of osteosarcoma is the presence of proliferating malignant cells producing an osteoid substance or material histologically indistinguishable therefrom (Dahlin and Unni 1986). While the majority of osteosarcomas are primary idiopathic neoplasms occurring in the first two and a half decades, they may also arise spontaneously against a background of Paget's disease of bone or as a consequence of therapeutic radiation for other tumors. In the Mayo Clinic series (Dahlin and Unni 1986), however, no patient developed osteosarcoma

---

K. William Harter, MD, Associate Professor and Vice Chairman, Department of Radiation Oncology, Georgetown University Medical Center, Vincent T. Lombardi Cancer Center, 3800 Reservoir Rd. NW, Washington, DC 20007, USA

from Paget's disease prior to the age of 30, thus excluding this etiology from discussion in the context of childhood. While the long latency period for radiation-associated osteosarcoma, 15.1 years in the Mayo Clinic series (Dahlin and Unni 1986), generally places the clinical presentation of such secondary tumors beyond the pediatric age group, enough cases are the apparent consequence of radiation in childhood to warrant further discussion (vide infra) (Dahlin et al. 1970; Nascimento et al. 1979; Hutter et al. 1962; Johnson and Dahlin 1959).

The cumulative experience employing radiation therapy in the treatment of osteosarcoma is rather limited. The tumor itself is somewhat rare, with an incidence in North America of less than 1000 cases annually (Dahlin and Unni 1986; Silverberg and Lubera 1987; Spjut and Ayala 1986). Additionally, the primary treatment modality historically has been surgery, principally amputation, as the predominant site of presentation is in the long bones of the extremities (82% of osteosarcomas in the Mayo series: Dahlin and Unni 1986). There is a predilection to present in the metaphyseal region of the long bones, and thus an anatomic association with regions of rapid bone growth in childhood and adolescence. In fact, according to Dahlin and Unni, nearly 50% of their osteosarcomas occurred in the region of the knee (distal femur, proximal tibia, proximal fibula) (Dahlin and Unni 1986). In the older age group (patients beyond 2½ decades), the incidence of osteosarcoma presenting in the long bones falls to 58% (Dahlin and Unni 1986). The past 15 years have seen the rapid evolution of limb-sparing surgery, allowing adequate extirpation of tumor with margins adequate for local control while permitting at least some functional preservation (Marcove and Rosen 1980; Campanacci et al. 1981; Simon et al. 1986; Malawer et al. 1985; Eilber et al. 1984). The ability to establish local-regional control of osteosarcoma without limb loss has solidified the selection of surgery as the treatment of choice in resectable lesions. Nevertheless, the past half century has seen the accumulation of sufficient clinical data to permit some analysis and conclusions regarding the utility of radiation therapy in osteosarcoma. Radiation can be applied in sites of anatomic presentation where surgical margins are inadequate or where surgical resection would prove to be functionally catastrophic. An analysis of the available clinical data, wherein radiation has been employed in the treatment of osteosarcoma, would therefore permit conclusions regarding efficacy, outcome, dose, technique, and complications for the current clinical setting.

20.1.2 Historical Experience

Throughout the first half of the twentieth century, amputation was the standard local therapy for osteosarcoma of the extremity. While this procedure is associated with excellent local-regional control (WEISENBURGER et al. 1981; JENKIN et al. 1972), the overwhelming majority of patients were seen to succumb to the persistent force of mortality of distant disease. Sir Stanford Cade observed in 1955 that while virtually all patients presenting with osteosarcoma were subjected to amputation, the long-term disease-free survival was only 20% (CADE 1955). His analysis is supported by the large Mayo Clinic retrospective series from 1967 (DAHLIN and COVENTRY 1967), which reported a 5-year survival rate of 20.3% for 408 patients (17.3% for 359 patients at 10 years). Cade inferred from his clinical data that the overwhelming majority of patients with osteosarcoma suffered the mutilation of amputation needlessly. Given the high probability of the rapid manifestation of metastatic disease to lung, he elected to treat patients with clinically localized disease using initial radiation as a holding action to select out patients with disseminated disease and thus spare this group of patients from amputation. The treatment protocol consisted of initial local radiation using a 2 MV Van de Graaff generator to deliver between 7000 and 8000 R at 1000 R per week. Treatment was apparently well tolerated and nearly all patients had either a complete or partial clinical response. A waiting period of 4–6 months was then undertaken, to allow for the manifestation of distant disease. Patients who had manifested metastatic disease (usually lung) were then excluded from further treatment, the remainder going on to amputation. Of 133 patients in this series, 29 were long-term disease-free survivors (21.8%); Cade concluded that there was no survival benefit to early amputation and that a majority of osteosarcoma patients could be spared unnecessary amputation. An interesting subset of

patients in this series, who had complete clinical resolution of disease and were free of metastases at the end of the waiting period, went on to refuse amputation. Although there seemed to be a fairly high incidence of subsequent local recurrence and/or metastatic disease in this group, some patients were apparently rendered permanently disease-free with radiation therapy alone.

This report spawned a number of further investigations. Between 1964 and 1981 a dozen similar clinical series were reported (FARRELL and REVENTOSA 1964; LEE and MACKENZIE 1964; VAN DEN BRENK et al. 1966; PHILLIPS and SHELINE 1969; SWEETNAM et al. 1971; CACERES and ZAHARIA 1972; JENKIN et al. 1972; ALLEN and STEVENS 1973; POPPE et al. 1968; JENKIN 1977; LEE 1971; BECK et al. 1976). Radiation treatment in these series was generally with low-energy megavoltage (cobalt 60 or 2 MV van de Graaff generator or low-energy linear accelerator). Doses ranged from 50 to 120 Gy and survival, for the most part, ranged between 12% and 22%. The consensus among the authors was that while radiation alone was not recommended for the treatment of osteogenic sarcoma, no advantage was gained by initial amputation. Interestingly, Gaitan-Yanguas (1981), reporting on 18 patients from Bogota, reported dose-response data based on pathologic analysis of postradiation amputations. There was significant variability in the radiation delivered to the 18 patients in this series. No patient had control of disease at less than 30 Gy. All patients had sterilization of tumor at doses greater than 100 Gy.

The recent phase II trial by the French Bone Tumor Study Group (1988) includes 16 patients with primary limb osteosarcoma treated definitively with radiation alone. They comprised 41% of the accrued patients; rationale for primary treatment with radiation was not offered. The local-regional outcome for this group of patients was rather disappointing. One of the patients progressed during treatment, requiring amputation. Two additional patients suffered local recurrence within 1 year. An additional ten patients required amputation 1–5 years after radiotherapy for "major post-radiotherapy dystrophic sequelae." Three of these ten patients were found to have persistent tumor on pathologic examination. The investigators note that 13 of 16 patients in the radiation group underwent amputation, and fear that two additional patients will require amputation for posttreatment complications. Therefore, local control, in this series of patients, is no better than 62% (10 of 16). Limb preservation was 18.7% at publication [3 of 16 with the stated possibility of ultimate limb preservation in 1 of 16 (6%)].

One may conclude, from the available data, that radiation therapy alone is not a suitable treatment modality in osteosarcoma. The long-term functional results in patients whose tumors were controlled by high dose of radiation (greater than 80–100 Gy) are seemingly suboptimal. Additionally, there appears to be no particular benefit to preoperative radiation therapy other than as a selection tool to avoid unnecessary amputation in patients who will develop metastatic disease. One British series looking at low-dose preoperative irradiation in the range of 10 Gy given prior to biopsy showed no apparent benefit (SWEETNAM 1974). Survival in this series was quoted at 20%, consistent with the overall clinical experience at that time.

20.1.3 Adjuvant Treatment: Chemotherapy

The middle 1970s provided a watershed in treatment outcome for patients with osteogenic sarcoma. The Mayo Clinic reported a dramatic increase in survival for patients treated there between 1972 and 1974 as compared to those treated prior to 1972 (TAYLOR et al. 1978). Since that time, over the past two decades, there has been an apparent marked increase in long-term disease-free survival for patients with osteogenic sarcoma. This improvement in survival has largely been attributed to the development and use of adjuvant chemotherapy, particularly with the agents methotrexate and doxorubicin (MALAWER et al. 1993). At about the same time that the Mayo Clinic group was noticing a marked improvement in treatment outcome, FRIEDMAN and CARTER (1972) undertook a large retrospective review, analyzing 1337 patients in 11 studies over the 25-year period from 1946 to 1971. Their analysis was consistent with that of Cade and the dozen or so subsequent radiation-surgical series showing an overall 5-year survival of less than 20%. As previously noted by Cade, approximately 50% of the patients developed metastatic disease (most often lung) without 6 months of initial surgery and 80% of patients ultimately developed metastatic and/or locally recurrent disease. A rationale for adjuvant chemotherapy trials was offered therein.

The temporal concomitance of improved outcome with the advent of adjuvant chemotherapy cannot be ignored. Several randomized trials are available for analysis. The Multi-Institutional Osteosarcoma Study (MIOS) (LINK 1986) analyzed 201 patients (36 randomized, 165 nonrandomized) who received either no adjuvant therapy or multi-agent chemotherapy with bleomycin, cyclophosphamide, dactinomycin, doxorubicin, and cisplatin. They reported 63% relapse-free survival in the chemotherapy group versus 12% in the control arm. UCLA randomized patients between no adjuvant therapy and treatment with bleomycin, cyclophosphamide, dactinomycin plus high-dose methotrexate, vincristine, and doxorubicin (EILBER et al. 1987). All patients received preoperative doxorubicin via arterial infusion and preoperative radiation therapy to a dose of 17.5 Gy in 3.5-Gy fractions. Eilber and colleagues found a striking difference at 2 years in both disease-free and overall survival. The control arm exhibited relapse-free survival of 20% compared to 55% in the adjuvant chemotherapy arm.

The Mayo group, after observing an increase in survival to 50% in the period 1972–1974 (*vide supra*) (TAYLOR et al. 1978), undertook a (small) randomized trial comparing surgery alone versus surgery plus high-dose methotrexate and vincristine. They found no difference between the arms, with survival in both groups being 52% at 2 years. Relapse-free survival was 40% in the chemotherapy arm and 44% in the control arm (EDMONSON et al. 1986).

There is not a logical hypothesis which would effect concordance among these randomized trials. Glatstein (personal communication, 1992) has argued cogently, however, that the dramatic increase in survival and disease-free survival for osteosarcoma may be largely illusory, reflective only of more precise staging employing CT scans, nuclear medicine bone scans, etc. He notes that the survival for the entire group of osteosarcoma patients has not altered materially in the past 25 years, but rather more patients have been pushed to higher stages by these improved scanning modalities, thus selecting out previously undetectable metastatic patients from early disease groupings.

A trend toward earlier diagnosis would contribute to this effect via the phenomenon of lead-time bias (zero-time shift) "which can extend the statistical length of a patient's survival without necessarily prolonging the duration of life" (FEINSTEIN et al. 1985). Earlier diagnosis can thus seem to prolong the period of survival, either disease-free or absolute, via the inclusion of a presymptomatic time period (in effect, predating the diagnosis with respect to historical controls) (HUTCHISON and SHAPIRO 1968; FEINLEIB and ZELEN 1969).

The net effect of earlier diagnosis and more precise clinical staging is to improve survival in early-stage disease by shifting to higher stages those patients with metastatic disease with concomitant improvement of survival of higher stages because of the subsequent inclusion therein of patients with minimal metastatic disease. Feinstein and colleagues at Yale have dubbed this the "Will Rogers phenomenon"[1] (FEINSTEIN et al. 1985).

At this time, however, routine use of adjuvant multiagent chemotherapy represents the "standard of care" for these patients.

20.1.4 Adjuvant Treatment: Radiation Therapy

Concomitant with early investigations in adjuvant chemotherapy, several trials were done evaluating the role of whole-lung irradiation as an adjuvant treatment in clinically localized osteosarcoma. Early pulmonary metastatic disease continues to be the dominant distant difficulty. Bilateral pulmonary irradiation has long been an integral part of the curative therapy for stage IV Wilms' tumor (WAGGET and KOOP 1970; LEMERLE et al. 1976; BALLANTINE et al. 1975; CASSADY et al. 1977; TEFFT 1977). While whole-lung irradiation has little clinical efficacy in metastatic osteosarcoma, some prolongation in survival has been effected with pulmonary treatment and/or high-dose local boost (JENKIN 1977; SUTOW et al. 1978; WEICHSELBAUM et al. 1976). Certainly, in the clinical setting, gross disease in osteosarcoma requires a higher radiation dose for local control than does Wilms' tumor (GAITAN-YANGUAS 1981; WEICHSELBAUM et al. 1977). However, the preponderance of cell culture data suggests that osteosarcoma cell lines have an intermediate radiation sensitivity (WEICHSELBAUM et al. 1976; FERTIL and MALAISE 1981; CARNEY et al. 1983; DEACON et al. 1984). Given the dose limitation in bilateral whole lung irradiation, it is therefore of interest to explore the use of radiation as an adjuvant agent intended to prevent pulmonary metastatic disease (i.e., to treat presumptive micrometastatic disease). Clinical studies to this end have been carried out by eight different groups between the years 1965 and 1988 (JENKIN et al. 1972; JENKIN 1977; LOUGHEED et al. 1965; NEWTON 1972; RAB et al. 1976; CACERES et al. 1978; NEWTON and

---

[1] William Penn Adair Rogers (1879–1935), American actor and humorist is purported to have offered the following comment about the migration westward during the Great Depression occasioned by the Dust Bowl. "When the Okies left Oklahoma and moved to California, they raised the average intelligence level in both states."

BARRETT 1978; BREUR et al. 1978; 1981; BREUR and VAN DER SCHUEREN 1978; ZAHARIA et al. 1986; BURGERS et al. 1988; French Bone Tumor Study Group 1988). The oldest of these studies, that of LOUGHEED et al. (1965), analyzed 15 Gy prophylactic irradiation of one lung in conjunction with dactinomycin. Of eight patients so treated, four developed metastases in the untreated lung, a fifth patient failing in the treated lung. Newton and co-workers (NEWTON 1972; NEWTON and BARRETT 1978) reported on 14 patients given initial local radiation with delayed amputation in conjunction with 19.5 Gy bilateral whole lung irradiation. They noted 43% survival (6 of 14 patients) at 4½ years. The Mayo Clinic group (RAB et al. 1976) randomized 53 patients with localized osteosarcoma to receive either 15 Gy of prophylactic lung irradiation with dactinomycin or no adjuvant therapy. Eleven of 26 patients in the adjuvant arm (42%) survived as compared with 10 of 27 (37%) receiving no adjuvant therapy, indicating no apparent benefit to the adjuvant treatment. The Bogota group (ZAHARIA et al. 1986) analyzed 36 patients given adjuvant therapy after definitive local surgery. Seven patients received 20 Gy whole lung irradiation, 29 patients receiving the same irradiation plus doxorubicin. In this nonrandomized study, a statistically significant survival benefit was noted for the doxorubicin group. The EORTC (BREUR et al. 1978; 1981; BREUR and VAN DER SCHUEREN 1978) reported on 86 patients, randomized between 17.5 Gy in ten fractions and control. Among the treated group, 23 of 44 (54%) were disease-free at 5 years compared with 17 of 42 (40%) in the control group. There was not a statistically significant difference in overall survival between the two groups, although disease-free survival favored the treated arm. In conjunction with SIOP, EORTC (BURGERS et al. 1988) conducted a follow-up study, randomizing 205 patients with localized osteosarcoma among three arms. Group I received 9 months of multiagent chemotherapy, with 20 of 65 patients surviving at 5 years (31%). Group II received 20 Gy of whole lung irradiation, 18 of 73 patients (24%) surviving at 5 years, and group III received 3 months of multiagent chemotherapy with 20 Gy whole lung irradiation, 13 of 67 patients (19%) surviving at 5 years. No statistical difference was noted between or among the treatment arms. Most recently, the French Bone Tumor Study Group (1988) incorporated lung irradiation (20 Gy in 2 weeks) into an adjuvant program, utilizing mitomycin C, vincristine, and methotrexate, alternating with doxorubicin, vincristine, dacarbazine, and Cytoxan. This phase II study reported 58% disease-free survival with a median follow-up of 5 years and was not designed to evaluate the efficacy of pulmonary irradiation.

While these studies (RAB et al. 1976; ZAHARIA et al. 1986; BURGERS et al. 1988) as will as the recent prospective analysis at the University of Florida (ELLIS et al. 1992) demonstrate that pulmonary irradiation can be delivered in the adjuvant setting with acceptable toxicity, the French Study (1988) did find clinically significant decrements in pulmonary function, perhaps because the radiation and chemotherapy were administered concomitantly. None of these studies demonstrates a statistically significant benefit to adjuvant pulmonary irradiation in terms of survival or disease-free survival (prevention of pulmonary metastases). Sufficient clinical experience has been accrued over the past 25 years to warrant discontinuation of clinical interest in the subject.

20.1.5 Osteosarcoma in Unusual Sites: Treatment and Results

20.1.5.1 Head and Neck

Primary osteosarcoma of the facial bones, particularly the mandible and maxilla, is associated with a much better prognosis than that of other sites (DAHLIN and UNNI 1986; CLARK et al. 1983; CHAMBERS and MAHONEY 1970; DE FRIES et al. 1970; AKBIYIK and ALEXANDER 1981; SUIT 1975). Although the average age of such patients is greater than that for conventional sites, 34.2 years in the recent Mayo Clinic series (DAHLIN and UNNI 1986; CLARK et al. 1983), these tumors do present in the pediatric/adolescent age group. In this series, most cases were primary idiopathic osteosarcoma, although 8.5% (8/84) were felt to arise from previous radiation and two (2.3%) from Paget's disease.

Analysis of the available clinical experience suggests that a combination of radiation therapy and wide local excision represents the optimal treatment for such a presentation. CHAMBERS and MAHONEY (1970) described 33 patients treated with high-dose preoperative radiation therapy (either brachytherapy or external beam) followed by wide surgical excision, which included the diseased portion of bone and adjacent soft tissues. Of the 33 patients, 23 (73%) survived at 5 years. Prognosis was better among their pediatric subgroup, with ten of 11 children as long-term survivors. In the Mayo Clinic group experience (CLARK et al. 1983) the 5-year survival rate was 36% overall. However, of the 64% of patients dead from disease, most suffered primary local recurrence. Treatments included limited surgery alone, radiation therapy, surgical salvage, and primary radical resection, sometimes followed by postoperative radiation therapy. This last subset of patients had a 5-year survival rate of 77% and forms the basis for their treatment recommendation. LIVOLSI (1977) reported five patients treated with surgery and postoperative radiation therapy with no long-term survivors. Other small series (DE FRIES et al. 1970; ABBIYAK and ALEXANDER 1981; SUIT 1975) report favorable outcome employing preoperative radiation therapy and surgery, sometimes combined with methotrexate-based chemotherapy.

The selection of preoperative or postoperative radiation therapy in osteosarcoma of the head and neck is likely moot. Certainly the argument that postoperative radiation is compromised by prolonged surgical healing has been obviated by the widespread contemporary usage of the myocutaneous flap graft. Preoperative radiotherapy and/or radio-chemotherapy may offer an advantage in terms of surgical facilitation. A recent Japanese report (HIRANO et al. 1992) describes 16 patients with osteosarcoma treated with preoperative chemotherapy and radiation. At resection and on pathologic analysis, a thick capsule formation was noted at the periosteal and parosteal region of the tumors. Similar clinical observations have been made previously at Stanford (MARTINEZ et al. 1985) and Memorial-Sloan Kettering (ROSEN et al. 1976, 1979). Although preoperative doses of radiation are customarily lower, the nature of surgical extirpation, employing en bloc resection of bone and soft tissue with graft placement, readily permits dose escalation.

Osteosarcoma of the skull, in contradistinction to maxillary or mandibular presentation, is associated with an extremely poor prognosis (DAHLIN and UNNI 1986; MALAWER et al. 1993). Only one long-term survivor was noted in the Mayo Clinic series of 21 patients reported. Both uncontrolled local disease and metastases were noted, the former a function of difficulty with three-dimensional surgical margins. In this admittedly rare presentation, preoperative chemo-radiotherapy might be employed to advantage.

20.1.5.2 Truncal and Vertebral

Central presentations of osteosarcoma pose therapeutic challenges similar to those of other mesenchymal tumors in this region, namely with difficulty with adequate resection and radiation dose limitation by critical normal structures. Lesions of the ilium and ischium/pubis account for less than 10% of all presentations (DAHLIN and UNNI 1986). As with extremity lesions, management of the primary disease is generally surgical. Hemipelvectomy is generally required, although selected lesions can be treated with limb-sparing internal hemipelvectomy (MALAWER et al. 1993). Even with adequate local treatment, however, metastatic disease is an overwhelming probability, making long-term survival quite rare (MARANGOLO et al. 1992).

Vertebral presentation is even less common, accounting for approximately 3% of all osteosarcomas (DAHLIN and UNNI 1986). Local control with primary irradiation therapy is extremely poor, given the dose limitation of the spinal cord (WIGG et al. 1981). A recent retrospective review from Memorial-Sloan Kettering analyzed the treatment results of 24 patients accrued over three-and-a-half decades (SUNDARESAN et al. 1988). As might be expected, they noted that surgical decompression and local radiation was uniformly unsuccessful. Rather, they recommended definitive resection of vertebral lesions in a two-stage procedure. Initial partial anterior spondylectomy should be followed by combination chemotherapy. In patients remaining free of metastatic disease, definitive resection via posterior approach with stabilization should be undertaken. Surgery is followed by external beam radiation to tolerance.

There has been some interest in the past decade in intraoperative radiation therapy as an adjunct to resection in central osteosarcoma (ABE et al. 1989; CALVO et al. 1991; YAMAMURO and KOTOURA 1993). Used in conjunction with surgical resection and postoperative external beam irradiation, single intraoperative doses in the range of 10–20 Gy seemed to offer some potential for benefit in terms of local control and disease-free survival.

There is also some evidence in support of the use of fast neutrons (ISHII et al. 1989), including two small clinical trials from Russia (MUSABAEVA et al. 1990; CHERNICHENKO et al. 1990). A group in Moscow (MUSABAEVA et al. 1990) reports five cases where fast neutrons were used as a local boost, this therapy being well tolerated. A larger study from Kiev (CHERNICHENKO et al. 1990) compared patients treated definitively with fast neutrons to those receiving limited surgery and conventional radiation with a survival benefit at 3 years in the neutron group.

20.1.5.3 Hand and Foot

A minuscule subset of patients (1%) (DAHLIN and UNNI 1986) will present with primary osteogenic sarcoma of the wrist, hand, ankle, or foot. While historically such distal lesions have been treated with amputation, there is ample clinical experience in soft part sarcomas and Ewing's tumor to support treatment with limited resection (affected bone and adjacent soft tissue) followed by high-dose radiation therapy (KINSELLA et al. 1983; KLIMAN et al. 1982; OKUNIEFF et al. 1986; POTTER et al. 1986; TEPPER et al. 1982). It has long been part of the conventional wisdom of clinical practice in orthopedics and radiation oncology that the hand and the foot are intolerant of high-dose radiation therapy, such treatment producing severe dysfunction. This is not borne out by recent experience (KINSELLA et al. 1983, 1984; KLIMAN et al. 1982; OKUNIEFF et al. 1986; POTTER et al. 1986; TEPPER et al. 1982) and is clearly erroneous (KINSELLA 1986). Therefore, if surgical extirpation of disease can be effected with neurovascular and tendon preservation, this should be undertaken, to be followed by adjuvant radiation in the range of 63 Gy. Interstitial implantation for afterloading sources at the time of surgery may also be considered.

20.1.6 Osteosarcoma and Secondary Oncogenesis

Secondary osteosarcoma as a late consequence of therapeutic irradiation is, by its very nature, almost always encountered in the adult age group. The predisposing therapy, however, often dates from the pediatric and adolescent age groups. Of 1274 osteosarcomas in the current Mayo Clinic series, 52 (4.2%) were encountered in previously irradiated bones (DAHLIN and UNNI 1986). The mean interval between radiation and diagnosis of subsequent osteosarcoma was 15.1 years (2.75–55 years). Thirty of the 52 patients (58%) had a latent period of greater than 20 years. While secondary oncogenesis is an extremely rare complication of curative radiation therapy in childhood malignancy (LI et al. 1975; KIM et al. 1978), the clinical irradiation of benign conditions in the young should be undertaken rarely and reluctantly.

There are several interesting reports of second cancers after radiation in the treatment of osteosarcoma. Recently, investigators at Stanford (HANCOCK et al. 1993) and Harvard-JCRT (MAUCH PM, personal communication) have noted the increased susceptibility of adolescent breast tissue to radiation carcinogenesis in the treatment of Hodgkin's disease. Previously, Cassady and colleagues reported a case of male breast cancer 30 years after chest radiation for metastatic osteosarcoma in childhood (THOMPSON et al. 1979). Subsequently, IVINS et al. (1987) noted that two of 13 adolescent females who received prophylactic lung irradiation in a previous clinical trial (RAB et al. 1976) developed bilateral breast cancer with a latency interval of approximately 15 years.

20.1.7 Palliation

External beam radiation therapy is an effective local palliative modality in osteosarcoma. Osteosarcoma is quite responsive to radiation [vide supra (WEICHSELBAUM et al. 1976; FERTIL and MALAISE 1981; CARNEY et al. 1983; DEACON et al. 1984)] and a satisfactory palliative result can be expected with customary short-course treatment regimens (JENKIN et al. 1972; CADE 1955; JENKIN 1977; WEICHSELBAUM et al. 1977). The best dose-response description for osteosarcoma comes from Sir Stanford Cade, who noted marked reduction in pain and swelling at the tumor site with a dose of 2000 R with daily fractions of 200 R (CADE 1955). A more rapid clinical response would be expected with the larger fraction sizes employed in palliative therapy.

20.1.8 Conclusion

The mainstay of local treatment in osteosarcoma remains surgical resection, with limb-sparing procedures replacing amputation in many extremity presentations. In the more difficult anatomic areas (head and neck, truncal and vertebral, hand, and foot) a more limited surgical approach with adjuvant radiation (preoperative or postoperative) will produce excellent local control and will maximize functional result. While there remains the potential for considerable debate about the relative efficacy of adjuvant chemotherapy in osteosarcoma [vide supra (TAYLOR et al. 1978; MALAWER et al. 1993; FRIEDMAN and CARTER 1972; LINK 1986; EILBER et al. 1987; EDMONSON et al. 1986; GLATSTEIN E, personal communication; FEINSTEIN et al. 1985; HUTCHISON and SHAPIRO 1968; FEINLEIB and ZELEN 1969)], such clinical investigation in improbable in the light of universal chemotherapeutic utilization in current clinical practice and current clinical trials. .

20.2 The Less Common Pediatric Sarcomas

20.2.1 Introduction

The soft part sarcomas account for approximately 7% of all childhood malignancies, the most common tumor of this group being rhabdomyosarcoma (YOUNG and MILLER 1975; see also Chap. 19). The remainder, accounting for 3% of childhood tumors (MISER et al. 1989) are comprised of a diverse group of 15 histopathologic subtypes (Table 20.1). Given that the medical literature contains fewer than 500 cases of pediatric soft part sarcomas distinct from rhabdomyosarcoma, conclusive clinical evidence for each distinct histology is quite limited. While some of these tumors are discernibly distinct in terms of age of presentation and/or clinical behavior, presentation, treatment, and outcome are quite similar between and among the many subtypes (HOROWITZ et al. 1986; SOLLACCIO et al. 1986; BRIZEL et al. 1988; RANEY 1987). Therapy is derived, by and large, from data and experience in adult soft tissue sarcomas. While these can hardly be said to be plentiful, they are an order of magnitude more common than comparable disease incidence in children. Such tumors presenting in the adolescent age group seem to have a similar behavior and prognosis to those found in older patients (MISER et al. 1989). Soft part sarcomas in infancy and early childhood, on the other hand, are possessed of a more benign clinical course (HOROWITZ et al. 1986; SOLLACCIO et al. 1986; BRIZEL et al. 1988; RANEY 1987).

There is no uniformity of staging for soft part sarcomas of childhood between and among the various reporting institutions. The American Joint Committee (AJC) Staging System (Table 20.2) (BEAHRS et al. 1992) permits a fine discrimination between stages due to its greatly detailed nature. Until recently, however, it has not been in widespread clinical use in the pediatric oncology arena. The Intergroup Rhabdomyosarcoma Study (IRS) Clinical Grouping System (Table 20.3) (RANEY et al. 1982) has perhaps been more commonly employed in the past. While the IRS system has been criticized for its dependence upon the extent of surgical resection,[2] it appears to function well as a framework in nonrhabdomyosarcoma soft part tumors. In general, children with small primary sarcomas who undergo complete resection with negative margins have an outstanding prognosis without

---

[2] In fact, the proposed staging system for IRS-IV has been reworked to resemble closely the AJC system (Table 20.2).

Table 20.1. The less common pediatric soft tissue sarcomas: histologic classification of nonrhabdomyosarcoma subtypes

Histology	Approximate percentage of non-RMS STS	Comment
Aleveolar soft-part sarcoma	1%–9%	Long clinical course with high mortality from distant disease
Angiosarcoma	< 1%	Highly unusual
Dermatofibrosarcoma protuberans	< 1%	Highly unusual
Epithelioid sarcoma	1%–3%	Rare extremity lesion
Fibrosarcoma	6%–18%	Bimodal–infants and adolescents
Hemangiopericytoma	< 5%	Usual presentation in adolescent extremity. Rare infant cases have a more benign course
Leiomyosarcoma	1%–2%	Truncal adolescent presentation often
Liposarcoma	1%–6%	Retroperitoneum and extremity in adolescents
Malignant fibrous histiocytoma	5%–10%	No age or site predilection in pediatric group
Malignant schwannoma	7%–30%	May be associated with von Recklinghausen's disease and/or include neurofibrosarcoma
Mixed mesenchymal sarcoma	< 1%	Highly unusual
Neurofibrosarcoma	5%–10%	Strong association with von Recklinghausen's disease in children
Spindle cell sarcoma	< 1%	Rarely encountered
Synovial sarcoma	15%–30%	Adeloscent presentation, extremity > trunk
Undifferentiated (sarcoma NOS/other)	5%–10%	Likely a "waste-basket diagnosis"

RMS, rhabdomyosarcoma; STS, soft tissue sarcoma; NOS, not otherwise specified

adjuvant therapy (Horowitz et al. 1986; Sollaccio et al. 1986; Brizel et al. 1988; Raney 1987). Patients with microscopic residual disease, while benefiting in terms of survival from postoperative radiation and (probably) from chemotherapy, do have a more intermediate prognosis. Gross residual disease augurs poorly for the potential for cure, and patients with metastatic disease do badly with near uniformity. Thus the clinical behavior of the soft part sarcomas is well described by the IRS system.

20.2.2 Clinical Experience and Results

While the Pediatric Oncologic Group (POG) is currently conducting a prospective multi-institutional trial to evaluate adjuvant chemotherapy and postoperative radiation therapy in childhood soft part sarcomas (Pizzo et al. 1983), currently available clinical experience exists as single-institution retrospective reviews of either general experience with soft part sarcomas or specific histologic subtypes. There are four reviews of general experience available for analysis: St. Jude's Hospital (Memphis) (Horowitz et al. 1986), University of Florida (Gainesville) (Sollaccio et al. 1986), Harvard Joint Center for Radiation Therapy (JCRT-Boston) (Brizel et al. 1988), and University of Pennsylvania (Children's Hospital of Philadelphia) (Raney 1987). Each study analyzes between 40 and 62 patients with varying histologies. While the case-mix among these institutions varies somewhat, overall results by (surgical) stage are relatively consistent. The St. Jude study (Horowitz et al. 1986) employing the IRS Clinical Grouping System analyzed 62 cases accrued over a 22-year period (1962–1983). Of this group, 50 patients had only local disease at time of diagnosis, 31 with complete resection (group I), 5 with micro-

Table 20.2. American Joint Committee staging system for soft tissue sarcomas (BEAHRS et al. 1992)

T	Primary tumor	
	T1	Tumor less than 5 cm
	T2	Tumor 5 cm or greater
G	Histologic grade of malignancy	
	G1	Low
	G2	Moderate
	G3	High
N	Regional lymph nodes	
	N0	No histologically verified metastases to regional lymph nodes
	N1	Histologically verified regional lymph node metastasis
M	Distant metastasis	
	M0	No distant metastasis
	M1	Distant metastasis

Stage I		
	Stage IA	Grade 1 tumor less than 5 cm in diameter with no
	G1T1N0M0	regional lymph node or distant metastases
	Stage IB	Grade 1 tumor 5 cm or greater in diameter with no
	G1T2N0M0	regional lymph node or distant metastases
Stage II		
	Stage IIA	Grade 2 tumor less than 5 cm in diameter with no
	G2T1N0M0	regional lymph node or distant metastases
	Stage IIB	Grade 2 tumor 5 cm or greater in diameter with no
	G2T1N0M0	regional lymph node or distant metastases
Stage III		
	Stage IIIA	Grade 3 tumor less than 5 cm in diameter with no
	G3T1N0M0	regional lymph node or distant metastases
	Stage IIIB	Grade 3 tumor 5 cm or greater in diameter with no
	G3T2N0M0	regional lymph node or distant metastases
Stage IV		
	Stage IVA	Tumor of any grade or size with histologically
	G1-3T12-2N1M0	verified metastasis to regional lymph nodes, but no distant metastases
	Stage IVB	Clinically diagnosed distant metastases
	G1-3T1-2N0-1M1	

scopic residuum (group II), and 14 with gross residual disease (group III). The remaining 12 patients were diagnosed with metastatic disease at presentation. Of the 31 patients in group I, 12 received adjuvant chemotherapy consisting of vincristine and cyclophosphamide +/– dactinomycin and two received postoperative radiation therapy. It is not entirely clear why certain patients were given adjuvant therapy and others were not, although leading possibilities include unspecified surgical concerns and time of presentation (adjuvant chemotherapy being available later in the series). Disease-free survival overall in group I was 84% (26 of 31). Kaplan-Meier analysis of survival showed no benefit to adjuvant postoperative therapy in group I ($P = 0.32$). Of the five patients in group II, however, two treated with surgery alone developed local recurrence while two treated with chemotherapy and one with chemotherapy plus radiation remained disease-free at 6 years. Of 14 patients in group III, only one survived; all of the 12 patients in group IV died of disease. Clearly, early favorable presentation and complete surgical resection are associated with improved outcome. More aggressive combined modality therapy may be of benefit in group III patients.

The Gainesville report (SOLLACCIO et al. 1986) analyzed 50 patients accrued over 24 years (1960–1983). This group employed their own staging system (Enneking) which roughly parallels the IRS system. Of 20 patients treated with surgery alone (favorable presentation), 90% survived at 5 years. In patients requiring adjuvant therapy (radiation 4,

Table 20.3. Intergroup Rhabdomyosarcoma Study: clinical grouping system (RANEY et al. 1982)

Group I	Localized disease, completely resected Regional nodes not involved A. Confined to muscle or organ of origin B. Contiguous involvement/infiltration outside the muscle or organ of origin, as through fascial planes
Group II	Regional disease A. Grossly resected tumor with microscopic residual disease. No evidence of gross residual tumor. No clinical or microscopic evidence of regional node involvement B. Regional disease, completely resected (regional nodes involved completely resected with no microscopic residual disease) C. Regional disease with involved nodes, grossly resected, but with evidence of microscopic residual disease
Group III	Incomplete resection or biopsy with gross residual disease
Group IV	Metastatic disease present at onset

chemotherapy 13, both 12) the survival at 5 years was 65%, implying benefit from adjuvant therapy in more advanced presentations. In stratifying the series by histologic grade, patients with low-grade lesions had a 92% survival rate at 5 years compared with 59% for high-grade lesions ($P = 0.04$). Synovial cell sarcoma had a strikingly poor outcome, with survival at 20% compared to 80% for all other histologies. This is somewhat worse than the St. Jude's series, where 8 of 18 patients (44%) with synovial cell sarcoma were long-term survivors (HOROWITZ et al. 1986).

The Harvard series (BRIZEL et al. 1988) analyzed 44 patients accrued over 15 years (1970–1984). Retrospective staging showed comparable results between the IRS and AJC systems in group stage I–III. All patients in this series received local radiation therapy, 43 in an adjuvant setting and one at the time of local recurrence. Patients were treated to initial volumes encompassing the entire surgical bed including the scar, using a median dose of 40 Gy. Reduced field boost was then added for a median total dose of 57.6 Gy (range 45–70 Gy). Ten-year overall survival was 100% in the 14 patients in IRS group I. Disease-free survival in this group was 83%. Of 15 patients in IRS group II, 11 survived at 10 years (1972%), disease-free survival being 62%. Of patients with gross residual disease (group III) 8 of 15 were alive at 10 years (54%) with disease-free survival reported at 34%. Of 44 patients, 26 received adjuvant chemotherapy with vincristine, actinomycin, cyclophosphamide +/– doxorubicin. Chemotherapy did not appear to affect outcome. Histologic subtype was not felt to be significant. In the analysis of patterns of failure, local recurrence was 30% (13 of 44), and a component of failure in 13 of 14 relapsed patients (local only, eight; distant only one; local + distant, five). Given the median radiation dose of 57.6 Gy, perhaps higher doses would be associated with improved local control. With the perspective of the St. Jude (HOROWITZ et al. 1986) and Florida (SOLLACCIO et al. 1986) experiences, however, the role for local adjuvant radiation in group I patients is not established.

Study from the Children's Hospital of Philadelphia (CHOP) (RANEY 1987; RANEY et al. 1986, 1987) show results largely in accord with those of other groups. The CHOP experience reinforces the favorable prognosis for children with soft part sarcomas who present with small tumors and have complete resection (IRS group I). The outcome for patients with gross residual disease was uniformly poor (RANEY 1987; RANEY et al. 1986, 1987). Synovial sarcoma was not associated with a worsened prognosis. While much of the CHOP series predates those of other institutions, thus temporally eliminating adjuvant chemotherapy and partially spanning the orthovoltage era of radiation, their data nevertheless underscore the importance of definitive surgical resection in early-stage disease and suggest the need for aggressive adjuvant therapy in more advanced presentations.

Several of the histologic subtypes, most particularly fibrosarcoma (SOULE and PRITCHARD 1977; STOUT 1962) and hemangiopericytoma (KAUFFMAN and STOUT 1960), exhibit distinct bimodal age distribution in infancy and adolescence. While there is no apparent histopathologic difference among the soft part sarcomas diagnosed in the very young, teenagers, and adults, the general sense of most authors is that the tumors of infancy, stage for stage, have a less aggressive clinical course. There is little appreciable difference in outcome or recommendations for therapy between adolescents and adults.

20.2.3 Conclusions

The nonrhabdomyosarcoma soft part sarcomas of childhood form an uncommon but important clinical subset in pediatric oncology. Overall, the outcome appears to be somewhat better than that from soft part sarcomas in the adult population, although this may be attributable in part to a more favorable clinical course in the very young. From the available clinical experience, local resection with negative margins appears to be the mainstay of therapy, particularly in patients with early disease (tumors less than 5 cm). In such cases (IRS group I), postoperative radiation therapy may not, for the most part, be necessary. Adjuvant chemotherapy may be of potential benefit in histologic high-grade lesions. In group II situations, local-regional control appears to be greatly enhanced with the addition of radiation therapy. While the role of chemotherapy remains undefined, as with group I, it may be of benefit in terms of distant disease. For patients with gross residual disease (group III), aggressive treatment with radiation and chemotherapy may possibly enhance prospects for survival. The utilization of brachytherapy at the time of surgical resection may well contribute to local control for patients with residual disease or those in whom the adequacy of resection margin is in question.

References

Abe M, Takahashi M, Shibamoto Y, Onok (1989) Application of intraoperative radiation therapy to refractory cancers. Ann Radiol (Paris) 32: 493–494

Akbiyik N, Alexander LL (1981) Osteosarcoma of the mandible treated with radiation therapy and surgery. J Natl Med Assoc 73: 355–356

Allen SEV, Stevens KR (1973) Preoperative irradiation for osteogenic sarcoma. Cancer 31: 1365–1366

Ballantine TVN, Wiseman NE, Filler RM (1975) Assessment of pulmonary wedge resection for the treatment of lung metastases. J Pediatr Surg 10: 329–337

Beahrs OH, Henson DE, Hutter RVP, Myers MH (eds) (1992) Manual for staging of cancer, 4th edn. J.B. Lippincott, Philadelphia, pp 127–132

Beck JC, Wara WM, Bovill EG, Phillips TL (1976) The role of radiation therapy in the treatment of osteosarcoma. Radiology 120: 163–165

Breur K, van der Schueren E (1978) Adjuvant therapy in the management of osteosarcoma, need for critical reassessment. Recent Results Cancer Res 68: 5–15

Breur K, Cohen P, Schweisguth O, Hart AM (1978) Irradiation of the lungs as an adjuvant therapy in the treatment of osteosarcoma of the limbs and EORTC randomized study. Eur J Cancer 14: 461–471

Breur K, Schweisguth O et al. (1981) Prophylactic irradiation of the lungs to prevent development of pulmonary metastases in patients with osteosarcoma of the limbs. NCI Monogr 56: 233–236

Brizel DM, Weinstein H, Hunt M (1988) Failure patterns and survival in pediatric soft tissue sarcoma. Int J Radiat Oncol Biol Phys 15: 37–41

Burgers JM, van Glabbeke M, Busson et al. (1988) Osteosarcoma of the limbs. Report of the EORTC-SIOP 03 trial 20781 investigating the value of adjuvant treatment with chemotherapy and/or prophylactic lung irradiation. Cancer 61: 1024–1031

Caceres E, Zaharia M (1972) Massive preoperative radiation therapy in the treatment of osteogenic sarcoma. Cancer 30: 364–368

Caceres E, Zaharia M, Moran M, Tejada F (1978) Adjuvant whole lung radiation with or without Adriamycin treatment in osteogenic sarcoma. Cancer Treat 62: 297–299

Cade S (1955) Osteogenic sarcoma: a study based on 133 patients. J R Coll Surg Edinb 1: 79–111

Calvo FA, Ortiz de Urbina D, Sierrasesumaga L et al. (1991) Intraoperative radiotherapy in the multidisciplinary treatment of bone sarcomas in children and adolescents. Med Pediatr Oncol 19: 478–485

Campanacci M, Bacci G, Bertoni F, Picci P, Minutillo A, Franceschi C (1981) The treatment of osteosarcoma of the extremities: twenty years' experience at the Instituto Ortopedico Rizzoli. Cancer 48: 1569–1581

Carney DN, Mitchell JB, Kinsella TJ (1983) In vitro radiation and chemotherapy sensitivity of established cell lines of human small cell lung cancer and its large cell morphologic variance. Cancer Res 43: 2806–2811

Cassady JR, Jaffe N, Filler RM (1977) The increasing importance of radiation therapy in the improved prognosis of children with Wilms' tumor. Cancer 39: 825–829

Chambers RG, Mahoney WD (1970) Osteogenic sarcoma of the mandible, current management. Am Surg 36: 463–471

Chernichenko VA, Tolstopiatov BA, Konovalenko VF, Monich AIU, Palivets AIU (1990) The combination treatment of malignant bone tumors using fast neutrons. Vopr Onkol 36(8): 970–973

Clark JR, Unni KK, Dahlin DC, Devine KD (1983) Osteosarcoma of the jaw. Cancer 51: 2311–2316

Dahlin DC, Coventry MB (1967) Osteogenic sarcoma: a study of 600 cases. J Bone Joint Surg [Am] 49: 101–110

Dahlin DC, Unni KK (1986) Bone tumors, 4th edn. Charles C. Thomas, Springfield, Ill.

Dahlin DC, Cupps RE, Johnson EW (1970) Giant cell tumor: a study of 195 cases. Cancer 25: 1061–1070

Deacon J, Peckham MJ, Steel GG (1984) The radio-responsiveness of human tumors and the initial slope of the cell-survival curve. Radiother Oncol 2: 317–323

De Fries HO, Perlin E, Leibel SA (1970) Treatment of osteogenic sarcoma of the mandible. Arch Otolaryngol 105: 358–359

Edmonson JH, Green SJ, Ivins IC et al. (1986) A controlled pilot study of high dose methotrexate as post-surgical adjuvant treatment for primary osteosarcoma. J Clin Oncol 2: 152–156

Eilber FR, Eckhardt J, Morton DL (1984) Advances in the treatment of sarcoma of the extremity: current status of limb salvage. Cancer 54: 2695–2701

Eilber F, Giuliano A, Eckardt J, Patterson K, Hoseley S, Goodnight J (1987) Adjuvant chemotherapy for osteosarcoma: a randomized prospective trial. J Clin Oncol 5: 21–26

Ellis ER, Marcus RB Jr, Cicale MJ et al. (1992) Pulmonary function tests after whole-lung irradiation and doxorubicin in patients with osteogenic sarcoma. J Clin Oncol 10: 459–463

Farrell C, Reventosa A (1964) Experience in treating osteosarcoma at the Hospital of University of Pennsylvania. Radiology 83: 1080–1083

Feinleib M, Zelen M (1969) Some pitfalls in the evaluation of screening programs. Arch Environ Health 19: 412–415

Feinstein AR, Sosin DM, Wells CK (1985) The Will Rogers phenomenon: stage migration and new diagnostic techniques as a source of misleading statistics for survival in cancer. Engl J Med 312: 1604–1608

Fertil B, Malaise EP (1981) Inherent cellular radiosensitivity as a basic concept for human tumor radiotherapy. Int J Radiat Oncol Biol Phys 7: 621–629

French Bone Tumor Study Group (1988) Age and dose of chemotherapy as major prognostic factors in a trial of adjuvant therapy of osteosarcoma combining two alternating drug combinations and early prophylactic lung irradiation. Cancer 61: 1304–1311

Friedman MA, Carter SK (1972) The therapy of osteogenic sarcoma: current status and thoughts for the future. J Surg Oncol 4: 482–610

Gaitan-Yanguas M (1981) A study of the response of osteogenic sarcoma and adjacent normal tissues to radiation. Int J Radiat Oncol Biol Phys 7: 593–595

Hancock SL, Tucker MA, Hoppe RT (1993) Breast cancer after treatment of Hodgkin's disease. J Nat Cancer Inst 85: 25–31

Hirano T, Iwasaki K, Kumashiro T, Sadamatsu T (1992) Encapsulation around malignant bone tumors after preoperative adjuvant treatment. Nippon Seikeigeka Gakkai Zasshi 66: 31–37

Horowitz ME, Pratt CB, Webber BL et al. (1986) Therapy for childhood soft tissue sarcomas other than rhabdomyosarcoma: a review of 62 cases treated at a single institution. J Clin Oncol 4: 559–564

Hutchison GB, Shapiro S (1968) Lead time gained by diagnostic screening for breast cancer. J Natl Cancer Inst 41: 665–673

Hutter VP, Worcester JN et al. (1962) Benign and malignant giant cell tumor of bone: a clinicopathological analysis of the natural history of the disease. Cancer 15: 653–690

Ishii T, Ando K, Koike S (1989) Biological effectiveness of fast neutrons on a murine osteosarcoma. Int J Radiat Oncol Biol Phys 16: 693–699

Ivins JC, Taylor WF, Wold LE (1987) Elective whole-lung irradiation in osteosarcoma treatment. Appearance of bilateral breast cancer in two long-term survivors. Skeletal Radiol 16: 133–135

Jaffe HL (1958) Tumors and tumorous conditions of the bone and joints. Lea and Febiger, Philadelphia

Jenkin RD (1977) Radiation treatment of Ewing's sarcoma and osteogenic sarcoma. Can. J. Surg 20: 530–536

Jenkin RDT, Allt WEC, Fitzpatrick PJ (1972) Osteosarcoma: an assessment of management with particular reference to primary irradiation and selective delayed amputation. Cancer 30: 393–400

Johnson EW Jr, Dahlin DC (1959) Treatment of giant cell tumor of bone. J Bone Joint Surg [Am] 41: 895–904

Kauffman SL, Stout AP (1960) Hemangiopericytoma in children. Cancer 13: 695–710

Kim JH, Chu FC, Woodard HQ, Melamed MR, Huvos A, Cantin J (1978) Radiation-induced soft tissue and bone sarcoma. Radiology 129: 501–508

Kinsella TJ (1986) Limited surgery and radiation therapy for sarcomas of the hand and foot. Int J Radiat Oncol Biol Phys 12: 2045–2046

Kinsella TJ, Loeffler JS, Fraass BA, Tepper J (1983) Extremity preservation by combined modality therapy in sarcomas of the hand and foot. An analysis of local control, disease-free survival and functional result. Int J Radiat Oncol Biol Phys 9: 1115–1119

Kinsella TJ, Lichter AS, Miser J, Gerber L, Glatstein E (1984) Local treatment of Ewing's sarcoma. Radiation therapy vs. surgery. Cancer Treat Rep 68: 695–701

Kliman M, Harwood AR, Jenkin RD (1982) Radical radiotherapy as primary treatment for Ewing's sarcoma distal to the elbow and knee. Clin Orthop 165: 233–238

Lee ES (1971) Treatment of bone sarcoma. Proc R Soc Med 64: 1179–1181

Lee ES, MacKenzie DH (1964) Osteosarcoma: a study of the value of preoperative megavoltage radiotherapy. Br J Surg 51: 252–274

Lemerle J, Voute PA, Tournade MF et al. (1976) Preoperative versus postoperative radiotherapy: single versus multiple courses of actinomycin D in the treatment of Wilm's tumor. Cancer 38: 647–654

Li FP, Cassady JR, Jaffe N (1975) Risk of second tumors and survivors of childhood cancer. Cancer 35: 1230–1235

Lichtenstein L (1977) Bone tumors, 5th edn. C.V. Mosby, St. Louis

Link MP (1986) The effect of adjuvant chemotherapy on relapse-free survival in patients with osteosarcoma of the extremity. N Engl J Med 314: 1600–1606

Livolsi VA (1977) Osteogenic sarcoma of the maxilla. Arch Otolaryngol 103: 485–488

Lougheed MN, Palmer JD et al. (1965) Radiation and regional chemotherapy in osteogenic sarcoma. In: Excerpta Medica International Congress Series 105: 1124–1128

Malawer MM, Sugarbaker PH, Lampert M, Baker AR, Gerber NL (1985) Report of ten patients and presentation of a modified technique for tumors of the proximal Humerus. The Tikhoff-Linberg procedure: Surgery 97: 518–528

Malawer MM, Link MP, Donaldson SS (1993) Sarcomas of bone. In: De Vita VT Jr, Hellman S, Rosenberg SA (eds) Cancer, principles and practice of oncology, 4th edn. J.B. Lippincott, Philadelphia, pp 1509–1566

Marangolo M, Tienghi A, Fiorentini G, Dazzi C, Graziani G, Priori T, Emiliani E (1992) Treatment of pelvic osteosarcoma. Ann Oncol 3 (Suppl 2): 21–39

Marcove RC, Rosen G (1980) En bloc resections for osteogenic sarcoma. Cancer 45: 3040–3044

Martinez A, Goffinet DR, Donaldson SS, Bagshaw MA, Kaplan HS (1985) Intra-arterial infusion of radiosensitizer (BUdR) combined with hypofractionated irradiation and chemotherapy for primary treatment of osteogenic sarcoma. Int J Radiat Oncol Biol Phys 11: 123–128

Miser JS, Triche TJ, Pritchard DJ, Kinsella TJ (1989) Ewing's sarcoma and the non-rhabdomyosarcoma soft tissue sarcomas of childhood. In: Pizzo PA, Poplack DG (eds) Principles and practice of pediatric oncology. J.B. Lippincott, Philadelphia, p 678

Musabaeva LI, Lantsman IV et al. (1990) Dose fractionation in photon and neutron therapy in the combined treatment of osteogenic sarcoma. Med Radiol (Moscow) 35(4): 27–32

Nascimento AG, Huvos AC, Marcove RC (1979) Primary malignant giant cell tumor of bone: a study of 8 cases and review of the literature. Cancer 44: 1393–1402

Newton KA (1972) Prophylactic irradiation of the lung in bone sarcoma. In: Price CHG, Ross FGM (eds) Bone: certain aspects of neoplasia. Butterworths, London, pp 307–311

Newton KA, Barrett A (1978) Prophylactic lung irradiation in the treatment of osteogenic sarcoma. Clin Radiol 29: 493–496

Nora FE, Unni KK, Pritchard DJ, Dahlin DC (1983) Osteosarcoma of extragnathic craniofacial bones. Mayo Clin Proc 58: 268–272

Okunieff P, Suit HD, Proppe KH (1986) Extremity preservation by combined modality therapy treatment of sarcomas of the hand and wrist. Int J Radiat Oncol Biol Phys 12: 1923–1930

Phillips TL, Sheline GE (1969) Radiation therapy of malignant bone tumors. Radiology 92: 1537–1545

Pizzo PA, Horowitz ME, Poplack DG, Hays DM, Kun LE (1993) Solid tumors of childhood. In: DeVita VT, Hellman S, Rosenberg SA (eds) Cancer principles and practice of oncology, 4th edn. J.B. Lippincott, Philadelphia, p 1784

Poppe E, Liverud K, Efskind J (1968) Osteosarcoma. Acta Chir Scand 134: 549–556

Potter D, Kinsella TJ, Glatstein E et al. (1986) High-grade soft tissue sarcomas of the extremities. Cancer 58: 190–205

Rab GT, Ivins JC, Childs DS, Cupps RE, Pritchard DJ (1976) Elective whole lung irradiation in the treatment of osteogenic sarcoma. Cancer 38: 939–942

Raney RB (1987) Soft tissue sarcoma in adolescence. In: Tebbi CK (ed) Major topics in adolescent oncology. Futura, Mount Kisco, pp 221–240

Raney RB, Ragab AH, Ruymann FB, Lindberg RD, Hays DM, Gehan EA, Soule EH (1982) Soft tissue sarcoma of the trunk in childhood, results of the Intergroup Rhabdomyosarcoma Study. Cancer 49: 2612–1616

Raney RB Jr, Allen A, O'Neill J, Handler SD, Uri A, Littman P (1986) Malignant fibrous histiocytoma of soft tissue in childhood. Cancer 57: 2198–2201

Raney RB, Schnaufer L, Ziegler M, Chatten J, Littman P, Jarrett P (1987) Treatment of children with neurogenic sarcoma. Experience at the Children's Hospital of Philadelphia 1958–1984. Cancer 59: 1–5

Rosen G, Murphy ML, Huvos AG, Gutierrez M, Marcove RC (1976) Chemotherapy, en bloc resection, and prosthetic bone replacement in the treatment of osteogenic sarcoma. Cancer 37: 1–11

Rosen G, Marcove RC, Caparros B, Nirenberg A, Kosloff C, Huvos AG (1979) Primary osteogenic sarcoma. The rationale for preoperative chemotherapy and delayed surgery. Cancer 43: 2163–2177

Silverberg E, Lubera J (1987) Cancer statistics. CA 37: 2–20

Simon MA, Aschliman MA, Thomas N, Mankin HJ (1986) Limb salvage treatment versus amputation for osteosarcoma of the distal end of the femur. J Bone Joint Surg 68: 1331–1337

Sollaccio RJ, Conrad C, Mendenhall NP et al. (1986) Soft tissue sarcoma in children: analysis of prognostic factors. Int J Radiat Oncol Biol Phys 12 (Suppl 1): 133

Soule EH, Pritchard DJ (1977) Fibrosarcoma of infants and children. A review of 110 cases. Cancer 40: 1711–1721

Spjut HJ, Ayala AG (1986) Skeletal tumors in childhood and adolescence. In: Finegold M (ed) Pathology of neoplasia in children and adolescence. WB Saunders, Philadelphia, pp 256–281

Stout AP (1962) Fibrosarcoma in infants and children. Cancer 15: 1028–1040

Suit HD (1975) Role of therapeutic radiology in cancer of bone. Cancer 35: 930–935

Sundaresan N, Rosen G, Huvos AG, Krol G (1988) Combined treatment of osteosarcoma of the spine. Neurosurgery 23: 714–719

Sutow WW, Gehan EA, Dyment PG, Vietti T, Miale T (1978) Multidrug adjuvant chemotherapy for osteosarcoma: interim report of the Southwest Oncology Group studies. Cancer Treat Rep 62: 265–270

Sweetnam R (1974) Tumors of bone and their management. Ann R Coll Surg Engl 54: 63–66

Sweetnan R, Knowelden J, Seedon H (1971) Bone sarcoma: treatment by irradiation, amputation, or a combination of the two. Br Med J 2: 363–367

Taylor WF, Ivins JC, Dahlin DC, Edmonson JH, Pritchard DJ (1978) Trends and variability in survival from osteosarcoma. Mayo Clin Proc 53: 695–700

Tefft M (1977) Radiation related toxicities in National Wilms' Tumor Study 1. Int J Radiat Oncol Biol Phys 2: 455–463

Tepper J, Rosenberg SA, Glatstein E (1982) Radiation therapy technique in soft tissue sarcomas of the extremity. Policies of treatment at the National Cancer Institute. Int J Radiat Oncol Biol Phys 8: 263–273

Thompson DK, Li FP, Cassady JR (1979) Breast cancer in a man 30 years after radiation for metastatic osteogenic sarcoma. Cancer 44: 2362–2365

van den Brenk HAS, Kerr RC et al. (1966) Results from tourniquet anoxia and hyperbaric oxygen techniques combined with megavoltage treatment of sarcomas of bone and soft tissues. Am J Roentgenol 96: 760–776

Wagget J, Koop CE (1970) Wilm's tumor preoperative radiotherapy and chemotherapy in the management of massive tumors. Cancer 26: 338–340

Weichselbaum RR, Epstein J, Little JB (1976) In vitro cellular radiosensitivity of human malignant tumors. Eur J Cancer 12: 47–51

Weichselbaum RR, Cassady JR, Jaffe N, Filler RM (1977) Preliminary results of an aggressive multimodality therapy for metastatic osteosarcoma. Cancer 40: 78–83

Weisenburger TH, Eilber FR, Grant TT, Morton DL, Mirra JJ, Steinberg M, Rickles D (1981) Multidisciplinary "limb salvage" treatment of soft tissue and skeletal sarcomas. Int J Radiat Oncol Biol Phys 7: 1495–1499

Wigg DR, Koschel K, Hodgson GS (1981) Tolerance of the mature human central nervous system to photon irradiation. Br J Radiol 54: 787–798

Yamamuro T, Kotoura Y (1993) Intraoperative radiation therapy for osteosarcoma. Cancer Treat Res 62: 177–183

Young JL, Miller RW (1975) Incidence of malignant tumors in U.S. children. J Pediatr 86: 245–258

Zaharia M, Caceres E, Valdivia S, Moran M, Tejada F (1986) Postoperative whole lung irradiation with or without Adriamycin in osteogenic sarcoma. Int J Radiat Oncol Biol Phys 12: 907–910

21 Retinoblastoma

J. Robert Cassady

CONTENTS

21.1   Introduction 319
21.2   Epidemiology 319
21.3   Molecular Genetics 319
21.4   Etiology 320
21.5   Pathology 320
21.6   Natural History and Clinical Features 321
21.7   Staging 321
21.8   Treatment 322
21.8.1   Surgery 323
21.8.2   Photocoagulation and Cryotherapy 324
21.8.3   Radiation Therapy 324
21.8.4   Chemotherapy 330
21.8.5   Treatment of Advanced Local or Metastatic
            Disease 330
21.9   Results 331
21.10   Complications 331
21.10.1 Somatic and Growth Effects 331
21.10.2 Cataract Formation 332
21.10.3 Keratitis and Keratoconjunctivitis 332
21.10.4 Vascular Effects 332
21.10.5 Dental Effects 332
21.10.6 Second-Tumor Formation 332
21.11   Future Prospects 333
            References 334

21.1 Introduction

Retinoblastoma (RB) represents the most common primary ocular tumor in childhood and is a significant cause of childhood blindness. The treatment of the child with RB exemplifies the dilemma of the pediatric radiation oncologist. On the one hand, treatment with radiation is highly effective both in obtaining local control of the neoplasm and, of equal importance, in preserving vision in the treated eye (s). However, these considerable accomplishments are purchased at a price which includes both cosmetic and possible functional visual deficits and, more seriously, the threat of a future "in field" second neoplasm which may ultimately lead to loss of life. It will

J. Robert Cassady, M.D., Professor and Head, Department of Radiation Oncology, The University of Arizona, Health Sciences Center, 1501 North Campbell Ave., Tucson, AZ 85724, USA

be the purpose of this chapter to briefly review the biology, molecular genetics, and natural history of this childhood malignancy as they influence radiation therapy (RT) policies and treatment decisions, discuss the many RT options that exist, and consider their rightful place in the treatment of this fascinating tumor.

21.2 Epidemiology

Approximately 200 new cases of RB are diagnosed each year in the United States. This translates into a frequency of roughly 1/20 000 ± 6000 live births, a figure which is relatively constant in most countries and nationalities (Schappert–Kimmijser et al. 1966; Banks 1969; Devesa 1975; Young et al. 1978). Exceptions include East Africa (e.g., Tanzania), where RB is said to represent the commonest solid tumor of childhood, Yemen (geographically close to East Africa), and the Yucatán Peninsula and Guatemala with its Mayan population (Jensen and Miller 1987).

The vast majority of newly diagnosed cases are felt to arise spontaneously, a feature that limits simple attempts at prevention or early diagnosis. Between 60% and 70% of new cases are unilateral and the overwhelming majority of these (~95%) have no positive family history. Approximately 20% of bilateral cases have a relevant family history. Therefore, in less than 10% of newly diagnosed cases will a positive family history be found (Green 1985). The foregoing has relevance to the radiation oncologist because a very small minority of unilateral cases (especially with a negative family history) present with useful, salvageable vision or, in the United States, with advanced but not metastatic disease outside the globe. The number of potential candidates for curative RT among all patients with RB is therefore limited.

21.3 Molecular Genetics

Hypotheses made by Knudson (1971, 1989) regarding RB and subsequently supported or confirmed in the past two decades have initiated an era of molecular biology in pediatric oncology. Homozygous loss in a retinal precursor cell of the RB gene located at the 13q14 locus appears to make development of RB by that cell highly likely or inevitable. In individuals in whom this gene is already deleted in one allele of every cell (e.g., offspring of patients with bilateral disease) a deletion of the RB gene of the other allele will likely cause tumor development. As the number of at risk precursor retinal cells exceeds the mutation frequency at the 13q14 locus, development of at least one tumor in these individuals is highly likely, thus simulating a classical mendelian autosomal dominant situation. However, the requirement for homozygosity at the 13q14 locus suggests in fact a recessive gene (ALLDERDICE et al. 1969; CAVENEE et al. 1983; DRYJA et al. 1984; KNUDSON 1989). The likelihood of simultaneous mutations (deletions) of both alleles at that locus is quite low, thus accounting for the observed rarity of the disease except in those with a known family history.

Only 5%–6% of offspring of patients with unilateral disease subsequently develop RB. This figure has been used by VOGEL (1979), who calculates that only 10%–12% of these patients have a germinal mutation which they will pass on to their offspring.

The RB gene has now been cloned and has been classed as a "tumor suppressor" gene. Its absence presumably allows lack of suppression of some aspect of cellular growth leading to tumor formation.

The relevance of these observations for the radiation oncologist lies in their implication for the retinal volume at risk for tumor development. In the rare spontaneous (no family history) unilateral tumor patient with vision in whom consideration for RT is given, localized approaches such as plaque treatment or particle therapy seem most appropriate as presumably only a single cell or small number of retinal cells are at risk. In the patient with bilateral, multifocal disease or with a positive family history, treatment of the entire retinal surface must be seriously considered.

21.4 Etiology

Although the precise etiology of RB is not known, the high frequency of this tumor observed in patients with known major loss of the 13q (long arm) 14 chromosome band – who present with mental retardation, low set ears, hypertelorism, micrognathia, and other less common anomalies – in combination with

more recent molecular data suggests that homozygous loss of this chromosomal segment is a necessary precursor to RB development (ALLDERDICE et al. 1969). This chromosomal loss may occur by many different mechanisms, including nondisjunction, mitotic recombination, deletion, and point mutation (CAVENEE et al. 1983). The precise cellular events leading to tumor development are not known at this time. However, loss of this chromosome, region in cells of nonretinal lineage apparently also predisposes at least some of them to tumor development as well (ABRAMSON et al. 1979, 1984).

21.5 Pathology

Retinoblastoma belongs to the group of malignancies that have been termed small blue cell tumors of infancy and childhood. Grossly, these tumors are "chalky white," friable lesions (GREEN 1985). Tumors which arise from the internal or external nuclear layers, the nerve cell layer, or the ganglion cell layer tend to grow towards the subretinal space, displace the retina inwards, are frequently associated with retinal detachment, and have been termed "exophytum type." Those arising from the inner retinal layers grow towards the vitreous have been termed "endophytum type" (REESE 1976; SANG and ALBERT 1982). Calcification (thought, by some, to be calcified DNA) (BERNARDINO and SALCEDA 1970) is very common and accounts in part for the gross appearance.

The tumor is composed of small round or polygonal cells with scanty cytoplasm and a relatively large, densely staining nucleus. Three types of cell arrangement have been described: the fleurette, the Homer-Wright rosette, and the Flexner-Wintersteiner rosette. The last-mentioned represents a radial arrangement of cells around a lumen which contains acid mucopolysaccharide similar to that surrounding rods and cones. It is generally only observed in RB. Fleurettes are so called because the cells contain abundant eosinophilic cytoplasm and their arrangement resembles the "fleur-de-lis" pattern. Homer-Wright rosettes also represent a radial arrangement of cells about dense intertwined fibrils but are not unique to RB (Ts'o et al. 1969; 1970; SHIELDS and AUGSBURGER 1981; SANG and ALBERT 1982).

PARKHILL and BENEDICT (1941) recognized three main categories of retinal tumors: (a) RB composed of highly undifferentiated cells, (b) neuroepithelioma showing partial differentiation with rosette formation, and (c) rare tumors composed primarily of astrocytes resembling gliomas of the brain and probably representing ocular extension of an optic glioma.

21.6 Natural History and Clinical Features

Leukokoria (cat's eye reflex) predominates as the cause of presentation for most children with RB. However, a significant number of children present because of unexplained strabismus or, due to a recognized family history, at the time of a routine screening examination. Unexplained strabismus in an infant or young child *must be considered RB until proven otherwise*. For unknown reasons, boys are more frequently affected than girls (1.15:1.0). Children with bilateral disease present at a mean age nearly 1 year earlier than those with unilateral disease (11 months vs 24 months)(GREEN 1985). It was this observation that led KNUDSON (1971) to postulate his "two-hit" hypothesis, speculating that only one additional event rather than two or more events was required for tumor formation in children with a positive family history. This critical hypothesis is now recognized as probably correct. In the United States, children rarely present with tumor outside the globe or with overt metastatic disease.

The differential diagnosis for RB is shown in Table 21.1. Visceral larva migrans (*Toxocara canis*) and Coats' disease, an autoimmune-like disease of the retina, present the most frequent difficulty, although in the past, when prolonged oxygen use at high levels was more common, retrolental fibroplasia was occasionally confused with RB.

Clinical examination of the child with RB should include thorough examination of the entire retinal surface of both eyes using indirect ophthalmoscopy with the child anesthetized. Leukokoria is noted due to both the whitish color of the neoplasm and the frequent presence of calcium. In addition, a careful neurologic examination should be performed in view of the potential for spread to the central nervous system via the optic nerve or the possibility of a pineal region

Table 21.1. Differential diagnosis for RB

1. Visceral larva migrans (*Toxocara canis*)
2. Granulomatous uveitis (toxoplasmosis)
3. Coats' disease (isolated retinal telangiectasia)
4. Angiomatosis retinae
5. Metastatic retinitis
6. Retrolental fibroplasia
7. Persistent hyperplastic primary vitreous
8. Retinal fold/retinal dysplasia
9. Massive retinal fibrosis

tumor, so-called "trilateral retinoblastoma." Lymph nodes should be assessed but will rarely contain tumor unless massive orbital disease is present or an orbital recurrence has developed post-enucleation. Care should be taken to look for any congenital anomalies that may be present.

Radiographic evaluation should include computed tomography (CT) of both eyes and orbits to assess intraocular extent and to determine whether any extraocular disease is present. Magnetic resonance imaging (MRI) with gadolinium enhancement should also be considered in view of the possibility of meningeal spread and also to image the remainder of the brain as trilateral retinoblastomas have, by now, been well documented in from 1% to 5% of children with hereditary bilateral RB (JAKOBIEC et al. 1977; BADER et al. 1982). Ocular ultrasonography should also be considered for the child likely to undergo RT in order to optimally assess the location of the lens in relation to other facial structures.

Laboratory studies should include a bone marrow aspirate and biopsy and examination of the cerebrospinal fluid with cytospin evaluation for tumor cells potentially spread by meningeal extension. Although usually performed in most clinics, these latter studies will have an extremely low yield and, in the absence of relatively marked intraocular or extraocular disease, their usefulness and cost-benefit ratio is a matter of controversy. Similarly controversial is catecholamine determination prior to treatment. Although elevated levels have been reported in children with RB, the initial presence or development of metastatic disease is extremely rare in the United States and thus routine performance of this test does not appear to be warranted.

21.7 Staging

In addition to the presence of metastatic disease and, to a lesser extent, intraocular tumor size, certain local features influence prognosis. They include extraocular disease, the presence of full-thickness choroidal invasion, scleral involvement, and the presence of optic nerve invasion (MERRIAM 1950; BROWN 1958; CARBAJAL 1958, 1959; ZIMMERMAN 1961; TAKTIKOS 1966; REDLER and ELLSWORTH 1973; ELLSWORTH 1974; LENNOX et al. 1975; STANNARD et al. 1979).

The influence of choroidal and optic nerve involvement on prognosis is shown in Table 21.2. REDLER and ELLSWORTH (1973) have demonstrated the importance of the volume of choroidal involvement for ultimate prognosis. All but one death in

Table 21.2. Correlation of extent of choroidal and optic nerve involvement with prognosis in RB (Brown 1958; Carbajal 1958, 1959; Zimmerman 1961; Redler and Ellsworth 1973)

	Range of survival
Choroidal involvement (n = 265)	
Superficial or small volume	57%–95%
Full thickness or massive	0%–44%
Optic nerve involvement (n = 576)	
No involvement	72.4%–91.6%
Invasion anterior to lamina cribrosa	83%–85%
Invasion posterior to lamina cribrosa	
Resection line negative	33%–55.6%
Resection line positive	19%–36%

Table 21.3. Prognostic staging systems for RB

St. Jude system (Pratt 1972)

Stage I: Tumor (unifocal or multifocal) confined to retina
   a) Occupying one quadrant or less
   b) Occupying two quadrants or less
   c) Occupying more than 50% of retinal surface

Stage II: Tumor (unifocal or multifocal) confined to globe
   a) With vitreous seeding
   b) Extending to optic nerve head
   c) Extending to choroid
   d) Extending to choroid and optic nerve head
   e) Extending to emissaries

Stage III: Extraocular extension of tumor
   a) Extending beyond cut end optic nerve (including subarachnoid extension)
   b) Extending through sclera into orbital contents
   c) Extending to choroid and beyond cut end of optic nerve (including subarachnoid extension)
   d) Extending through sclera into orbital contents and beyond cut end of optic nerve (including sub arachnoid extension)

Stage IV: Distant metastases
   a) Extending through optic nerve to brain
   b) Blood-borne metastases to soft tissue (s) and bone (s)
   c) Bone marrow metastases

Proposed system

Stage I: Tumor confined to retina, no vitreous seeding present. If eye is enucleated, there is no evidence of optic nerve or choroidal involvement and the sclera is not affected.

Stage II: Tumor confined to orbit. Vitreous seeding present. If eye is enucleated, there is involvement of the choroid and/or optic nerve; however, massive extension through the choroid and/or tumor at cut end of optic nerve not present. There may be minimal scleral involvement.

Stage III: Massive choroid involvement present and/or tumor at cut end of optical nerve. Massive scleral involvement present.

State IV: Distant metastases present beyond orbit.

Table 21.4. Reese-Ellsworth grouping system: probability of tumor control with vision (Reese and Ellsworth 1963)

Group I
   a) Solitary tumor, less than 4 disk diameters (dd)[a] in size, at or behind equator
   b) Multiple tumors < 4 dd in size at or behind equator

Group II
   a) Solitary tumor, 4–10 dd at or behind the equator
   b) Multiple tumors, 4–10 dd all at or behind equator

Group III
   a) Any lesion anterior to the equator
   b) Solitary tumor larger than 10 dd behind the equator

Group IV
   a) Multiple tumors, some larger than 10 dd
   b) Any lesion extending anteriorly to the ora serrata

Group V
   a) Massive tumors involving more than half the retina
   b) Vitreous seeding

[a] 1 disk diameter = approximately 1.5 mm

their series occurred in patients with massive involvement (>270 mm^3).

It is important to recognize that a substantial decrease in survival occurs only with relatively massive choroidal involvement or, when irradiation is used postoperatively, with optic nerve involvement posterior to the lamina cribrosa.

At this time, no uniformly accepted staging system which has prognostic relevance has been adopted. Table 21.3 shows two proposed systems. One represents the system currently in use at St. Jude Children's Research Hospital (Pratt 1972) while the other is a proposal of the author.

Reese and Ellsworth (1963) developed a widely used grouping system to assess the probability of retention of useful vision and tumor control following treatment with irradiation (Table 21.4) Tumor size, number, location and the presence of vitreous seeding are variables considered to be relevant. More frequent failure to control anteriorly placed tumors is felt by many to be a function of radiation technique e.g., underdosing due to use of a lateral field approach with lens sparing) rather than an inherent increase in radioresistance in more anteriorly placed tumors (Weiss et al. 1975; Salmonsen et al. 1979; Foote et al. 1989).

21.8 Treatment

The ideal treatment approach for RB would make possible routine tumor control, cause no retinal, lens, or structural (i.e., bone, muscle, teeth) damage or growth arrest, and not be associated with an increased risk of second tumor development. In fact an "ideal" approach would prevent second tumors not only in the orbital region but elsewhere, especially in the child with bilateral disease or a known family history. Unfortunately, no such treatment currently exists and the oncologist must therefore utilize surgery, radiation therapy, cryotherapy, photocoagulation, and, in advanced cases, chemotherapy in an optimum fashion.

21.8.1 Surgery

Most children with RB present with unilateral disease and useful vision is rarely present or possible. For this group surgical enucleation with removal of as long a segment of the optic nerve as possible is recommended. Similarly, many children with bilateral disease will have extensive disease in one of the two eyes affected, with no useful vision in that eye. Enucleation also represents the most appropriate treatment of the blind eye in this setting. Except for the infrequent patient with optic nerve, scleral, extraocular, or metastatic disease (vide infra),

additional systemic treatment with chemotherapy or local orbital postoperative radiation treatment is not warranted. Enucleation is also indicated for any eye in which conservative treatment with radiation or cryotherapy or photocoagulation followed by RT has failed or in which a complication has occurred, eliminating useful vision (e.g., vitreous hemorrhage, retinal vascular damage, rubeosis iridis leading to glaucoma); in the latter context enucleation is especially appropriate if the complication has occurred within 2 years of treatment and obscures retinal visualization (ELLSWORTH 1969, 1977).

Orbital exenteration is rarely required in the United States except for the extremely rare child with massive ocular and extraocular tumor or children in whom a local, postenucleation orbital recurrence has occurred.

In addition to surgery, other proven treatment modalities include both photocoagulation and cryotherapy as well as RT. The role of chemotherapy in the curative treatment of RB is uncertain and will be discussed later. Although dramatic and even complete responses have been reported, primarily in patients with metastatic disease, only anecdotal reports attest to the long-term durability of these responses.

Table 21.5. Results of photocoagulation treatment for RB[a] (ABRAMSON 1989)

	No. of tumors		No. cured	% cured	Significance
Size (dd)					
0–1	72	(26%)	70	97	
>1<2	98	(35%)	70	72	
>2<3	50	(18%)	29	59	
>3<4	23	(8%)	9	39	$P < 0.0001$
>4<5	13	(5%)	6	46	
>5	22	(8%)	9	41	
Location					
Ant. to equator	81		67	83	
Equator	123		84	68	$P < 0.0001$
Post. to equator	74		44	60	
Elevation					
Low	201		162	81	$P < 0.0001$
High	76		33	43	

[a] 85/281 tumors failed photocoagulation
47/85 enucleated
10/85 cured with cryotherapy
20/85 cured with ^{60}Co plaque

Nature of tumor (new, old, etc.) not a significant variable for success.
47/85 (55%) of failures evident within 6 months of photocoagulation.
23/196 cured tumors (12%) required additional treatment for new postphotocoagulation tumors, etc.

21.8.2 Photocoagulation and Cryotherapy

Photocoagulation and cryotherapy are relatively noninvasive techniques that offer, with radiation, the potential for tumor control with preservation of useful vision. Although photocoagulation was introduced into the RB clinic before cryotherapy, the latter technique has largely supplanted it.

The use of photocoagulation as a significant treatment modality for RB was first reported by MEYER-SCHWICKERATH (1954, 1979). With this approach, the operator identifies the tumor site and then, using a laser apparatus, coagulates the entire periphery (+ margin) of the retina immediately adjacent to the tumor in a circumferential pattern. In this way, blood supply to the tumor from lateral vessels is eradicated and tumor control obtained. However, should a more posterior blood supply exist, it may escape coagulation and continue to function and permit tumor persistence and growth.

In cryotherapy, access for the cryotherapy probe to the more posterior portions of the globe is first obtained surgically followed by identification of the tumor(s) by indirect ophthalmoscopy. Multiple freeze-thaw cycles are then applied to the tumor site and adjacent retina using the probe. Both these techniques cause damage to the treated retina and the efficacy of both is tumor size related. An increasing incidence of recurrence is obtained for tumors larger than 3–4 disk diameters (dd) (Tables 21.5, 21.6).

Because of retinal or nerve damage, neither of these approaches is appropriate for tumors located on or near the macula or close to the optic nerve head. The eye which contains multiple (>2) and/or large tumors is also not best approached primarily by these techniques (LINCOFF 1968; NADEL and LINCOFF 1968; NEEL and DE SANTO 1973; ABRAMSON 1989).

21.8.3 Radiation Therapy

A number of effective radiation modalities are available. The ideal approach should deliver an adequate and homogeneous dose to the entire tumor volume and negligible radiation to surrounding structures (especially the lens) and be capable of rapid, precise, and repeated treatment (ARMSTRONG 1974). It is the task of the radiation oncologist to best approximate this ideal goal utilizing available modalities.

Radioactive plaques of varying sizes utilizing ^{60}Co or ^{125}I, high-energy particle beams, and external beam photons generally produced by a linear accelerator or betatron all have a place in management of this tumor. A large number of clinical settings are possible and no single treatment approach is optimum for all cases.

It must be emphasized that the rationale for use of RT in children with an intact globe is to preserve sight. Should no sight be present in an eye, enucleation is the preferred treatment.

Table 21.6. Results of cryotherapy treatment for RB[a] (ABRAMSON 1989)

	No. of tumors	No. cured	% cured	Size range and average size (dd)	Comment
New tumor	21	20	95	0.25–5 Mean 1.5	16 cured with 1 session 4 with 2 sessions Mean follow-up = 47 mo
New post-irradiation tumor	27	23	85	0.5–3 Mean 1.0	16 cured with 1 session 5 cured with 2 sessions Mean follow-up = 46 mo
Old post-irradiation tumors (local failures)	39	35	90	0.25–5 Mean 1.5	22 cured with 1 session 6 cured with 2 sessions Mean follow-up = 40 mo
Vitreous base	29	0	0	0.25–5	Mean follow-up = 32 mo

[a] Of 113 pts (mean follow-up = 40 months, range 4–144), 105 survive (93%). Authors found that tumor size and location (vitreous base) were prognostic variables and noted "tumors larger than 3–4 dds were rarely cured with cryotherapy alone."

Table 21.7. Results of radioactive plaque treatment for RB (STALLARD 1962; BRADY et al. 1988; AMENDOLA et al. 1989)

Author	Patients	Eyes	Tumor control	Useful vision	Cataract	Death
STALLARD	104	111	62 (56%)	50 (45%)	6	7
AMENDOLA et al. Primary cases	16	16	14 (3 required replaquing)	14 vitreous Hemorrhage in one case	2	0
AMENDOLA et al.	20	20	16	10 Five additional with poor vision	3	1

[a] 33/62 with one tumor and 52/62 with one application (1 tumor in 28, 2 in 14, 3 in 7, and 4 in 3)

21.8.3.1 Plaque Treatment

In this technique, selection and preparation of an appropriately constructed plaque is followed by surgery to gain access to the posterior sclera. Tumor location is determined by mechanical pressure in combination with indirect ophthalmoscopy. Following scleral placement and suturing of a "dummy" plaque with confirmation of proper location, the radioactive plaque is secured and then left in place for an appropriate time.

Historically, direct radon seed implantation into RB was first undertaken by MOORE (MOORE et al. 1931). Following this, his younger associate STALLARD (1962) utilized ^{60}Co plaques to treat a large series of patients. Variable results, dependent on tumor size, location, and number combined with radiation protection problems associated with ^{60}Co, caused concern (STALLARD 1955). The rapid and successful development of megavoltage external beam photon treatment devices combined with these concerns brought this technique into relative disfavor until recently, when it has been revived by use of the more readily shielded ^{125}I and other radioisotopes with similar properties.

Table 21.7 depicts Stallard's results as well as those of more recent series (STALLARD 1962; BRADY et al. 1988; AMENDOLA et al. 1989). It is notable that two-thirds of Stallard's successes occurred in tumors smaller than 1 cm (6–7 dd) and half involved treatment of a single tumor. General agreement exists that patients with large tumors (> 6–7 dd), multiple (> 2) tumors, vitreous seeding, or tumor location at the macula, optic nerve head, or anterior to the equator

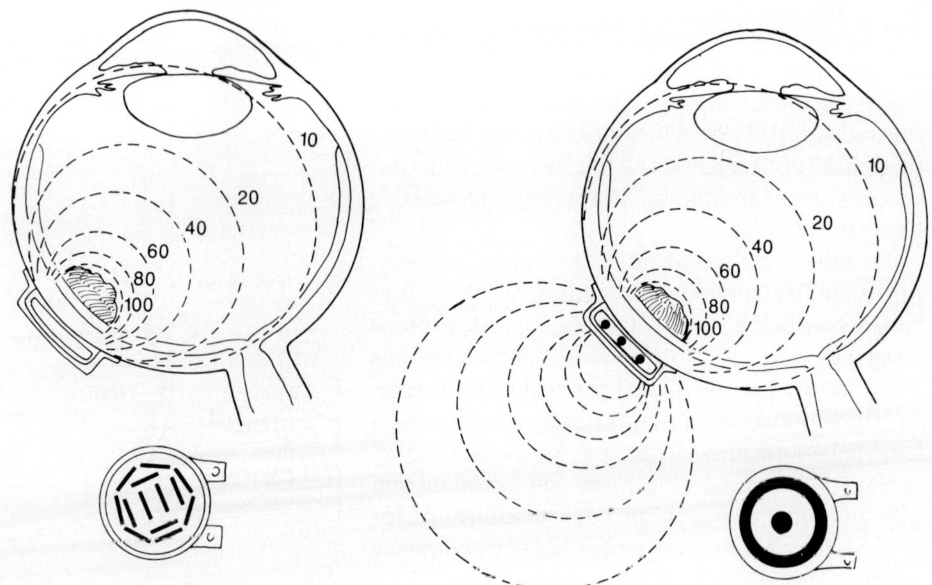

Fig. 21.1. Isodose distributions for ^{60}Co (*left*) and ^{125}I (*right*) eye plaques. A significant scleral (and retinal vascular) dose is delivered by both isotopes but because of the lower energy of the ^{125}I photons, considerably greater shielding of normal tissues from irradiation is possible with this isotope. Lens dose is also appreciable with both isotopes

are best treated with external beam radiation approaches. Anterior location is a relative contraindication for plaque treatment primarily because of the lens dose that will be delivered with subsequent risk of cataract formation and possibly glaucoma. It is equally clear that isotopes such as ^{125}I are superior to ^{60}Co or ^{192}Ir due to shielding considerations that can limit radiation to the uninvolved retina and other anteriorly placed structures and deliver virtually no radiation to more posterior orbital structures.

Most commonly, a dose at the apex of the tumor of approximately 40 Gy is delivered in 2–4 days. Due to inverse square considerations (Fig. 21.1), an apex dose of this magnitude often results in a scleral (and potential retinal vascular) dose of 160–200 Gy.

The selection criteria previously noted combined with the potential tumor-bearing volume of the retina at risk limit indications for plaque treatment to the rare patient with small, spontaneous unilateral involvement or patients who have developed limited local failure resistant to cryotherapy approaches following external beam RT (EBRT). Although AMENDOLA et al. (1989) have reported results from the use of plaque treatment in bilaterally affected patients, most patients had previously been subjected to unilateral enucleation (8/10) and/or had developed limited failure after EBRT.

21.8.3.2 Electron Beam and Particle Treatment

Few clinical reports are available detailing results of charged particle treatment. In part, this paucity of data is due to the fact that the location of existing proton and stripped nuclei facilities have not been hospital based until recently and thus necessary support services (e.g., anesthesia) have been unavailable (Armstrong 1974).

Results of treatment are also unclear. MUNZENRIDER (1989) has indicated that four patients with RB have been treated with protons using the Harvard cyclotron. Tumor recurrence was noted in one patient treated for recurrent disease, and three infants with primary disease have not been followed for an adequate period. MCCORMICK et al. (1988) have used electrons in conjunction with photons; however, in later treatment plans devised, the electron component has been relatively minor.

Published electron-only treatment plans have had significant inhomogeneities and the number of children treated by these approaches and their outcome

is not known (GRIEM et al. 1968; ARMSTRONG 1974). Therefore, at this time, the role of charged particle treatment in relation to external beam photon techniques is a minor one.

Much more straightforward is the usefulness of electron beam treatment in postenucleation orbital treatment when scleral, extraocular extension or optic nerve involvement has been present, substantially increasing the risk of local recurrence. In these instances, electron beam therapy should be the major or only radiation modality in order to minimize the volume of normal tissue exposed to moderate or high doses of radiation.

21.8.3.3 External Beam Approaches

Prior to a consideration of available external beam treatment techniques, anatomic relationships must be considered. Figure 21.2 demonstrates a representative globe and orbit. Of particular importance is the proximity of the meninges sheathing the optic nerve to the posterior globe and the proximity of the anteriormost retina (ora serrata) to a vertical plane tangent to the posterior lens (< 1–3 mm).

As most irradiated children will be less than 24 months of age at the time of treatment, the minimum interglobe separation between the two eyes will be less than 4 cm and therefore reliance on an ipsilateral lateral field will ensure substantial irradiation to

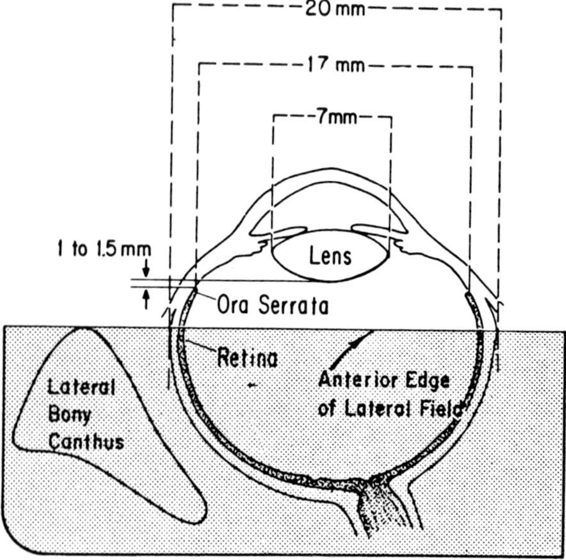

Fig. 21.2. Representation of an infant's eye demonstrating several critical relationships between the globe and bony landmarks and lens and retinal anatomy

the contralateral eye (if present). McCormick et al. (1988) have proposed a pair of vertical oblique wedged photon fields with an ipsilateral 11 MeV electron field to address this issue for the patient with unilateral disease.

21.8.3.4 External Beam Treatment Techniques

Prior to the development of megavoltage equipment, two equally weighted orthovoltage fields were used (ipsilateral lateral and contralateral oblique nasal) (Sagerman et al. 1969). Doses used were in excess of 80 Gy and, although tumor control was obtained in many children, visual changes precluded a useful functional result. Subsequently, use of a high-energy (> 4 MV) linear accelerator or betatron delivering a D-shaped ipsilateral lateral field became standard practice until recently (Bagshaw and Kaplan 1966; Cassady et al. 1969). With this lateral field approach, the child is generally sedated or anesthetized and the anterior field border is placed at or just anterior (2–3 mm) to the bony canthus. The remaining three field edges are placed to ensure adequate coverage of orbital structures. Using table rotation or a split-field approach to avoid divergence into the con-

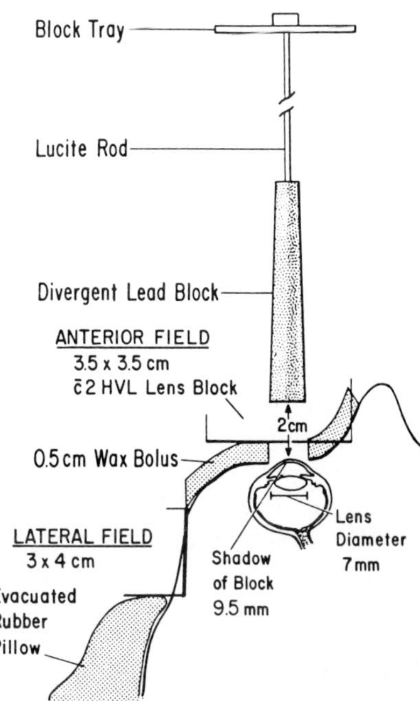

Fig. 21.3. "Hanging divergent lens block" technique proposed by Weiss et al. to accomplish irradiation (to hopefully adequate, although lower doses) to the anterior retina. The technique is appropriate only when the treated child is anesthetized and immobilized and is utilized for potentially microscopic disease anterior to the equator

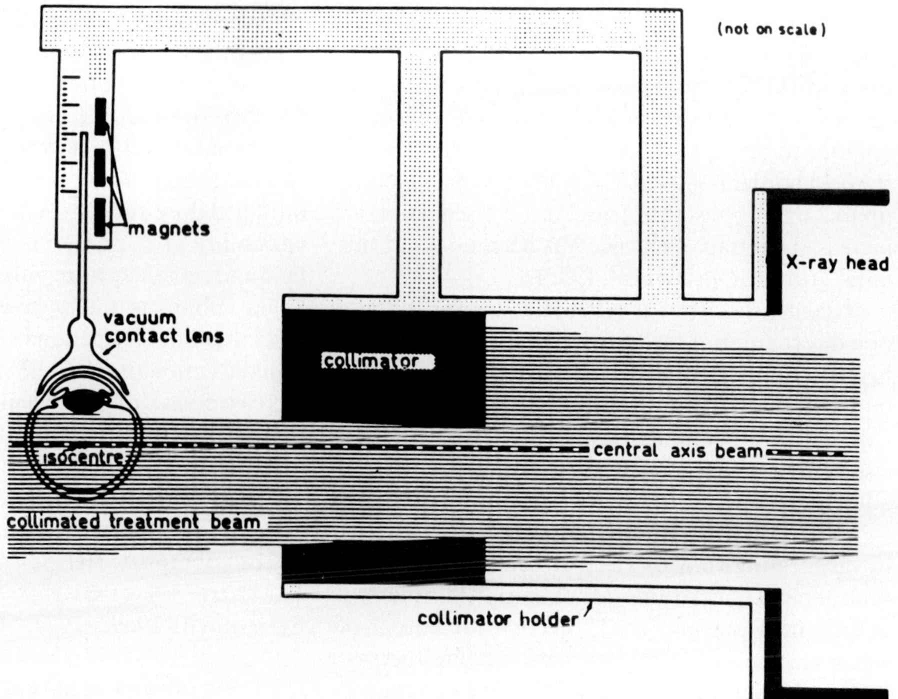

Fig. 21.4. Contact lens positioning device proposed by Schipper's Utrecht group and Harnett et al. The device is used with an anesthetized child and the anterior, split-field border position varies depending on the extent of anterior tumor (see text)

tralateral lens (if present), 35–45 Gy was delivered, most commonly in large (> 3 Gy) fractions thrice weekly.

Although ocular tumor control by Reese-Ellsworth group and dose was analyzed, no distinction was made between true in-field failure and either marginal failure or new tumor development (anterior to the equator) (Cassady et al. 1969). Weiss et al. (1975) first drew attention to the frequency of anterior "failures" and their report was subsequently confirmed by Salmonsen et al. (1979). Beginning with these reports, new external beam treatment techniques have been devised, with varying success, in an attempt to adequately irradiate the retina anterior to the equator. Weiss et al. proposed use of a supplemental anterior field (~14 Gy) with a divergent "hanging" central lens block in addition to the standard lateral field (~35 Gy) and routine anesthesia for daily (5 days/week) treatment (Fig. 21.3). In addition to the complexity of setup for daily treatment, the radiation inhomogeneity of this approach potentially represented a disadvantage (Weiss et al. 1975). The Utrecht group of Schipper and, subsequently, Harnett et al. implemented use of a complex contact lens treatment device linked to the linear accelerator in order to accurately and reproducibly ensure adequate retinal coverage using a split-field lateral field approach (Fig. 21.4) (Schipper 1983; Schipper et al. 1985; Harnett et al. 1987). Anesthesia has been routinely used and daily fraction sizes have been reduced to less than 3 Gy. The center of the field (anterior irradiation field border) has been placed close to the posterior lens border except when retinal involvement anterior to the equator exists. With anterior tumor, the field border is moved anteriorly and may include up to 3 mm of posterior lens. As a consequence, an increased cataract incidence has been noted in this latter group (Schipper et al. 1985).

Recently, Foote et al. (1989) have noted that use of a direct anterior field (no lens sparing) leads to a higher relapse-free survival, thus confirming the importance of anterior underdosing in tumor control. However, cataract formation, a complication less easily managed in children of this age than in adults, occurred in virtually all patients treated.

McCormick modified the approach of Weiss et al. by substituting a 6-MeV electron beam with a 1.2-cm central block for the anterior photon field. A lateral photon field was also used, the anterior border of which is uncertain. Children were not anesthetized and results were suboptimal with poor local control and a relatively high incidence of cataracts due presumably to patient motion during treatment. The substitution of an electron field also did not improve homogeneity within the tumor volume, variations of 30%–90% being reported (McCormick et al. 1988).

Thus, no ideal approach exists. It must also be noted that appropriate careful follow-up of children following treatment with a "classical" lateral field approach will almost always permit cryotherapeutic control of new tumors or marginal failures that may develop (Abramson 1989).

In our experience, however, the approach of Weiss et al. (1975) has led to a decrease in anterior recurrences and no significant increase in complications. We do not favor use of a direct, unshielded anterior field as it assures a usually avoidable cataract, and we have similar concerns about the increased cataract incidence observed when the anterior field border subtends 1–3 mm of posterior lens. Adequacy of dose distribution in very anterior tumors in this latter approach is also of concern.

21.8.3.5 Dose-Response Data

Scantly data exist plotting local control as a function of radiation dose or tumor size (or patient age). This problem is magnified by the multifocal nature of this tumor, the possibility of new tumor formation, and the frequent use of postirradiation cryotherapy when any concern exists regarding possible tumor regrowth. Cassady et al. (1969) demonstrated no advantage to radiation doses exceeding 40 Gy (> 3 Gy Fx), but did not distinguish between true and marginal failures or new tumor development. More recently, Abramson (1989) has constructed a modified dose-response curve based on known dose variability at the anterior border of the treatment field and correlated this with tumor status (Fig. 21.5). While subject to many caveats, this approach suggests that dose reduction below 25 Gy with conventional fractionation would likely be attended by an increased rate of true local failure even for small tumors. Similarly, as results obtained in patients with group V disease are dismal (vide infra), larger volumes of tumor are likely to require relatively larger radiation doses if a reasonable local control rate is to be obtained (Reese and Ellsworth 1963; Taktikos 1966; Bagshaw and Kaplan 1966; Ellsworth 1969, 1977; Cassady et al. 1969; Thompson et al. 1972; Lennox et al. 1975; Weiss et al. 1975; Salmonsen et al. 1979; Gagnon et al. 1980; Shields and Augsburger 1981; Abramson et al. 1981a,b; Schipper 1983; Migdal 1983; Schipper

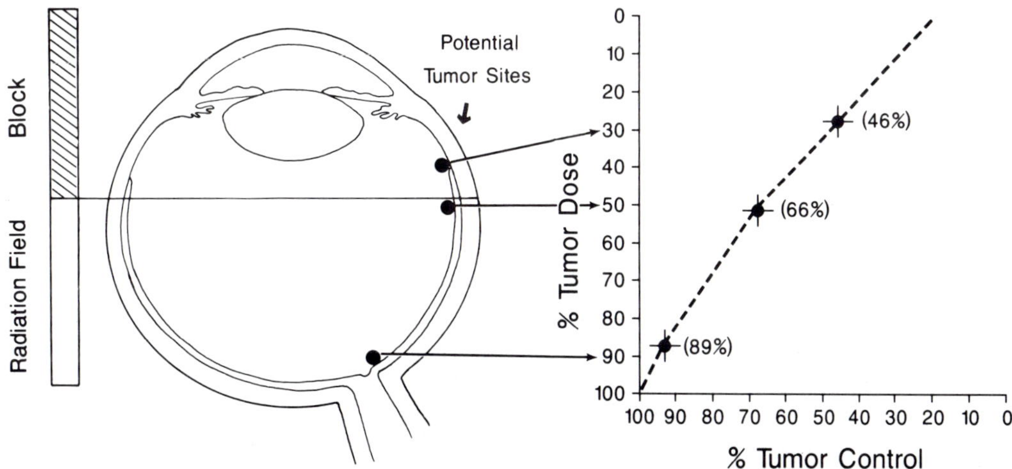

Fig. 21.5. Dose-response curve constructed by Abramson (1989) based on estimated dose delivered by a classic lateral split-field approach where the nondivergent central beam point has been placed about 5 mm *behind* the posterior lense to eliminate (or markedly decrease) the risk of cataract

et al. 1985; ABRAMSON 1985; MONGE et al. 1986; HARNETT et al. 1987; McCORMICK et al. 1988; FOOTE et al. 1989).

A possible treatment decision tree for patient management is presented in Fig. 21.6. Several points deserve additional comment. Most ophthalmologists, radiation oncologists, and perhaps parents will prefer enucleation for spontaneous, unilaterally affected children with group V disease even if vision is present. The most optimistic data suggest that less than one-third of children with group V disease will have tumor control with useful vision following conservative treatment with radiation (ABRAMSON et al. 1981b). The probability of metachronous tumor

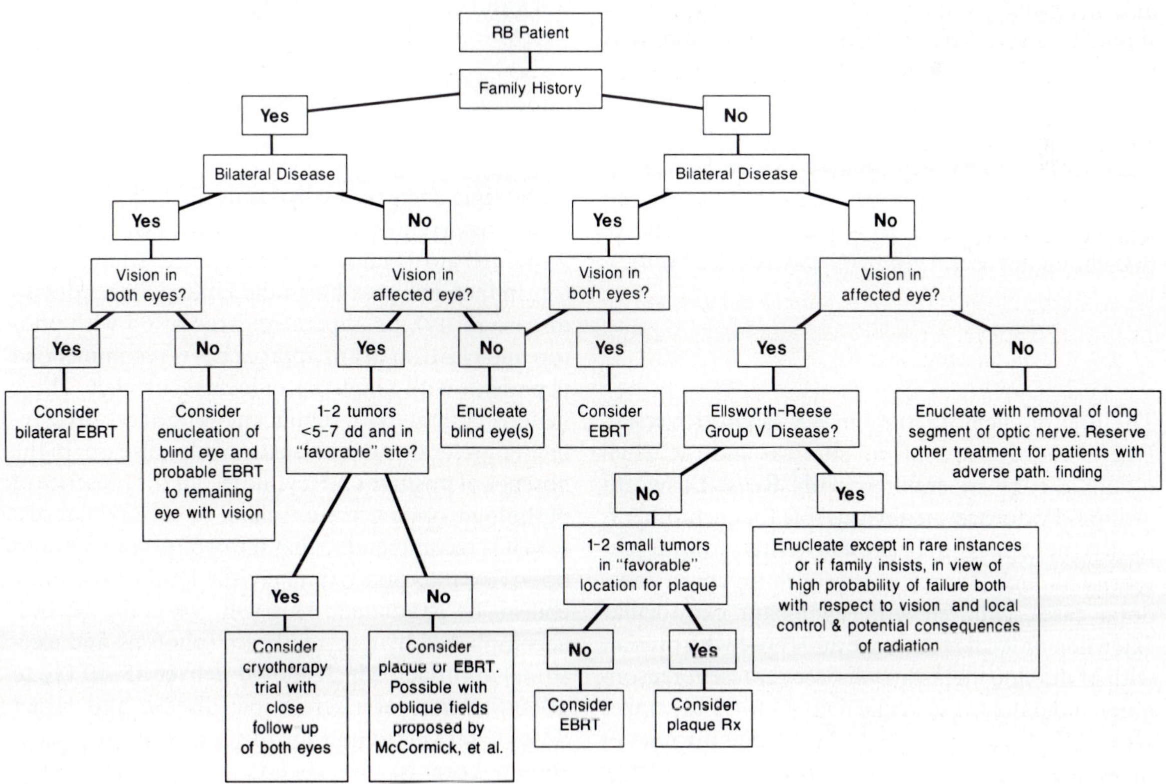

Fig. 21.6. Possible decision tree for treatment of a child with RB. Choices are felt to represent the most probable and optimum therapeutic choice utilized in the United States today

development in the contralateral eye is very low and therefore the possible gain – binocular vision in less than one-third of all treated children (vs unilateral vision) – must be weighed against the potential long-term risks of irradiating an infant. Should functional and treatment results be significantly improved by the introduction of new approaches, this decision point may be reversed.

As noted in the discussion, most children with bilateral disease will have multiple tumors or tumor size and location that favor EBRT. Obviously some eyes in these patients will require initial enucleation because of blindness and a small minority of eyes will be amenable to more local treatment approaches with cryotherapy or plaque treatment.

Tumor recurrence in an eye previously treated with adequate doses of EBRT may be managed in a variety of ways (ELLSWORTH 1969, 1977; CASSADY et al. 1969; SALMONSEN et al. 1979; ABRAMSON et al. 1981b; MIGDAL 1983; ABRAMSON 1989; AMENDOLA et al. 1989). Limited local failure, marginal failure of tumors at or anterior to the equator, or new (90% anterior) tumors are usually best managed initially by cryotherapy in an attempt to preserve vision (SALMONSEN et al. 1979; ABRAMOSN 1989). Should this approach fail but tumor be limited in extent and in a favorable location then strong consideration should be given to plaque treatment or perhaps particle irradiation (AMENDOLA et al. 1989). Should failure be generalized or massive in an eye, enucleation is strongly advised both to prevent possible tumor spread (and fatality) and because a second course of EBRT rarely accomplishes tumor control and almost invariably leads to retinal vascular damage that eliminates useful vision (CASSADY et al. 1969).

21.8.4 Chemotherapy

The role of chemotherapy in RB is controversial. Due to the almost uniform survival and the usual visual salvage in children with Reese-Ellsworth group I–IV disease, an obvious role for chemotherapy does not appear to be present in this group at present. Although efficacy is unproven except in anecdotal cases, children with significant extraocular extension or local recurrence and those who present with or develop metastatic disease represent reasonable candidates for systemic therapy (St. Jude stages III and IV, Cassady stages II–IV). No uniformity of opinion exists for children with an intermediate stage of disease (e.g., those with Reese-Ellsworth group Vb). An adjuvant effect has been claimed for this

group when treated with routine chemotherapy but this is currently unproven and, due to the high cure rate (> 85%–90%) with no adjuvant therapy and the infrequency of the disease, is likely to remain so (ELLSWORTH 1974; HOWARTH et al. 1980; FREEMAN et al. 1980; WHITE 1983; KINGSTON et al. 1987). Visual salvage is currently rarely accomplished with conventional irradiation regimens in Vb disease and it is possible that preirradiation chemotherapy might reduce tumor bulk sufficiently to permit such irradiation to be more effective. Earlier attempts using the single alkylating agent triethylenemelamine failed and we know of no recent result with positive data for this approach using multiple agents (CASSADY et al. 1989; HAYE et al. 1987).

Systemic drugs shown to be effective against neuroblastoma will generally demonstrate efficacy for RB. Thus multiple alkylating agents, vinca alkyloid derivatives, anthracyclines, and platinum derivatives have all been used with variable degrees of efficacy. As a single agent, cyclophosphamide has appeared to be most effective and one of the more encouraging reports for children who present with or develop metastatic disease concerns the initial promising results using high-dose chemotherapy with this agent and bone marrow transplantation (GEE and GRAHAM-POLE 1990; EKERT et al. 1982).

21.8.5 Treatment of Advanced Local or Metastatic Disease

Pathologic factors predisposing to a high rate of local recurrence have been discussed earlier. Although no randomized controlled studies exist (or, in fact, are possible in the United States due to disease rarity), postoperative irradiation with photon and electron beam approaches is recommended in patients with a high risk of local recurrence. These include patients with significant optic nerve involvement or scleral or orbital, extraocular disease. In the absence of positive CSF cytology but the presence of pathologic optic nerve or scleral or extraocular disease it is recommended that the orbital contents and optic nerve to approximately the level of the optic chiasm be irradiated. This will generally be best accomplished by a mixed beam (photons and electrons) approach which should deliver 45–50 Gy to potential sites of microscopic disease and larger doses (~ 60 Gy) to any site of residual gross disease should cure be the goal (CASSADY et al. 1969; ELLSWORTH 1974; STANNARD et al. 1979; HUNGERFORD et al. 1987).

The development of metastases almost always signals an ultimately fatal course. Should local signs or symptoms mandate urgent alleviation of tumor effects or should resistance to initially effective systemic agents be evident, then palliation of bone, lymph node, or locally recurrent tumor is indicated. We would recommend palliative regimens similar to those given for neuroblastoma, e.g., 21–30 Gy in 2.5-to 3-Gy fractions.

21.9 Results

In the United States, more than 85%–90% of all children who present with RB are cured. Thus virtually 100% of children with group I–IV globe-limited disease survive. Between 85% and 90% of all patients with group V disease survive and only in this group and the small group (in the United States) of children who currently present with extraocular disease is any appreciable mortality seen (BAGSHAW and KAPLAN 1966; CASSADY et al. 1969; THOMPSON et al. 1972; GAGNON et al. 1980; ABRAMSON et al. 1981a,b; SCHIPPER 1983; MIGDAL 1983; ABRAMSON 1985; SCHIPPER et al. 1985; MONGE et al. 1986; HARNETT et al. 1987).

Table 21.8 presents expected probability of tumor control with vision both as a function of a primary course of EBRT and after one or more courses of salvage therapy (i.e., cryotherapy, subsequent plaque treatment, etc.).

It is of note that a sizable fraction of children with ultimately preserved useful vision require additional treatment, usually with cryotherapy. As noted in the discussion of dose and local control, not all of these "failures" are definite or "proven" and it is unclear from the published literature what fraction represent new tumors. The high failure rate in children with group V disease has been previously noted. In this group, due to the frequent presence of vitreous seeds,

hypoxia may play a significant role in failure and results are currently in need of improvement.

Treatment of gross recurrent orbital disease is rarely successful. Most of these patients will already have central nervous system or distant metastases which are rarely controlled by systemic therapy. CASSADY et al. (1969) reported survival in 17 of 33 patients with residual or recurrent orbital disease. However, many of these patients were treated in the immediate postoperative period because of concern regarding residual microscopic disease. HUNGERFORD et al. (1987) reported no local recurrences following postoperative irradiation (50 Gy/5 weeks) to the orbit in eight patients with probable residual microscopic orbital or optic nerve disease. Several orbital recurrences were reported by these authors when adjuvant irradiation was not given to patients with similar risk factors. LENNOX et al. (1975) reported survival in 22 of 33 patients with optic nerve involvement. All five children with extraocular disease died in this series. The effect of treatment with irradiation cannot be ascertained in this series. Other than anecdotal reports of this type, few data exist on the true orbital recurrence rate in unirradiated patients with high-risk features for local recurrence.

21.10 Complications

Despite in vitro demonstration of an apparently increased cellular sensitivity to irradiation, with the exception of second tumor development, children with RB have not been shown to suffer excessive soft tissue or somatic complications following treatment with irradiation as have children with certain other genetic diseases such as ataxia telangiectasia (WEICHSELBAUM et al. 1978; WEICHSELBAUM and LITTLE 1980).

Table 21.8. Results of EBRT (BAGSHAW and KAPLAN 1966; ABRAMSON et al. 1981a, b; MIGDAL 1983; ABRAMSON 1985; SCHIPPER et al. 1985; HARNETT et al. 1987; FOOTE et al; 1989)

Reese-Ellsworth group	No. treated	No. Requiring additional cryotherapy, photocoagulation or RT	No. with enucleation	No. with vision
I	74	31	5	69
II	32	16	5	27
III	50	26	17	32
IV	27	22	18	9
V	56	48	42	14
	239	143 (60%)	87 (36%)	151 (63%)

21.10.1 Somatic and Growth Effects

Children receiving orthovoltage irradiation manifested considerable facial effects following treatment, including a saddle-nose deformity and temporal depression. Although some degree of temporal depression is evident following megavoltage treatment and children have relatively "dolichocephalic" heads, these changes are usually not overtly striking, especially when symmetrical, and generally require no management. As major effects on bone growth in the child are generally demonstrated after 25–30 Gy of megavoltage treatment, such changes are not surprising.

21.10.2 Cataract Formation

The lens is highly susceptible to cataract formation, even with relatively low doses of radiation. Therefore it is also not surprising to note virtually uniform cataract formation after direct *en face* treatment with radiation doses in excess of 25 Gy, with cataract development usually occurring between 18 and 36 months following irradiation. When fractionated (1.5–2 Gy/Fx) treatment is delivered at conventional dose rates, nearly 100% of eyes so treated will manifest a cataract (MERRIAM and FOCHT 1957; EGBERT et al. 1978; HOWARTH et al. 1980; FOOTE et al. 1989).

Although feasible, treatment of a cataract appears to be more difficult and less efficient in the very young child and ABRAMSON has drawn attention to the regular amblyopia that results when a cataract is present in one eye while the other "sees" normally. For all these reasons, attempts to avoid this complication should be made in most cases (BROOKS et al. 1990; ABRAMSON D.H., personal communication, 1990).

Cataract formation is quite uncommon following "classical" EBRT approaches where the anterior field border lies ~2 mm posterior to the posterior lens. Of 54 eyes in which the posterior 1-3 mm of lens were irradiated to doses exceeding 30 Gy, 18 developed cataracts (SCHIPPER et al. 1985).

Similarly, cataract formation has been noted following plaque treatment, especially after two applications and/or when anterior tumor locations have been treated (AMENDOLA et al. 1989).

21.10.3 Keratitis and Keratoconjunctivitis

Keratitis and keratoconjunctivitis are extremely uncommon when a lateral field approach has been used or when only a minor (<35%) fraction of the total treatment (40–50 Gy) has come from an anterior field. However, they are reported with some frequency when a direct anterior field is used primarily, especially if no attempt is made to "open the eye" that is being treated by retracting the lids (FOOTE et al. 1989). Failure to do so will eliminate conjunctional surface sparing of dose from a megavoltage beam, and when macroscopic tumor deposits and/or vitreous seeding necessitate such an anterior approach, such lid retraction should always be done (as in orbital rhabdomyosarcoma) to minimize this complication.

21.10.4 Vascular Effects

Cumulative radiation doses exceeding 70–75 Gy commonly produce some degree of retinal vascular damage, often with hemorrhage. These effects can be visually devastating and are the second most common cause of visual loss from irradiation after cataract formation. Although very mild changes may be noticeable in time after fractionated doses totaling 40–50 Gy, they will seldom be responsible for significant visual loss (CASSADY et al. 1969; CHAN and SCHUKOVSKY 1976; ABRAMSON 1989).

Due to inverse square considerations, tumor apex doses of 40 Gy accomplished by plaque treatment potentially deliver much larger (4–5x) doses to a small volume of retinal vasculature, and thus such treatment may be followed by hemorrhage (BRADY et al. 1988; AMENDOLA et al. 1989).

21.10.5 Dental Effects

Due to the anatomic configuration of the orbit and the cephalad position of unerupted maxillary tooth buds, these incipient teeth may be treated by either a lateral or anteriorly directed orbital field and result in failure of tooth eruption. With knowledge of this possibility, appropriate shielding and/or beam angulation can generally avoid this problem (DOLINE et al. 1980).

21.10.6 Second-Tumor Formation

Figure 21.7 demonstrates the cumulative frequency of second tumors in patients with RB noted by ABRAMSON et al. (1988). It is of note that the incidence curves for irradiated and unirradiated patients are parallel although the latent period prior to development of a second tumor is roughly 5 years shorter in

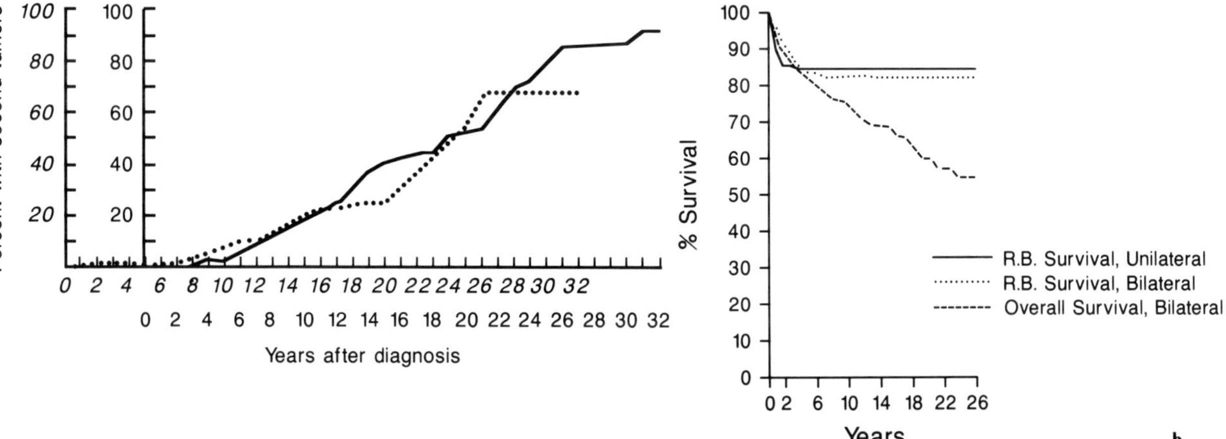

Fig. 21.7. a Abramson's actuarial incidence of second tumor curve in both unirradiated (*solid line*) and irradiated (*dotted line*) children. Although the latent period is approximately 5 years shorter in the irradiated group, the cumulative frequency steadily increases in a parallel fashion in both groups. **b** Survival curves demonstrating similar survival from RB for unilaterally and bilaterally affected patients but progressively decreasing survival for bilateral patients after 5 years due to second tumor formation

the irradiated group. Osteosarcomas predominate, followed by a variety of other sarcomas and melanoma (SAGERMAN et al. 1969; SCHIFTER et al. 1983; MEADOWS et al. 1985; DRAPER et al. 1986; ABRAMSON et al. 1988; ROARTZ et al. 1988; TRABOULSI et al. 1988).

JAKOBIEC et al. (1977) and BADER et al. (1982) have also drawn attention to the frequent development of a primitive neuroectodermal tumor arising in the region of the pineal gland ("trilateral" RB) in patients with hereditary RB. The incidence of this problem has been estimated at 1%–5% in these patients. To date, all such cases have proved fatal despite aggressive treatment in many.

Molecular studies of osteosarcomas in both RB and non-RB patients have shown deletions in the 13th chromosome, which suggests that the RB gene acts as a general tumor suppressor gene and, when absent, the type of malignancy that develops may relate more to the tissue or cell type sustaining the "second hit" than to the chromosome defect itself (DRYJA et al. 1986). In this model any agent, including irradiation capable of inducing mutations, will have the potential to also induce a second tumor. As mutations also occur spontaneously, in time the probability that a "second hit" mutation will occur at the 13 q 14 locus in some cells, leading to malignancy, is very high – a presumption supported by ABRAMSON et al.'s data (1988).

At this time, the risk of fatal second tumor development poses an overall higher mortality risk for children with hereditary RB than their retinoblastoma (ABRAMSON 1989). This highlights the need, in addition to treating the tumor, to correct the molecular genetic defect in these children in the future.

21.11 Future Prospects

Although remarkable advances have occurred in the past three to four decades, several aspects of RB treatment are currently suboptimal. The need to address the generalized molecular genetic problem and second tumor risk in hereditary patients has been noted.

Although most patients in the United States present with disease limited to the globe, this is not the situation in many areas of the world where the disease incidence is higher and death rates are substantial. In addition to educational and public health approaches, the need for more consistently effective and durable systemic therapy is clear. Development of such therapy would also likely improve control and functional likelihood in children with group V disease, who are currently suboptimally treated in the United States. The problem of drug access to vitreous seeds remains, however, and clinical trials of altered fractionation and/or use of newer, more effective hypoxic cell sensitizers are needed. It also seems likely that autologous marrow transplant will find a real place in treatment of locally recurrent or metastatic disease (GRIER et al. 1986).

Newer approaches such as photodynamic therapy using hematoporphyrin derivative and laser light appear worthy of investigation and may find a place in treatment.

A general pattern that has frequently recurred in pediatric oncology has been the substitution of systemic therapy for irradiation after its efficacy has been confirmed. It seems likely that a similar approach will be tried with RB; however, whether this substitution will ultimately prove less toxic than irradiation is questionable.

References

Abramson DH (1985) Treatment of retinoblastoma. In: Blodi FC (ed) Retinoblastoma. (Contemporary issues in Ophthalmology). Churchill Livingstone, New York, pp 63–93

Abramson DH (1989) The focal treatment of retinoblastoma with emphasis on xenon arc photocoagulation. Act Ophthalmol 67 [Suppl 194]: 1–63

Abramson DH, Ronner HJ, Ellsworth RM (1979) Second tumors in non-irradiated bilateral retinoblastoma. Am J Ophthalmol 87: 624–627

Abramson DH, Ellsworth RM, Tretter P, Javitt J, Kitchen FD (1981a) Treatment of bilateral groups I–III retinoblastoma with bilateral radition. Arch Ophthalmol 99: 1761–1762

Abramson DH, Ellsworth RM, Tretter P, Adams K, Kitchen FD (1981b) Simultaneous bilateral radiation for advanced bilateral retinoblastoma. Arch Ophthalmol 99: 1763–1766

Abramson DH, Ellsworth RM, Kitchen FD, Tung G (1984) Second non-ocular tumors in retinoblastoma survivors. Are they radiation induced? Ophthalmology 91: 1351–1355

Abramson DH, Ellsworth RM, Kitchen FD, Tung G (1988) Second nonocular tumors in retinoblastoma survivors. Are they radiation-induced? Ophthalmology 91: 1351–1355

Allderdice PW, Davis JG, Miller OJ et al. (1969) The 13q-deletion syndrome. Am J. Hum Genet 21: 449–512

Amendola BE, Markoe AM, Augsburger JJ et al. (1989) Analysis of treatment results in 36 children with retinoblastoma treated by scleral plaque irradiation. Int J Radial Oncol Biol Phys 17: 63–70

Armstrong DI (1974) The use of 4–6 MeV electrons for the conservative treatment of retinoblastoma. Br J Radiolo 47: 326–331

Bader JL, Meadows AT, Zimmerman LE, Rorke LB, Voute P, Champion LAA, Miller RW. (1982) Bilateral retinoblastoma with ectopic retinoblastoma: trilateral retinoblastoma. Cancer Genet Cytogenet 5: 203–213

Bagshaw MA, Kaplan HS (1966) Supervoltage linear accelerator radiation therapy. VII: retinoblastoma. Radiology 86: 242–246

Banks CN (1969) Inheritance of retinoblastoma. Br J Ophthalmol 53: 212–213

Bernardino V Jr, Salceda SR (1970) DNA precipitation. Arch Ophthalmol 84: 547

Brady L, Markoe AM, Amendola BE et al. (1988) The treatment of primary intraocular malignancy. Int J Radiol Oncol Biol Phys 15: 1355–1361

Brooks HL, Meyer D, Schields JA, Balas AG, Nelson LB, Fontanesi J (1990) Removal of radiation-induced cataracts in patients treated for retinoblastoma. Arch Ophthalmol 108: 1701–1708

Brown DH (1958) The clinicopatholgy of retinoblastoma. Am J Ophthalmol 45: 391–402

Carbajal UM (1958) Observations in retinoblastoma. Am J Ophthalmol 45: 391–402

Carbajal UM (1959) Metastases in retinoblastoma. Am J Ophthalmol 48: 47–69

Cassady JR, Sagerman RH, Tretter P, Ellsworth RM (1969) Radiation therapy in retinoblastoma. Radiology 93: 405–409

Cavenee WK, Dryja TP, Phillips RA et al. (1983) Expression of recessive alleles by chromosomal mechanisms in retinoblastoma. Nature 305: 779–784

Chan RC, Schukovsky LJ (1976) Effects of irradiation on the eye. Radiology 120: 673–675

Devesa SS (1975) The incidence of retinoblastoma. Am J Ophthalmol 80: 263–265

Doline S, Needleman HL, Peterson RA, Cassady JR (1980) The effect of radiotherapy in the treatment of retinoblastoma upon the developing dentition. J Pediatr Ophthalmol 17: 109–113

Draper GJ, Sanders BM, Kingston JE (1986) Second primary neoplasms in patients with retinoblastoma. Br J Cancer 53: 661–671

Dryja TP, Cavenee W, White R, et al. (1984) Homozygosity of chromosome 13 in retinoblastoma. N Engl J Med 310: 550–553

Dryja TP, Rappaport, JM, Epstein J, et al. (1986) Chromosome 13 homozygosity in osteosarcoma without retinoblastoma. Am J Hum Genet 38: 59–66

Egbert PR, Donaldson SS, Moazed K, Rosenthal AR (1978) Visual results and ocular complications following radiotherapy for retinoblastoma. Arch Ophthalmol 96: 1826–1830

Ekert H, Ellis, WM, Waters KD, et al. (1982) Autologous bone marrow rescue in the treatment of advanced tumors of childhood. Cancer 49: 603–609

Ellsworth RM (1969) Practical management of retinoblastoma. Trans Am Ophthalmol Soc 67: 462–534

Ellsworth RM (1974) Orbital retinoblastoma. Trans Am Ophthalmol Soc 72: 79–88

Ellsworth RM (1977) Retinoblastoma. Mod Probl Ophthalmol 18: 94–100

Foote RL, Genetson BR, Schombert PJ, Buskirk SJ, Robertson DM, Earle JD (1989) External beam irradiation for retinoblastoma: patterns of failure and dose-response analysis. Int J Radiol Biol Phys 16: 823–830

Freeman CR, Esseltine DL, Whitehead VM, Chevalier L, Little JM (1980) Retinoblastoma: the case for radiotherapy and for adjuvant chemotherapy. Cancer 46: 1913–1918

Gagnon JD, Ware CM, Moss WT, Stevens KR (1980) Radiation management of bilateral retinoblastoma: the need to preserve vision. Int J Radiat Oncol Biol Phys 6: 669–673

Gee AP, Graham-Pole J (1990) Use of bone marrow purging and bone marrow transplantation for neuroblastoma. In: Pochedly C (ed) Neuroblastoma: tumor biology and therapy CRC Press, pp 317–332

Green DM (1985) Diagnosis and management of malignant solid tumors in infants and children. In: Green DM (ed) Retinoblastoma. Martinus Nijhoff, Boston, pp 90–128

Griem ML, Ernest JT, Rozenfeld ML, Newell FW (1968) Eye lens protection in the treatment of retinoblastoma with high energy elections. Radiology 90: 351–352

Grier HE, Weinstein HJ, Revesz T, et al. (1986) Cytogenetic evidence for the involvement of erythroid progenitors in a child with therapy-linked myelodysplasia. Br J Hematol 64: 513–519

Harnett AN, Hungerford JL, Lambert GD, et al. (1987) Improved external beam radiotherapy for the treatment of retionoblastoma. Br J Radiol 60: 753–760

Haye C, Desjardins L, Schlienger P, Zucker JM, Laurent M (1987) Treatment of bilateral retinoblastoma stage V at the Curie Foundation – 33 cases. Ophthalmic Pediatr Genet 8: 73–76

Howarth C, Meyer D, Husta HO, Johnson WW, Shanks E, Pratt C (1980) Stage related combined modality treatment of retinoblastoma. Cancer 45: 851–858

Hungerford J, Kingston J, Plowman N (1987) Orbital recurrence of retinoblastoma. Ophthalmic Pediatr Genet 8: 63–68

Jakobiec FA, Ts'o MOM, Zimmerman LE, Davis P (1977) Retinoblastoma and intracranial malignancy. Cancer 39: 2048–2058

Jensen RD, Miller RW (1987) Retinoblastoma: epidemiologic characteristics. N Engl J Med 283: 307–311

Kingston JR, Hungerford JL, Plowman PN (1987) Chemotherapy in metastatic retinoblastoma. Ophthalmic Pediatr Genet 8: 69–72

Knudson AG, Jr (1971) Mutation and cancer: statistical study of retinoblastoma. Proc Nat Acad Sci USA 68: 820–823

Knudson AG, Jr (1989) Hereditary cancers disclose a class of cancer genes. Cancer 63: 1888–1891

Lennox EL, Draper GJ Sanders BM (1975) Retinoblastoma: a study of natural history and prognosis. Br Med J 3: 731–734

Lincoff H (1968) A report of freezing of intraoculars. Mod Probl Ophthalmol 7: 348–358

McCormick B, Ellsworth R, Abramson D et al. (1988) Radiation therapy for retinoblastoma: comparison of results with lens-sparing versus lateral beam techniques. Int J Radial Oncol Biol Phys 15: 567–574

Meadows AT, Baum E, Fossati-Bellani F et al. (1985) Second malignant neoplasms in children: an update from the late-efforts study group. J Clin Oncol 3: 532–537

Merriam GM (1950) Retinoblastoma: an analysis of 17 autopsies. Arch Ophthalmol 44: 71–108

Merriam GR, Focht EF (1957) A Clinical study of radiation cataracts and the relationship to dose. AJR 77: 759–785

Meyer-Schwickerath G (1954) Licht Koagulation. Graefes Arch Ophthalmol 156: 44–50

Meyer-Schwickerath G (1979) Indications and limitations of light coagulation of the retina. Trans Am Acad Ophthalmol Otolaryngol 63: 725–738

Migdal C (1983) Bilateral retinoblastoma: the prognosis for vision. Br J Ophthalmol 67: 592–595

Monge OR, Flage T, Hatlevoll R, Vermond H (1986) Sight saving therapy in retinoblastoma. Experience with external megavoltage radiotherapy. Acta Ophthalmol 64: 414–420

Moore RF, Stallard HB, Milner JG (1931) Retinal gliomata treated by radon seeds. Br J Ophthalmol 105: 673–696

Munzenrider JE (1989) Particle treatment of the eye. Refresher course syllabus #107, p 7

Nadel A, Lincoff H (1968) Cryosurgical treatment of eye tumors. Geriatrics 23: 89–97

Neel HB, De Santo LW (1973) Cryosurgical control of cancer: effects of freeze rates, tumor temperatures and ischemia. Am Otol Rhinol Larynogil 82: 716–723

Parkhill EM, Benedict WL (1941) Gliomas of the retina: histopathologic study. Am J Ophthalmol 24: 1354–1373

Pratt, CG (1972) Management of malignant solid tumors in children. Pediatr Clin North Am 19: 1141–1155

Redler LD, Ellsworth RM (1973) Prognostic importance of choroidal invasion in retinoblastoma. Arch Ophthalmol 90: 294–296

Reese AB (1976) Tumors of the eye, 3rd edn. Harper & Row, Hagerstown, pp 90–124

Reese AB, Ellsworth RM (1963) The evaluation and current concept of retinoblastoma therapy. Trans Am Acad Ophthalmol Otolaryngol 67: 164–172

Roartz JD, McLean IW, Zimmerman LE (1988) Incidence of second neoplasms in patients with bilateral retinoblastoma. Ophthalmology 95: 1583–1587

Sagerman RH, Cassady JR, Tretter P et al. (1989) Radiation–induced neoplasia following external-beam therapy for children with retinoblastoma. AJR 105: 529–535

Salmonsen PC, Ellsworth RM, Kitchen FD (1979) The occurrence of new retinoblastomas after treatment. Ophthalmology 86: 837–840

Sang DN, Albert DM (1982) Retinoblastoma: clinical and histopathologic features. Hum Pathol 13: 133–147

Schappert-Kimmijser J, Hemmes GD, Nijland R (1966) The heredity of retinoblastoma. Ohthalmologica 151: 197–213

Schifter S, Vendelgo L, Jensen OM, Kaae S (1983) Ewing's tumor following bilateral retinoblastoma. Cancer 52: 1746–1749

Schipper J (1983) An Accurate and simple method for megavoltage radiation therapy of retinoblastoma. Radiother Oncol 1: 31–41

Schipper J, Tan KEWP, Van peperzeel HA (1985) Treatment of retinoblastoma by precision megavoltage radiation therapy. Radiother Oncol 3: 117–132

Shields JA, Augsburger SJ (1981) Current approaches to the diagnosis and management of retinoblastoma. Surv J Ophthalmol 25: 347–372

Stallard HB (1955) Multiple islands of retinoblastoma. Br Ophthalmol 39: 241–243

Stallard HB (1962) The conservative treatment of retinoblastoma. The Doyne memorial lecture 1962. Trans Ophthalmol Soc UK 82: 473–535

Stannard C, Lipper S, Sealy R, Sevel, D (1979) Retinoblastoma: correlation of invasion of the optic nerve and choroid with prognosis and metastasis. Br J Ophthalmol 63: 560–570

Taktikos, A (1966) Investigation of retinoblastoma with special reference to histology and prognosis. Br J Ophthalmol 50: 225–234

Thompson RW, Small RC, Stein JJ (1972) Treatment of retinoblastoma. AJR 114: 16–23

Traboulsi EI, Zimmerman L, Manz HJ (1988) Cutaneous malignant melanoma in survivors of hereditable retinoblastoma. Arch Ophthalmol 106: 1059–1061

Ts'o MOM, Fine BS, Zimmerman LE (1969) The Flexner-Wintersteiner rosettes in retinoblastoma. Arch Pathol 88: 664–671

Ts'o MOM, Zimmerman LE, Fine BS (1970) The nature of retinoblastoma. I. Photoreceptor differentiation: a clinical and histopathologic study. Am J Ophthalmol 69: 339–349

Vogel F (1979) Genetics of retinoblastoma. Hum Genet 51: 1–54

Weichselbaum RR, Little JB (1980) Familial retinoblastoma and ataxia-telangiectasis. Human models for the study of DNA damage and repair. Cancer 45: 775–779

Weichselbaum RR, Nove J, Little JB (1978) X-ray sensitivity of diploid fibroblasts from patients with hereditary or sporadic retinoblastoma. Proc Natl Acad Sci USA 75: 3962–3964

Weiss DR, Cassady JR, Petersen R (1975) Retinoblastoma: a modification in radiation therapy technique. Radiology 114: 705–708

White L (1983) The role of chemotherapy in the treatment of retinoblastoma. Retina 3: 194–199

Young JL, Heise HW, Silverberg E, Myers MH (1978) Cancer incidence, survival and mortality for children under 15 years of age. American cancer Society Bulletin, New York

Zimmerman LE (1961) The registry of Ophthalmic pathology: past, present and future. Trans Am Acad Ophthalmol Otolaryngol 65: 51–113

22 Langerhans Cell Histiocytosis

KENNETH L. MCCLAIN, JOHN J. HUTTER, and J. ROBERT CASSADY

CONTENTS

22.1   Introduction 337
22.2   Etiology and Incidence 337
22.3   Pathology and Biology 338
22.4   Immunology of Langerhans Cells and
       Defects in LCH 339
22.5   Clinical Manifestations 340
22.6   Patient Evaluation 340
22.7   Solitary Bone Lesions 340
22.8   Multiple Lesions 341
22.9   Natural History and Prognosis 342
22.10   Therapy 343
22.10.1 Radiation Therapy 344
22.10.2 Bone Marrow Transplantation 346
       References 346

22.1 Introduction

A panel of experts representing the Histiocyte Society has suggested that the original terminology for the various syndromes in the "histiocytosis X" category (eosinophilic granuloma, Letterer-Siwe disease, and Hand-Christian-Schüller syndrome) be discarded and replaced by the term Langerhans cell histiocytosis (LCH) (CHU et al. 1987). This is because the proliferative cell which causes these entities is known to be the Langerhans cell.

This chapter will deal only with the Langerhans cell histiocyte diseases. The benign but aggressive non-Langerhans cell histiocytoses should not be treated with radiation therapy. Malignant histiocytosis is rarer than the LCH syndromes in children and will not be covered here.

KENNETH L. MCCLAIN, M.D., Ph.D. Associate Professor, Department of Pediatrics, Baylor College of Medicine, Texas Childern's Hospital, 6621 Fannin Street MC 3-3320, Houston, TX 77030-2299, USA
JOHN HUTTER, M. D., Associate Professor, Department of Pediatrics, Arizona Health Sciences Center, University of Arizona, 1501 N. Campbell Ave., Tucson, AZ 85724, USA
J. ROBERT CASSADY, M. D., Professor and Head, Department of Radiation Oncology, The University of Arizona, Health Sciences Center, 1501 North Campbell Ave., Tucson, AZ 85724, USA

22.2 Etiology and Incidence of LCH

There is no known etiology of LCH. One group of investigators has suggested the possibility of a transmissible (viral?) agent (ATHANASIU et al. 1970; NASTAC et al. 1970). Phenol extracts of tissue from bone lesions of LCH patients were injected into mice. Cell suspensions were made from the lungs of the mice and assayed for cytopathic effect on primary human embryo cultures. The presence of syncytia and nuclear changes were taken as evidence of a transmissible agent. On the basis of immuno-fluorescence studies it was claimed that the cytopathic effect did not result from mouse antigens or mouse viruses. The sera of eosinophilic granuloma or leukemia patients reacted with the extracts of the original eosinophilic granulomas. Since then no specific studies have been published to further elucidate these findings.

A genetic propensity for LCH has not been definitively shown. However, there are several reports in the literature of familial occurrences (SCHOECK et al. 1963; MILLER 1966; KATZ et al. 1991). The earlier reports relied on the histologic tools and criteria of the era, so there could be some doubt as to the diagnoses. However, many of these earlier cases seem to be "classical cases," as do monozygotic twins with biopsy identification of Birbeck granules (KATZ et al. 1991). If one is to believe the clinical diagnoses, there are at least ten sibships with what was called Letterer-Siwe disease. The caveats stated by KATZ and co-workers in relation to confusion with the non-Langerhans cell histiocytoses are appropriate. However, known HLA type propensities in LCH patients and the identified immunologic abnormalities make familial cases very likely.

The frequency of congenital anomalies constitutes further evidence for genetic/embryologic abnormalities in LCH patients (SHEILS and DOVER 1989). It was reported that 23% of LCH patients had major anomalies, including malformations of the central nervous system and renal, vertebral, genitourinary, and several other categories of malformations, compared to 13% of patients with bone tumors or 15% of a control group.

Although LCH may appear at all ages from birth through adulthood, over half will be diagnosed between the ages of 1 and 15 years (BERRY et al. 1986). In a recent study from Denmark the incidence rate of LCH was reported as 5.4/million (CARSTENSON and ORNVOLD 1991). By comparison, AUSTIN et al. (1988) reported incidences per million children of 47.8 for all acute leukemias, 5.6 for acute nonlymphocytic leukemia, 6.5 for Hodgkin's disease and 7.9 for Wilms' tumor (AUSTIN et al. 1988). It has been estimated that approximately 1200 new cases of LCH are seen annually in the United States (LAVIN and OSBAND 1987).

22.3 Pathology and Biology

The abnormal cell in LCH is a bone marrow-derived member of the dendritic histiocytes, also called the Langerhans cell, which contains characteristic five-layered Birbeck granules seen by electron microscopy (EM) (FAVARA 1981) (Fig. 22.1). In skin lesions many cells have these granules, but in other organs the infiltration is often by histiocytes of bone marrow origin which do not contain Birbeck granules. Langerhans cells also stain with monoclonal antibodies to the CD1a (T6) epitope of lymphocytes (MURPHY et al. 1981). The major problem with this marker is the need for fresh- or snap-frozen tissue. Two other markers for the Langerhans cells are peanut agglutinin (PNA) and S-100, which can be used with paraffin-embedded material (MC-CLELLAND and CHU 1988). PNA produces dense cell surface and paranuclear staining of the LCH cells.

Although PNA staining also occurs in Reed-Sternberg cells of Hodgkin's lymphoma and interdigitating reticulum cells of normal lymph nodes, it is very useful in differentiating non-Langerhans cell histiocytes, which are negative. The S-100 stain is almost as useful as PNA and suffers only from marking normal Langerhans cells and some cases of malignant histiocytosis. Most importantly, the histiocytes found in the non-Langerhans cells histiocytoses (virus-associated hemophagocytic syndrome or familial erythrophagocytic lymphohistiocytosis and juvenile xanthogranuloma) are negative.

It is important to use EM and S-100 or PNA staining on suspected LCH specimens because of the variability of results. In a study by YE et al. (1990) on 27 cases of LCH, the S-100 was reactive in 88.5% and PNA in 75%, while EM was positive for Birbeck granules in 47% of cases. Of the negative cases on EM, four were from bone lesions, five from lymph nodes, and one from an ear canal scraping. New reagents are being tried to further aid diagnostic assessments. LUKSCH et al. (1989) used a novel antibody KP1 (CD28) which reacts with LCH cells but not with normal Langerhans cells. It was positive in 18 of 22 cases. Other antibodies used included: anti-CD45 (lymphocyte cell adhesion) (3/22 positive), PNA (21/21 positive), S-100 (21/21 positive), HLA-DR (16/22 positive) and CD30 (Ki 1) (0/22 positive). Most experts agree that to establish the diagnosis of LCH, identification by EM of Birbeck granules or staining of Langerhans cells with one of the two special stains or the CD1a marker is necessary.

Histologically the proliferation of LCH cells in solitary bone lesions (formerly eosinophilic granuloma) reveals Langerhans cells with eosinophils, neu-

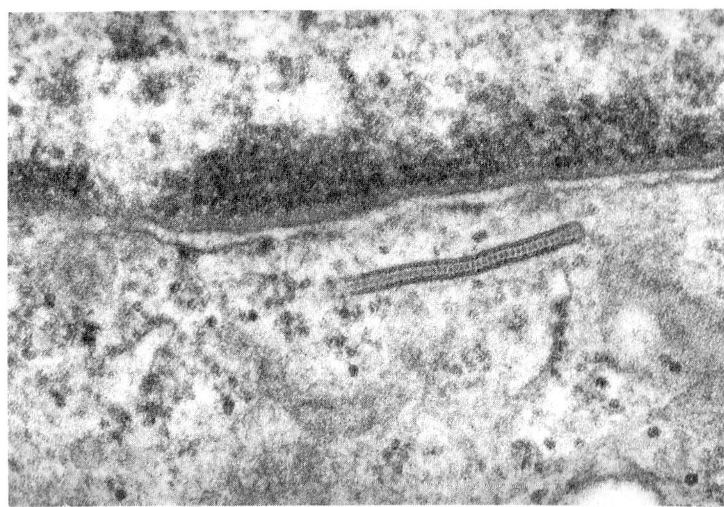

Fig. 22.1. Electron micrograph of a Langerhans cell from a lymph node showing the diagnostic pentalaminar Birbeck granule. (Courtesy of Hal Hawkins, MD, PhD, Texas Children's Hospital)

trophils, lymphocytes, plasma cells, and fibroblasts (FAVARA 1981). Sometimes syncytia of Langerhans cells are formed. In the skin the Langerhans cells accumulate at the epidermal-dermal junction. There may be local destruction and an infiltration of lymphocytes, eosinophils, and neutrophils. The Langerhans cells do not form multinucleated giant cells or cohesive sheets as readily in the skin lesion. When lymph nodes or the spleen are involved, sinusoidal infiltration by Langerhans cells usually does not efface normal architecture. The thymus is often abnormal in LCH patients. Dysplastic changes and loss of Hassall's corpuscles with infiltration of histiocytes and fibroblasts are commonly seen. Liver and lung infiltrations involve the sinusoids of the liver and interstitial areas of the lung. Fibrosis in both organs is a late sequela.

Although it is generally agreed that LCH is not a malignant disease by morphologic criteria, there have been some conflicting data in the literature from flow cytometric studies. RABKIN et al. (1988) studied 36 LCH patients and found only normal DNA content. MCLELLAND et al. (1989) looked for aneuploidy in nine biopsies from six patents with LCH. They found a normal DNA content in all specimens. However, ORNVOLD et al. (1990) found that 2 of 26 biopsy specimens from 18 children had DNA indices of 1.5 (aneuploid). Both of the patients had disseminated disease without organ dysfunction and responded well to prednisone treatment. They had no evidence of disease with follow-up times of 1 and 10 years. It is generally concluded that LCH is not a malignant process, and the aneuploidy would seem to represent an unstable clone in the aforementioned two patients.

Histologic proof of LCH proliferation is essential since osteomyelitis and cranial fasciitis may simulate the "classical" lesions (ADLER and WONG 1986) or multifocal osteomyelitis (BJORKSTEN et al. 1978). Disseminated tuberculosis has also been reported in an infant who was at first suspected of having LCH (SCHUSTER et al. 1985).

22.4 Immunology of Langerhans Cells and Defects in LCH

The Langerhans cells is a distinct member of the antigen-processing cells, which include monocytes or histiocytes. Like other antigen-processing cells, Langerhans cells produce a stimulating factor for T lymphocytes called Interleukin-1 (IL-1) which is necessary for the activation and response of T cells (LEIKIN 1987). The activated T cells in turn produce interleukin-2, which stimulates other T-cells. Feedback stimulation on Langerhans cells (or other histiocytes) results from production of interferon-γ and prostaglandin E_2 (PGE_2) by the T cells.

Another element in the cycle of responses is tumor necrosis factor (TNF), which is stimulated by IL-1. TNF increases the expression of HLA-A and -B antigens and Langerhans cells and thus may explain their excessive proliferation. Somewhere in the interactive cycle a regulatory element is lost such that the histiocytes proliferate locally or diffusely. Elaboration of PGE-2 and IL-1 by LCH cells in culture has been reported (ARENZANA-SEISDEDOS et al. 1986). When the mononuclear cells of LCH patients are stimulated with lipopolysaccharide (LPS), they release more IL-1 than do normal mononuclear cells (BURGIO et al. 1990). It is likely that these factors, as well as TNF, play a role in resorption of bone.

Other leukocytes may also play a role in tissue destruction. Eosinophils from a patient with disseminated LCH were shown to have excessive degranulation (ZABUCCHI et al. 1991). Extracellular release of eosinophil peroxidase to surrounding cells was found in a bony lesion and the peripheral blood.

There is abundant evidence of immunologic abnormalities in patients with LCH. Thymic dysplasia, involution, and dysmorphic changes have been well documented (NEWTON et al. 1987). Elevation of at least one type of immunoglobulin is found in 75% of patients, with most having high IgM (LAHEY et al. 1985; NESBIT et al. 1981). Although lymphocyte mitogenic responses are normal in most patients, the number of suppressor T cells is often low. A larger series has confirmed that the percent and absolute numbers of suppressor cells are decreased (SHANNON and NEWTON 1986). Circulating lymphocytes may be spontaneously cytotoxic to cultured human fibroblasts as well as have a decrease in the number of suppressor T cells (OSBAND et al. 1981). Such defects can be corrected in vitro by thymic extract. This information has provided the impetus for therapeutic trials with thymic extracts (CECI et al. 1981; OSBAND et al. 1981). It is because of the suppressor T-cell abnormality that polyclonal B-cell activation, with hypergammaglobulinemia, occurs in these patients when they are infected. Low levels of serum thymic factor and the presence of an inhibitor to it have been documented in patients with LCH (CONSOLINI et al. 1987). Chemotactic defects and a preponderance of HLA types have also been found (TOOMOKA et al. 1986). The chemotactic response was 25% of controls despite equivalent immunoglobulin and complement concentrations. No inhibitors of chemotaxis were identified. In LCH cases 54% had Bw61 and 45% Cw7 HLA phenotypes, compared to 20% and 18% respectively in a control group.

Although intriguing, the immunologic abnormalities in patients with LCH are not consistent and sometimes spontaneously improve. Additional immunologic defects probably exist which are yet to be fully explained (see a more inclusive summary in LEIKIN 1987).

These theoretical constructs may apply in vivo, but in vitro data are conflicting. When Langerhans cells were put into culture with granulocyte-macrophage stimulating factor (GM-CSF), IL-I, or TNF, there was no stimulation of Langerhans cells (KOLENIK et al. 1990). In fact, the CD1-positive cells decreased from 30% to 10% after 3 days.

Recently YU et al. (1990) reported that LCH cells had less functional activity on a per cell basis than did normal epidermal Langerhans cells. It was concluded that LCH cells are functionally defective rather than suffering from a suppressive effect of cytokines.

Whenever a high incidence of neoplasms occurs in the context of a particular disease, one may suspect that disease has an associated immunodeficiency. Such is the case for LCH. Although an actual incidence of malignancies is not established, several series and case reports suggest the association may be real. GREENBERGER et al. (1981) reported that 5 of 127 patients developed malignant diseases after LCH. Malignancies included anaplastic thyroid carcinoma, acute myelogenous leukemia, hepatocellular carcinoma, undifferentiated leukemia, and papillary-follicular thyroid carcinoma. It is likely that these were secondary effects of radiotherapy and cytotoxic chemotherapy including alkylating agents and is one reason why the routine use of x-ray therapy and certain drugs may not be advisable. Sometimes the occurrence of a malignancy with LCH is after chemotherapy for a primary malignancy. SHANLEY et al. (1990) reported a patient treated with only chemotherapy for Hodgkin's disease who subsequently developed pulmonary LCH. It is important to note the patient had "smoker's macrophages" in the lung biopsy specimen. Many people who develop pulmonary LCH are smokers. Other associations of malignancy and LCH are equally complex, with more than one underlying reason for immune deficiency (MAHONEY et al. 1989). EGELER et al. (1990) reported a case of T-cell leukemia with LCH and reviewed the literature through 1991. They found 53 case reports of LCH and malignancy. Thirty-six of these cases involved malignant lym-

phoma and LCH, with 70% of the diagnoses being made concomitantly. Thirteen cases were associated with acute leukemia; eight of these were monocytic leukemia. LCH preceded the leukemia in six cases and was simultaneous with it in five.

22.5 Clinical Manifestations

Clinical syndromes of LCH should now be identified according to the degree or number of organ systems involved, e.g., Langerhans cell histiocytosis – solitary skull lesion instead of "eosinophilic granuloma." The original descriptions of what we now call LCH concentrated on the varying clinical presentations of soft tissue, bone alone, or multiorgan involvement. In general, more diffuse disease and a younger age at diagnosis suggest a worse prognosis (GREENBERGER et al. 1981).

22.6 Patient Evaluation

A complete evaluation should include a thorough history and physical examination; complete blood count, including platelet determination; measurement of serum bilirubin, alanine aminotransferase, and albumin; bone marrow aspiration and biopsy (when abnormalities of the peripheral blood count are present); x-ray survey of the complete skeleton and chest; bone scan; spinal tap (if clinically indicated); careful monitoring of intake and output, serum and urine osmolality; and biopsy of an affected site for confirmatory histologic diagnosis (BROADBENT et al. 1989a). Although a specific immune system evaluation is not routinely done in all patients, it may be of interest to determine immunoglobulin levels, helper and suppressor T-cell subsets, and natural killer cell function or numbers, and to perform mitogen studies in order to evaluate lymphocyte proliferative responses.

22.7 Solitary Bone Lesions

The most benign form of LCH is that which involves solitary bone lesions, frequently occurring as one or more well-circumscribed lesions in the skull (Fig. 22.2). The patient presents because of pain or swelling over the affected region. Often the defects are easy to palpate. Any bone in the body can be involved, but the most common sites are skull (40%), femur (13%), ribs (13%), pelvis (12%), vertebrae

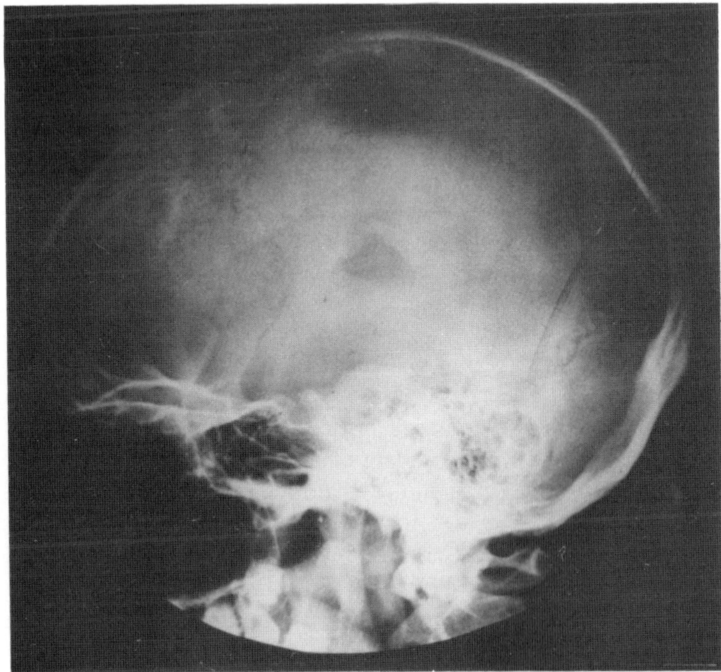

Fig. 22.2. Lytic skull lesions in a child with multifocal Langerhans cell histiocytosis. (Courtesy of Milton Wagner, MD, Texas Children's Hospital)

(9%), and mandible (8%) (SLATER and SWARM 1980). Orbital lesions can cause marked proptosis. Other symptoms and signs include headache, fever, loose teeth, and stiff neck. These children are usually seen between 1 and 9 years of age with peaks of incidence in the second to third and seventh to eighth years of life (SLATER and SWARM 1980).

The radiographic appearance of the lytic bone lesions is almost diagnostic in children. However, a biopsy or curettage is necessary for histologic confirmation. Radionuclide imaging with technetium or gallium can be helpful, but is not markedly better than plain radiography (SCHAUB et al. 1987). False-negative bone scans were observed in 19 of 27 children who had skull lesions and 10 of 15 who had disease in other sites detected by plain radiographs. Gallium scans were positive in each of two cases. Mild elevations of the erythrocyte sedimentation rate and leukocytosis may be the only other abnormalities.

When LCH affects vertebra they may collapse ("vertebral plana"). The thoracic vertebrae are involved most often, followed in frequency by lumbar and cervical vertebrae (KIEFFER et al. 1969). Neurologic manifestations secondary to spinal cord or nerve root compression from vertebral lesions have been described in 2% – 10% of lesions involving the cervical or upper thoracic vertebrae (BOLLINI et al. 1991). Spinal cord compression usually results from soft tissue extension of LCH rather than disease confined to bone. It has been suggested that vertebral forms of LCH, such as vertebra plana, which are confined to bone and produce no vertebral instability require no treatment (JOUVE et al. 1991).

22.8 Multiple Lesions

Patients with multiple lesions fall into two clinical groups: those who have disease limited to bone and/or soft tissue whose disease is not aggressive, and those with diffuse disease that progresses despite multiple therapeutic trials. There are no prognostic clues from the initial presentation which will help the clinician predict the outcome of a particular patient (BERRY and BECTON 1987). Many of these children are first seen with a seborrheic rash of the scalp and periauricular regions which mimics "cradle cap" or eczema. Draining ears may at first appear to be routine chronic otitis externa. A characteristic erythematous, maculopapular rash is commonly found on the abdomen, groin, or trunk. Gingival hypertrophy and gingivitis also may be seen. Hepatosplenomegaly (LEBLANC et al. 1981), anemia, thrombocytopenia (MCCLAIN et al. 1983), and pulmonary disease (BASSET et al. 1978; STANFORD et al. 1971) make the diagnosis more obvious clinically, but the diagnostic Langerhans cells must be confirmed histologically by methods previously mentioned. Infiltration of the thyroid and pancreas associated with dysfunction has been reported. Of the children presenting with generalized LCH, most will be less than 5 years of age and have involvement of the bone (100%), skin (88%), liver (71%), lung (54%), lymph nodes (42%), spleen (25%), pituitary (25%), bone marrow (18%), and central nervous system (16%) (BERRY and BECTON 1987).

Central nervous system involvement with LCH may result from the primary disease process or may be secondary to treatment, usually in the pituitary-hypothalamic axis. Such patients may have diabetes insipidus and growth and sexual developmental abnormalities (BRAUNSTEIN and KOHLER 1981). Endocrinopathies caused by the LCH disease process most often involve the hypothalamus or posterior pituitary and are believed to result from Langerhans cell infiltration. However, pathologic changes in the pituitary or hypothalamus are not necessarily evident in patients with diabetes insipidus who die of their disease (GRAMATOVICI and D'ANGIO 1988). The most common endocrinopathy is diabetes insipidus, which occurs in approximately 30%–40% of children with multisystem disease (DEAN et al. 1986; DUNGER et al. 1989; MCLELLAND et al. 1990). Patients with proptosis may also be at higher risk for diabetes insipidus. Diabetes insipidus may not be evident at initial presentation and may develop during the first 4 years after diagnosis (DUNGER et al. 1989). Magnetic resonance imaging (MRI) with gadolinium enhancement provides excellent images by revealing a thickened pituitary stalk, a thickened infundibulum, or a thickened median eminence of the hypothalamus without the bright posterior pituitary signal seen in normals (ARICO et al. 1991). Evaluation of the CNS by MRI has demonstrated high signal foci in the hypothalamus on T2-weighted images which subsequently disappear after therapy (MOORE et al. 1989). Others have reported that computed tomography (CT) images are more useful for detecting mass lesions. In contrast to diabetes insipidus, clinically significant growth hormone deficiency is uncommon in children with LCH. Although patients with LCH and diabetes insipidus may have abnormal growth hormone responses to exercise, arginine, hypoglycemia, or L-dopa/propranolol, the incidence of children exhibiting growth retardation to the extent that growth hormone therapy is required appears to be quite low (DEAN et al. 1986). DEAN et al. have suggested that growth hormone deficiency is not a common complication of LCH unless direct hypothalamic/pituitary irradiation has been administered. Responses to growth hormone therapy have been observed

in children with LCH who have developed short stature secondary to growth hormone deficiency (BRAUNSTEIN et al. 1975).

Six patients with cerebellar signs and learning disabilities have been reported (BROADBENT and NESBIT 1990). A biopsy of two showed histiocytic infiltration of non-Langerhans cells. Imaging studies of the others showed atrophy, demyelination, or ventricular enlargement.

22.9 Natural History and Prognosis

Langerhans cell histiocytosis is considered a reactive process and the concept that some forms of LCH are a malignancy is now generally believed to be incorrect (BROADBENT et al. 1989a). Treatment strategies should be based on an understanding of the natural history of LCH and designed to reduce the immediate and long-term complications of the disease.

The observation that the prognosis for children with histiocytosis X is related to the extent of organ involvement and dysfunction (LAHEY 1975) has been confirmed in several large retrospective reviews of LCH (GREENBERGER et al. 1981; BERRY et al. 1986; GADNER et al. 1987; RANEY and D'ANGIO 1989; MCLELLAND et al. 1990). The Lavin-Osband modification of the Lahey staging system is outlined in Table 22.1. It is important to note that the prognostic criteria for visceral organ involvement in LCH are based on clinical evidence of abnormal liver, pulmonary, and/or hematopoietic organ *function* and not merely on the histologic or imaging detection of LCH in a visceral organ.

A younger age at onset of the illness is often considered an unfavorable prognostic variable in children with histiocytosis X. In general, LCH with multiple severe organ dysfunction as well as the non-LCH forms of fulminant aggressive histiocytosis occur in children less than 3 years of age. However, there are localized benign forms of LCH that occur during infancy which have an excellent prognosis. A specific example is a localized cutaneous form of LCH which appears at the time of birth or during the first several months of life and which heals spontaneously with no therapeutic intervention (ROPER and SPRAKER 1985; HANSEN 1991).

Children with LCH confined to bone usually do well and often require minimal or no therapeutic intervention. Radiologic evidence of healing of LCH bone lesions includes change from a nontrabecular to a trabecular pattern, the development of sclerosis,

Table 22.1. Lavin-Osband modification of the Lahey staging system

Variable	No. of points
Age at presentation	
< 2 years	1
> 2 years	0
Number of organs involved	
< 4	0
> 4	1
Presence of organ dysfunction[a]	
Yes	1
No	0
Stage	Total points
I	0
II	1
III	2
IV	3

[a] Definition of organ dysfunction:
Liver. Liver dysfunction is defined as being present if there is hypoproteinemia (< 5.5 g/dl total protein and/or less than 2.5 g/dl albumin), edema, ascites, or hyperbilirubinemia (total serum bilirubin greater than 1.5 mg/dl).
Lung. Lung dysfunction is defined as being present if there is tachypnea, dyspnea, cyanosis, cough, pneumothorax, or pleural effusion. (The presence of radiographic abnormalities without symptoms is *not* considered evidence of pulmonary dysfunction.)
Hematopoietic. Hematopoietic dysfunction is defined as existing if there is anemia (hemoglobin less than 10 g/dl), leukopenia (white blood cell count less than 4000/mm^3), neutropenia (neutrophil count less than 1500/mm^3), or thrombocytopenia (platelet count less than 100000/mm^3), (The presence of increased abnormal histiocytes in the bone marrow without accompanying hematologic changes is *not* considered evidence of hematopoietic dysfunctions.)

and the loss of distinct margins. Early radiographic changes of healing may be evident in 3 months but complete resolution of bony abnormalities may take 12–15 months (ALEXANDER et al. 1988; BOLLINI et al. 1991). Radiographic resolution of LCH bony lesions may be incomplete. In a review of 38 bone lesions in 18 patients, complete resolution was noted in 22 of 38 (58%) lesions (ALEXANDER et al. 1988). The rate of healing and time course of healing of LCH bone lesions appear to be similar for the various therapeutic options (observation, surgery, chemotherapy, radiation therapy) that have been used in the management of bony LCH (SARTORIS and PARKER 1984; WOMER et al. 1985; BOLLINI et al. 1991). Children less than 3 years of age at the onset of LCH bony lesions are more likely to have multifocal bony disease and also to develop disease recurrence at a site distant from the initial lesions. Recurrences are rare (less than 10%) in children with solitary bone lesions at onset. However, the development of recurrence per se in the absence of evidence of organ dysfunction does not influence ultimate survival adversely in chil-

dren with LCH (RANEY and D'ANGIO 1989). Recurrences are most likely to be observed within the first several years. In most children the disease appears to eventually "burn out" and no new lesions evolve on long-term follow-up. However, the description of disease reactivation greater than 10 years after onset (GRIMM et al. 1981) underscores the extremely variable disease history for LCH.

In contrast to the excellent long-term survival observed for children with LCH without visceral organ involvement, the prognosis for patients less than 2 years of age with organ dysfunction remains poor. Despite current therapeutic interventions, many of these latter patients have progressive organ dysfunction and die within 2 years of diagnosis (BERRY et al. 1986; RANEY and D'ANGIO 1989; McLelland et al. 1990).

22.10 Therapy

Current therapeutic approaches to LCH should be directed at control of major clinical signs and symptoms. As children with LCH who do not have major organ dysfunction have an excellent prognosis for survival, therapeutic options should be considered which control clinically significant disease but also minimize potential late sequelae of therapy. Recent reviews have emphasized both the need for an individualized approach to children with LCH (RANEY and D'ANGIO 1989) and the value of a conservative approach to treatment (McLelland et al. 1990).

Children with LCH confined to skin or bone usually require no treatment unless symptomatic or at risk for fracture or deformity. Solitary painful bone lesions are usually treated surgically by curettage or excision. Lesions in crucial weight-bearing bones may require autologous bone grafting (RANEY and D'ANGIO 1989). Intralesional corticosteroids have also been used by some in the management of bone lesions (COHEN et al. 1980; McLELLAND et al. 1990). Major symptoms may result from the soft tissue mass component of an LCH bone lesion rather than the bony component itself. Examples include the massive proptosis associated with orbital disease and extradural spinal cord compression secondary to soft tissue extension from a vertebral lesion (HAGGSTORM 1988; JOUVE et al. 1991; BOLLINI et al. 1991). Surgical decompression has been utilized in patients with vertebral lesions who have signs and symptoms of cord compression (SWEASEY and DAUSER 1989). Treatment of orbital soft tissue lesions has included intralesional injection of methylprednisolone (WIRTSCHAFTER et al. 1987).

Chemotherapy should be considered as an option in children with cutaneous, skin, or bony LCH who also have systemic fever, weight loss, or failure to thrive (RANEY and D'ANGIO 1989). Chemotherapy is also indicated in children with visceral organ involvement. However, some children with LCH with organ dysfunction receiving chemotherapy continue to progress rapidly. The overall mortality for children with LCH with organ dysfunction is 30%–70% (GADNER et al. 1987; RANEY and D'ANGIO 1989; McLELLAND et al. 1990). Multiagent chemotherapy utilized in LCH has included corticosteroids, vinca alkaloids, alkylating agents, and antimetabolites. McLELLAND et al. (1990) have suggested that the results of using short courses of single-agent prednisolone compare favorably with other reports where more aggressive therapy was employed.

The semisynthetic epipodophyllotoxin etoposide has recently been described to induce remissions in children with symptomatic LCH (BROADBENT et al. 1989b; VIANA et al. 1991). However, recurrences have been observed after etoposide therapy and this agent should be used judiciously due to concerns regarding its leukemogenic potential.

Therapeutic approaches directed at immune modulation in children with LCH have included calf thymic extract (OSBAND et al. 1981; CECI et al. 1988) and interferon-α (SATO et al. 1990). Resolution of organ dysfunction has recently been described in children with multisystem LCH who were treated with cyclosporine (MAHMOUD et al. 1991b). Further understanding of immunologic abnormalities associated with forms of LCH may help to better define those patients who may benefit from immunologic intervention.

Certain patients with LCH hepatic involvement may develop end-stage liver failure secondary to sclerosing cholangitis. Liver transplantation has been employed successfully in children with LCH and slowly evolving progressive liver failure (CONCEPCION et al. 1991; MAHMOUD et al. 1991a). Allogeneic bone marrow transplantation has been employed in multisystem disease LCH (STOLL et al. 1990). (see Sect. 22.10.2)

22.10.1 Radiation Therapy

Although radiation therapy was in the past the principal nonsurgical treatment option for LCH, its role has markedly decreased due both to a change in treatment philosophy and to the development of systemic agents with significant activity and, in some cases, less long-term toxicity.

Rather than approach LCH as a malignant entity, a practice common during the 1950s and 1960s, appreciation of its generally "nonmalignant" character and its usually indolent nature coupled with a growing appreciation of long-term toxic effects of therapy has tempered therapeutic intervention. Thus, rather than actively pursuing every manifestation of the disease regardless of its symptomatic or functional significance, restrained and more selective use of available treatment options is the current philosophy at many centers. Overall this translates into a policy whereby attempts are made to achieve minimum morbidity from both the disease and its treatment in the child. We favor a conservative individualized approach to children with LCH. Therapy is indicated only for symptomatic patients and the aggressivity of therapy should be based on the degree of soft tissue compromise of neurologic function, organ dysfunction, and progression of *visceral* disease despite conservative therapy.

Children and young adults requiring radiation therapy usually present in limited clinical settings. Older children, often more than 5 years of age, frequently present with monostotic bone lesions (BERRY et al. 1990). Although radiation treatment is rarely necessary, occasionally the juxtaneural location of such lesions and/or progression despite surgical treatment with or without steroid injection will make irradiation a feasible treatment option. Alternatively, a short course of systemic prednisone and/or vinblastine may represent another treatment option in some children.

Somewhat younger children (18 months to 5–6 years) more commonly demonstrate symptomatic multisite disease which may benefit from irradiation when LCH soft tissue involvement threatens vision, hearing, CNS, or spinal cord functions (LAVIN and OSBAND 1987; CASSADY 1987; RANEY and D'ANGIO 1989). Rarely, lung and/or multisite disease may warrant wide-field (including TBI) low-dose fractionated treatment (GRIFFIN 1977). Very young children and infants (birth to 2 years) generally manifest more aggressive multisystem disease, often with significant organ dysfunction (LAVIN and OSBAND 1987; GREENBERGER et al. 1981; LIPTON 1983). These children clearly fall into a poorer prognostic group and have most commonly been approached with multiagent cytotoxic chemotherapy. Despite this more aggressive treatment, children with Lipton or

Lavin/ Osband stage IV disease usually succumb (no survivors in LIPTON's series) and allogeneic or perhaps autologous (purged) bone marrow transplantation may be warranted and incorporate total body irradiation (LIPTON 1983; STOLL et al. 1990).

Finally, older adolescents and young adults represent a separate group. They usually manifest relatively indolent disease with bone, lung, and/or CNS disease which may benefit from irradiation. Unlike younger children, local recurrence after usual childhood radiation doses (6–12 Gy) have been noted more frequently in this group (CASSADY 1987; SELCH and PARKER 1990). Primary (in contrast to concurrent) lung involvement, perhaps related to smoking, is seen occasionally, in contrast to its virtual absence in children (KOMP and BOM 1991).

22.10.1.1 Radiotherapeutic Considerations

The radiation oncologist will most commonly be asked to consider treatment of a bony site which is usually symptomatic. For unknown reasons, certain sites such as the mastoids, mandible, orbit, calvarium, and vertebrae appear to be involved with greater than expected frequency. In most instances radiation therapy will not be necessary (BERRY et al. 1990). In accessible sites, local curettage, perhaps augmented by injection of methylprednisolone (40–160 mg), will usually result in healing (COHEN et al. 1980). Immediate post-operative radiation therapy should not be administered in these cases even when incomplete curettage has occurred as many such lesions will nevertheless heal uneventfully (BERRY et al. 1990; Halperin et al. 1989). Pediatric Oncology Group Study 8047 determined that only 3 of 23 children with bony LCH treated surgically showed disease progression, and at least two required radiation (Berry et al. 1990).

Radiation should be reserved for sites that are surgically less easily accessible (paravertebral mass producing neurologic symptoms, orbit, mandible, functionally risky site in long bone) or recurrent and/or progressive sites after attempted surgery. Usually 6–10 Gy will be adequate, and even lower doses (e.g., 4.5 Gy) have been successful (SELCH and PARKER 1990; GREENBERGER et al. 1981; SMITH et al. 1973). GREENBERGER et al. (1981) and others have demonstrated the absence of a dose-response relationship in children with this condition. For lesions in certain sites (e.g. the mandible, rarely the calvarium), electron beam treatment will limit normal tissue exposure. Electron beam treatment should also be utilized

for the very rare patient requiring treatment of skin or lymph node disease.

GREENBERGER et al. (1979) demonstrated reversal of pitressin requirements in four patients with diabetes insipidus and reduction in four others. Three of four patients irradiated with 1 week of onset of symptoms had complete reversal of symptoms and replacement medication. In contrast, drug requirements when symptoms had been present for longer than 2 weeks were rarely reversible. This experience has recently been corroborated by the group at the Mayo Clinic (MINEHAN et al. 1991) who irradiated 28 patients with diabetes insipidus and LCH and noted a response in 36% (10/28), which was complete in 22% (six patients). Five of six complete responders were irradiated within 14 days of onset of symptoms. Others have reported that pituitary function does not routinely improve with the administration of radiation therapy shortly after the onset of diabetes (GRAMATOVICI and D'ANGIO 1988; DUNGER et al. 1989). It also remains unclear whether aggressive or maintenance systemic therapy has any role in the reduction of diabetes insipidus in LCH (MCCLELLAND et al. 1990). Unfortunately, most patients reported in the literature fall into the delayed diagnosis group. The delay in diagnosis question is also confounded by the observation that diabetes insipidus in LCH may not necessarily be present at diagnosis and may evolve over months to years following the initial onset of LCH. Rarely, involvement of the meninges/suprasellar region is the first manifestation of LCH (this is more common in older patients in our experience), and, with a differential diagnosis of suprasellar germinoma, astrocytoma, and craniopharyngioma, stereotaxic or open biopsy followed by irradiation may be warranted. In the initial counseling of parents of children with LCH it is therefore extremely important to discuss this disease site and the symptoms that might suggest its involvement, emphasizing the importance of early diagnosis and treatment. With such patients, 6–10 Gy in three to five daily fractions using a two- or three-field approach or coronal-arc technique is desirable. If coronal arcs are used it is important to position the child so that no exit radiation reaches the thyroid gland.

A very controversial issue is the necessity or desirability of irradiation of the pituitary-suprasellar region when symptoms/signs have been present for longer than 2–4 weeks. A similar irradiation approach has been considered for such cases to prevent further growth and worsening neurologic or neuroendocrine manifestations. Several reports document more extensive evidence of CNS LCH in association with long-standing CNS disease and diabetes insipidus in unirradiated patients (BRAUNSTEIN et al. 1973; RANSOM and MURPHY 1977). Symptomatically these children may manifest ataxia and tandem gait disturbances as well as other cerebellar symptoms. Decreased cognition has also been documented (BRAUNSTEIN et al. 1973). It is likely that these symptoms are caused by unimpaired growth of CNS LCH and are therefore preventable by early treatment (BERRY and BECTON 1987). Others recommend careful follow-up without immediate treatment in such cases (KOMP and BOM 1991). It has also been suggested that hypothalamic/pituitary irradiation therapy may increase the frequency of growth hormone abnormalities in LCH (DEAN et al. 1986).

Fractionated low-dose wide-field irradiation approaches without autologous/allogeneic bone marrow transplantation support have been successfully utilized in anecdotal patients who have manifested progressive disease (especially of the lung) despite cytotoxic chemotherapy (GRIFFIN 1977). A total of 1.5–1.6 Gy in eight to ten fractions in 4–5 weeks has been recommended. Reportedly, hemibody irradiation has been more effective in cases without long-standing nodular pulmonary involvement (HALPERIN et al. 1989).

22.10.1.2 Volume

When focal lesions in bone or in the suprasellar region are to be treated, the treatment margin beyond the radiographic lesion should be quite limited as these lesions are usually sharply circumscribed and non-infiltrative.

22.10.1.3 Dose

As noted earlier, reviews of children (usually < 10 years) treated in the past have failed to demonstrate a clear dose-response relationship, the rate of local control being nearly uniform at radiation doses of 6–12 Gy (CASSADY 1987; GREENBERGER et al. 1979, 1981; SELCH and PARKER 1990; HALPERIN et al. 1989; SMITH et al. 1973; RICHTER and D'ANGIO 1981). We have, however, treated three young adults (>15 years) with this condition who have developed local failure in the treatment site, and we have also been told of many other similar cases. Recently SELCH and PARKER (1990) reported 12 failures of 41 adults (0/15 children) treated with usual doses of 6–15 Gy (5/17 in bone). The actuarial risk of local failure in treated

adults is unclear; however, Selch and Parker noted local failures at 4 years and stated that all soft tissue local failures occurred after 2 years.

For these reasons, we feel that LCH in adults is less radiocontrollable at doses of 6–15 Gy and recommend radiation doses of 20–25 Gy for this group. Whether this will ultimately result in improved control is uncertain; however, growth consequences of these somewhat larger doses will generally not be a long-term problem.

22.10.2 Bone Marrow Transplantation

Substantial mortality is documented in patients with Lipton or Osband stage IV disease (GREENBERGER stage IIIA) despite improvements in systemic therapy and support (CASSADY 1987; LIPTON 1983; LAVIN and LAVIN/OSBAND 1987; Ringdon et al. 1987; MCLELLAND et al. 1990). These infants (< 24 months and usually <12 months) often manifest overwhelming systemic disease with involvement of skin, liver, spleen, bone marrow, and, less symptomatically, lung and bone. Severe disturbances in hematologic parameters are common.

To date, at least two children have undergone successful allogeneic bone marrow transplant utilizing conditioning chemotherapy and fractionated total body irradiation (2 Gy b.i.d × 3; total dose, 12 Gy) (STOLL et al. 1990; RINGDEN et al. 1987). Both these children had progressive disease resistant to conventional therapy.

As extensive bone marrow involvement is usual in this group of children, development of effective purging techniques would make autologous transplant approaches feasible and significantly increase the number of children eligible for transplantations.

References

Adler R, Wong CA (1986) Cranial fasciitis simulating histiocytosis. J Pediatr 109: 85–88.

Alexander JE, Seibert JJ, Berry DH, Glasier CM, Williamson SL, Murphy J (1988) Prognostic factors for healing of bone lesions in histiocytosis X. Pediatr Radiol 18: 326–332.

Arenzana-Seisdedos F, Barbey S, Virelizier JL, Kornprobst M, Nezelof C (1986) Histiocytosis X Purified (T6+) cells from bone granuloma produce interleukin 1 and prostaglandin E2 in culture. J Clin Invest 77: 326–329

Arico M, Maghnier M, Villa A (1991) Central nervous system involvement in Langerhans cell histiocytosis: evidence for a diagnostic and prognostic role of MR imaging. Seventh Annual Meeting of the Histiocyte Society, Chicago, Ill., 10 September 1991

Athanasiu P, Hozoc M, Lungu VS, Stoian MM, Ionescu T, Nastac E (1970) Experimental investigations in human eosinophilic granuloma. Note II. Morphologic and immunofluorescent study of cells infected in vitro with the agents isolated from three clinical cases. Rev Roum D'Inframicrobiol 7: 125–129

Austin DF, Flannery J, Greenberg R et al. (1988) The SEER Program 1973–1982. In: Parkin DM Stiller CA, Draper GJ, Bieber CA, Terracini B, and Young JL (ed) International incidence of childhood cancer. Lyon, IARC

Basset F, Corrin B, Spencer H et al. (1978) Pulmonary histiocytosis-X. Am Rev Respir Dis 118: 811–820

Berry DH, Becton DL (1987) Natural history of histiocytosis-X. Hematol Oncol Clin North Am 1: 23–24.

Berry DH, Gresik MV, Humphrey GB, Starling K, Vietti T, Boyett J, Marcus R (1986) Natural history of histiocytosis X: a Pediatric Oncology Group study. Med Pediatr Oncol 14: 1–5.

Berry DH, Gresik M, Maybee D, Marcus R (1990) Histiocytosis in bone only. Med Pediatr Oncol 18: 292–294

Bjorksten B, Gustavson KH, Eriksson B, Lindholm A, Nordstrom S (1978) Chronic recurrent multifocal osteomyelitis and pustulosis palmoplantaris. J Pediatr 93: 227–231

Bollini G, Jouve JL, Gentet JC, Jacquemier M, Bouyala JM (1991) Bone lesions in histiocytosis X. J Pediatr Orthop 11: 469–477

Braunstein GD, Kohler PO (1981) Endocrine manifestations of histiocytosis. Am J Pediatr Hematol Oncol 3: 67–75

Braunstein GD, Whitaker NJ, Kohler PO (1973) Cerebellar dysfunction in Hand-Schüller-Christian disease. Arch Intern Med 132: 387

Braunstein GD, Raiti S, Hansen JW, Kohler PO (1975) Response of growth-retarded patients with Hand-Schüller-Christian disease to growth hormone therapy. N Engl J Med 292: 332–333

Broadbent V, Nesbit ME (1990) Clinical problems of the central nervous system in LCH. Second Nikolas Symposium, Astir Palace Hotel, Vouliagmeni, Greece, 4–7 May 1990

Broadbent V, Gadner H, Komp DM, Ladisch S (1989a) Histiocytosis syndromes in children: II. Approach to the clinical and laboratory evaluation of children with Langerhans cell histiocytosis. Med Pediatr Oncol 17: 492–495

Broadbent V, Pritchard J, Yeomans E (1989b) Etoposide (VP16) in the treatment of multisystem Langerhans cell histiocytosis (histiocytosis X). Med Pediatr Oncol 17: 97–100

Burgio GB, Arico M, Marconi M, Lanfranchi A, Caseli D, Ugazio AG (1990) Spontaneous NBT reduction by monocytes as a marker of disease activity in children with histiocytosis. Br J Haematol 74: 146–150

Carstenson H, Ornvold K (1991) The epidemiology of Langerhans cell histiocytosis in children in Denmark, 1975–89. Seventh Annual Meeting of the Histiocyte Society, Chicago Ill., 10–12 September 1992.

Cassady JR (1987) Radiation therapy in the management of histiocytosis-X. Hematol Oncol Clin North Am 1: 123–129

Ceci A, deTerlizzi M, Toma MG (1988) Heterogeneity of immunological patterns in Langerhans's histiocytosis and response to crude calf thymic extract in 11 patients. Med Pediatr Oncol 16. 111–115.

Chu T, D'Angio GJ, Favara BE, Ladisch S, Nesbit ME, Pritchard J (1987) Histiocytosis syndromes in children. Lancet II: 41–42

Cohen M, Zornoza J, Cansir A, Murray JA, Wallace S (1980) Direct injection of methylprednisolone sodium succinate in the treatment of solitary eosinophilic granuloma of bone: a report of 9 cases. Radiology 136: 289–293

Concepcion W, Esquivel CO, Terry A, Nakazato P, Garcia-Kennedy R, Houssin D, Cox KL (1991) Liver transplantation in Langerhans cell histiocytosis (histiocytosis X). Semin Oncol 18: 24–28

Consolini R, Cini P, Ceci B, Bottone E (1987) Thymic dysfuction in histiocytosis-X. Am J Pediatr Hematol Oncol 9: 146–148

Dean HJ, Bishop A, Winter JSD (1986) Growth hormone deficiency in patients with histiocytosis X. J Pediatr 109: 615–618

Dubowy RL, Rossman MJ, Kanzer MD et al. (1985) Severe cerebellar degeneration and delayed onset ataxia in histiocytosis-X. Pediatr Res 19: 216a

Dunger DB, Broadbent V, Yeoman E, Seckl JR, Lightman SL, Grant DB, Pritchard J (1989) The frequency and natural history of diabetes insipidus in children with Langerhans cell histiocytosis. N Engl J Med 321: 1157–1163

Egeler RM, Neglia JP, Puccetti DM, Brennan CA, Nesbit ME (1990) Association of malignancy with langerhans cell histiocytosis. Seventh Annual Meeting of the Histiocyte Society, Chicago, Ill., 10–12 September 1990.

Favara BE (1981) The pathology of "histiocytosis". Am J Pediatr Hematol Oncol 3: 45–56

Gadner H, Heitger A, Ritter J, Gobel U, Janka GE, Kuhl J, Bode U, Spaar HJ (1987) Langerhanszell-Histiozytose im Kindesalter-Ergebnisse der DAL-HX 83 Studie. Klin Padiatr 199: 173–182

Gramatovici R, D'Angio GJ (1988) Radiation therapy in soft-tissue lesions in histiocytosis X (Langerhans cell histiocytosis). Med Pediatr Oncol 16: 259–262

Greenberger JS, Cassady JR, Jaffe N et al. (1979) Radiation therapy in patients with histiocytosis: management of diabetes insipidus and bone lesions. Int J Radiat Oncol Biol Phys 5: 1749–1755

Greenberger JS, Crocker AC, Vawter G (1981) Results of treatment of 127 patients with systemic histiocytosis (Letterer-Siwe syndrome, Schüller-Christian syndrome and multifocal eosinophilic granuloma. Medicine 60: 311–338

Griffin TW (1977) The treatment of advanced histiocytosis-X with sequential hemibody irradiation. Cancer 39: 2435–2436

Grimm RA, Muss HB, Patterson RB, Weathers DR, White JP, Medford HM (1981) Reactivation of Hand-Schuller-Christian disease six and thirteen years after discontinuation of systemic therapy. Med Pediatr Oncol 9: 17–21

Haggstrom JA, Brown JC, Morsh PW (1988) Eosinophilic granuloma of the spine; MR demonstration. J Comput Assist Tomogr 12: 344–345

Halperin EC, Kun LE, Constine LS, Tarbell NJ (1989) Langerhan's cell histiocytosis. In: Halperin EC, Kun LE, Constine LS, Tarbell LS (eds) Pediatric radiation oncology. Raven, New York, pp 321–38

Hansen RC (1991) Childhood histiocytosis syndromes. 6: 161–198

Jouve JL, Bollini G, Jacquemier M, Bouyala JM (1991) 15 cases of vertebral involvement of histiocytosis X in children. Review of the literature. Ann Pediatr (Paris) 38: 167–174

Katz AM, Rosenthal D, Jakubovic HR, Pai RKM, Quinonez GE, Sauder DN (1991) Langerhans cell histiocytosis in monozygotic twins. Acad Dermatol 24: 32–37

Kieffer SA, Nesbit ME, D'Angio GJ (1969) Vertebra plana due to histiocytosis x serial studies. Acta Radiol 8: 241–250

Kolcnik S, Ding T, Longley J (1990) Granulocyte macrophage-colony stimulating factor (GM-CSF) decreases CDla expression by human Langerhans cells and increases proliferation in the mixed epidermal cell-lymphocyte reaction (MELR). J Invest Dermatol 95: 359–362

Komp DM, Bom LP (1991) Langerhans cell histiocytosis. In: Mossar AR, Schimpff SC, Robson MC (eds) Comprehensive textbook of oncology, 2nd edn. Williams and Wilkins, Baltimore, pp 1582–1586

Lahey ME (1975) Histiocytosis X – an analysis of prognostic factors. J Pediatr 87: 184–188

Lahey ME, Heyn R, Ladisch S et al. (1985) Hypergammaglobulinemia in histiocytosis X. J Pediatr 107: 572–574

Lavin PT, Osband ME (1987) Evaluating the role of therapy in histiocytosis-X: clinical studies, staging and scoring. Hematol Oncol Clin North Am 1: 35–47

Leblanc A, Hadchouel M, Jehan M et al. (1981) Obstructive jaundice in children with histiocytosis-X. Gastroenterology 80: 134–139

Leikin SL (1987) Immunobiology of histiocytosis-X. Hematol Oncol Clin North Am 1: 49–61

Lipton JM (1983) The pathogenesis, diagnosis and treatment of histiocytosis syndromes. Pediatr Dermatol 1: 112–120

Luksch R, Soligo D, Cerri A, Fina L, Berti E, Lambertenghi-Deliliers G (1989) Bone marrow monocytes in histiocytosis X acquire some phenotypic features of Langerhans cells in long term bone marrow cultures. Virchows Arch [A] 416: 43–49

Mahmoud H, Gaber O, Wang W, Whitingston G, Vera S, Murphy SB (1991a) Successful orthotopic liver transplantation in a child with Langerhans cell histiocytosis. Transplantation 51: 278–280

Mahmoud HH, Wang WC, Murphy SB (1991b) Cyclosporine therapy for advanced Langerhans cell histiocytosis. Blood 77: 721–725

Mahoney DH, McClain KL, Hanson IC, Taylor LD, Steuber CP (1989) Acquired immune deficiency myelodysplasia, and acute nonlymphocytic leukemia (q21;q26) in a child with Langerhans cell histiocytosis. Am J Pediatr Hematol Oncol 11: 153–157

McClain K, Ramsay NKC, Robinson L, Sundberg RD, Nesbit ME Jr (1983) Bone marrow involvement in histiocytosis X. Med Pediatr Oncol 11: 167–171

McLelland J, Chu AC (1988) Comparison of peanut agglutinin and S100 stains in the paraffin tissue diagnosis of Langerhans cell histiocytosis. Br J Dermatol 119: 513–519

McLelland J, Newton JA, Malone M, Complejohn RS, Chu AC (1989) A flow cytometric study of Langerhans cell histiocytosis. Br J Dermatol 120: 485–491

McLelland J, Broadbent V, Yeomans E, Malone M, Pritchard J (1990) Langerhans cell histiocytosis: the case for conservative treatment. Arch Dis Child 65: 301–303

Miller DR (1966) Familial reticuloendotheliosis: concurrence of disease in five siblings. Pediatrics 38: 986–994

Minehan KJ, Chen MG, Zimmerman D et al. (1991) Radiation therapy for diabetes insipidus caused by Langerhans cell histiocytosis (abstract). Int J Radiat Oncol Biol Phys 21(Sl):169

Moore JB, Kulkarni R, Crutcher DC, Bhimani S (1989) MRI in multifocal eosinophilic granuloma: staging disease and monitoring response to therapy. Am J Pediatr Hematol Oncol 11: 174–177

Murphy GF, Bhan AK, Sato S, Mihm MC Jr, Harrist TJ (1981) A new immunologic marker for human Langerhans cells. N Engl J Med 304: 791–792

Nastac E, Athanasiu P, Lungu M et al. (1970) I. Experimental investigations in human eosinophilic granuloma. Note I. Phenolic extracts of nucleic acids from bone granulomatous tissue, pathogenic for mice. Rev Roum D'Inframicrobiol 7: 149–154

Nesbit ME, O'Leary M, Dehner LP, Ramsay NKC (1981) The immune system and the histiocytosis syndromes. Am J Pediatr Hematol Oncol 3: 141–149

Newton WA, Hamoudi AB, Shannon BT (1987) Role of the thymus in histiocytosis-X. Hematol Oncol Clin North Am 1: 63–74

Ornvold K, Carstensen H, Larsen JK, Christensen IJ, Ralfkiaer E (1990) Flow cytometric DNA analysis of lesions from 18 children with langerhans cell histio-cytosis (histiocytosis X). Am J Pathol 136: 1301–1307

Osband ME, Lipton JM, Lavin P et al. (1981) Histiocytosis-X: demonstration of abnormal immunity, T-cell histamine-H$_2$-receptor deficiency, and successful treatment with thymic extract. N Engl J Med 304: 146–153

Rabkin MS, Wittwer CT, Kjeldsberg CR, Piepkorn MW (1988) Flow-cytometric DNA content of histiocytosis X (Langerhans cell histiocytosis). Am J Pathol 131: 283–289

Raney RB Jr, D'Angio GJ (1989) Langerhans' cell histiocytosis (histiocytosis X): experience at the Children's Hospital of Philadelphia, 1970–1984. Med Pediatr Oncol 17: 20–28

Ransom JL, Murphy SB (1977) Histiocytosis-X: abnormal cerebrospinal fluid cytology in extra-hypothalmic central nervous system involvement. South Med J 70: 1367

Richter MP, D'Angio GJ (1981) The role of radiation therapy in the management of children with histiocytosis-X. Am J Pediatr Hematol Oncol 3: 161–163

Ringdon O, Ahstrom L, Lownquist B et al. (1987) Allogenic BMT in a patient with chemotherapy-resistant progressive histiocytosis-X. N Engl J Med 316: 733–735

Roper SS, Spraker MK (1985) Cutaneous histiocytosis syndromes. Pediatr Dermatol 3: 19–30

Sartoris DJ, Parker BR (1984) Histiocytosis X: rate and pattern of resolution of osseous lesions. Radiology 152: 679–684

Sato Y, Ikeda Y, Ito E, Miyano T, Kawauchi K, Yokoyama M, Kamata Y (1990) Histiocytosis X: successful treatment with recombinant interferon-alpha A. Acta Paediatr Jpn 32: 151–154

Schaub T, Ash JM, Gilday DL (1987) Radionuclide imaging in histiocytosis X. Pediatr Radiol 17: 397–404

Schoeck VW, Peterson RDA, Good RA (1963) Familial occurrence of Letterer-Siwe disease. Pediatrics 32: 1055–1062

Schuster JD, Rakusan TA, Chonmaitree T, Box QT (1985) Tuberculous osteitis of the skull mimicking histiocytosis X. J Pediatr 105: 269–271

Selch MT, Parker RG (1990) Radiation therapy in the management of Langerhan's cell histiocytosis. Med Pediatr Oncol 18: 97–102

Shanley DJ, Lerud KS, Luetkehans TJ (1990) Development of pulmonary histiocytosis X after chemotherapy for Hodgkin's disease. Am J Roentgenol 155: 741–742

Shannon BT, Newton WA (1986) Suppressor-cell dysfunction in children with histiocytosis-X. J Clin Immunol 6: 510–518

Sheils C, Dover G (1989) Frequency of congenital anomalies in patients with histiocytosis X. Am J Hematol 31: 91–95

Slater JM, Swarm OJ (1980) Eosinophilic granuloma of bone. Med Pediatr Oncol 8: 151–64

Smith DG, Nesbit ME, D'Angio GJ et al. (1973) Histiocytosis-X: role of radiation therapy with special reference to dose levels employed. Radiology 106: 419–422

Stanford W, Spivey C, Lindberg EF et al. (1971) Eosinophilic granuloma of the lung. Ann Thorac Surg 11: 299

Stoll M, Freund M, Schmid H, Deicher H, Riehm H, Poliwoda H, Link H (1990) Allogeneic bone marrow transplantation for Langerhans' cell histiocytosis. Cancer 66: 284–288

Sweasey TA, Dauser RC (1989) Eosinophilic granuloma of the cervicothoracic junction. Case report. J Neurosurg 71: 942–944

Toomoka Y, Torisu M, Miyazaki S, Goya N (1986) Immunological studies on histiocytosis X. I. Special reference to the chemotactic defect and the HLA antigen. J Clin Immunol 6: 355–362

Viana MB, Oliveira BM, Silva CM, Leite VHR (1991) Etoposide in the treatment of six children with Langerhans cell histiocytosis (histiocytosis X). Med Pediatr Oncol 19: 289–294

Wirtschafter JD, Nesbit M, Anderson P, McClain K (1987) Intralesional methylprednisolone for Langerhans' cell histiocytosis of the orbit and cranium. J Pediatr Ophthalmol Strabismus 24: 194–197

Womer RB, Raney RB Jr, D'Angio GJ (1985) Healing rates of treated and untreated bone lesions in histiocytosis X. Pediatrics 76: 285–288

Ye F, Huang SW, Dong HJ (1990) Histiocytosis X: S-100 protein, peanut agglutinin, and transmission electron microscopy study. Am J Clin Pathol 94: 627–631

Yu R, Morris J, Chu A (1990) Allo-antigen presenting capacity of Langerhans cell histiocytosis cells. Seventh annual Meeting of the Histiocyte, Society, Chicago, Ill., 10–12 September 1990

Zabucchi G, Soranzo MR, Menegazzi R, Cattin L, Vecchio M, Lanza F, Patriarca P (1991) Eosinophilic granuloma of the bone in Hand-Schüller-Christian disease: extensive in vivo eosinophil degranulation and subsequent binding of release eosinophil peroxidase (EPO) to other inflammatory cells. J Pathol 163: 225–231

23 Epithelial Carcinomas in the Child

K. William Harter

CONTENTS

23.1   Introduction 351
23.2   Thyroid Cancer 351
23.3   Nasopharyngeal Cancer 354
23.4   Adrenal Carcinoma 357
23.5   Colorectal Carcinoma 360
23.5.1 Epidemiology and Etiology 360
23.5.2 Presentation and Prognosis 361
        References 363

23.1 Introduction

Malignancies derived from epithelial tissues account for the overwhelming majority of tumors in the adult population (American Cancer Society 1991). Such cancers are extremely rare in the pediatric age group (Young et al. 1981), representing less than 5% of all childhood malignancies. The infrequency with which such carcinomas are encountered in patients less than 18 years of age has thus far precluded prospective, systematic evolution of therapy. In general, treatment strategies are adapted from those in use for adults. Etiologic factors in childhood cancer include genetic predisposition (Sherlock et al. 1975; Reed and Neel 1955; McKusick 1964; Bussey 1970; Stemper et al. 1975; Haggitt and Pitcock 1970; Lynch et al. 1973), environmental factors and exposures (Correa and Haenszel 1978; Howell 1975; Wynder and Shigematsu 1967; Pratt and George 1982; Pratt et al. 1977; Odone et al. 1982; Rao et al. 1985; Caldwell et al. 1981), ionizing radiation (Duffy and Fitzgerald 1950; Fjalling et al. 1986; Winship and Rosvoll 1961), and possibly Epstein-Barr virus (Klein et al. 1974; Huang et al. 1978; Henle and Henle 1976; Naegele et al. 1982). Potential causation is, of course, inapparent in many cases. When identified, such risk factors do not appear to have an influence upon clinical outcome, other than perhaps mitigating toward earlier diagnosis in those patients with recognizable clinical syndromes which put them at increased risk for malignancy.

Generalization as to clinical outcome in the pediatric age group is difficult vis-à-vis their adult counterparts. Certain cancers, such as nasopharyngeal cancer, may have a slightly better prognosis in childhood, perhaps attributable to more aggressive management. Platinum-based multiagent chemotherapy has been in common use for more than a decade in conjunction with definitive radiation therapy. Other tumors such as large bowel cancer seem less favorable in childhood, perhaps owing to later diagnosis at a more advanced stage due to a low index of clinical suspicion (Pratt and George 1982; Pratt et al. 1977; Odone et al. 1982; Rao et al. 1985; Exelby and Frazell 1969; Winship and Rosvoll 1970; Block et al. 1970; Harness et al. 1971). Prevention, other than the avoidance of toxic chemicals and needless irradiation, is not yet a utile clinical tool.

23.2 Thyroid Cancer

Thyroid carcinomas are uncommon in childhood, accounting for between 1.5% and 3% of malignancies in the age group (Duffy and Fitzgerald 1950; Winship and Rosvoll 1961, 1970; Exelby and Frazell 1969; Block et al. 1970; Harness et al. 1971; Liechty et al. 1972; Kirkland et al. 1973; Rallison et al. 1975; Buckwalter et al. 1975; Scott and Crawford 1976). The disease affects females preferentially, at nearly a 2:1 ratio (Duffy and Fitzgerald 1950; Winship and Rosvoll 1961, 1970; Exelby and Frazell 1969; Block et al. 1970; Harness et al. 1971; Liechty et al. 1972; Kirkland et al. 1973; Rallison et al. 1975; Buckwalter et al. 1975; Scott and Crawford 1976). Modal incidence from infancy through adolescence is bell shaped, with the peak at between 7 and 12 years of age (Duffy and Fitzgerald 1950; Winship and Rosvoll 1961,1970; Exelby and Frazell 1969; Winship and Rosvoll 1970; Block et al. 1970; Harness et al. 1971; Liechty

K. William Harter, M.D., Associate Professor and Vice Chairman, Department of Radiation Oncology, Georgetown University Medical Center, 3800 Reservoir Rd. NW, Washington, DC 20007, USA

et al. 1972; KIRKLAND et al. 1973; RALLISON et al. 1975; BUCKWALTER et al. 1975; SCOTT and CRAWFORD 1976). This age incidence peak corresponds to the latency/induction period observed for radiation-induced thyroid malignancy following treatment for a variety of benign conditions in infancy and early childhood (HEMPELMANN 1968; HEMPELMANN et al. 1975; REFETOFF et al. 1975; McCONAHEY and HAYLES 1976; FAVUS et al. 1976; GREENSPAN 1977; MAXON et al. 1977; SCHNEIDER et al. 1978, 1980; KAPLAN et al. 1983). This is in contradistinction to the latency period for thyroid carcinoma of approximately 20 years noted in the atomic bomb survivors (Hirsoshima and Nagasaki) (KERR 1978; PARKER et al. 1973, 1974) and in tinea capitis patients who received scalp irradiation for epilation (Israel and New York) (MODAN et al. 1977; SHORE et al. 1976). The fallout studies from the Marshall Islands also noted a latency period for thyroid carcinoma of about two decades (CONRAD 1977).

Risk of thyroid cancer is increased dramatically in patients receiving therapeutic radiation for malignant disease of childhood. The study by the Late Effects Study Group (LESG) (TUCKER et al. 1991) indicated that the risk is greatest following radiation treatment for neuroblastoma, Wilms' tumor, and lymphoma (both non-Hodgkin's and Hodgkin's disease). The average latency period was about a decade, corresponding to the induction period of treatment of benign disease in infancy and early childhood. Of importance is the LESG observation that doses to the thyroid in excess of 2 Gy carried a risk of thyroid cancer 13 times greater than that in patients receiving lesser doses to the thyroid. Analysis of the postradiation thyroid malignancy data suggests that the dose range for induction is between 6 cGy (tinea capitis) and 15 Gy (neuroblastoma, lymphoma). Children receiving lower doses in a single exposure tend to have a lower overall incidence with a longer latency period (tinea capitis, atomic fallout). Patients receiving higher doses of fractionated therapeutic irradiation are seen

to have a shorter latency period resulting in the manifestation of thyroid malignancy in childhood and adolescence.

The incidence of thyroid carcinoma in childhood has declined over the past 30 years (SCOTT and CRAWFORD 1976; HEMPELMANN 1968; HEMPELMANN et al. 1975; REFETOFF et al. 1975; McCONAHEY and HAYLES 1976; FAVUS et al. 1976; GREENSPAN 1977; MAXON et al. 1977; SCHNEIDER et al. 1978, 1980; KAPLAN et al. 1983). This temporal reduction corresponds to the discontinuation of radiation therapy for benign disease in infancy and childhood. Of course, the majority of cases of thyroid carcinoma in childhood are not radiation associated. While previous radiation may have accounted for as much as 35% of childhood thyroid cancers in the past (DUFFY and FITZGERALD 1950), even then the preponderance of cases was spontaneous and idiopathic. With the virtual elimination of childhood irradiation for all but malignant conditions, the proportion of primary idiopathic cases is increasing concomitant with the overall in incidence.

A minority of cases of childhood thyroid cancer are of familial origin. In particular, medullary carcinoma of the thyroid, arising from the calcitonin-secreting cells (C cells), is associated with three distinct genetic syndromes. Two are subgroups of multiple endocrine neoplasia (MEN) syndromes, MEN IIa and MEN IIb (CANCE and WELLS 1985; NORTON et al. 1979). The remainder of hereditary cases are found in the familial medullary thyroid carcinoma group (FARNDON et al. 1986). Overall, these account for approximately 20% of all medullary thyroid carcinomas in childhood, inherited as an autosomal dominant trait (WELLS 1990). The overwhelming preponderance of nonmedullary thyroid cancer in children is not genetically linked. There are some data for familial clusterings of papillary carcinoma and possible genetic linkage with both Gardner's syndrome and familial polyposis of the colon (PHADE et al. 1981; LOTE et al. 1980; BELL and MAZZAFERRI 1993).

Table 23.1. Histology and incidence of thyroid carcinoma in children and adults

	Papillary and/or mixed	Follicular	Medullary	Anaplastic
Age at diagnosis (children)	< 7 yrs	> 7 yrs	Any	Any
% Incidence (children)	70	20	5–10	Rare
% Incidence (adults)	70–75	15	5	< 5

The histologic subtypes of thyroid carcinoma are identical in the adult and pediatric patient populations. Incidence of histologic subtype is also quite similar between the two populations, with the majority of cases being papillary and/or mixed papillary follicular. Pure follicular carcinoma accounts for 15%–20% of cases in both groups and medullary carcinoma for 5%–10%; anaplastic carcinoma is equally uncommon in both populations (Table 23.1). There are prognostic differences by age, however. Perhaps because of a tendency toward better differentiation in the younger age group, survival at 10 years is reported in the range of 80%–85% in children compared to 60% in adults (EXELBY and FRAZELL 1969; WINSHIP and ROSVOLL 1970; BLOCK et al. 1970; HARNESS et al. 1971; LIECHTY et al. 1972). This differential does not hold true for the anaplastic or undifferentiated carcinoma, which is rapidly fatal in both age groups (WINSHIP and ROSVOLL 1961; SHVERO et al. 1988).

The majority of cases will present with either anterior cervical adenopathy or a palpable thyroid nodule. These two physical findings are encountered jointly in about half the cases. Typically, thyroid cancer patients in the pediatric age group are euthyroid at the time of presentation. Further evaluation would include nuclear medicine scanning with radioiodine (OZAKI et al. 1983), the likelihood being that identification of a cold nodule will lead to a diagnosis of malignancy. In patients at particular risk for medullary carcinoma, baseline serum calcitonin assay can be obtained. Fine needle aspiration (FNA) is the preferred method of biopsy. It must be remembered, however, that a negative FNA is valueless and open biopsy of either a thyroid nodule or a cervical lymph node should be undertaken in that instance (WALFISH et al. 1977a,b; MILLER et al. 1985; MILLER 1979).

The primary therapy for all but anaplastic thyroid cancers is surgical extirpation. Extent of surgical resection is dictated by both histology and anatomic spread of malignancy. The role for total thyroidectomy is limited to medullary carcinoma and to patients with clinically obvious bilateral disease (WILLIAMS et al. 1966; MELVIN and TASHJIAN 1968; HILL et al. 1973; WOLFE et al. 1973). The overwhelming majority of cases of pediatric thyroid cancer are best managed with subtotal thyroidectomy (lobectomy plus isthmus) or occasional local excision of an isolated nodule) FARRAR et al. 1980; CHRISTENSEN et al. 1983; OZAKI et al. 1983; SIERK et al. 1990; BLOCK 1981; BREAUX and GUILLAMONDEGUI 1980; WEBER and CLARK 1985; COHN et al. 1984). Such limited surgery

is clearly adequate for local control and avoids the potential morbidity of hypoparathyroidism and recurrent laryngeal nerve injury, which are risked in total thyroidectomy (FARRAR et al. 1980; CHRISTENSEN et al. 1983; OZAKI et al. 1983; SIERK et al. 1990; BLOCK 1981; BREAUX and GUILLAMONDEGUI 1980; WEBER and CLARK 1985; COHN et al. 1984). In patients presenting with lymphadenopathy, conservative dissection of the neck is also recommended. The classical radical neck dissection does not appear to be of therapeutic benefit, and limited resection of gross disease sparing neurovascular structures is most appropriate. Because of the tendency for pediatric papillary carcinoma to involve lymph nodes of the superior mediastinum, these should be explored extending inferiorly from the isthmus chain.

In the pediatric age group, all patients should be evaluated for radioiodine treatment (OZAKI et al. 1983) in the adjuvant setting. The relatively high risk of pulmonary metastatic disease (20%–25%), which is inapparent on CT scan, is a strong argument in favor of such evaluation (SIERK et al. 1990; MAZZAFERRI and YOUNG 1981; YOUNG et al. 1980; MAZZAFERRI et al. 1977). Therefore, while the overwhelming majority of patients will be treated postoperatively with thyroid replacement resulting in thyroid-stimulating hormone (TSH) suppression, all patients should be scanned postoperatively and those with evidence of metastatic disease treated aggressively with radioiodine (OZAKI et al. 1983). Well over half of patients with metastatic thyroid cancer can be rendered permanently free of disease with isotope therapy (BEIERWALTES et al. 1982; BEIERWALTES 1978; MAXON et al. 1983, 1992; SAMAAN et al. 1983, 1985, 1992; BROWN et al. 1984; VAN NOSTRAND et al. 1986; SMITH et al. 1985). Depending upon dose, side-effects may include transient suppression of bone marrow seen at 6 weeks posttreatment, and rare late complications, including pulmonary fibrosis and fertility compromise (BEIERWALTES et al. 1982; BEIERWALTES 1978; MAXON et al. 1983, 1992; SAMAAN et al. 1983, 1985, 1992; BROWN et al. 1984; VAN NOSTRAND et al. 1986; SMITH et al. 1985). Rare cases of secondary leukemia are also reported (LEEPER 1985).

The role of external beam radiation therapy is limited to patients with close surgical margins in whom there is no radioactive iodine uptake, patients with gross residual disease after surgery, and a few unfortunate patients with anaplastic carcinoma. Patients with close surgical margins (less than 3 mm) are at increased risk for local recurrence (SIMPSON et al. 1988). Such patients are to be considered for treatment with radioiodine (OZAKI et al. 1983), which has been shown to enhance local control greatly. Patients without radioiodine uptake should be considered for postoperative external beam therapy to the surgical bed with doses of 45–50 Gy. Patients with gross residual disease after surgery can also be treated with external beam radiation if radioiodine uptake is not demonstrated or if the bulk of the residuum precludes isotope therapy (SIMPSON et al. 1988; SIMPSON and CARRUTHERS 1978; KIM and LEEPER 1983, 1987). The rare pediatric patient with anaplastic thyroid carcinoma can be treated with combination therapy employing doxorubicin and external beam radiation therapy, given concomitantly. A treatment protocol from Memorial-Sloan Kettering employs weekly doxorubicin ($10 \mu g/m^2$) concomitant with daily external beam radiation therapy in 2 Gy fractions to 50 Gy. Local control rates in anaplastic carcinoma and also in bulk disease from other thyroid cancers is reported to be approximately 70%–75% (LEEPER 1985; KIM and LEEPER 1983, 1987). The use of twice-daily fractionation may further enhance local control (KIM and LEEPER, 1987). Unfortunately, all patients with anaplastic thyroid carcinoma will succumb to distant disease.

There does not seem to be prognostic or therapeutic difference in the management of radiation-induced thyroid carcinoma compared with the primary idiopathic variety (HEMPELMANN 1968; HEMPELMANN et al. 1975; REFETOFF et al. 1975; MCCONAHEY and HAYLES 1976; FAVUS et al. 1976; GREENSPAN 1977; MAXON et al. 1977; SCHNEIDER et al. 1978, 1980; KAPLAN et al. 1983; BLOCK 1976). Radiation-induced cancers often are clinically inapparent and found only at autopsy in patients who have died of other causes. In children with clinically apparent cancer, subtotal thyroidectomy or local resection is recommended in spite of the high incidence of bilaterality/multifocality in these tumors. No difference in outcome was noted at 12 years in a prospective study at the University of Wisconsin in patients receiving limited resection versus total thyroidectomy (DEACONSON et al. 1986). As with cases of primary idiopathic thyroid cancer in the pediatric age group, postoperative adjuvant therapy generally is thyroid replacement to suppress TSH. The recommendations for isotope therapy with radioiodine (OZAKI et al. 1983) are the same as for the non-radiation-associated group.

Conclusions: Over the past 30 years, the incidence of radiation-associated thyroid carcinoma in childhood has decreased and no longer accounts for one-third of cases in childhood. The overall decrease in incidence of thyroid cancer in the past 30 years is directly attributable to a reduction in the radiation-associated incidence, which in turn is related to the cessation of indiscriminate radiation therapy for benign conditions in infancy and early childhood. While the histology and proportional incidence of thyroid cancer are similar in children and adults, clinical outcome is better in the pediatric age group, perhaps due to a higher proportion of well-differentiated cancers. The primary management of thyroid cancer in the child is surgical with local resection or subtotal thyroidectomy (lobectomy plus isthmus) as the standard of care. Total thyroidectomy is limited to cases of medullary carcinoma and those cases with clinically obvious bilateral disease. In the postoperative state, all patients are given exogenous hormone to suppress TSH. Radioactive iodine is used in the therapy of residual, recurrent, or metastatic disease and in patients with close surgical margins. External beam radiation (with or without concomitant doxorubicin) is used in patients with indication for adjuvant therapy who do no have radioiodine uptake. Additionally, patients with bulky residual or recurrent disease and patients with anaplastic carcinoma are candidates for combined modality therapy.

23.3 Nasopharyngeal Cancer

Primary cancer of the nasopharynx is uncommonly found in the pediatric/adolescent age group, amounting to perhaps 5% of all reported cases (COUNTER et al. 1980; SNOW 1975). Etiologic factors derived from epidemiologic studies suggest linkage with Epstein-Barr virus (EBV), diet, and genetic predisposition (KLEIN et al. 1974; HUANG et al. 1978; HENLE and HENLE 1976; NAEGELE et al. 1982; MILLER 1980; HENDERSON et al. 1976; YU et al. 1986; OLD et al. 1966; ZUR HAUSEN et al. 1970; FAHRACUS et al. 1988; CHAN et al. 1983; SIMONS et al. 1976). Identified endemic geographic regions include Southern China, North Africa, and certain populations clustered along the Arctic Circle. Common among peoples in these regions is the practice of curing fish and meat with salt, associated with the carcinogenic chemical family of the nitrosamines (YU et al. 1986). Linkage with EBV is more direct, in that the overwhelming majority of patients with nasopharyngeal carcinoma have elevated anti-EBV titers (OLD et al. 1966). Subsequently, the EBV genome has been identified within nasopharyngeal cancer cells (ZUR HAUSEN et al. 1970; FAHRACUS et al. 1988; CHAN et al. 1983) and EBV-associated proteins have been shown to induce malignant transformation of lymphocyte-derived cell lines in vitro (Zur Hausen et al. 1970; FAHRACUS et al. 1988). Genetic studies of nasopharyngeal cancer patient populations among the Chinese have identified several gene-antigen loci which are associated with an increased risk of the disease. Of particular interest in children is the B17 antigen (CHAN et al. 1983), which seems to correlate with increased disease risk in a younger-age population (CHAN et al. 1983). In North America, there is some evidence for increased risk of nasopharyngeal carcinoma among black teenagers (GREEN et al. 1977; EASTON et al. 1980).

Carcinoma of the nasopharynx was first described as a discrete histopathologic entity simultaneously by investigators in Germany (SCHMINCKE 1921) and France (REGAUD 1921) in 1921. Currently, the World Health Organization subdivides the histopathology into three subtypes: keratinizing squamous cell carcinoma, nonkeratinizing carcinoma, and undifferentiated carcinoma with lymphoid infiltrate (lymphoepithelioma). Lymphoepitheliomas are most common and are most closely associated with viral, dietary and genetic risk factors. Analysis of the case-mix in North America, however, demonstrates a higher incidence of keratinizing squamous cell carcinoma (which is not associated with EBV) than in the geographic locales where the disease is endemic (GREEN et al. 1977; EASTON et al. 1980).

The most common presentation of nasopharyngeal carcinoma is adenopathy in the neck, frequently bilateral. Neck disease is present at diagnosis in between 71% and 91% of all patients, depending on the series. This adenopathy is often accompanied by nasal obstruction/stuffiness and symptoms of otitis media. Clinical staging (TNM) is based upon the extent of the primary tumor and the extent and size of neck disease (Table 23.2). In all reported series where such data are available, there is a significant difference in prognosis between patients with T1-T2 primaries and those with T3-T4 (Table 23.3). While one may postulate with regard to differences in tumor biology between those patients presenting with limited primary disease and those with locally advanced cancers, the most important factor appears to be direct tumor burden. This hypothesis is strengthened by data from a recent combined analysis of cases of childhood nasopharyngeal carcinoma from Stanford and M.D. Anderson (INGERSOLL et al.

Table 23.2. A.J.C. staging of nasopharyngeal cancer (BEAHRS et al. 1992)

Primary tumor		
T0		No evidence of primary tumor
Tis		Carcinoma in situ
T1		Tumor confined to one site of nasopharynx or tumor visible (positive biopsy only)
T2		Tumor involving two sites (both postero-superior and lateral walls)
T3		Extension of tumor into nasal cavity or oropharynx
T4		Tumor invasion of skull, cranial nerve involvement, or both
Nodal involvement		
N0		No clinically positive node
N1		Single clinically positive homolateral node 3 cm or less in diameter
N2		Single clinically positive homolateral node more than 3 cm but not more than 6 cm in diameter, or multiple clinically positive homolateral nodes, none more than 6 cm in diameter
	N2a	Single clinically positive homolateral node more than 3 cm but not more than 6 cm in diameter
	N2b	Multiple clinically positive homolateral nodes, none more than 6 cm in diameter
N3		Massive homolateral nodes, bilateral nodes, or contralateral nodes
	N3a	Clinically positive homolateral nodes, none more than 6 cm in diameter
	N3b	Bilateral clinically positive nodes
	N3c	Contralateral clinically positive nodes only
Distant metastasis		
M0		No evidence of metastasis
M1		Distant metastasis present

1990). Patients with T3-T4 primary lesions were stratified by N stage at presentation (N0-N1 versus N2-N3). Reported 5-year disease-free survival was 71% in six patients with T3-T4, N0-N1 disease as opposed to 46% in 37 patients with T3-T4, N2-N3 presentation.

An overview of published data from the past two decades (Table 23.3) indicates that children with nasopharyngeal carcinoma may have a slightly better prognosis than their adult counterparts. While this may be due, in part, to more aggressive management and the frequent use of neoadjuvant chemotherapy based on 5-fluorouracil and cisplatin, no direct evidence exists at the present time to support this explanation. In the Stanford-M.D. Anderson analysis (INGERSOLL et al. 1990) patients receiving adjuvant chemotherapy had a somewhat better outcome at 5 years (60% for the chemotherapy group versus 50% for those receiving radiation alone) but this was not statistically significant. Data from St.

Table 23.3. Selected series of nasopharyngeal carcinoma in childern and adolescents

Institution	Author (year)	No. of pts.	Grouping T stage		Survival (%)		
			T1–T2	T3–T4	T1–T2	T3–T4	(overall)
M.C.V.	Pick et al. (1974)	9	5	4	–	–	4/9 (44%)
U.S. Carolina	LaNasa et al. (1974)	1	0	1	–	0/1 (0%)	0/1 (0%)
M.D. Anderson	Fernandez et al. (1976)	10	2	8	2/2 (100%)	4/8 (50%)	6/8 (75%)
Penn	Snow (1977)	7	–	–	–	–	4/7 (57%)
U. Athens (Greece)	Papavasiliov et al. (1977)	22	–	–	–	–	11/22(50%)
Salah Aziz (Tunisia)	Ellouz et al. (1978)	82	15	67	8/15	20/67	28/82 (34%)
Pitt	Deutsch et al. (1978)	7	–	–	–	–	1/7 (14%)
Royal Marsden	Counter et al. (1980)	39	–	–	–	–	18/39 (46%)
Princess Margaret	Berry et al. (1980)	25	12	13	8/12	5/13	13/25 (52%)
Memorial-Sloan Kettering	Jereb et al. (1980)	16	8	8	2/8 (25%)	0/8 (0%)	2/16 (12%)
C.C.S.G.	Jenkin et al. (1981)	109	41	68	30/41 (73%)	23/68 (34%)	53/190 (49%)
Ann Arbor	Baker et al. (1981)	10	8	2	–	–	5/10 (50%)
N.C.I. Milan	Lombardi et al. (1982)	20	8	12	7/8 (88%)	1/12 (8%)	8/20 (40%)
Emory	Vita et al. (1983)	27	11	16	8/11 (82%)	6/16 (38%)	14/27 (52%)
Gonzalez-Martinez (San Juan, P.R.)	Morales et al. (1984)	17	9	8	3/9 (33%)	0/8 (0%)	3/17 (18%)
S.U.N.Y.-Downstate	Bass et al. (1985)	6	1	5	1/1	0/5 (0%)	1/16 (17%)
Children's Hosp. (Costa Rica)	Lobo-Sanahuja et al. (1986)	22	12	10	–	–	13/22 (59%)
St. Mary's (Manchester, U.K.)	Roper et al. (1986)	18		–	–	–	7/18 (39%)
N.C.I. Milan	Gasparini et al. (1988)	12	0	12	–	9/12 (75%)	9/12 (75%)
Cancer Hosp. Beijing (China)	Qin et al. (1988)	67	–	–	–	–	43/67 (64%)
St. Jude	Pao et al. (1989)	27	–	–	–	–	16/27 (59%)
Queen Mary (Hong Kong)	Sham et al. (1990)	71	–	–	–	–	27/71 (38%)
Sun Yat-Sen U. (China)	Wvang (1990)	53	–	–	–	–	11/53 (21%)
Stanford & M.D. Anderson	Ingersoll et al. (1990)	56	13	43	8/13 (61%)	21/43 (49%)	29/56 (52%)

Jude (Pao et al. 1989), N.C.I. Milan (Gasparini et al. 1988), St. Mary's Hospital (Manchester, UK) (Roper et al. 1986), and the National Children's Hospital of Costa Rica (Lobo-Sanahuja et al. 1986) all suggest survival benefit with the addition of chemotherapy, particularly in advanced disease. The Children's Cancer Study Group (Jenkin et al. 1981) and Princess Margaret Hospital (Berry et al. 1980) found no survival benefit to chemotherapy in their analyses. One is left, therefore, only with an impression of possible improved efficacy. Given the observation that disease outcome is influenced negatively by an increasing volume of disease (either primary or nodal, vide supra), the addition of chemotherapy in advanced presentations would appear logical. However, proper prospective randomized data would be welcome to confirm or refute this observation.

Recommendations for treatment of nasopharyngeal carcinoma with radiation are similar in children and adults. The initial treatment volume should encompass the nasopharynx with adequate margins in three dimensions, thus encompassing the posteri-or nasal cavity, posterior maxillary sinus, and base of skull. The entire sphenoid sinus, the gasserian ganglion, and cavernous sinus should be encompassed in the initial treatment volume and carried to a dose sufficient for microscopic disease. In presentations of T4 disease, higher doses to the base of skull and intracranial structures which are either affected or at risk, are required. Using sequentially reducing fields, total dose to areas of gross disease should be in the range of 65–70 Gy. Dose reductions for age or chemotherapy are not recommended. There is no age-related dose-response curve in this disease and patients receiving chemotherapy generally have more advanced and bulkier tumor burdens, requiring higher doses.

The use of brachytherapy as a boost following external beam treatment of the nasopharyngeal primary is not well documented in children. Data in adults from Massachusetts General Hospital (MGH) (Wang 1990) are quite persuasive of the utility of intracavitary cesium treatment in T1-T3 lesions. Local control of 93% was observed in T1 and

T2 lesions after brachytherapy boost compared with 60% (T1) and 68% (T2) after external beam treatment only. Twelve patients with T3 primaries had uniform (100%) local control after brachytherapy compared with 64% of 20 patients treated with external beam alone. The implant procedure employs two pediatric endotracheal tubes placed under fluoroscopic guidance through the nares into the nasopharynx with the cuff balloon inflated both to fix position and to increase the distance between sources and mucosa. Each tube is afterloaded with 20 mg radium-equivalent of cesium. A dose of 7 Gy is delivered at 0.5 cm below the vault mucosa with a dose rate of approximately 1.2 Gy/h (WANG et al. 1975). The group at Georgetown have described a similar technique using high-dose rate iridium after-loading (TROOST and THOMAS 1992). A 2-mm semirigid Teflon catheter is inserted into each naris and then placed in the nasopharynx under direct visualization with the catheter tip anchored in the mucosa of the posterior wall. A boost dose of 5 Gy is delivered at a depth of 0.5 cm beneath the mucosa over a period of several minutes. The entire procedure takes about half an hour and can be performed on an outpatient basis.

Twice-daily fractionation is also not well documented in the child. Wang (1990) makes a strong case for using 1.6-Gy fractions twice daily, reporting improved local control in both T1-T2 lesions (80% b.i.d. vs 60% q.d.) and T3-T4 lesions (60% b.i.d. vs 37% q.d.). This is sometimes combined with brachytherapy.

Nasopharyngeal carcinoma represents one of the few clinical situations in which local/regional recurrence can be retreated with definitive doses of radiation with a reasonable probability of clinical cure. Data in adults from MGH demonstrate a 40% actuarial survival at 5 years for early recurrent lesions (T1-T2), 15% for T3-T4 (WANG 1990). Recommended technique is 40 Gy external beam via arc rotation followed by two sessions of brachytherapy treatment of 10 Gy each. The retreatment of recurrent disease in children should include platinum-based chemotherapy (PAO et al. 1989).

The late consequences of definitive radiation treatment for nasopharyngeal carcinoma in childhood include xerostomia with concomitant risk to teeth and gingiva, as well as the possibility of fibrosis of the soft tissues of the neck and masseter muscles. Most patients will develop a rise in TSH (CHEN et al. 1989) within 10 years of treatment, many requiring exogenous hormone replacement. Abnormalities in growth hormone and luteinizing hormone have also

been described (CHEN et al. 1989; BLACKLAY et al. 1986). At least one case of hypopituitary dwarfism following radiotherapy for nasopharyngeal carcinoma has been described (TAN and KUNARATNAM 1966). Patients undergoing reirradiation for recurrent disease are at extremely high risk for hormonal complications and overt central nervous system injury if survival is sufficiently long (WANG 1990).

Conclusions: Nasopharyngeal carcinoma is uncommon in childhood and adolescence, accounting for approximately 5% of all nasopharyngeal cancers. Risk factors include Epstein-Barr virus, diet including salt-cured fish and meat, and genetic predisposition (at least in the Chinese). Treatment should be undertaken with definitive radiation therapy to doses in the range of 65–70 Gy. Adverse clinical outcome correlates with bulk of disease (both primary and nodal). While multiagent platinum-based chemotherapy is frequently given to children with nasopharyngeal carcinoma, no direct evidence is available to support its use. Potential benefit from adjuvant chemotherapy would seem likely, however, in advanced disease (T3-T4 and/or N2-N3) and in the definitive retreatment of recurrent malignancy. Children cured of nasopharyngeal carcinoma are more likely to have hypothalamic-pituitary hormonal abnormalities and comprehensive endocrine follow-up is mandatory.

23.4 Adrenal Carcinoma

Primary adenocarcinoma of the adrenal cortex is exceedingly rare in childhood, accounting for but a fraction of 1% of all childhood cancers (American Cancer Society 1991; YOUNG et al. 1981). Virtually all pediatric cases will present prior to the age of 8 years, the majority, in fact, being seen before 6 years of age. The disease has a bimodal distribution with the second age peak occurring in adults in the fifth decade of life. There are ample data to support the assertion that adrenocortical carcinoma is a different disease in children than in adults. Among the adult population, approximately two-thirds of patients will present with hormonal symptomatology (COHN et al. 1986). The incidence of presenting hormonal manifestation is much higher in children, being nearly uniform (EPELMAN et al. 1991; RIBEIRO et al. 1990; NEBLETT et al. 1987). There is a female predominance of nearly 2:1 in incidence in childhood. Virilization is manifested in most females, many male children presenting with precocious puberty. The incidence of feminizing tumors in males, along with precocious puberty in females, is much less common (EPELMAN et al. 1991; RIBEIRO et al. 1990; NEBLETT et al. 1987). Concomitant with these sex hormone manifestations, Cushing's syndrome is frequently noted. Unlike presentations in the adult, Cushing's syndrome is rarely noted in the child as an isolated finding. Urinary steroids, particularly 17 ketosteroids and 17 hydroxycorticosteroids, are usually elevated, but this does not discriminate specifically between malignant and benign adrenal tumors. It does appear, however, that serum levels of sulphated pregnenolone and/or pregn-5-ene-3 B, 20 α-diol, possibly together with free 11-deoxycortisol, may provide a fairly precise preoperative clinical differentiation (GRONDAL and CURSTEDT 1991).

Further evidence for the fundamental etiologic difference of adrenocortical carcinoma in children and adults has come from chromosomal analysis. In adults, most adrenocortical carcinomas are sporadic, and a recent report noted that tumor DNA analysis from six adult cases showed no loss of heterozygosity in chromosome 11. In contradistinction, tumor DNA from five childhood cases showed loss of heterozygosity in four of five, suggesting a different oncogenic mechanism (BRUGIERES et al. 1991). Adrenal carcinoma in childhood has also been linked to a number of genetic syndromes, most recently the Li-Fraumeni . syndrome (LFS) (WARNEFORD et al. 1991, 1992; THORESEN 1992; MALKIN 1993). In LFS, adrenocortical carcinoma has thus far accounted for 10% of all childhood neoplasms, all presenting in the first decade (MALKIN 1993). Most malignancies in this syndrome are associated with point mutations of the tumor-suppressor gene p53, although over-expression of the retinoblastoma susceptibility gene (RB) has also been reported (WARNEFORD et al. 1991). Malignancy of the adrenal cortex has also been associated with hemihypertrophy, Beckwith-Wiedeman syndrome, Conn syndrome and the MEN syndromes (GREEN et al. 1993; SIRINELLI et al. 1989; SHE et al. 1980; OGITA et al. 1989; FRASCH et al. 1992).

The histopathologic diagnosis of malignant adrenal tumors is not difficult, although clinical data are useful in the distinction from benign adenomas. Clinically, malignant tumors are generally much larger than adenomas and have a propensity for local spread and invasion to the adjacent kidney and surrounding retroperitoneum. Malignant cells are characterized by pleomorphism and a large number of mitoses (STEWART et al. 1974; VAN SLOOTEN et al. 1985). The number of mitoses appears to be the most significant prognostic variable distinguishing low-grade from high-grade tumors. A recent report from Stanford on 42 cases of adrenocortical carcinoma noted that patients whose tumors had more than 20 mitoses per 50 high power fields (hpf) had a median survival of 14 months whereas patients whose carcinomas had 20 or less had a median survival of 58 months. Thus, prevalence of mitotic figures can be used as the major criterion for grade differentiation with good correlation to clinical outcome (WEISS et al. 1989). Surprisingly, DNA ploidy has been shown not to be useful as a discriminating factor between malignant and benign lesions (CIBAS et al. 1990). Flow cytometry data from adenomas and carcinomas demonstrate that both malignant and benign tumors can be aneuploid and that clinical outcome in cases of malignancy does not correlate with diploid or aneuploid characteristics.

At presentation, in addition to the clinical manifestations of sex hormone abnormalities, patients will have evidence of abdominal mass. Characteristics indicative of malignancy can be identified with ultrasonography, computed tomography (CT), and magnetic resonance imaging (MRI) (PRANDO et al. 1990; HUSSAIN et al. 1985; ROUCAYROL et al. 1986). Malignant tumors are seen by ultrasonography to be circumscribed and hypoechoic, often characterized by the "Scar sign" (radiating linear echoes)(PRANDO et al. 1990). Findings on CT, which correlate with malignancy, include tumor size, contrast enhancement, and consistency (HUSSAIN et al. 1985). Images from MRI show a markedly reduced lipid/water ratio in carcinomas as compared benign lesions (ROUCAYROL et al. 1986). These imaging techniques will also assess functioning of the contralateral kidney (if ipsilateral nephrectomy is required) and image the inferior vena cava for tumor thrombus. Thoracic CT and bone scan are necessary to survey for metastatic disease. Bone marrow aspiration and biopsy is not routinely recommended but should be undertaken if bone marrow abnormality is suspected from the hemogram.

Complete surgical extirpation is the single most important therapeutic maneuver in potentially curative treatment (EPELMAN et al. 1991; RIBEIRO et al. 1990; NEBLETT et al. 1987; STEWART et al. 1974; MAGEE et al. 1987; PERCARPIO and KNOWLTON 1976; LEFEVRE et al. 1983; HENLEY et al. 1983; ZABBO et al. 1987; TELANDER et al. 1986; BODIE et al. 1989; SCHIER et al. 1988; CHUDLER and KAY 1989; BORRELLI et al. 1989; GODINE et al. 1990; MARKOE et al. 1991; RANEY et al. 1983). While it may be argued that surgical cure is a self-fulfilling prophesy, in that resectable lesions are biologically more favorable and/or diagnosed at an earlier stage, the fact remains that patients with metastatic disease are not cured by additional therapies (RIBEIRO et al. 1990; NEBLETT et al. 1987; LEFEVRE et al. 1983; ZABBO et al. 1987; BODIE et al. 1989; BORRELLI et al. 1989). Considerable pessimism surrounds the use of radiation therapy in pediatric adrenal cancer. As no systematic trials have been carried out, however, analysis of radiotherapeutic efficacy is often undertaken in patients with advanced disease with predictably poor results. A careful examination of available data suggests a clear role for radiation in the adjuvant setting in patients with large tumors, local invasion, and/or positive lymph nodes following gross total resection. The irradiation of gross residual disease also offers some promise.

Adrenocortical carcinoma has been shown to spread by direct extension, frequently involving regional lymph nodes. Such local regional extension can involve adjacent kidney, retroperitoneum, and even inferior vena cava (GODINE et al. 1990). Patients with disease which is sufficiently localized to permit en bloc primary resection have a probablity of long-term disease-free survival in the range of 45%–68% (RIBEIRO et al. 1990; LEFEVRE et al. 1983; HENLEY et al. 1983; BODIE et al. 1989). The Cleveland Clinic (BODIE et al. 1989) reported long-term survival in 18 of 40 (45%) patients after primary resection. In the Mayo Clinic series, 21 of 31 patients (68%) were seen to survive long-term. Data from the Institut Gustave-Roussy (LEFEVRE et al. 1983) showed 20 of 35 (60%) surgical survivors while 17 of 26 patients (65%) from St. Jude (RIBEIRO et al. 1990) were apparent surgical cures. The majority of patients in these series who were not cured succumbed to distant disease. However, some patients in each series were found to have local recurrence after curative resection.

While the Cleveland Clinic report states that radiation therapy was not of benefit in patients with metastatic disease, it was not employed in either the 40 patients with localized disease or an additional 12 patients who were found to have regional disease without metastases. The St. Jude and Mayo groups both suggest the possibility of adjuvant radiation. Radiotherapy was given to 11 patients at Gustave-Roussy, all of whom had advanced bulk disease. Only one response was documented, in that the patient was converted to resectability and was surviving NED at 19 years.

Two patients from the Royal Manchester Children's Hospital were given postoperative radiation therapy following incomplete excision (STEWART et al. 1974). One died promptly of metastatic disease and another was reported NED at 1 year. An additional four patients received postoperative radiotherapy after resection (15–30 Gy), all of whom were NED from 1 to 12 years postoperatively. Specific indications for the radiation were not given, however. At the Christie Hospital and Holt Radium Institute, also in Manchester, of 15 patients with adrenal cortical carcinoma nine received postoperative radiation therapy. Of this group, absolute survival at 10 years was 33% (MAGEE et al. 1987). The group at Hahnemann (MARKOE et al. 1991) reported on five patients treated postoperatively for either local invasion or positive lymph nodes. They noted a median survival in this group of between 3 and 7 years and suggested possible benefit to adjuvant radiotherapy in patients with resected local-regional disease. Five patients at Children's Hospital of Philadelphia (RANEY et al. 1983) underwent resection for localized disease. None received radiation and one of five developed a local recurrence treated with mitotane (op'DDD), subsequently dying of distant disease. One may conclude that the local-regional pattern of spread exhibited by adrenocortical carcinoma in conjunction with the established (albeit difficult to quantify) risk of local recurrence after gross total resection argues strongly for adjuvant radiation therapy. The available clinical data appear to support this. Additionally, preoperative radiotherapy may promote resectability in some patients. The occasional patient with gross residual disease may also be controlled.

Adjuvant radiation in childhood adrenal cancer is not without risk, however. Reports of radiation-associated second tumors include pancreatic carcinoma, renal cell carcinoma, and sarcoma of the breast (MAGEE et al. 1987; ANDLER et al.1978; SQUIRE et al. 1988).

Currently, most patients with recurrent or residual disease receive chemotherapy (LEFEVRE et al. 1983). While such treatment doses not offer the potential for cure, response rates approaching 40% have been reported with mitotane (op'DDD) (LEFEVRE et al. 1983; EPELMAN et al. 1990; CAPDEVILA-SANCHEZ et al. 1993). Significant prolongation of median survival is also reported. Responses to cisplatin, ketoconazole, and streptozotocin have also been reported (CROCK and CLARK 1989; HARINARAYAN et al. 1991).

Conclusions: Primary adenocarcinoma of the adrenal cortex is a rare spontaneous tumor in childhood, although it is seen with considerably more frequency in association with several clinical syndromes, most prominently the Li-Fraumeni syndrome, accounting for 10% of all childhood malignancies therein. The disease is encountered before the age of 8 years (most commonly before 6 years) and it has a different oncogenic mechanism involving chromosome 11 than the adult presentation (age peak fifth decade). In contradistinction to adults, most children present with sex hormone manifestations (virilization, feminization, or precocious puberty) which may or may not be associated with Cushing's syndrome. Treatment is primarily surgical but a role of adjuvant radiation therapy is suggested by the local-regional nature of the pattern of spread as well as by the propensity for local recurrence. This is supported to some extent by the clinical experience with radiation therapy.

23.5 Colorectal Carcinoma

23.5.1 Epidemiology and Etiology

Carcinoma of the colon and rectum is extremely rare in childhood and adolescence, accounting for a tiny proportion of malignancy in this age group (BIRCH et al. 1980; SMITH et al. 1976; RAMAKUMAR et al. 1963). A retrospective survey of admissions to Rajendra Hospital in Patiala, India from 1958 through 1961 revealed one colon carcinoma in 12 760 children admitted (RAMAKUMAR et al. 1963). The surveillance, epidemiology, and end results (SEER) data show less than 100 new cases per year of colorectal carcinoma in patients in the first and second decades (YOUNG et al. 1981). The median age at presentation is 15 years (PRATT and GEORGE 1982; KOH and JOHNSON 1986; LEWIS et al. 1990) with a preponderance of cases being diagnosed in African Americans (American Cancer Society 1991; KOH and JOHNSON 1986; CHABALKO and FRAUMENI 1975; ELLIOT and STEVEN 1984). Fraumeni's group at the National Cancer Institute noted in their epidemiologic survey that in fact the incidence of colorectal cancer was rising among young African Americans and that the patterns and incidence of the disease suggested an environmental influence (CHABALKO and FRAUMENI 1975). The majority of cases in the United States are reported from the Mississippi Valley (PRATT and GEORGE 1982; PRATT et al. 1977; ODONE et al. 1982). In line with Fraumeni's environmental postulate, at least one study has identified a high incidence of exposure to pesticides and herbicides among pediatric colorectal patients (CALDWELL et al. 1981).

Adolescents suffering from ulcerative colitis or Crohn's disease also appear to be at increased risk for colorectal malignancy. Endoscopy surveillance reports from Sweden, Finland, Ireland, and the United States all note a significant incidence of dysplasia (range 10.8%–22%), and approximately 10% of these patients will go on to develop large bowel cancer (ALLEN et al. 1985; ARNOT et al. 1977; ARVANITIS et al. 1990; BEDIKIAN et al. 1981; BELL and MAZZAFERRI 1993; BIRCH et al. 1980; BUCK et al. 1992; BULLOW 1984; BUSSEY 1970; CHABALKO and FRAUMENI 1975; CORREA and HAENSZEL 1978; DONALDSON et al. 1971; ELLIOTT and STEVEN 1984; ERBE 1976; FOCHIOS et al. 1986; GIARDELLO et al. 1987; HEIMANN et al. 1986; HRABOVSKY et al. 1984; JEGHERS et al. 1949; KARNER–HANUSCH et al. 1989; KOH and JOHNSON 1986; KORLEITZ et al. 1990; LEIDENIUS et al. 1991; LEIJONMARCK et al. 1990; LEWIS et al. 1990; LIPKIN et al. 1981; LYNCH et al. 1973; LYNCH et al. 1985; RAMAKUMAR et al. 1963; SCHRODER et al. 1983; SHERLOCK et al. 1975; SMITH MA et al. 1976; STEMPER et al. 1975; TAGUCHI et al. 1991; WATNE et al. 1983; WOOLRICH et al. 1992). Not all cancers were preceded by a biopsy of dysplasia, however. In ulcerative colitis patients managed with colectomy and ileorectal anastomosis, no postoperative rectal carcinomas were encountered, although nearly half the patients ultimately required completion proctectomy because of progressive inflammation or dysplasia (LEIJONMARCK et al. 1990). In Crohn's disease of the large bowel, a recent study noted that 18 of 356 patients (5%) manifested rectal dysplasia, of whom two progressed to frank carcinoma. Four other cancers were diagnosed in patients without rectal dysplasia (KORELITZ et al. 1990).

A small but significant number of pediatric colorectal cancers are found in association with several genetic syndromes (SHERLOCK et al. 1975; REED and NEEL 1955; McKUSICK 1964; BUSSEY 1970; STEMPER et al. 1975; HAGGITT and PITCOCK 1970; LYNCH et al. 1973). The best known is perhaps familial polyposis, an autosomal dominant genetic defect expressed phenotypically 80% of the time (SHERLOCK et al. 1975; LIPKIN et al. 1981). This figure corresponds to the rate of neoplasm in untreated patients with the syndrome (ERBE 1976). A retrospective review of 132 patients from the Cleveland Clinic showed that 64 patients (58%) died of colorectal carcinoma (ARVANITIS et al. 1990). Patients treated with subtotal colectomy and ileoproctostomy have manifested a very high rate of subsequent rectal cancers following this rectum-sparing procedure. Subsequent incidence of rectal cancer was 50% among patients undergoing subtotal colectomy for large bowel malignancy. The incidence of rectal cancer in such patients undergoing subtotal colectomy without a diagnosis of malignancy was less than 15% (HEIMANN et al. 1986; WATNE et al. 1983; HRABOVSKY et al. 1984; BULOW 1984). This argues strongly for total proctocolectomy in familial polyposis patients with a diagnosis of malignancy. Sphincter-sparing surgery with close observation is probably appropriate for prophylactic colectomy without malignancy.

Gardner's syndrome, encompassing polyposis, exostoses, and multiple cysts, is a variant of familial polyposis with a much lower incidence (LIPKIN et al. 1981). Oldfield's syndrome, multiple cysts and polyposis, is another related syndrome which can predispose to large bowel cancer (OLDFIELD 1954). Patients with Turcot's syndrome have been reported to have colorectal carcinomas in a background of polyposis in association with either glioma or glioblastoma (TURCOT et al. 1959; GOLDTHORN et al. 1983; SCHRODER et al. 1983; OBERLIN et al. 1991). The Peutz-Jegher's syndrome is yet another autosomal dominant hereditary disease characterized by hamartomatous polyps of the gastrointestinal tract and mucocutaneous melanin deposits. The associated incidence of gastrointestinal carcinomas is less than 15% (JEGHERS et al. 1949; BUCK et al. 1992; GIARDIELLO et al. 1987). There are additionally two hereditary syndromes associated with colorectal cancer which do not involve polyposis. Hereditary site-specific colon cancer (Lynch syndrome I) manifests itself as early-onset proximal colonic cancer with family members often developing neoplasia in essentially the same region of the large bowel (LYNCH et al. 1973, 1985; ARNDT et al. 1977; KARNER-HANUSCH et al. 1989). The cancer family syndrome (Lynch syndrome II) also includes early-onset proximal colonic cancer with site specificity as well as other associated extracolonic adenocarcinomas (particularly endometrial carcinoma) (LYNCH et al. 1973, 1985; ARNDT et al. 1977; KARNER-HANUSCH et al. 1989).

Iatrogenic causes of colonic carcinogenesis include ureterosigmoidoscopy for severe epispadias or congenital bladder exstrophy (BRISTOL 1981; SHELDON et al. 1983; HARZMANN et al. 1986; STRACHAN et al. 1987) and second malignancies following treatment for other childhood cancers (KUSHNER et al. 1988; CACAVIO et al. 1989; BLATT et al.

1992). The development of colon carcinoma at the anastomotic site following ureterosigmoidostomy is a well-recognized phenomenon. Interestingly, even if the urine is subsequently rediverted into an ileal conduit, the risk of carcinogenesis remains. The mechanism for cancer induction is somewhat controversial, with some authors implicating the introduction of nitrosamines in the large bowel and others postulating an etiology of hyperplasia secondary to the procedure itself (BRISTOL 1981; SHELDON et al. 1983; HARZMANN et al. 1986; STRACHAN et al. 1987). In survivors of childhood cancer, colorectal second cancers have been described following treatment for Hodgkin's disease (KUSHNER et al. 1988), rhabdomyosarcoma (CACAVIO et al. 1989), and Wilms' tumor (BLATT et al. 1992).

23.5.2 Presentation and Prognosis

Colorectal carcinoma in childhood and adolescence generally presents at an advanced stage and carries a much worse prognosis than the adult counterpart (ODONE et al. 1982; RAO et al. 1985; SMITH et al. 1976; KOH and JOHNSON 1986; LEWIS et al. 1990; ELLIOT and STEVEN 1984; KELSH and AVERY 1978; ANDERSSON and BERGDAHL 1976; KARLIN 1981; BEDIKIAN et al. 1981; PRATT et al. 1987, 1992; PRITCHARD and McCULLOCH 1986; ROSE et al. 1988; TAKAI and YAMAMURA 1988; TAGUCHI et al. 1991; SOBERMAN and LEONIDAS 1991). Unfortunately, the most common clinical presentation is that of crampy abdominal pain, often with palpable abdominal mass. This can be associated with anemia, weight loss, and ultimately rectal bleeding (KELSH and AVERY 1978; ANDERSSON and BERGDAHL 1986; KARLIN 1981). Clinical diagnostic evaluation should include a barium enema, abdominal-pelvic CT scan, and possible ultrasonography. A recent report suggests increased discrimination for abdominopelvic masses in the adolescent with MRI (SOBERMAN and LEONIDAS 1991). Chest x-ray and CT scan of the chest should also be obtained because of the high propensity for pulmonary metastases in advanced presentation.

Unfortunately, the overwhelming majority of young patients present with Dukes stage C or D disease (Table 23.4). In the St. Jude series (PRATT et al. 1992), 42 of 46 patients were in stage C or D. Long-term survival was less than 10% in these patients. The M.D. Anderson Hospital noted that 96% of their young patients had transmural invasion and that the 5-year survival was 25%–30% overall (BEDIKIAN et al. 1981). In a series of 29 patients reported from Osaka

Table 23.4. Staging of colorectal cancer

Dukes	Astler-Coller	TNM	Description
A	A	T1 N0 M0	Lesion limited to submucosa, nodes negative
B	B1	T2 N0 M0	Lesion into muscularis; nodes negative
	B2	T2 N0 M0	Lesion transmural, nodes negative
C	C1	T2 N1 M1	Lesion into muscularis; nodes positive
	C2	T2 N1 M0	Nodes positive, lesion transmural
D	D	T3 N1 M1	Metastases to liver, lung, bone; tumor unresectable

(TAKAI and YAMAMURA 1988), only 14 were able to undergo potentially curative resection, with three long-term survivors (21%). Overall survival in the series was 10%. There is a predilection for presentation in the right and transverse colon (BEDIKIAN et al. 1981; PRATT et al. 1987), which may also be a contributing factor to delayed diagnosis.

Although well established in the adult population, the role of CEA and CA 19-9 is somewhat controversial. A report from the University of Tennessee (KOH and JOHNSON 1986) found that all childhood colorectal carcinomas in their series were CEA positive and that active tumor and tumor regrowth were well correlated with rising serum CEA levels. A subsequent report from St. Jude (ANGEL and PRATT 1992), however, notes relatively poor specificity and sensitivity for both CEA and CA 19-9 in the clinical follow-up of childhood colorectal cancer.

There is widespread agreement upon the need for earlier diagnosis, but also for more aggressive therapy given the frequency of late-stage presentation (SMITH et al. 1976; KARLIN 1981; ANGEL and PRATT 1992). No separate analyses or trials exist for therapy in the young. As a consequence, recommendations for treatment are generally adapted from the adult population. Clearly, primary surgical resection is essential in patients with local regional disease. In patients without metastatic disease who undergo potentially curative resection, the risk of local recurrence in Astler-Coller stages B_2, C_1, and C_2 is sufficiently high to warrant the addition of postoperative radiation therapy (GUNDERSON and SOSIN 1974). Careful simulation and treatment planning including barium meal for small-bowel delineation and four-field treatment in the prone position are essential for optimal delivery of adjuvant radiation doses in the abdomen (HARTER 1992). Treatment to the previous volume of gross disease plus adjacent

draining lymph nodes should be carried to 45 Gy followed by a reduced field boost of a further 9 Gy to the primary tumor volume (HARTER 1992). Concomitant sensitizing chemotherapy based on 5-fluorouracil should also be administered. Additional adjuvant chemotherapy is also recommended (DONALDSON et al. 1976).

Conclusions: Colorectal carcinoma in childhood and adolescence is an extremely rare neoplasm, the SEER data suggesting an incidence of less than 100 cases per year in the United States. There is a postulated environmental etiology and some geographic and toxologic evidence to support this. The majority of cancers are spontaneous but some are associated with syndromes of genetic abnormality and/or familial predisposition. The overwhelming majority of patients present in an advanced stage, perhaps because of a low index of clinical suspicion. Because of this, prognosis is generally rather poor. Treatment recommendations borrowed from the adult population include surgery and concomitant radiation and chemotherapy for resectable local-regional disease. Adjuvant chemotherapy should also be considered.

References

Allen DC, Biggart JD, Pyper PC (1985) Large bowel mucosal dysplasia and carcinoma in ulcerative colitis. J Clin Pathol 38: 30–43
American Cancer Society (1991) Cancer facts and figures 1991. American Cancer Society, New York
Andersson A, Bergdahl L (1976) Carcinoma of the colon in children. A report of six new cases and a review of the literature. J Pediatr Surg 11: 967–971
Andler W, Havers W et al. (1978) Renal cell carcinoma following radiation therapy for an adrenal cortical carcinoma. J Pediatr 93: 634–636

Angel CA, Pratt CB (1992) Carcinoembryonic antigen and carbohydrate 19-9 antigen as markers for colorectal carcinoma in children and adolescents. Cancer 69: 1487–1491

Arndt RD, Kositchek RJ, Boasberg PD (1977) Colon carcinoma and the cancer family syndrome. JAMA 237: 2847–2848

Arvanitis ML, Jagelman DG et al. (1990) Mortality in patients with familial adenomatous polyposis. Dis Colon Rectum 38: 639–642

Baker SR, McClatchey KD (1981) Carcinoma of the nasopharynx in childhood. Otolaryngol Head Neck Surg 89: 555–559

Bass IS, Haller JO et al. (1985) Nasopharyngeal carcinoma. Clinical and radiographic findings in children. Radiology 156: 651–654

Beahrs OH, Henson DE, Hutter RVP, Myers MH (eds) (1992) Manual for staging of cancer, 4th edn. J.B. Lippincott, Philadelphia, pp 34–35

Bedikian AY, Kantarjian H et al. (1981) Colorectal cancer in young adults. South Med J 74: 920–924

Beierwaltes WH (1978) The treatment of thyroid carcinoma with radioactive iodine. Semin Nucl Med 8: 79–94

Beierwaltes WH, Nishiyama RH et al. (1982) Survival time and "cure" in papillary and follicular thyroid carcinoma with distant metastases: statistics following University Michigan therapy. J Nucl Med 23: 561–568

Bell B, Mazzaferri EL (1993) Familiar adenomatous polyposis (Gardner's syndrome) and thyroid carcinoma. A case report and review of the literature. Dig Dis Sci 38: 185–190

Berry MP, Smith CR et al. (1980) Nasopharyngeal carcinoma in the young. Int J Radiat Oncol Biol Phys 6: 415–421

Birch JM, Marsden HB, Swindell R (1980) Incidence of malignant disease in childhood: a 24-year review of the Manchester Children's Tumour Registry data. Br Cancer 42: 215–223

Blacklay A, Grossman A et al. (1986) Cranial irradiation for cerebral and nasopharyngeal tumours in children: evidence for the production of a hypothalamic defect in growth hormone release. J Endocrinol 108: 25–29

Blatt J, Olshan A et al. (1992) Second malignancies in very-long-term survivors of childhood cancer. Am J Med 93: 57–60

Block MA (1976) Surgery of the irradiated thyriod gland for possible carcinoma. Criteria, technique and results. In: Degroot LJ, Frohman LA, Kaplan EL, Refetoff S (eds) Proceedings of radiation-associated thyroid carcinoma conference held at the University of Chicago, 30 September–1 October 1976. Grune and Stratton, New York, p 539

Block MA (1981) Primary treatment of well-differentiated thyroid cancer. J Surg Oncol 16: 279–288

Block MA, Horn RC, Miller JM (1970) Hazards in the diagnosis and management of certain thyroid nodules in children. Am J Surg 120: 447–451

Bodie B, Novick AC et al. (1989) The Cleveland Clinic experience with adrenal cortical carcinoma. J Urol 141: 257–260

Borrelli D, Ingenito A et al. (1989) Surgical management of adrenal cortical carcinoma. Ital J Surg Sci 99: 69–74

Breaux EP, Guillamondegui OM (1980) Treatment of locally-invasive carcinoma of the thyroid: How radical? Am J Surg 140: 514–517

Bristol JB (1981) Ureterosigmoidostomy and colon carcinogenesis. Science 214: 351

Brown AP, Greening WP et al. (1984) Radioiodine treatment of metastatic thyroid carcinoma: the Royal Marsden Hospital experience. Br J Radiol 57: 323–327

Brugieres L, Henry I et al. (1991) Loss of heterozygosity for chromosome 11 markers in childhood and adult adrenocortical carcinoma (meeting abstract). Proceedings of the Annual Meeting of the American Society of Clinical Oncology 10: A183

Buck JL, Harned RK, Lichtenstein JE, Sobin LH (1992) Peutz-Jeghers syndrome. Radiographics 12: 365–378

Buckwalter JA, Thomas CG, Freeman JB (1975) Is childhood thyroid cancer a lethal disease? Ann Surg 181: 632–639

Bulow S (1984) The risk of developing rectal cancer after colectomy and ileorectal anastomosis in Danish patients with polyposis coli. Dis Colon Rectum 27: 726–729

Bussey HJR (1970) Gastrointestinal polyposis. Gut 11: 970–978

Cacavio A, Ghavimi G, Mandell L, Exelby P (1989) Late effects of therapy in long-term survivors of rhabdomyosarcoma (meeting abstract). Proceedings of the Annual Meeting of the American Society of Clinical Oncology 8: A1996

Caldwell GC, Cannon SB, Pratt CB, Arthur RD (1981) Serum pesticide levels in childhood colorectal carcinoma patients. Cancer 48: 774–778

Cance WG, Wells SA Jr (1985) Multiple endocrine neoplasia type IIa. Curr Probl Surg 22: 1–56

Capdevila-Sanchez J, Pavia-Sesma C et al. (1993) Carcinoma suprarenal virilizante: exeresisy tratamiento con op'DDD, Seguido de Curacion. Annales Espanoles de Pediatrica 38: 351–354

Chabalko JJ, Fraumeni JF (1975) Colorectal cancer in children. Epidemiologic aspects. Dis Colon Rectum 18: 1–3

Chan SH, Day HE et al. (1983) HLA and nasopharyngeal carcinoma in Chinese: a further study. Int J Cancer 32: 171–176

Chen MS, Lin FJ et al. (1989) Prospective hormone study of hypothalamic-pituitary function in patients with nasopharyngeal carcinoma after high dose irradiation. Jpn J Clin Oncol 19: 265–270

Christensen SB, Ljungberg O, Tibblin S (1983) Surgical treatment of thyroid carcinoma in a defined population 1960–1977. Evaluation of the results after a conservative surgical approach. Am J Surg 14: 349–354

Chudler RM, Kay R (1989) Adrenocortical carcinoma in children. Urol Clin North Am 16: 469–479

Cibas ES, Medeiros LJ et al. (1990) Cellular DNA profiles of benign and malignant adrenocortical tumors. Am J Surg Pathol 14: 948–955

Cohn KH, Backdahl M et al. (1984) Biologic considerations and operative strategy in papillary thyroid carcinoma. Arguments against the routine performance of total thyroidectomy. Surgery 96: 957–971

Cohn K, Gottesman L, Brennan M (1986) Adrenocortical carcinoma. Surgery 100: 1170–1175

Conard RA (1977) A summary of thyroid findings in Marshallese 22 years after exposure to radioactive fallout. In: DeGroot LJ, Frohman LA, Kaplan EL, Refetoff S (eds) Proceedings of radiation-associated thyroid carcinoma conference held at the University of Chicago, 30 September–1 October 1976. Grune and Stratton, New York, pp 241–257

Correa P, Haenszel W (1978) The epidemiology of large bowel cancer. Adv Cancer Res 26: 1–141

Counter RT, Linares L, Shaw HJ, Dalley VM (1980) Cancer of the nasopharynx in under 21-year-olds, a review. Clin Oncol 6: 213–220

Crock PA, Clark AC (1989) Combination chemotherapy for adrenal carcinoma: response in a 5½ year old male. Med Pediatr Oncol 17: 62–65

Deaconson TF, Wilson SD, Cerletty JM, Komorowski RA (1986) Total or near total thyroidectomy versus limited resection for radiation-associated thyroid nodules. A twelve-year follow-up of patients in a thyroid screening program. Surgery 100: 1116–1120

Deutsch M, Mercado R, Parsons JA (1978) Cancer of the nasopharynx in children. Cancer 41: 1128–1133

Donaldson MH, Taylor P, Rawitscher R, Sewell JB (1971) Colon carcinoma in childhood. Pediatrics 48: 307–312

Duffy BJ Jr, Fitzgerald PJ (1950) Thyroid cancer in childhood and adolescence: report of 28 cases. J Clin Endocrinol 10: 1296–1308

Easton JM, Levine PH, Hyams VJ (1980) Nasopharyngeal carcinoma in the United States. A pathologic study of 177 U.S. and 30 foreign cases. Arch Otolaryngol 106: 88–91

Elliot MS, Steven DM (1984) Carcinoma of the colon and rectum in patients under 30 years of age. South Afr Med J 66: 129–131

Ellouz R, Cammoun M, Ben-Attia R, Bahi J (1978) Nasopharyngeal carcinoma in children and adolescents in Tunisia. Clinical aspects and the paraneoplastic syndrome. IARC Scientific Publications 20: 115–129

Epelman S, Gorender EF, Lopes LF, Bianchi A (1990). The role of op'DDD in childhood adrenal carcinoma (meeting abstract). Proceedings of the Annual Meeting of the American Society of Clinical Oncology 9: A1148

Epelman S, Gorender EF, Spindola-Castro A, Bianchi A (1991) High incidence of adrencortical carcinomas in Sao Paulo (meeting abstract). Proceedings of the Annual Meeting of the American Society for Clinical Oncology 10-A1109

Erbe RW (1976) Current concepts in genetics, inherited gastrointestinal-polyposis syndromes. N Engl J Med 294: 1101–1104

Exelby PE, Frazell EL (1969) Carcinoma of the thyroid in children. Surg Clin North Am 49: 249–259

Fahraeus R, HL et al. (1988) Expression of Epstein-Barr virus-encoded proteins in nasopharyngeal carcinoma. Int J Cancer 42: 329–338

Farndon JR, Leight GS et al. (1986) Familial medullary thyroid carcinoma without associated endocrinopathies: a distinct clinical entity. Br J Surg 73: 278–281

Farrar WB, Cooperman M, James AG (1980) Surgical management of papillary and follicular carcinoma of the thyroid. Ann Surg 92: 701–704

Favus MJ, Schneider AB et al. (1976) Thyroid cancer occurring as a late consequence of head and neck irradiation. N Engl J Med 294: 1019–1025

Fernandez CH, Cangir A, Samaan NA, Rivera R (1976) Nasopharyngeal carcinoma in children. Cancer 37: 2787–2791

Fjalling M, Tisell L et al. (1986) Benign and malignant thyroid nodules after neck irradiation. Cancer 58: 1219–1224

Fochios SE, Sommers SC, Korelitz BI (1986) Sigmoidoscopy and biopsy in surveillance for cancer and ulcerative colitis. J Clin Gastroenterol 8: 249–254

Frasch W, Gnekow A et al. (1992) Nebennierenrinden-Karzinom, Eine Seltene Ursache Eines Conn-Syndroms im Kindesalter. Monastsschr Kinderheilkd 140: 95–101

Gasparini M, Lombardi F et al. (1988) Combined radiotherapy and chemotherapy in stage T3 and T4 nasopharyngeal carcinoma in children. J Clin Oncol 6: 491–494

Giardiello FM, Welsh SB et al. (1987) Increased risk of cancer in the Peutz-Jeghers syndrome. N Engl J Med 316: 1511–1514

Godine LB, Berdon WE, Brasch RC, Leonidas JC (1990) Adrenocortical carcinoma with extension into inferior vena cava and right atrium. Report of 3 cases in children. Pediatr Radiol 20: 166–168

Goldthorn JF, Powars D, Hays DM (1983) Adenocarcinoma of the colon and rectum in the adolescent. Surgery 93: 409–414

Green DM, Breslow NE, Beckwith JB, Norkool P, (1993) Screening of children with hemihypertrophy, aniridia, and Beckwith-Wiedemann syndrome in patients with Wilms' tumor: a report from the National Wilms' Tumor Study. Med Pediatr Oncol 21: 188–192

Green MH, Fraumeni JF, Hoover R (1977) Nasopharyngeal cancer among young people in the United States. Racial variations by cell type. J Natl Cancer Inst 58: 1267–1270

Greenspan FS (1977) Radiation exposure on thyroid cancer. JAMA 237: 2089–2091

Grondal S, Curstedt T (1991) Steroid profile in serum. Increased levels of sulphated pregnenolone and pregn-5-ene-3β,20α-diol in patients with adrenocortical carcinoma. Acta Endocrinol (Copenh) 124: 381–385

Gunderson LL, Sosin H (1974) Areas of failure found at reoperation (Second or symptomatic look) following "curative surgery" for adenocarcinoma of the rectum. Clinical pathologic correlation and implications for adjuvant therapy. Cancer 34: 1278–1283

Haggitt RC, Pitcock JA (1970) Familial juvenile polyposis of the colon. Cancer 26: 1232–1238

Harinarayan CV, Gupta S et al. (1991) Clinical utility of Ketoconazol in cases of adrenocortical carcinoma. Indian J Cancer 28: 896–201

Harness JK, Thompson NW, Nishiyama RH (1971) Childhood carcinoma. Arch Surg 102: 278–284

Harter KW (1992) Principles of radiotherapy in gastrointestinal cancer. In: Ahlgren JD, Macdonald JS (eds) op cit, pp 51–59

Harzmann R, Kopper B, Carl P (1986) Karzinominduktion durch Harnab-oder-umleitung "uber Darmabschnitte? Urologe 25: 698–703

Heimann TM, Bolnick K, Aufses AH Jr (1986) Results of surgical treatment for familial polyposis coli. Am J Surg 15: 276–278

Hempelmann LH (1968) Risk of thyroid neoplasms after irradiation in childhood. Science 160: 159–163

Hempelmann LH, Hall WJ et al. (1975) Neoplasms in persons treated with x-rays in infancy. J Natl Cancer Inst 55: 519–530

Henderson BE, Louie E et al. (1976) Risk factors associated with nasopharyngeal carcinoma. N Engl J Med 295: 1101–1106

Henle G, Henle W (1976) Epstein-Barr virus-specific IgA serum antibodies as an outstanding feature of nasopharyngeal carcinoma. Int J Cancer 17: 1–8

Henley DJ, van Heerden JA et al. (1983) Adrenal cortical carcinoma: a continuing challenge. Surgery 94: 926–931

Hill CS, Ibanez ML et al. (1973) Medullary (solid) carcinoma of the thyroid gland. Medicine (Baltimore) 52: 141–171

Howell MA (1975) Diet as an etiological factor in the development of cancers of the colon and rectum. J Chronic Dis 28: 67–80

Hrabovsky EE, Watne AL, Carrier JM (1984) Changing management in familial polyposis. Role of ileoanal endorectal pull-through. Am J Surg 147: 130–133

Huang DP, Ho JHC et al. (1978) Presence of BBNA in nasopharyngeal carcinoma and control patients tissues related to EBV serology. Int J Cancer 22: 266–274

Hussain S, Beldegrun A et al. (1985) Differentiation of malignant from benign adrenal masses. Predictive indices on computed tomography. Am J Roentgenol 144: 61–65

Ingersoll L, Woo SY, Donaldson S et al. (1990) Nasopharyngeal carcinoma in the young. A combined M.D. Anderson and Stanford Experience. Int J Radiat Oncol Biol Phys 99: 881–887

Jeghers H, McKusick VA, Katz JH (1949) Generalized intestinal polyposis and melanin spots of the oral mucosa, lips and digits. N Eng J Med 241: 993–1005

Jenkin RD, Anderson JR et al. (1981) Nasopharyngeal carcinoma – a retrospective review of patients less than 30 years of age. A report from the Children's Study Group. Cancer 47: 360–366

Jereb B, Huvos A, Steinherz P, Unao A (1980) Nasopharyngeal carcinoma in children. Review of 16 cases. Int J Radiat Oncol Biol Phys 6: 487–491

Kaplan MM, Garnick MB et al. (1983) Risk factors for thyroid abnormalities after neck irradiation for childhood cancer. Am J Med 74: 272–280

Karlin DA (1981) Adenocarcinoma of the large bowel in patients less than 40 years of age. Cancer Bull 33: 35–36

Karner-Hanusch J, Feil W, Schiessel R (1989) Das familiäre Kolonkarzinom. Wien Klin Wochenschr 101: 125–129

Kelsh JM, Avery FW (1978) Primary carcinoma of the rectum in a 13-year-old patient. North Carolina Med J 39: 423–424

Kerr GD (1978) Organ dose estimates for the Japanese atomic bomb survivors. Oakridge National Laboratory Report 5436. National Technical Information Service, Springfield, VA, pp 1–46

Kim JH, Leeper RD (1983) Combination Adriamycin and radiation therapy for locally-advanced carcinoma of the thyroid gland. Int J Radiat Oncol Biol Phys 9: 565–567

Kim JH, Leeper RD (1987) Treatment of locally-advanced thyroid carcinoma with combination doxorubicin and radiation therapy. Cancer 60: 2372–2375

Kirkland RT, Kirkland JL et al. (1973) Solitary nodules in 30 children and report of a child with a thyroid abscess. Pediatrics 51: 85–90

Klein G, Giovanella BC et al. (1974) Direct evidence for the presence of Epstein-Barr virus, DNA and nuclear antigen in malignant epithelial cells from patients with poorly differentiated crcinoma of the nasopharynx. Proc Natl Acad Sci 71: 4747–4751

Koh SJ, Johnson WW (1986) Cancer of the large bowel in children. South Med J 79: 931–935

Korelitz BI, Lauwers GY, Sommers SC (1990) Rectal mucosa Dysplasia in Crohn's disease. Gut 31: 1382–1386

Kushner BH, Zauber A, Tan CT (1988) Second malignancies after childhood Hodgkin's disease. The Memorial Sloane-Kettering Cancer Center experience. Cancer 62: 1364–1370

LaNasa JJ, Putney JF (1974) Nasopharyngeal malignancy in childhood. South Med J 67: 1363–1364

Leeper RD (1985) Thyroid cancer. Med Clin NOrth Am 69: 1079–1096

LeFevre M, Gerard-Gerard-Marchant R et al. (1983) Adrenal cortical carcinoma in children: 42 patients treated from 1958 to 1980 at Villejuif. Cancer Treatment Res 17: 265–276

Leidenius M, Kellokumpu I et al. (1991) Dysplasia and carcinoma in long-standing ulcerative colitis: an endoscopic and hostologic surveillance programme. Gut 32: 1521–1525

Leijonmarck CE, Lofberg R, Ost A, Hellers G (1990) Long term results of ileorectal anastomosis in ulcerative colitis in Stockholm County. Dis Colon Rectum 33: 195–200

Lewis CT, Riley WE, Georgeson K, Warren JH (1990) Carcinoma of the colon and rectum in patients less than 20 years of age. South Med J 83: 383–385

Liechty RD, Safaie-Shirazi S, Soper R T (1972) Carcinoma of the thyroid in children. Surg Gynecol Obstet 134: 595–599

Lipkin M, Winawer SJ, Sherlock P (1981) Early identification of individuals at increased risk for cancer of the large intestine. Part I. Definition of high risk populations. Clin Bull 11: 13–21

Lobo-Sanahuja F, Garcia I, Carranza A, Camacho A (1986) Treatment and outcome of undifierentiated carcinoma of the nasopharynx in childhood. A thirteen year experience. Med Pediatr Oncol 14: 6–11

Lombardi F, Gasparini M et al. (1982) Nasopharyngeal carcinoma childhood. Med Pediatr Oncol 10: 243–250

Lote K, Andersen K, Nordal E, Brennhovd IO (1980) Familiar occurrence of papillary thyroid carcinoma. Cancer 46: 1291–1297

Lynch HT, Giurgis H et al. (1973) Genetics and colon cancer. Arch Surg 106: 669–675

Lynch HT, Kimberling W et al. (1985) Hereditary non-polyposis colorectal cancer (Lynch syndromes I and II). Cancer 56: 934–938

Magee BJ, Gattamanei HR, Pearson D (1987) Adrenal cortical carcinoma: survival after radiotherapy. Clin Radiol 38: 587–588

Malkin D (1993) The Li-Fraumeni syndrome. In: DeVita VT Jr, Hellman S, Rosenberg SA (eds) Principles and Practice of oncology updates, vol 7. J.B. Lippincott, Philadelphia, pp 1–14

Markoe AM, Serber W, Micaily B, Brady LW (1991) Radiation therapy for adjunctive treatment of adrenal cortical carcinoma. Am J Clin Oncol 14: 170–174

Maxon HR, Thomas SR et al. (1977) Ionizing radiation and the induction of clinically significant disease in the human thyroid gland. Am J Med 63: 967–978

Maxon HR, Thomas SR et al. (1983) Relation between effective radiation dose and outcome of radioiodine therapy for thyroid cancer. N Engl J Med 309: 937–941

Maxon HR, Englaro EE et al. (1992) Radioiodine-131 therapy for well-differentiated thyroid cancer. A quantitative radiation dosemetric approach: outcome and validation in 85 patients. J Nucl Med 33: 1132–1136

Mazzaferri EL, Young RL (1981) Papillary thyroid carcinoma: a ten-year follow-up report of the impact of therapy in 576 patients. Am J Med 70: 511–518

Mazzaferri EL, Young RL et al. (1977) Papillary thyroid carcinoma: the impact of therapy in 576 patients. Medicine (Baltimore) 56: 171–196

McConahey WM, Hayles AB (1976) Radiation to the head, neck, and upper thorax of the young and thyroid neoplasia. Proc Inst Med Chic 31: 91–92

McKusick VA (1964) Genetics and large bowel caner. Am J Dig Dis 19: 954

Melvin KEW, Tashjian AH (1968) The syndrome of excessive thyrocalcitonin produced by medullary carcinoma of the thyroid. Proc Natl Acad Sci 59: 1216–1222

Miller D (1980) The etiology of nasopharyngeal cancer and its management. Otolaryngol Clin North Am 13: 167–175

Miller JM, Hamburger JI, Kini SR (1979) Diagnosis of thyroid nodules. Use of fine needle aspiration and needle biopsy. JAMA 241: 481–484

Miller JM, Kini SR, Hamburger JI (1985) The diagnosis of malignant follicular neoplasms of the thyroid by needle biopsy. Cancer 55: 2812–2817

Modan B, Ron E, Werner A (1977) Thyroid neoplasms in a population irradiated for scalp tinea in childhood. In: DeGroot LJ, Frohman LA, Kaplan EL, Refetoff SR (eds) Radiation associated thyroid carcinoma. Grune and Stratton, New York, pp 449–457

Morrison P, Busch A et al. (1981) Cancer of the nasopharynx in young patients. J Surg Oncol 27: 181–185

Naegele RF, Champion J et al. (1982) Nasopharyngeal carcinoma in American children. Epstein-Barr virus-specific antibody titer and prognosis. Int J Cancer 29: 209–212

Neblett WW, Frexes-Steed M, Scott HW Jr (1987) Experience with adrenocortical neoplasms in childhood. Am Surg 53: 117–125

Norton JA, Froome LC, Farrell RE, Wells SA Jr (1979) Multiple endocrine neoplasia type IIb. The most aggressive form of medullary thyroid carcinoma. Surg Clin North Am 59: 109–118

Oberlin O, Brugieres L et al. (1991) Childhood cancer in siblings (meeting abstract). Med Pediatr Oncol 99: 395

Odone V, Chang L et al. (1982) The natural history of colorectal carcinoma in adolescents. Cancer 49: 1716–1720

Ogita S, Tokiwa K et al. (1989) Adrenocortical carcinoma in a child with congenital hemihypertrophy. Z Kinderchir 44: 166–168

Old LJ, Boyse EA et al. (1966) Precipitating antibody in human serum to an antigen present in cultured Burkitt's lymphoma cells. Proc Natl Acad Sci 56: 1699–1704

Oldfield MC (1954) The association of familial polyposis of the colon with multiple sebaceous cysts. Br J Surg 41: 534–541

Ozaki O, Notsu T, Hirai K, Mori T (1983) Differentiated carcinoma of the thyroid gland. World J Surg 7: 181–185

Pao WJ, Hustu HO et al. (1989) Pediatric nasopharyngeal carcinoma. Long term follow-up of 29 patients. Int J Radiat Oncol Biol Phys 17: 299–305

Papavasiliou C, Pavlatou M, Pappas J (1977) Nasopharyngeal cancer in patients under the age of 30 years. Cancer 40: 2312–2316

Parker LN, Belsky JL et al. (1973) Thyroid carcinoma diagnosed between 13 and 26 years after exposure to atomic radiation. A study of the ABCC-JNIH adult health care study population, Hiroshima and Nagasaki 1958-1971. Atomic Bomb Casualty Commission Technical Report PR 5–73. Hiroshima Atomic Bomb Casualty Commission, Washington, D.C.

Parker LN, Belsky JL et al. (1974) Thyroid carcinoma after exposure to atomic radiation. Ann Intern Med 80: 600–604

Percarpio B, Knowlton AH (1976) Radiation therapy of adrenal cortical carcinoma. Acta Radiol Ther Phys Biol 15: 288–292

Phade VR, Lawrence WR, Max MH (1981) Familial papillary carcinoma of the thyroid. Arch Surg 116: 836–837

Pick T, Maurer HM, McWilliams NB (1974) Lympho-epithelioma in childhood. J Pediatr 84: 96–100

Prando A, Wallace S et al. (1990) Sonographic findings of adrenal corticocarcinomas in children. Pediatr Radiol 20(3): 163–165

Pratt CB, George SL (1982) Epidemic colon cancer in children and adolescents. In: Correa P, Haenszel W (eds) Epidemiology of cancer of the digestive tract. Martinus Nijhoff, The Hague, pp 127–146

Pratt CB, Terrell W, Shanks E (1976) Carcinoma of the colon on adolescents: treatment with vincristine, methyl CCNU and 5-fluorouracil. Proceedings of the American Association for Cancer Research 17: 25

Pratt CB, Rivera G et al. (1977) Colorectal carcinoma in adolescents. Implications regarding etiology. Cancer 40 (Supplt): 2464–2472

Pratt CB, Parham DM, Rao BN, Fleming ID (1987) Adolescent colon carcinoma, colonic polyps and neurofibromatosis (meeting abstract). Proceedings of Annual Meeting of the American Association for Cancer Research 28: 254

Pratt CB, Rao BN et al. (1992) Colon carcinomas in adolescence (meeting abstract). Proceedings of the Annual Meeting of the American Association for Cancer Research 33: A1550

Pritchard J, McCulloch W (1986) Carcinomas and other very rare tumours in children. In: Voute PA, et al. (eds) Cancer in children. Clinical management, 2nd edn. Springer, New York Berlin Heidelberg, pp 348–357

Qin DX, Hu YH, Yan JH et al. (1988) Analysis of 1379 patients with nasopharyngeal carcinoma treated by radiation. Cancer 61: 1117–1124

Rallison ML, Dobyns BM et al. (1975) Thyroid nodularity in children. JAMA 233: 1069–1072

Ramakumar L, Sood SC, Diwan SP (1963) Childhood malignancies: a statistical survey. Indian J Child Health 12: 490–495

Raney RB Jr, Meadows AT, D'Angio GJ (1983) Adrenocortical carcinoma in children. Experience at the Children's Hospital of Philadelphia, 1961–1980. Cancer Treatment Res 17: 303–305

Rao BN, Pratt CB et al. (1985) Colon carcinoma in children and adolescents: a review of 30 cases. Cancer 55: 1322–1326

Reed TE, Neel JV (1955) A genetic study of multiple polyposis of the colon. Am J Hum Genet 7: 236–259

Refetoff S, Harrison J et al. (1975) Continuing occurrence of thyroid carcinoma after radiation to the head and neck in infancy and childhood. N Engl J Med 292: 171–175

Regaud C (1921) Lympho-epitheliome de l'hypopharynx traite par la roentgentherapie. Bull Soc Franc Otorhinolaryngol 34: 209–214

Ribeiro RC, Sandrini-Neto RS et al. (1990) Adrenocortical carcinoma in children: a study of 40 cases. J Clin Oncol 8: 67–74

Roper HP, Essex-Cater A et al. (1986) Nasopharyngeal carcinoma in children. Pediatr Hematol Oncol 3: 143–152

Rose RH, Axelrod DM, Aldea PA, Beck AR (1988) Colorectal carcinoma in the young. A case report and review of the literature. Clin Pediatr 27: 107–108

Roucayrol JC, Leroy-Willig A, Courtieu J, Luton JP (1986) Mise en evidence par spectroscopie RMN a 1.5 tesla des changements de la proportion lipides/eau en pathologie du cortex surrenalien. Comptes Rendus Des Seances de la Societe de Biologie et de Ses Filiales. 180: 677–682

Samaan NA, Maheshwari YK et al. (1983) Impact of therapy for differentiated carcinoma of the thyroid: an analysis of 706 cases. J Clin Endocrinol Metab 56: 1131–1138

Samaan NA, Schultz PN, Haynie TP, Ordonez NG (1985) Pulmonary metastasis of differentiated thyroid carcinoma: treatment results in 101 patients. J Clin Endocrinol Metab 60: 376–380

Samaan NA, Schultz PN et al (1992) The results of various modalities of treatment of well-differentiated thyroid carcinomas: a retrospective review of 1599 patients. J Clin endocrinol Metab 75: 714–720

Schier F, Hauss J, Vetter H, Zurwonne F (1988) Lokalisationsdiagnostiche und postoperative Ergebnisse bei hormonproduzierenden Tumoren der Nebennirerinde – Übersicht – Über 51 Fälle. Z Kinderchir 43(4): 262–266

Schmincke A (1921) Über lymphoepitheliale Geschwulste. Beitr Pathol Anat

Schneider AB, Favus MJ et al. (1978) Incidence, prevalence and characteristics of radiation induced thyroid tumors. Am J Med 64: 243–252

Schneider AB, Pinsky S, Bekerman C, Ryo UY (1980) Characteristics of 108 thyroid cancers detected by screening in a population with a history of head and neck irradiation. Cancer 46: 1218–1227

Schroder S, Moehrs D et al. (1983) The Turcot syndrome. Report of an additional case and review of the literature. Dis Colon Rectum 26: 533–538

Scott MD, Crawford JD (1976) Solitary thyroid nodules in childhood: Is the incidence of thyroid carcinoma declining? Pediatrics 58: 521–525

Sham JS, Poon YF, Wei WI, Choy D (1990) Nasopharyngeal carcinoma in young patients. Cancer 65: 2606–2610

She Y, Wu X, Wang R (1980) Chung Hua Hsiao Erh Wai Ko Tsa Chih 1(3): 162–164

Sheldon CA, McKinley CR, Hartig PR, Gonzalez R (1983) Carcinoma at the site of ureterosigmoidostomy. Dis Colon Rectum 26: 55–58

Sherlock P, Lipkin M, Winauer SJ (1975) Predisposing factors in carcinoma of the colon. Adv Intern Med 20: 121–150

Shore RE, Albert RE, Pasternak BS (1976) Follow-up study of patients treated by x-ray epilation for tinea capitis. Arch Environ Health 31: 17–28

Shvero J, Gal R et al. (1988) Anaplastic thyroid carcinoma: a clinical, histologic and immunohistochemical study. Cancer 62: 319–325

Sierk AE, Askin FB, Reddick RL, Thomas CG Jr (1990) Pediatric thyroid cancer. Pediatr Pathol 10: 877–893

Simons MJ, Wee GB et al. (1976) Immunogenetic aspects of nasopharyngeal carcinoma. IV. Increased risk in Chinese of nasopharyngeal carcinoma associated with a Chinese-related HCA profile. J Natl Cancer Inst 57: 977–980

Simpson WJ, Carruthers JS (1978) The role of external radiation in the management of papillary and follicular thyroid cancer. Am J Surg 136: 457–460

Simpson WJ, Panzarella T et al. (1988) Papillary and follicular thyroid cancer. Impact of treatment in 1578 patients. Int J Radiat Oncol Biol Phys 14: 1063–1075

Sirinelli D, Silberman B et al. (1989) Beckwith-Wiedemann syndrome and neural crest tumors. A report of two cases. Pediatr Radiol 99: 242–245

Smith LE ((1992) Colorectal cancer surgical approach. In: Ahlgren JD, Macdonald JS (eds) Gastrointestinal oncology. J.B. Lippincott, Philadelphia, p 299

Smith MA, Golding RL, Katz A (1976) Carcinoma of the colon in child. South Afr Med J 50: 879–880

Smith R, Blum C, Benua RS, Fawwaz RA (1985) Radioactive iodine treatment of metastatic thyroid carcinoma with clinical thyrotoxicosis. Clin Nucl Med 10: 874–875

Snow JB Jr (1975) Carcinoma of the nasopharynx in children. Ann Otolaryngol 84: 817–826

Snow JB (1977) Neoplasms of the nasopharynx in children. Otolaryngol Clin North Am 10: 11–24

Soberman N, Leonidas JC (1991) Magnetic resonance imaging in the diagnosis of adolescent colorectal carcinoma. Pediatr Radiol 21: 531–532

Socolow EL, Hashizume A, Neriishi S, Niitani R (1963) Thyroid carcinoma in man after exposure to ionizing radiation. A summary of the findings in Hiroshima and Nagasaki. N Engl J Med 268: 406–410

Squire R, Bianchi A, Jakate SM (1988) Radiation-induced sarcoma of the breast in a female adolescent. Case report with histologic and therapeutic considerations. Cancer 61: 2444–2447

Stemper TJ, Kent TH, Summers RW (1975) Juvenile polyposis and gastrointestinal carcinoma. Ann Intern Med 83: 639–646

Stewart DR, Morris-Jones PH, Jooleys A (1974) Carcinoma of the adrenal gland in children. J Pediatr Surg 9: 59–67

Strachan JR, Rees HC, Cox R, Woodhouse CR (1987) Mucin changes adjacent to carcinoma following ureterosigmoidostomy. Eur Urol 13(6): 4–9

Taguchi T, Suita S et al. (1991) Carcinoma of the colon in children: a case report and review of 41 Japanese cases. J Pediatr Gastroenterol Nutr 12: 394–399

Takai S, Yamamura M (1988) Carcinoma of the colon in children: report of a case and review of the literature. Jpn J Surg 18: 341–345

Tan BC, Kunaratnam N (1966) Hypopituitary dwarfism following radiotherapy for nasopharyngeal carcinoma. Clin Radiol 17: 302–304

Telander RL, Wolf SA et al. (1986) Endocrine disorders of the pancreas and adrenal cortex in pediatric patients. Mayo Clin Proc 61: 459–466

Thoresen SO (1992) Li-Fraumeni Syndromet og p53-genet. Tidsskrift Nor Laegeforen 112: 887–889

Troost T, Thomas DS (1992) Nasopharyngeal brachytherapy under direct visualization. Meeting abstract, the Third International Conference of Head and Neck Cancer, San Francisco

Tucker MA, Morris-Jones PH et al. (1991) Therapeutic radiation at a young age is linked to secondary thyroid cancer. Cancer Res 51: 2885–2888

Turcot J, Despies JP, St. Pierre F (1959) Malignant tumors of the central nervous system associated with familial polyposis of the colon. Report of 2 cases. Dis Colon Rectum 2: 465–468

Van Nostrand D, Neutze J, Atkins F (1986) Side effects of "rational dose" iodine 131 therapy for metastatic welldifferentiated thyroid carcinoma. J Nucl Med 27: 1519–1527

Van Slooten H, Schaberg A et al. (1985) Morphological characteristics of benign and malignant adrenocortical tumors. Cancer 55: 766–772

Vita HC, Mendiondo OA et al. (1983) Nasopharyngeal carcinoma in the second decade of life. Radiology 148: 253–256

Walfish PG, Hazani E et al. (1977a) Combined ultrasound and needle aspiration cytology in the assessment and management of hypofunctioning thyroid nodule. Ann Intern Med 87: 270–274

Walfish PG, Hazani E et al. (1977b) A prospective study of combined ultrasonography and needle aspiration biopsy in the assessment of the hypofunctioning thyroid nodule. Surgery 82: 474–482

Wang CC (1990) Radiation therapy for head and neck neoplasms: indications, techniques and results, 2nd edn. Yearbook Medical, Chicago, pp 280–281

Wang CC, Busse J, Gitterman M (1975) A simple afterloading applicator for intracavitary irradiation for carcinoma of the nasopharynx. Radiology 115: 737–738

Warneford S, Townsend M et al. (1991) Over-expression of the retinoblastoma gene in a familial adrenocortical carcinoma. Cell Growth differentiation 2: 439–445

Warneford SG, Witton LJ et al. (1992) Germ-line splicing mutation of the p53 gene in a cancer-prone family. Cell Growth Differentiation 3: 839–846

Watne AL, Carrier JM et al. (1983) The occurrence of carcinoma of the rectum following ileoproctostomy for familial polyposis. Ann Surg 997: 550–554

Weber CA, Clark OH (1985) Surgery for thyroid disease. Med Clin North Am 69: 1097–1115

Weiss LM, Medeiros LJ, Vickery AL Jr (1989) Pathologic features of prognostic significance in adrenocortical carcinoma. Am J Surg Pathol 13: 202–206

Wells SA Jr (1990) Multiple endocrine neoplasia type II. Recent Results Cancer Res 118: 70–78

Williams ED, Brown CL, Doniach I (1966) Pathological and clinical findings in a series of 67 cases of medullary carcinoma of the thyroid. J Clin Pathol 19: 103–113

Winship T, Rosvoll RV (1961) Childhood thyroid carcinoma. Cancer 14: 734–743

Winship TH, Rosvoll RV (1970) Thyroid carcinoma in childhood; final report on a 20-year study. Clin Proc Children's Hosp Natl Med Center 26: 327–338

Wolfe HJ, Melvin KE et al. (1973) C-cell hyperplasia preceding medullary thyroid carcinoma. N Engl J Med 289: 437–441

Woolrich AJ, DaSilva MD, Korelitz BI (1992) Surveillance in the routine management of ulcerative colitis: the predictive value of low grade dysplasia. Gastroenterology 103: 431–438

Wuang TB (1990) Cancer of the nasopharynx in childhood. Cancer 66: 968–971

Wynder EL, Shigematsu T (1967) Environmental factors of cancer of the colon and rectum. Cancer 20: 1520–1561

Young RL, Mazzaferri EL, Rahe AJ, Dorfman SG (1980) Pure follicular thyroid carcinoma impact of therapy in 214 patients. J Nucl Med 21: 733–737

Young YL, Percy CL, Asire AJ (eds) (1981) Surveillance, epidemiology and end results incidence and mortality data, 1973–1977. National Cancer Institute Monograph 57. United States Government Printing Office, Washington, D.C.

Yu MC, JHC, Lai SH, Henderson BE (1986) Cantonese-style salted fish as a cause of nasopharyngeal carcinoma. Report of a case-control study in Hong Kong. Cancer Res 46: 956–961

Zabbo A, Straffon RA, Montie JE (1987) Adrenocortical carcinoma. In: Javadpour N (ed) Principles and management of adrenal cancer. Springer, New York Berlin Heidelberg pp 113–120

Zur Hausen H, Schulte-Holthausen H et al. (1970) Epstein-Barr virus DNA in biopsies of Burkitt's tumors and anaplastic carcinoma of the nasopharynx. Nature 228: 1056–1059

24 Unusual Neoplasms of Childhood

J. Robert Cassady

CONTENTS

24.1 Introduction 369
24.2 Aggressive Fibromatosis 369
24.2.1 Hormonal Treatment 370
24.2.2 Cytotoxic Chemotherapy............... 370
24.2.3 Radiation Therapy 370
24.3 Juvenile Nasopharyngeal Angiofibroma 371
24.3.1 Surgical Treatment..................... 372
24.3.2 Radiation Therapy 372
24.3.3 Chemotherapy 373
24.4 Plasma Cell Granuloma 373
24.4.1 Treatment.......................... 373
24.5 Giant Cell Tumor and
       Aneurysmal Bone Cyst 374
24.5.1 Treatment 374
       References 376

24.1 Introduction

The radiation oncologist may be consulted for a number of unusual tumors which are generally considered to be benign in the classical sense – that is, they do not develop metastases – but which may be locally aggressive and result in death or considerable disability if not managed properly.

24.2 Aggressive Fibromatosis

The specific nature of aggressive fibromatosis, a rare tumor-like condition, is uncertain (Das Gupta et al. 1969; Greenberg et al. 1981; Reitamo et al. 1982; Häyry et al. 1982; Rock et al. 1984; Kiel and Suit 1984; Posner et al. 1989). Also known as desmoid tumors and musculoaponeurotic fibromatosis, these lesions consist of histologically benign appearing fibroblasts with no or extremely rare mitoses and relatively abundant collagen (Reitamo 1983). Typically the lesions have an infiltrative border and

J. Robert Cassady, M.D., Professor and Head, Department of Radiation Oncology, The University of Arizona, Health Sciences Center, 1501 North Campbell Ave., Tuscon, AZ 85724, USA

they are occasionally multifocal; they may achieve an extremely large size, invade bone and neurovascular structures, and extend widely along fascial planes but they only rarely develop metastases (Greenberg et al. 1981; Kiel and Suit 1984; Posner et al. 1989; Lopez et al. 1990). From 25% to 30% of patients will give a history of prior trauma (Häyry et al. 1982; Lopez et al. 1990) often surgical in nature, and patients with certain genetic conditions such as Gardner's syndrome and, in our experience, children with supernumerary toes appear to be particularly prone to develop aggressive fibromatosis (Eagel et al. 1989). A Finnish study noted a high frequency of associated bony abnormalities (Reitamo et al. 1982).

Whether the lesions represent a true neoplasm (clonally derived) or a disordered healing process is uncertain (Reitamo et al. 1982; Suit 1990). They represent less than 0.25% of all tumors and are seen primarily in children and adults less than 50 years old (Pack and Erlich 1944; Greenberg et al. 1981; Reitamo et al. 1982). Although they may appear virtually anywhere, they tend to occur in certain locations such as the shoulder/neck area, the abdominal wall, and the feet/ankle areas with relative frequency (Das Gupta et al. 1969; Greenberg et al. 1981; Reitamo et al. 1982; Rock et al. 1984) (Table 24.1). About 10% of cases are multifocal (Rock et al. 1984).

Imaging studies of these lesions, such as CT or MRI, may be extremely helpful in localizing tumor extent; however, these studies should not be overly relied upon as, due to their infiltrative ability, the true extent of the tumors may be much greater than is visualized.

Surgery is the mainstay of treatment and, except where surgical resection will result in unacceptable cosmetic and/or functional loss, should be the initial and usually the only treatment (Das Gupta et al. 1969; Rock et al. 1984). Although overt local recurrences have been noted in 10%–60% of cases reported in the literature following surgery (Pack and Erlich 1944; Musgrove and McDonald 1948; Hunt et al. 1960; Dahn et al. 1963; Enzinger and

Table 24.1. Extra-abdominal primary sites of aggressive fibromatosis ($n = 266$) (DAS GUPTA et al. 1969; ROCK et al. 1984)

Site	No. of cases	%
Lower neck and shoulder	19	7
Upper extremity	88	33
Feet and lower extremity	89	33
Pelvis and trunk	57	21
Miscellaneous	13	5

SHIRAKI 1967; BRASFIELD and DAS GUPTA 1969; DAS GUPTA et al. 1969; ROCK et al. 984), the frequency of recurrence is related to the ability of the surgeon to obtain free margins (DAS GUPTA et al. 1969; ROCK et al. 1984; POSNER et al. 1989). However, not all patients with microscopic or even grossly positive margins following surgery will develop clinical recurrence (ENZINGER and SHIRAKI 1967; MARKHEDE et al. 1986; SUIT 1990). SUIT (1990) has reported that 81% of 21 lesions resected with positive margins and followed *without* other therapy have not recurred clinically. Although data are scanty controversial, lesions in children appear to be somewhat more aggressive in terms of both likelihood of recurrence and probability of control; the likelihood of subsequent (third) recurrence seems greater after a second post-surgical recurrence has been noted (LOPEZ et al. 1990).

Unfortunately, local recurrences occur with relative frequency and may involve or extend to anatomic sites that make them technically unresectable or resectable only with major cosmetic/functional consequences such as an amputation (LEIBEL et al. 1983). In these instances, three options are available to the pediatric oncologist: hormonal therapy, cytotoxic chemotherapy, and radiation.

24.2.1 Hormonal Treatment

Tamoxifen and progesterone have been utilized in patients with fibromatosis in an attempt to induce regression (LANARI 1983; KINZBRUNNER et al. 1983; WADDELL et al. 1983; KLEIN et al. 1987; EAGEL et al. 1989). Variable results have been reported, primarily in patients with desmoid tumors complicating preexisting Gardner's syndrome.

Use of these agents is based in the observation that estrogens appear to stimulate growth and tumors may appear after pregnancy or contraceptive use. Estrogen receptors have been noted in desmoids (KLEIN et al. 1987).

Complete responses are rare and although partial responses were noted in 8 of 11 patients in one series

(LANARI 1983), most series demonstrate less favorable results and responses are often of short duration and, at most, partial (KLEIN et al. 1987; EAGEL et al. 1989).

24.2.2 Cytotoxic Chemotherapy

More encouraging are scattered recent reports documenting several patients, primarily children, who have been treated with a number of cytotoxic drug regimens, of which VAC appears to have been most effective, and who have experienced complete regression sustained in some instances for several years (STEIN 1977; HUTCHINSON et al. 1979; RANEY et al. 1987; WEISS and LACKMAN 1989; GOEPFERT et al. 1982). Several patients have required consolidation surgery and/or irradiation, and recurrences after chemotherapy alone or in combination with other therapy have been documentated (RANEY et al. 1987; WEISS and LACKMAN 1989; GOEPFERT et al. 1982). Toxicity, especially to adriamycin containing regimens has been significant (GOEPFERT et al. 1982).

Although the number of cases with documented sustained responses are few in number, reports are quite encouraging and for the very young child in whom adequate doses of irradiation would produce major growth or development abnormalities, a trial of chemotherapy (e.g., VAC) seems warranted. In children or young adults who are to be irradiated in any case, the added toxicity engendered by addition of cytotoxic chemotherapy is not justified in view of the excellent results achieved by irradiation alone (vide infra).

24.2.3 Radiation Therapy

Collectively many patients described in numerous reports from centers through the United States and Europe now attest to the efficacy of irradiation in control of unresectable or post-surgical recurrent aggressive fibromatosis (GREENBERG et al. 1981; LIBEL et al. 1983; ROCK et al. 1984; KEIL and SUIT 1984; BARTELINK and KEUS 1986; RANEY et al. 1987; LOPEZ et al. 1990; SUIT 1990).

Uniform agreement exists that, when treatment is contemplated, wide margins are necessary to minimize the risk of marginal recurrence or geographic miss (GREENBERG et al. 1981; LEIBEL et al. 1983; SUIT 1990). Agreement also exist on the often-noted slow time to complete response demonstrated by these tumors during and following irradiation

Table 24.2. Local control of agressive fibromatosis by radiation therapy in eight recent series (Greenberg et al. 1981; Leibel et al. 1983; Kiel and Suit 1984; Bartelink and Keus 1986; McCollough et al. 1988; Atahan et al. 1989; West et al. 1989; Sherman et al. 1990)

	Dose		
	< 40 Gy	40.1–55 Gy	> 55 Gy
Local control	1/4 (25%)	47/60 (78%)	71/84 (85%)
Site of failure			
Local	2/3	5/13	10/13[a]
Marginal	1/3	8/13	3/13

[a] 2/10 failures occurred at the 50-Gy dose point

(Greenberg et al. 1981; Sherman et al. 1990). Regression periods of 24–36 months are common and periods of response of up to 60 months have been reported (Sherman et al. 1990).

The minimum dose necessary to achieve local control is somewhat controversial (Greenberg et al. 1981; Suit 1990; Sherman et al. 1990). General agreement exists that tumor volume correlates poorly with probability of local control, an argument against fibromatosis being a classical neoplasm (Leibel et al. 1983; Rock et al. 1984; Bartelink and Keus 1986; Maralbell et al. 1988; Suit 1990). Table 24.2 depicts control achieved at three dose ranges in eight series (148 sites) reported in the literature. As noted, a large majority of reported cases have been treated with total radiation doses in excess of 50 Gy. It is also notable that 12 of 29 reported recurrences were marginal in nature, a testament to the need for wide fields with adequate margins (Leibel et al. 1983). At this time, we favor treatment plans that deliver 54–58 Gy in 1.8- to 2-Gy fractions to the primary tumor volume using a shrinking field approach delivering 45 Gy to sites of potential microscopic extension. We have also noted the efficacy of accelerated fractionation approaches (1.2–1.5 Gy b.i.d.) both for tumor control and for long-term normal tissue outcome. Although scanty data exist, Suit's recommendation to deliver somewhat larger total doses (60–65 Gy) to recurrent (vs primary) tumors and those where surgical salvage of relapse would be devastating or impossible seems reasonable (Suit 1990).

24.3 Juvenile Nasopharyngeal Angiofibroma

Juvenile nasopharyngeal angiofibroma (JNA) is a histologically benign but locally aggressive and potentially lethal tumor of adolescence. It accounts for 0.5% of all head and neck neoplasms (Batsakis 1979). Although girls have been reported with this lesion, the diagnosis of JNA in a girl should always be questioned as males are overwhelmingly more frequently affected (>20:1). Affected patients present at an average age of 14–16 years (Jereb et al. 1970; Snow 1977; Briant et al. 1978; Antonelli et al. 1987; Duvall and Morcano 1987; Spector 1988; Cuyler 1988).

Nasal bleeding and obstruction (nasal "stuffiness" and adenoidal speech) are the primary symptoms in almost all children. As uncontrolled biopsy or excessive instrumentation of these lesions can have serious or potentially fatal consequences due to massive blood loss, knowledge of the characteristics of the lesion is essential for the pediatric oncologist.

Tumors arise from the roof of the posterior nares and nasopharynx and frequently extend anteriorly in the nasal cavity(s). The characteristic growth pattern of JNA has been very well described by Neel et al. (1973) and more recently by Duvall and Morcano (1987), who noted that submucosal growth occurs initially laterally and anteriorly, where it may cause flattening of the turbinates. Subsequent growth occurs in the nasopharynx proper with expansion through the sphenopalatine foramen into the pterygopalatine fossa, where continued growth causes characteristics anterior bowing of the posterior wall of the maxillary antrum as well as distortion of the pterygoid plates.

With continued expansion the lesion extends laterally through the pterygomaxillary fissure into the temporal and infratemporal fossa, where it may present as a cheek mass. Extension may occur into the orbit or infracranially through the sphenoid sinus or orbital fissure.

The etiology of JNA is unknown and *no* convincing or consistent endocrine pattern has been recognized despite the prevalence of adolescent males. Testosterone receptors have been noted on tumor tissue (Antonelli et al. 1987).

In addition to careful physical examination and nasopharyngoscopy, imaging studies including CT and MRI are essential for optimum visualization of tumor extent. The lesions are intensely vascular and angiography may be important both for surgical removal and for presurgical embolization procedures (Antonelli et al. 1987; Economon et al. 1988; Close et al. 1989; Maharaj and Fernandez 1989; Andrews et al. 1989). CT has generally replaced angiography for determining the extent of the lesions (Duvall and Morcano 1987). In studies where children have routinely undergone appropriate imaging

Table 24.3. JNA Staging System (CHANDLER et al. 1984)

Stage I	Tumor confined to nasopharynx and/or nasal fossa
Stage II	Tumor extending into sphenoid sinus and/or pterygomaxillary fossa
Stage III	Tumor beyond stage II limits, extending into one or more of the following structures: maxillary sinus, ethmoid, orbit, infratemporal fossa, cheek, palate
Stage IV	Tumor with intracranial extension

studies prior to surgical intervention, approximately one in five has been shown to have intracranial extension (WARD et al. 1974; ECONOMON et al. 1988; ANDREWS et al. 1989).

Metastases are virtually unreported and although isolated reports comment on the frequency of children who are fair and have red hair, the significance of this observation is unknown (SCHIFF 1959).

The modified staging system of Chandler is most commonly utilized (CHANDLER et al. 1984) (Table 24.3).

24.3.1 Surgical Treatment

The great majority of all cases should be managed with surgical removal performed by a surgical team with broad experience in pediatric practice and removal of these lesions. The importance of surgical experience cannot be overstated. Both from the standpoint of successful tumor removal and in view of the possible morbidity (including stroke) and mortality that may occur with attempted resection, surgical technique is critical (ANTONELLI et al. 1987; ECONOMON et al. 1988; CHOSE et al. 1989; MAHARAJ and FERNANDEZ 1989; ANDREWS et al. 1989).

Presurgical embolization in the radiology department is commonly performed prior to surgical removal in an attempt to minimize blood loss at surgery. Nevertheless, blood loss may exceed 1.5–2 liters and careful anesthetic monitoring and fluid and blood replacement are essential.

From the anecdotal nature of much of the literature, with results of varying treatment philosophies and surgical skills being presented, it is not possible to accurately estimate the number of cases initially inappropriate for attempted surgical removal; one can only say that they should be less than 1 in 5 cases and will likely be less than 1 in 10 or 20 (ECONOMON et al. 1988; ANDREWS et al. 1989). We therefore do not agree with the philosophy and approach of CUMMINGS et al. (1954) and BRIANT et al. (1978), who advocate almost routine radiotherapeutic treatment

for these lesions regardless of their size. Currently, improvements in surgical technique, blood bank practices, pediatric anesthesia, and presurgical radiologic techniques have made surgery in the hands of experts a much more successful and safe venture than past surgical reports document (ANTONELLI et al. 1987; ECONOMON et al. 1988; CLOSE et al. 1989; ANDREWS et al. 1989).

24.3.2 Radiation Therapy

Despite the above-mentioned surgical advances, an occasional patient will be seen in whom the size and/or extent of disease either at initial presentation or (as is more frequent in our experience) at the time of recurrence poses substantial risks for attempted (re)removal. In these children, radiation therapy represents a highly effective and, certainly in the short term, safer alternative. Approximately 15%–20% of surgically treated patients will develop a recurrence (DUVALL and MORCANO 1987; ANTONELLI et al. 1987; SPECTOR 1988; ECONOMON et al. 1988; MAHARAJ and FERNANDEZ 1989; ANDREWS et al. 1989).

Significant numbers of children have been treated with irradiation and reported in the literature. Most commonly 34–36 Gy has been delivered in 1.8- to 2-Gy fractions by opposed lateral fields sometimes supplemented by an anterior fields (JEREB et al. 1970; WARD et al. 1974; BRIANT et al. 1978; CUMMINGS 1980; BENGHIAT 1986; ECONOMON et al. 1988; McGAHAN et al. 1988; ROBINSON et al. 1989; FIELDS et al. 1990). Meticulous preradiation imaging of tumor extent is critical as many of the reported failures following irradiation have been geographic (marginal) misses due to under appreciation of the true extent of the lesion (BRIANT et al. 1978; CUMMINGS et al. 1984). Tumor extension into sites such as the orbit, anterior cranial fossa, or nasal cavity may also necessitate elaborate treatment planning prior to irradiation to ensure minimal normal tissue consequences.

McGAHAN et al. (1988) reported apparent true recurrence in four of five children initially treated with 32 Gy in 16 2-Gy fractions. They and others with similar experience have therefore advocated somewhat higher doses and report no failures at doses of 40 Gy or more. In the series reported by FIELDS et al. (1990), two patients failed in the nasal area at 50 and 52 Gy; however, in view of the location of the failure it is unclear whether these failures represent geographic misses or true local failures.

All authors draw attention to the *slow* response to irradiation exhibited by JNA and stress that persistence, even for periods of 12–24 months, without signs of growth should *not* be considered a failure of treatment but warrants further careful follow-up (JEREB et al. 1970; BRIANT et al. 1978; CUMMINGS 1980; CUMMINGS et al. 1984; ROBINSON et al. 1989; FIELDS et al. 1990).

Successful regression following appropriate irradiation occurs in more than 80% of treated cases so long as cautions about tumor extent and slow resolution are borne in mind.

To date, complications reported following irradiation include eight second tumors [thyroid carcinoma (NED), basal cell carcinoma (NED), and six sarcomas], two cataracts, and some degree of caries and xerostomia in treated patients (CUMMINGS 1980; CHEN and BAUER 1983; CUMMINGS et al. 1984; Andrews et al. 1989).

24.3.3 Chemotherapy

Ancedotal reports exist detailing the response of JNA to multiagent cytotoxic regimens – most commonly VAC (GOEPFERT et al. 1982). Due to the small number of reported cases, minimal follow-up, and relative infrequence, to date, of reports of significant morbidity following irradiation, the relative place of this cytotoxic approach in the management of the rare child who cannot be managed with surgery is not known. Therapy with hormonal agents (estrogen, testosterone) is generally not recommended (ANTONELLI et al. 1987).

24.4 Plasma Cell Granuloma

Plasma cell granuloma is a rare lesion of unknown etiology. Aggressive local behavior may occur throughout the body; however, most cases have occurred in the pulmonary parenchyma (BAHADORI and LIEBOW 1973). A vast array of names, many misleading, have been used, including inflammatory pseudotumor, sclerosing hemangioma, histiocytoma, and xanthogranuloma (BUSELL et al. 1976; TOMITA et al. 1980; PETTINATO et al. 1990). BAHADORI and LIEBOW (1973) wrote the initial, definite pathologic reports and described many of this tumor's clinical features.

Although plasma cell granuloma may occur in both children and adults, it is seen more frequently in young people (two-thirds of patients are less than 30 years old) and accounts, in childhood, for nearly 60% of all benign pulmonary masses and nearly 20%

of all primary pulmonary masses (HARTMAN and SHOCHAT 1983; PETTINATO et al. 1990). It is exceeded in frequency only by bronchial adenomas and the rare (usually *non*squamous) bronchial carcinoma as the cause of a pulmonary mass in childhood (HARTMAN and SHOCHAT 1983). Although children with prior malignancies have developed plasma cell granuloma, no clear association is evident with this or any other feature (PETTINATO et al. 1990). Recent studies have shown plasma cells in affected lesions to be polyclonal in nature (MURAOKO et al. 1985; PETTINATO et al. 1990).

Although uncommon, the lesion may reach great size and extend proximally into the mediastinum or even into the contralateral lung and, because of its sclerosing nature, it may engulf, narrow, or obliterates structures such as the esophagus, great vessels, trachea, bronchi, and lung. As such, if untreated or not controlled, it has caused death (BAHADORI and LIEBOW 1973; HOOVER et al. 1977; MANDELBAUM et al. 1981; KIRKPATRICK 1982; MONZON et al. 1982; HARTMAN and SHOCHAT 1983; PETTINATO et al. 1990; LAUFER et al. 1990).

Modern imaging studies such as CT and MRI have made possible much more accurate identification of the lesion's true extent than could be achieved with the previously utilized plain films and tomography, and are essential prior to attempted removal.

Metastases are not known, nor are any consistent associations with any recognized organism apparent (BAHADORI and LIEBOW 1973).

24.4.1 Treatment

The overwhelming majority of cases will be cured by surgical excision with adequate free margins (BAHADORI and LIEBOW 1973; KIRKPATRICK 1982; MONZON et al. 1982). This endeavor may require removal of a segment or lobe or even a pneumonectomy (KIRKPATRICK 1982). However, incomplete removal is not infrequently accompanied by local recurrence and extension (BAHADORI and LIEBOW 1973; MANDELBAUM et al. 1981; KIRKPATRICK 1982). An occasional child or young adult may also present with a lesion which has already invaded the mediastinum and technically cannot be removed or in whom removal can only be accomplished at high risk for both survival and function. This latter group of children may have further progression/extension of tumor controlled or eliminated by moderate doses of radiation (HOOVER et al. 1977; MEHTA et al. 1982;

KIRKPATRICK 1982; IMPERATO et al. 1986). Radiation doses of 35–40 Gy using 1.5- to 1.8-Gy fractions have been successful (HOOVER et al. 1977; IMPERATO et al. 1986). Even case reports documenting "failure" of radiation report lack of further extension/progression 2 years following treatment (MEHTA et al. 1980). As in many benign conditions, tumor "response" and decrease in size may occur extremely slowly and a substantial evident mass may be present 12 or more months after treatment (MEHTA et al. 1980; KIRKPATRICK 1982; IMPERATO et al. 1986). The goal of irradiation in the occasional treated case should be the cessation of further growth and progression. Although steroids have been used, we know of no reports confirming their efficacy, nor do we know of any reports confirming the efficacy of cytotoxic chemotherapy in childhood cases.

24.5 Giant Cell Tumor and Aneurysmal Bone Cyst

Although different in many respects, these two primary bone tumors are considered together as the indications for treatment with irradiation are virtually identical.

Giant Cell Tumor (GCT) is a rare (<5% of all primary bone tumors) tumor of unknown etiology which most commonly affects the epiphyseal and metaphyseal region of the long bones of the knee (JAFFE 1954; DAHLIN et al. 1970). The primary sites of 1332 cases are shown in Fig. 24.1 (SHANKMAN et al. 1988). Presentation is very rare before age 14 and most very young patients are girls (PICCI et al. 1983; CARRASCO and MURRAY 1989). The median age at presentation is 30–35 years (MCGRATH 1972).

Radiographically, a lytic process is seen which is long bones is centered at the epiphysis but with extension to the metaphysis and articular surface. MRI has been stated to be the best imaging modality because of its excellent contrast resolution. MRI permits excellent visualization of both intraosseous and extraosseous tumor.

Although rarely multifocal and usually considered "benign," all of these tumors are locally aggressive and tend to recur and invade bone and soft tissues if incompletely removed; furthermore, on occasion patients present with or subsequently develop metastases, usually to the lungs (HUTTER et al. 1962; GOLDENBERG et al. 1970). Even lesions that are extremely benign in microscopic appearance may demonstrate metastases (MALONEY et al. 1989). Wound seeding with later soft tissue recurrence fol-

lowing attempts at curettage and removal have been reported (EXARCHOU et al. 1989).

In contrast, aneurysmal bone cysts (ABCs) are lesions of uncertain pathogenesis which most commonly occur in the second decade of life (>50%) (LICHTENSTEIN 1957; JAFFE 1958). Most are considered to be primary lesions although up to 30% occur in association with another bony process (including osteosarcoma) which may only be noted on careful pathologic examination (BIESECKER et al. 1970; JOHNSON et al. 1988).

Workup of these lesions should be similar to that for GCT. Although most ABCs, like GCT, arise in bones of the extremities, they may develop in the spine, pelvis, sacrum, sphenoid, or calvarium, where surgical removal may be hazardous or functionally destructive (BIESECKER et al. 1970; JOHNSON et al. 1988; WARREN and HARRIS 1988; CYBALSKI et al. 1989).

24.5.1 Treatment

Treatment for both lesions should be surgical in almost all cases (BELL et al. 1983; SEIDER et al. 1986).

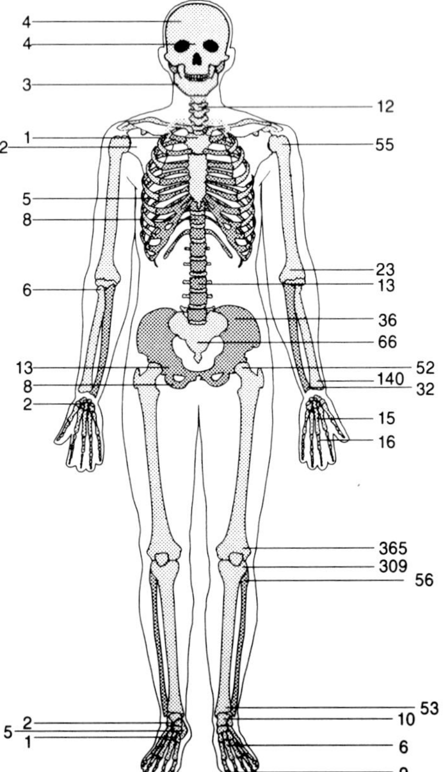

Fig. 24.1. Primary site of GCT in 1332 cases reviewed by SHANKMAN et al. (1988). The predominance of lesions occurring about the knee is striking although it is also evident that GCT may appear in either the appendicular or the axial skeleton

If no significant functional loss occurs, excisional removal and grafting and/or placement of a prosthesis is associated with the highest likelihood of local control. Treatment with bone curetting and grafting is associated in both lesions with a significant incidence of local recurrence which relates in part to the completeness of initial removal (NOBLER et al. 1968; BIESECKER et al. 1970; MCGRATH 1972; EXARCHOU et al. 1989). In most series, local recurrence rates range from 10% to 40%. although higher rates have been noted (GOLDENBERG et al. 1970).

Several recent series have been published confirming the ability of properly applied megavoltage irradiation, either as an adjunct to incomplete surgical removal or as a primary therapy, to control these lesions (NOBLER et al. 1968; CASSADY 1979; BELL et al. 1983; SEIDER et al. 1986; CHEN et al. 1986; DANGAARD et al. 1987; SHANKMAN et al. 1988; WARREN and HARIS 1988; SCHWARTZ et al. 1989; MILLION 1989; MAEDA et al. 1989; YAN et al. 1989). Cases so treated have been those considered "difficult" in view of the functionally destructive or disfiguring surgery necessary for removal or because recurrence (sometimes extensive) had developed after one or more initial surgical attempts at removal. Thus location of these irradiated lesions has been atypically centered in the base of the skull, the spine, the sacrum, and the pelvis (CASSADY 1979; BELL et al. 1983; SEIDER et al. 1986; SCHWARTZ et al. 1989).

Tumor doses of 5–30 Gy in 1–15 fractions have been successfully used with ABC and, so long as the entire lesion has been adequately encompassed, radiation doses of 20–30 Gy are usually successfully (NOBLER et al. 1968; MILLION 1989; MAEDA et al. 1989). GCT requires higher doses in order to obtain a high rate of local control. Although a dose of 35 Gy was used successfully in many cases reported by Bell et al. from the Princess Margaret Hospital, fraction size in several of these patients was more than 2 Gy and, using more conventional fractionation, most authors recommend 45–50 Gy for spinal lesions and somewhat larger doses for lesions of the sacrum, etc. (CASSADY 1979; BELL et al. 1983; SIEDER et al. 1986; SCHWARZT et al. 1989; MILLION 1989).

CASSADY (1979), BELL et al. (1983), and others have noted the frequent finding of apparent "growth" and increased size of the lucent bone defect immediately following radiation therapy. Coupled with transiently impaired bony healing due to radiation therapy, "healing" of these lesions and development of sclerosis in the treated site may take many months or even more than a year to develop. However, symptoms of pain or mass effect usually resolve by the end of treatment or shortly thereafter.

In addition to usual concerns regarding use of radiation in childhood (e.g., growth disturbance, late second tumors), two particular concerns exist regarding radiation treatment of ABC and GCT, namely the high failure rate detailed by early reports when radiation was utilized (BRADSHAW 1964; DAHLIN et al. 1970; GOLDENBERG et al. 1970; MCGRATH 1972) and the possible "induction" of a malignant GCT by treatment with irradiation (MNAYMNEH et al. 1964; GOLDENBERG et al. 1970; MCGRATH 1972). While each of these concerns is to some extent valid, they do not collectively eliminate radiation therapy as a reasonable treatment option in all cases of ABC and GCT.

Table 24.4. Results of modern radition therapy for "difficult" GCTs of bone, as reported in six recent series[a]

Author	No. of patients	Surgery + XRT	XRT only after biopsy	Recurrence	Comments
CHEN et al. (1986)	17[b]	–	–	3	–
MILLION (1989)	10	5	5	1(S + XRT)	Follow-up 2–6 years
BELL et al. (1983)	14	10 (5 with gross recurrence)	4	1(S + XRT p recur)	Recurrence in pt. with inadequate coverage by
SCHWARTZ et al. (1989)	13	6 (4 with recurrence)	7	2(XRT)	XRT1 "recurrence" in pt. with nobony healing after 5 months; therefore resected and currently NED
DANGAARD et al. (1987)	10	10 (2 with recurrence)	0	3	All recurrences with < 39 Gy, 2/3 with orthovoltage
SEIDER et al. (1986)	10	8	2	3	2/3 recurrences < 39 Gy
	74	–	–	13	

S, surgery; XRT, radiation therapy
[a] It is notable that no case of malignant transformation to a malignant GCT occured in any of these cases although one patient did develop a fibrosarcoma in the radiation field following orthovoltage treatment
[b] Treated with > 35 Gy

Most reports detailing frequent local failures following radiation therapy are from the orthovoltage era, when frequent courses of low-dose treatment were utilized with inadequate (by current standards) evaluation of true tumor extent. Failures are thus not surprising.

Compilation of the results from six recent series of GCT treated with modern equipment demonstrates an overall control rate of 82% (61/74) (Table 24.4) (BELL et al. 1983; SEIDER et al. 1986; CHEN et al. 1986; DANGAARD et al. 1987; SCHWARTZ et al. 1989; MILLION 1989). Some failures in this group occurred in patients who were treated with less than 40 Gy. Results with ABC, using doses of 20–30 Gy are at least as good, and in one series of 12 patients, 11 were controlled (92%) (NOBLER et al. 1968).

While induction of a late second bone tumor is a well-recognized risk of radiation therapy, induction of "malignant transformation" in a GCT is more controversial. HUTTER et al. (1962) could not ascertain an elevated risk of malignant degeneration in irradiated patients. Most reports of this occurrence were published in an era when pathology of bone tumors was less sophisticated and patients were treated with repeated courses of low-dose orthovoltage treatment. In the modern series noted earlier, although a fibrosarcoma occurring many years after orthovoltage treatment was documented (BELL et al. 1983) and patients with metastases were treated, no clear instance of a *radiation-induced malignant GCT* was noted with follow-up periods extending more than a decade.

The foregoing results indicate that although surgical management should be relied on in the great majority of patients, should disease extent or recurrence entail possible amputation, major neurologic disability (spine or sacral lesion), or disfigurement (lesion of face or skull), then radiation should be considered and when properly used should results in a very high success rate.

References

Andrews JC, Fisch U, Valavanis A, Aeppli U, Makek MS (1989) The surgical management of extensive nasopharyngeal angiofibromas with infratemporal fossa approach. Laryngoscope 99: 429–437

Antonelli AR, Cappiello J, DiLorenzo D, Donajo CA, Nicolai P, Orlandini A (1987) Diagnosis, staging and treatment of juvenile nasopharyngeal angiofibroma (JNA). Laryngoscope 97: 1319–1325

Atahan IL, Akyol F, Zorlu F, Gurkaynak M (1989) Radiotherapy in the management of aggressive fibromatosis. Br J Radiol 62: 854–856

Bahadori IL, Liebow AA (1973) Plasma cell granulomas of the lung. Cancer 31: 191–208

Bartelink H, Keus R (1986) The role of radiotherapy in the treatment of desmoid tumors. Radiother Oncol 7: 1–5

Batsakis JG (1979) Tumors of the head and neck, 2nd edn. Williams and Wilkins, Baltimore, pp 291–312

Bell RS, Harwood AR, Goodman SB, Fornasier VL (1983) Supervoltage radiotherapy in the treatment of difficult giant cell tumors of bone. Clin Orthop 174: 208–216

Benghiat A (1986) Juvenile nasopharyngeal angiofibroma treated by radiotherapy. J Laryngol Otol 100: 351–356

Biesecker JL, Marcove RC, Huvos AG, Mike V (1970) Aneurysmal bone cysts: a clinicopathologic study of 66 cases. Cancer 26: 615–625

Bradshaw JD (1964) The values of x-ray therapy in the management of osteoclastoma. Clin Radiol 15: 70

Brasfield RD, Das Gupta TK (1969) Desmoid tumors of the anterior abdominal wall. Surgery 65: 241–253

Briant TDR, Fitzpatrick PJ, Berman J (1978) Nasopharyngeal angiofibroma: a twenty year study. Laryngoscope 88: 1247–1251

Busell R, Wang N-S, Seemayer TA, Ahmed MN (1976) Endobrochial plasma cell granuloma (xanthomatous pseudotumor). Hum Pathol 7: 411–426

Carrasco CH, Murray JA (1989) Giant cell tumors. Ortho Clin North Am 20: 395–404

Cassady JR (1979) Radiation therapy in less common primary bone tumors. In: Jaffe N (ed) Bone tumors in children. Progress in pediatric hematology and oncology, vol II. PSG, Littleton, MA/USA pp 205–214

Chandler JR, Goulding R, Moskowitz L et al. (1984) Nasopharyngeal angiofibroma: staging and management. Am Otol Rhinol Laryngol 93: 322–329

Chen KTK, Bauer FW (1983) Sarcomatous transformation of nasopharyngeal angiofibroma. Cancer 49: 369–371

Chen ZX, Gu DZ, Yu ZH, Qian TN, Huang YR, Hu YH, Gu XZ (1986) Radiation therapy of giant cell tumor of bone: Analysis of 35 patients. Int J Radiat Onco Biol Phys 12: 329–334

Close LG, Schaefer SD, Mickey BE, Manning SC (1989) Surgical management of nasopharyngeal angiofibroma involving the cavernous sinus. Arch Otolaryngol Head Neck Surg 115: 1091–1095

Cummings BJ (1980) Relative risk factor in the treatment of juvenile nasopharyngeal angiofibroma. Head Neck Surg 3: 21–26

Cummings BJ, Blend R, Kaenet et al. (1984) Primary radiation therapy for juvenile nasopharyngeal angiofibroma. Laryngoscope 94: 1599–1605

Cuyler JP (1988) Treatment options for angiofibroma. J Otolaryngeal 17: 214–218

Cybalski GR, Anson J, Gleason T, Homsi MF, Reys MG (1989) Aneurysmal bone cyst of thoracic spine: treatment by excision and segemental stabilization with luque rods. Neurosurgery 24: 273–276

Dahlin DC, Cupps RE, Johnson EW (1970) Giant cell tumor: a study of 195 cases. Cancer 25: 1061–1070

Dahn I, Johnson N, Lundh G (1963) Desmoid tumors, a series of 33 cases. Acta Chir Scand 126: 305–314

Dangaard S, Johansen HF, Barfod G, Lanstein G, Schidt T, Lund B (1987) Radiation treatment of giant cell tumors of bone (osteoclastoma). Acta Onco 26 [Fasc 1]: 41–43

Das Gupta TK, Brasfield RD, O'Hara J, (1969) Exrtraabdominal desmoids: a clinicopathological study. Am Surg 170: 109–121

Duvall AJ, Morcano AE (1987) Juvenile nasopharyngeal angiofibroma: diagnosis and treatment. Otolaryngol Head Neck Surg 97: 534–540

Eagel BA, Zentler-Munro P, Smith IE (1989) Mesenteric desmoid tumors in Gardner's syndrome – review of medical treatments. Postgrad Med J 65: 497–501

Economon TS, Abemayer E, Ward PH (1988) Juvenile nasopharyngeal angiofibroma: an update of the UCLA experience, 1960–1985. Laryngoscope 98: 170–175

Enzinger FM, Shiraki M (1967) Musculoaponeurotic fibromatosis of shoulder girdle (extra-abdominal desmoid). Analysis of thirty cases. Cancer 20: 1131–1140

Exarchou E, Maris J, Assimakopoulos A (1989) Soft tissue recurrence of osteoclastoma. J Bone Joint Surg [Br] 71: 432–433

Fields JN, Halverson KJ, Devineni VR, Simpson JR, Perez CA (1990) Juvenile nasopharyngeal angiofibroma: efficacy of radiation therapy. Radiology 176: 263–265

Goepfert H, Cangir A, Ayala AG, Eftekhari F (1982) Chemotherapy of locally aggressive head and neck tumors in the pediatric age group: Desmoid fibromatosis and nasopharyngeal angiofibroma

Goldenberg RR, Campbell CJ, Bonfiglio M (1970) Giant cell tumor of bone. J Bone Joint Surg [Am] 52: 619–664

Greenberg HM, Goebell R, Weichselbaum RR, Greenberger JS, Chaffey JT, Cassady JR (1981) Radiation therapy in the treatment of aggressive fibromatoses. Int J Radiat Oncol Biol Phys 7: 305–310

Hartman GE, Shochat SJ (1983) Primary pulmonary neoplasms of childhood; a review. Am Thor Surg 36: 108–119

Häyry P, Reitamo JJ, Tötterman S, Hopfner-Hallikainen D, SiVula A (1982) The desmoid tumor. II. Analysis of factors possibly contributing to the etiology and growth behavior Am J Clin Pathol 77: 674–680

Hoover SV, Granston AS, Koch DF, Hudson TR (1977) Plasma cell granuloma of the lung: response to radiation therapy. Report of a single case. Cancer 39: 123–125

Hunt R, Thomas N, Morgan HC, Ackerman LV (1960) Principles in the management of extra-abdominal desmoids. Cancer 13: 825–836

Hutchinson RJ, Norris DG, Schnaufer L (1979) Chemotherapy: a successful application in abdominal fibromatosis. Pediatrics 63: 157–159

Hutter RVP, Worcester J, Francis K et al. (1962) Benign and malignant giant cell tumor of bone. Cancer 15: 653–690

Imperato JP, Folkman J, Sagerman RH, Cassady JR (1986) Treatment of plasma cell granuloma of the lung with radiation therapy: a report of two cases and a review of the literature. Cancer 57: 2127–2129

Jaffe HL (1954) Giant cell tumor (osteoclastoma) of bone: its pathologic delineation and the inherent clinical implications. Ann Surg 13: 343–355

Jaffe HL (1958) Tumors and tumorous conditions of the bones and joints. Lea and Febiger, Philadelphia, pp 54–62

Jereb B, Änggård A, Båryd I (1970) Juvenile nasopharyngeal angiofibroma. Acta Radiol Ther Phys Biol 9: 302–310

Johnson TE, Bergin DJ, McCord CD (1988) Aneurysmal bone cyst of the orbit. Opthalmology 95: 86–89

Kiel KD, Suit HD (1984) Radiation therapy in the treatment of aggressive fibromatoses (desmoid tumors). Cancer 54: 2051–2055

Kinzbrunner B, Ritter S, Domingo J, Rosenthal CS (1983) Remission of rapidly growing desmoid tumors after tamoxifen therapy. Cancer 52: 2201–2204

Kirkpatrick JA (1982) Case records of the Massachusetts General Hospital, case 10-1982. N Engl J Med 306: 596–602

Kleien WA, Miller HH, Anderson M, DeCosse JJ (1989) The use of indomethacin, sulindac, and tamoxifen for the treatment of desmoid tumors associated with familial polyposis. Cancer 60: 2863–2868

Lanari A (1983) Effect of progesterone on desmoid tumors (aggressive fibromatosis) (letter). N Engl J Med 309: 1523

Laufer L, Cohen Z, Mares AJ, Maor E, Hirsch M (1990) Pulmonary plasma-cell granuloma. Pediatr Radiol 20: 289–290

Leibel SA, Wara WM, Hill DR, Bovill EG, DeLorimer AA, Beckstead JH, Phillips TL (1983) Desmoid tumors: local control and patterns of relapse following radiation therapy. Int J Radiat Oncol Biol Phys 9: 1167–1171

Lichtenstein L (1957) Aneurysmal bone cyst: observation on fifty cases. J Bone Joint Surg [Am] 39: 873–882

Lopez R, Kemalyan N, Moseley HS, Denuis D, Vetto RM (1990) Problems in diagnosis and management of desmoid tumors. Am J Surg 159: 450–453

Maeda M, Tateishi H, Takaiwa H, Kinoshita G, Hatano N, Nakano K (1989) High energy, low-dose radiation therapy for aneurysmal bone cyst: report of a case. Clin Orthop 243: 200–203

Maharaj D, Fernandez CMC (1989) Surgical experience with juvenile nasopharyngeal angiofibroma. Am Otol Rhinol Laryngol 98: 269–272

Maloney WJ, Vaughan LM, Jones HH, Ross J, Nagel DA (1989) Benign metastasizing giant-cell tumor of bone: report of three cases and review of the literature. Clin Orthop 243: 208–215

Mandelbaum I, Brashear RE, Hull MT (1981) Surgical treatment and course of preliminary pseudotumor (plasma cell granuloma). Thorac Cardiovasc Surg 82: 77–82

Markhede G, Lundgren L, Bjurstam N, Berlin O, Stener B (1986) Extra-abdominal desmoid tumors. Acta Orthop Scand 57: 1–7

McCollough WM, Parson JT, Million RR, Enneking WF, Springfield DS (1988) Aggressive fibromatosis. Int J Radiat Oncol Biol Phys 15 [Suppl 1]: 186

McGahan RA, Durrance FY, Parke RB, Easley JD (1988) The treatment of advanced juvenile nasopharyngeal angiofibroma. Int J Radiat Oncol Biol Phys 159 [Suppl 1]: 217

McGrath PJ (1972) Giant-cell tumor of bone: an analysis of fifty-two cases. J Bone Joint Surg [er] 54: 216–228

Mehta J, Desphande S, Stauffer JL, Stanford R, Fernandez E (1980) Plasma cell granuloma of the lung: endobronchial presentation and absence of response of radiation therapy. South Med J 73: 1198–1201

Million RR (1989) The myth regarding bone or cartilage involvement by cancer and the likelihood of cure by radiotherapy. Head and Neck 11: 30–40

Miralbell R, Mankiu H, Zuckerberg LR, Stracker M, Suit HD (1989) Desmoid tumors: MGH experience 1970–1985. Int J Radiat Oncol Biol Phys 15 [Suppl 1]: 187

Mnaymneh WA, Dudely HR, Mnaymneh LG (1964) Giant-cell tumor of bone. J Bone Joint Surg [Am] 16: 63–75

Monzon CM, Gilchrist GS, Burgert EO, O'Connell EJ, Telander RL, Hoffman AD, Li C-Y (1982) Plasma cell granuloma of the lung in children. Pediatrics 70: 268–274

Muraoka S, Sato T, Takahashi T, Ando M, Shimoda A (1985) Plasma cell Granuloma of the lung with extra-pulmonal extension: immunohistochemical and electron microscopic studies. Acta Pathol Jpn 35: 933–944

Musgrove JE, McDonald JR (1948) Extra-abdominal Desmoid tumors. Arch Pathol 45: 513–540

Neel HB, Whicker JH, Devine KD (1973) Juvenile angiofibroma – review of 120 cases. Am J Surg 126: 547–560

Nobler MP, Higinbotham NL, Phillips RF (1968) The cure of aneurysmal bone cyt: irradiation superior to surgery in an analysis of 33 cases. Radiology 90: 1185–1192

Pack GT, Erlich HE (1944) Neoplasms of anterior abdominal wall with special consideration of desmoid tumors; experience with 391 cases and collective review of the literature. Int Abstr Surg 79: 177–198

Pettinato G, Manivel JC, DeRosa N, Dehner LP (1990) Inflammatory myofibroblatic tumor (plasma cell granuloma): clinicopathologic study of 20 cases with immunohistochemical and ultrastructural observations. Am J Clin Pathol 94: 538–546

Picci P, Manfrini M, Zucchi V et al. (1983) Giant cell tumor of bone in skeletally immature patients. J Bone Joint Surg [Am] 65: 486–490

Posner MC, Shiu MH, Newsome JL, Hajdu SI, Gaynor JJ, Brennan MF (1989) The desmoid tumor – not a benign disease. Arch Surg 124: 191–196

Raney B, Evans A, Granowetter L, Schnaufer L, Uri A, Littman P (1987) Non-surgical management of children with recurrent or unresectable fibromatosis. Pediatrics 79: 394–398

Reitamo JJ (1983) The desmoid tumor: choice of treatment results amd complications. Arch Surg 118: 1318–1322

Reitamo JJ, Häyry P, Nykyri E, Saxen E (1982) The desmoid tumor. I. Incidence, sex, age, and anatomical distribution in the Finnish population. Am J Clin Pathol 77: 665–673

Robinsen ACR, Khoury GG, Ash DV, Daly BD (1989) Evaluation of response following irradiation of juvenile angiofibromas. Br J Radiol 62: 245–247

Rock MG, Pritchard DJ, Reiman HM, Sonle EH, Brewster RC (1984) Extra-abdominal desmoid tumors. J Bone Joint Surg [Am] 66: 1369–1374

Schiff M (1959) Juvenile nasal angiofibroma: A theory of pathogenesis. Laryngoscope 69: 981

Schwartz LH, Okunieff PG, Rosenberg A, Suit HD (1989) Radiation thearpy in the treatment of difficult giant cell tumors. Int J Radiat Oncol Biol Phys 17: 1085–1088

Seider MJ, Rich TA, Ayala AG, Murray JA (1986) Giant cell tumor of bone: treatment with radiation therapy. Radiology 161: 537–540

Shankman S, Greenspan A, Klein MJ, Lewis MM (1988) Giant cell tumor of ischium: a report of two cases and review of the literature. Skeletal Radiol 17: 46–51

Sherman NE, Ronsdahl M, Evans H, Zagars G, Oswald MJ (1990) Desmoid tumors: a 20 year radiotherapy experience. Int J Radiat Oncol Biol Phys 19: 37–40

Snow JB Jr (1977) Neoplasms of the nasopharynx in children. Otolaryngol Clin North Am 10: 11–24

Spector JG (1988) Management of juvenile angiofibromata. Laryngoscope 8: 1016–1026

Stein R (1977) Chemotherapeutic response in fibromatosis of the neck. J Pediatr 90: 482–483

Suit HD (1990) Radiation dose and response of desmoid tumors. Int J Radiat Oncol Biol Phys 19: 225–227

Tomita T, Dixon A, Watanabe I, Mantz F, Richany S (1980) Sclerosing vascular variant of plasma cell granuloma. Hum Pathol 11: 197–202

Waddell WR, Gerner RF, Reich MP (1983) Nonsteroidal anti-inflammatory drugs and tamoxifen for desmoid tumors and carcinoma of the stomach. J Surg Oncol 22: 197–211

Ward PH, Thompson R, Calcaterra T, Kadin MR (1974) Juvenile angiofibroma: a more rational therapeutic approach based upon clinical and experimental evidence Laryngoscope. 84: 2181–2194

Warren NP, Harris NH (1988) Juxta-articular aneurysmal bone cyst. J R Soc Med 81: 291–292

Weiss AJ, Lackman RD (1989) Low dose chemotherapy of desmoid tumors. Cancer 64: 1192–1194

West CB, Shagets FW, Mansfield MJ (1989) Non-surgical treatment of aggressive fibromatosis in the head and neck. Otolaryngol Head Neck Surg 101: 338–343

Yan S-C, Xu Q-M, Lin J-R (1989) Diagnosis and treatment of giant cell tumor in the thoracic spine. J Surg Oncol 40: 128–131

25 Future Prospects in Childhood Cancer

J. Robert Cassady

CONTENTS

25.1 Will Radiation Therapy Be Utilized
in the Treatment of Children with Cancer
Two Decades from Now? 379
25.2 What Changes May Be Expected in
Current Practice? 379

Even a cursory review of most chapters in this book illustrates the rapid and wide-ranging changes that have occurred in pediatric oncology practice during the past 2 decades. Should a pediatric radiation oncologist attempt to treat children today with 1970s' "state-of-the-art" therapy, that person would clearly be woefully out-of-date and require substantial reeducation. Thus, it might be said that the only constant in pediatric oncology practice has been change combined with ongoing attempts to optimize results.

25.1 Will Radiation Therapy Be Utilized in the Treatment of Children with Cancer Two Decades from Now?

The answer to this question is somewhat uncertain, but is probably, "yes". Despite major advances (with corresponding reductions in the use of radiation therapy) in utilization of chemotherapy in the leukemias, non-Hodgkin's lymphomas, Hodgkin's disease, Wilms' tumor, and other pediatric neoplasms, and despite a better understanding of the relatively benign natural history of certain classes of patients with neuroblastoma, there are still, unfortunately, many childhood tumors such as brain tumors, rhabdomyosarcoma, other soft tissue and bone sarcomas, retinoblastomas, and certain neuroblastomas that continue to represent highly fatal

neoplasms if not properly managed and that are not currently well managed with surgery and/or chemotherapy only. Thus, for at least the next decade, it seems likely that radiation therapy will continue to play a major role in certain childhood tumors.

25.2 What Changes May Be Expected in Current Practice?

It is likely that there will be continuing change and increased discrimination in risk group analysis. As better histopathologic discrimination in Wilms' tumor permitted significant reductions in treatment intensity and/or elimination of a treatment modality (i.e., radiation therapy) in favorable histology early-stage patients, it seems likely that similar but additional separations in other tumors will occur in the future.

It has been previously noted that children with stage I neuroblastoma do not appear to benefit from either adjuvant chemotherapy of radiation treatment. It *may* be similarly found that children with stage T1N0M0 Wilms' tumor (Cassady stage) require only appropriate surgical treatment. This hypothesis is currently being tested at the Children's Hospital and the Dana Farber Cancer Center in Boston. Thus, the current approach to limit therapy to essentials irrespective of modality will continue, as will a parallel approach to substitute less toxic agents/modalities where and when possible.

Similarly, utilization of modern molecular and histopathologic techniques may permit significant improvements in categorization of tumor behavior and aggressiveness. Tumor ploidy and N-myc copy number in children with neuroblastoma are two obvious examples which are currently being tested and examined. It is likely that the diagnostic and risk group assessment benefits of the current explosion of knowledge in the molecular characteristics of pediatric tumors will yield substantial benefit in cancer treatment with greater rapidity than revolutionary treatment approaches such as gene therapy.

J. Robert Cassady, M.D., Professor and Head, Department of Radiation Oncology, The University of Arizona, Health Sciences Center, 1501 North Campbell Ave., Tucson, AZ 85724, USA

Many if not most childhood cancers have a substantial genetic etiologic component that not only predisposes the child to develop a certain tumor but also increases the long-term risks of most non-surgical cancer treatment approaches. Better knowledge of cell regulation and function at a molecular level may permit substantial reduction in risk when these therapies are necessary and may also permit a molecular approach to tumor prevention which would have vast benefit not only to children but to adult survivors of cancer as well. Studies of this type are likely in the future of pediatric oncology.

Current sophisticated approaches which are being developed and improved in radiation oncology such as radiosurgery (especially fractionated approaches), three-dimensional treatment planning with conformal treatment approaches, hospital-based particle treatment, and sophisticated brachytherapy and intraoperative radiation approaches, designed to minimize the volume of normal tissue irradiated to significant doses, seem likely to be utilized with increasing frequency in pediatric practice as the developing child should be the patient who will *most* benefit from the normal tissue sparing these approaches allow. It seems likely to this investigator that many, if not most, pediatric brain tumor patients requiring irradiation will ultimately receive their treatment by fractionated stereotaxic approaches with significant benefit. Examples such as craniopharyngioma, optic glioma, brain stem gliomas, and medulloblastoma "boosts" come immediately to mind. It is also likely that altered fractionation approaches will be of benefit to the child in terms of both improved tumor control (e.g., rhabdomyosarcoma) and reduced normal tissue damage.

Proliferating normal tissues which, when damaged, produce the developmental toxicity seen after radiation treatment have not been well studied from a radiobiologic standpoint. It may be that alterations in fractionation techniques will allow substantial minimization of damage without jeopardizing tumor control with radiation. This clearly represents an area in which further study is possible and is warranted.

Finally, it is also possible that currently less conventional treatment approaches will provide substantial benefit to the patient from both improved tumor control and normal tissue preservation. Included in this latter category are radioactively tagged monoclonal antibodies against tumor-associated antigens and certain photodynamic treatment approaches.

If the history of prior advances in oncologic treatment is any indication, improved approaches will continue to be pioneered in the treatment of children with cancer and then be introduced for adult treatment. Thus pediatric oncology will continue to represent the oncologic "test tube" of treatment advances.

Subject Index

ABVD 28
accelerated atherosclerotic narrowing 30
acoustic neuromas 245
actinomycin D 4, 13, 17, 32, 36, 80, 81, 82, 256
– and radiation 80
acute cerebral edema 134
acute encephalopathy 135
acute lymphoblastic leukemia (ALL) 87–95, 133, 141
– bone marrow transplantation 95
– intensification therapy 88
– intrathecal chemotherapy 91
– prevention of CNS disease 89
– – after relapse 93
– principles of therapy 88
– radiation
– – cranospinal 94
– – efficacy 94
– remission induction 88
– treatment factors 88
acute nonlymphocytic leukemia (ANLL) 99–110
– biology 100
– bone marrow transplantation 102
– chemotherapy 102
– clinical presentation 101
– CNS irradiation, complications 108
– cytogenetics 100
– diagnosis 101
– etiology 99
– extramedullary lesions, treatment 107
– FAB classification 100
– leukostasis, treatment 107
– pathogenesis 99
– radiation therapy 105
– treatment 102
– – complications 108
adrenal carcinoma 357–360
ALL see acute lymphoblastic leukemia
α 204
alveolar tumors 282
amenorrhea 39
anaplastic 254
astrocytomas 244

anesthesia 2, 3
aneurysmal
– bone cyst 374–376
– dilatation, fusiform 139
angiofibroma, juvenile nasopharyngeal 371–373
– chemotherapy 373
– radiation therapy 372
– surgical treatment 372
animal tumor studies 79
aniridia 7, 251
ANLL see acute nonlymphocytic leukemia
Ann Arbor staging system, Hodgkin's disease 154
anthracycline 28
ara-C, high-dose 135
arteriovenous malformations 244
Askin's tumor 283
astrocytomas 239, 242
– anaplastic 244
ataxia telangiectasia 10
atherosclerotic vascular disease 29
avascular necrosis 19

Beckwith-Wiedemann syndrome 10, 176, 251
behavior, treatment effects 145
β-hCG> 204
biologically effective dose 116
Birbeck granules 338
bladder
– radiation related normal tissue effects 39
– toxicity 39
Bloom's syndrome 10, 99
blueberry muffin 101
bone, growing 16
bone marrow 15
– radiation related normal tissue effects 15
bone marrow transplantation 33
– acute lymphoblastic leukemia 95
– acute nonlymphocytic leukemia 102
– Langerhans cell histiocytosis 346
– neuroblastoma 188
– Non-Hodgkin's lymphoma 129
– total body irradiation 115–121
brain stem glioma 215

– epidemiology 215
– pathology 217
– prognostic factors 215
– therapy 217
– – radiation therapy 217
– – surgery 217
brain tumors 68, 109
– malignant 197–210
breast
– cancer 282
– hypoplastic development 42
– radiation related normal tissue effects 42
Burkitt's lymphoma 124
– geographic and ethnic variation 8

calcification, dystrophic 138
calcitonin 352
cancer family syndrome 361
cancer prevention 69
cardiac dysfunction 168
cardiotoxicity 28
cardiovascular system, radiation related normal tissue effects 27
catecholamine metabolic pathway 177
Cavitron 243
cell cycle effects 76
cerebellar vermis 198
cerebral neuroblastoma 202
Chang staging system 198, 199
chemotherapeutic agents
– and total body irradiation 120
– toxic effects 4
chemotherapy
– acute nonlymphocytic leukemia 102
– combination with radiation 145
– high-dose 134
– intrathecal, acute lymphoblastic leukemia 91
– and irradiation 4
– juvenile nasopharyngeal angiofibroma 373
– medulloblastoma 201
– neuroblastoma 183
– osteosarcoma 307
– retinoblastoma 330
– rhabdomyosarcoma 286

chloromas 101
choroid plexus tumors 230
chromosomal
- abnormalities,
  neuroblastoma 176
- alterations 62
chromosomes translocation
  t(11;22) 265
chronic myelogenous leukemia
  (CML) 63
cisplatin 27, 120
clear cell sarcoma 254
clonogenic assays 79
CNS disease, prevention in ALL 89
CNS embryonal neuroepithelial
  tumors 201–204
- cerebral neuroblastoma 202
- ependymoblastoma 202
- medulloepithelioma 202
- pineoblastoma 202
- PNET 202
CNS functions, effect of
  therapy 133–146
- cognitive impairment 140
- experimental studies 144
- iatrogenic toxicity, clinical
  manifestations 134
- myelopathy 139
- radiation tolerance, determinants 144
- treatment effects of
  behavior 145
Coats' disease 321
cognitive impairment 140
colorectal carcinoma 360–362
combining chemotherapy and radiation 145
congenital
- anomalies 10
- bladder extrophy 361
coronary artery disease 29
craniopharyngiomas 230–232
craniospinal irradiation 104
Crohn's disease 360
cryotherapy, retinoblastoma 324
Cushing syndrome 360
cyclophosphamide 120
cytotoxic agents 3

damage
- interaction
- - doxorubicin and radiation 82
- - models 80
- - radiation and chemotherapeutic
  agents 75–85
- repair
- - potential lethal 77
- - radiation 77
- sublethal 76
dental complications 21
- teeth, radiation related normal
  tissue effects 21

- tooth agenesis 21
- tooth development, delayed or arrested 21
desmoid tumor 5
development, radiation related normal tissue effects 31
developmental toxicity 4
diabetes insipidus 345
diastematomyelia 240
diencephalic syndrome 227
DNA sequence analysis 57
dose
- biologically effective 116
- fractionation 118
- incidence relationship, age 144
- rate, influence 119
Down's syndrome (trisomy 21) 10,
  99
doxorubicin 13, 28, 82
Drash syndromes 251
drug-radiation interaction 13, 32,
  134
- radiation related normal tissue effects 32
dry eyes 24
dystrophic calcification 138

ear, radiation related normal tissue
  effects 26
ecogenetics 7
edema, acute cerebral 134
enamel dysplasia 21
encephalopathy, acute 135
endocrine disturbances 227
endocrine effects, radiation related
  normal tissue effects 42
eosinophilic granuloma 337
ependymoblastoma 202
ependymomas 239, 244
- supratentorial 225, 226
- - epidemiology 221
- - etiology 221
- - evaluation 222
- - prognostic factors 222
epidermoids 245
epispadias 361
epithelial carcinomas 351–363
esophageal motility 34
esophagus, radiation related normal
  tissue effects 34

Ewing's sarcoma (tumor) 1, 5, 57,
  265–278, 283
- complications 275
- diagnosis 266
- geographic and ethnic variation 8
- leg-length discrepancies 275
- pathologic fractures 275
- PNET of bone 265
- prognostic features 266, 273
- treatment 267–273

extramedullary leukemia 101
eye(s)
- dry 24
- radiation related normal tissue effects 23

FAB classification, ANLL 100
familial cancer 56
Fanconi's anemia 10, 99
fetal alcohol syndrome 176
fibromatosis, aggressive 369
- cytotoxic chemotherapy 370
- hormonal treatment 370
- radiation therapy 370
fibroplasia, retrolental 321
Flexner-Wintersteiner rosette 320
fluorescence in situ hybridization
  (FISH) 58
fraction size 145
fractions, time between 145
FSH, elevated serum 40
fusiform aneurysmal dilatation
  139

Gardner's syndrome 352, 361, 369
gastrointestinal tract, radiation
  related normal tissue effects 34
gene
- amplification 64
- loss 64
genetic advances 55–70
germ cell
- dysfunction 41
- tumor(s) 204–208
- - intracranial 204
germinoma 133
giant cell tumor 374–376
gliomas 144
- supratentorial 221–224
- visual pathway 226–230
- - complications 229
- - epidemiology 226
- - evaluation 227
- - management 227
- - pathology 227
- - radiation technique 229
- - symptoms 227
gonadal
- failure 39
- injury 170
granulocytic sarcoma 107
growth
- delay 227
- hormone deficiency 44
- radiation related normal tissue
  effects 31

Hand-Christian-Schüller syndrome 337
HD see Hodgkin's disease
hearing loss, high frequency 26
heart 27

– radiation related normal tissue effects 27
hemangioblastomas 244
hematopoietic tissues, radiation related normal tissue effects 15
hemihypertrophy 7
hepatoblastoma 10
Hirschsprung's disease 176
Hodgkin's disease (HD) 3, 8, 18, 29, 151–171
– combined modality therapy 171
– diagnosis 154
– epidemiology 151
– etiology 151
– lymphangiography 155
– pathology 153
– patterns of involvement and spread 153
– radiotherapy 156–170
– – complications 166
– staging 154
– – evaluation 154
Homer-Wright rosette 320
hormonal treatment, fibromatosis 370
hydantoin syndrome 176
hyperparathyroidism 44
hypogonadism 45
hypopigmentation 13
hypoplastic breast development 42
hyposplenism 16
hypothalamic dysfunction 44
hypothyroidism 42, 43
hypothyroidism/hypoadrenalism 45

iatrogenic
– neurotoxicity 133
– toxicity, clinical manifestations 134
immobilization 2, 3
immunodeficiency syndrome 10
intelligence tests 133
intracranial germ cell tumor 204
intramedullary tumors 242–244
irradiation (see also radiation), craniospinal 104

keratitis 24, 332
keratoconjunctivitis 332
kidney 251
– malignant rhabdoid tumor 254
– radiation related normal tissue effects 36
Klinefelter's syndrome 10
kyphosis 246

Langerhans cell histiocytosis 241, 337–346
– biology 338
– bone lesions, solitary 340
– clinical manifestations 340
– diabetes insipidus 345

– etiology 337
– immunology 339
– incidence 337
– pathology 338
– patient evaluation 340
– therapy 343
– – bone marrow transplantation 346
– – radiation therapy 344
– – – dose 346
late focal necrosis 137
leg length discrepancies, radiation related 20
Letterer-Siwe-disease 337
leukemia 8, 140
– extramedullary 101
– incidence 8
– total body irradiation 115–121
leukoencephalopathy, delayed necrotizing 134, 136
leukostasis 107
Leydig-cell injury 40
Lhermitte sign 168
– subacute 139
Li-Fraumeni syndrome 62, 282, 360
ligase-mediated PCR 57
linear quadratic models 116
lipomas 240, 245
liver, radiation related normal tissue effects 34
lordosis 246
lung volume 31
lungs, radiation related normal tissue effects 31
lymphangiography 154
lymphoepithelioma 355
lymphoma 8
– bone 128
– total body irradiation 115–121
Lynch syndrome I 361
Lynch syndrome II 361

medullary carcinoma 352
medulloblastoma 3, 133, 197–201
– treatment 199
– – chemotherapy 201
– – radiation therapy 200
medulloepithelioma 202
meningioma 144, 245
meta-iodobenzylguanidine 178
methotrexate 145
– high-dose intravenous 135
– parenteral 141
MIBG 242
microangiopathy, mineralizing 138
molecular biology 55–70
multidrug resistant mammalian cells 83
muscle and soft tissue, radiation related normal tissue effects 22
musculoskeletal tissues, radiation related normal tissue effects 16

myelopathy 139
myocardial infarction 29
myocardium 28

N-*myc* copy 67
nasopharyngeal cancer 354–357
National Wilms' Tumor Study 28, 32, 36, 254
– results 258
NB see neuroblastoma
necrosis
– late focal 137
– parenchymal 136
nerve sheath tumors 245
nesidioblastosis 176
neuroblastomas (NB) 5, 7, 10, 67, 175–191, 239, 240
– cerebral 202
– chromosomal abnormalities 176
– epidemiology 175
– etiology 176
– evaluation 176
– natural history 176
– pathology 178
– prevention 191
– prognostic features 178
– staging 178
– therapy 180
– – bone marrow transplantation 188
– – chemotherapy 183
– – radiation therapy 184–188
– – – dose 186
– – – volume 187
– – surgery 181
neurofibromatosis 9, 176, 226, 251, 282
– type I 245
– type II 245
neuromas, acoustic 245
neuropsychological sequelae, ALL 108
neuropsychometric tests 133
neurotoxicity, radiation-induced 134
Non-Hodgkin's lymphoma (NHL) 123–130
– advanced disease 126
– bone marrow transplantation 129
– Burkitt's lymphoma 124
– central nervous system 127
– – prophylaxes 127
– – relapse 127
– localized disease 126
– lymphoma of bone 128
– staging 125
nonrhabdomyosarcoma 312, 314
normal tissue assays 79
normal tissue effects, radiation related 13–46
– bladder 39
– bone marrow 15

normal tissue effects (cont.)
- breast 42
- cardiovascular system 27
- development 31
- drug-radiation interactions 32
- ear 26
- endocrine effects 42
- esophagus 34
- eye 23
- gastrointestinal tract 34
- growth 31
- heart 27
- hematopoietic tissues 15
- kidney 36
- liver 34
- lungs 31
- muscle and soft tissue 22
- musculoskeletal tissues 16
- olfactory mucosa 25
- oral cavity 22
- ovary 39
- parathyroid 44
- pitutary/hypothalamus references 46
- pulmonar toxicity after bone marrow transplantation 33
- radiation injury, chronic 31
- radiation pneumonitis 31
- reproductive organs 39
- salivary glands 22
- skin 14
- small bowel 35
- special sensory organs 23
- spleen 16
- taste buds 26
- testis 40
- teeth 21
- thyroid 42
- urinary tract 36
- vessels, large 30
normal tissue toxicity 5

Oldfield's syndrome 361
olfactory mucosa, radiation related normal tissue effects 25
oligodendrogliomas 224, 225
oncogenes 56, 59, 60
oophoropexy 155
optic nerve injury 25
oral cavity, radiation related normal tissue effects 22
osteonecrosis 26
osteosarcoma 1, 305 - 315
- chemotherapy, adjuvant 307
- radiation therapy, adjuvant 308
- unusual sites
-- head 309
-- neck 309
-- truncal 309
-- vertebral 309
osteosarcomas 333
otitis media, serous 26

ovarian function 39
ovary, radiation related normal tissue effects 39

p-glycoprotein 84
p53 61
parathyroid, radiation related normal tissue effects 44
parenchymal necrosis 136
pericarditis 27
pericardium 27
peripheral neuroepithelioma 57
Perlman syndromes 251
Peutz-Jegher's syndrome 361
Philadelphia chromosome 55, 63
photocoagulation, retinoblastoma 324
pineal
- parenchymal tumors 204
- region, tumors 204 - 208
- tumor, geographic and ethnic variation 8
pineoblastoma 202
pituitary adenomas 232
pituitary/hypothalamus references, radiation related normal tissue effects 46
plasma cell granuloma 373, 374
PNET 198
- of bone 265
pneumonitis 168
point mutations 62
polyposis, familial 352, 361
precocious puberty 45, 227
prevention 7
primitive neuroectodermal tumor see PNET
puberty, precocious 227
pulmonar toxicity after bone marrow transplantation, radiation related normal tissue effects 33
pulmonary
- function 32
- morbidity 31

radiation (therapy) (see also irradiation; total body irradiation)
- ANLL 105, 108
- brain stem glioma 217
- cataract 23
- and chemotherapy
-- combination 145
-- concurrent 3
- cranospinal, ALL 94
- damage (see also damage), repair of sublethal 77, 81
- enteritis 35
- esophagitis 34
- fibromatosis 370
- hepatitis 34
- Hodgkin's disease 156 - 170
- injury, chronic 31

- juvenile nasopharyngeal angiofibroma 372
- Langerhans cell histiocytosis 344, 346
- medulloblastoma 200
- necrosis 5
- nephropathy 36
- neuroblastoma 184 - 188
- neurotoxicity 134
- osteosarcoma 308
- pneumonitis 31
- retinoblastoma 324
- retinopathy 24
- rhabdomyosarcoma 287 - 297
- sensitivity 75
- tolerance, determinants 144
- toxicity 5
- visual pathway gliomas 229
- Wilms' tumor 257, 261
radiation-recall phenomena 22
ras gene 100
RB see retinoblastoma
recombinant DNA techniques 57
renal
- artery stenosis 38
- dysfunction 120
reproductive organs, radiation related normal tissue effects 39
restriction endonuclease 57
retinoblastoma (RB) 3, 7, 9, 66, 319 - 346
- cataract formation 331
- clinical features 321
- complications 331
- dental effects 332
- epidemiology 319
- etiology 320
- growth effects 331
- keratitis 332
- keratoconjunctivitis 332
- molecular genetics 319
- natural history 321
- pathology 320
- second tumor formation 8, 332
- staging 321
- treatment 322 - 330
-- chemotherapy 330
-- cryotherapy 324
-- decision tree 329
-- metastatic disease 330
-- photocoagulation 324
-- radiation therapy 324
-- surgery 323
- trilateral 333
- vasclular effects 332
retinoblastoma susceptibility gene 65
retrolental fibroplasia 321
rhabdoid tumor of the kidney, malignant 254
rhabdomyosarcoma (RMS) 281 - 300

– alveolar tumors 282
– bladder 294
– cataract formation 299
– complications 298
– embryonal histology 282
– epidemiology 281
– etiology 282
– evaluation 283
– extremity 295
– larynx 293
– lymph node involvement 283
– middle ear 292
– molecular genetic studies 283
– nasopharynx 290
– natural history 283
– orbit 289
– paratesticular 293
– pathology 283
– prostate 294
– staging 284, 285
– treatment 285–297
– – chemotherapy 286
– – – VAC 286
– – radiation therapy 287–297
– trunk 296
– vagina 293

salivary glands, radiation related normal tissue effects 22
scoliosis 246
– radiation related 18
second tumors 143
seminoma 29
Shimada system 179
skin, radiation related normal tissue
  effects 14
small bowel, radiation related normal
  tissue effects 35
small-round-cell sarcomas 265
smell acuity 26
soft tissue sarcomas 312
somnolence 135
– syndrome, subacute 135
Southern blot procedure 58
special sensory organs, radiation
  related normal tissue effects 23
spinal cord
– injury 247
– tumors 239–248
– – astrocytomas 242
– – bone growth 246
– – clinical presentation 241
– – complications of therapy 246
– – ependymomas 244
– – epidemiology 239
– – epidermoids 245
– – evaluation 241
– – intramedullary
    tumors 242–244

– – lipomas 245
– – meningiomas 245
– – nerve sheath tumors 245
– – pathology 240
– – spinal cord injury 247
– – teratomas 245
– – vascular lesions 244
spleen, radiation related normal
  tissue effects 16
staging
– Hodgkin's disease 154
– neuroblastoma 178
– Non-Hodgkin's lymphoma
  125
– retinoblastoma 321
– rhabdomyosarcoma 284, 285
– Wilms' tumor 254
strabismus 321
sublethal damage 76
supratentorial
– ependymomas see ependymomas
– gliomas 221–224
surgery
– brain stem glioma 217
– juvenile nasopharyngeal
  angiofibroma 372
– neuroblastoma 181
– retinoblastoma 323

taste
– acuity 26
– buds, radiation related normal
  tissue effects 26
TBI see total body irradiation
teeth see dental complications
telangiectasia 13
teratomas 245
testis 40
therapy-induced second
  malignancy 133
thyroid
– cancer 351–354
– dysfunction 42, 167
– radiation related normal tissue effects 42
tinea capitis 143
tooth see dental complications
total body irradiation
  (TBI) 115–121
– chemotherapeutic agents 120
– dose effect factor 117
– dose fractionation 118
– dose rate 119
– effective doses 116
– linear quadratic models 116
– regimes, comparison 117
– therapeutic gain factor 117
toxic effect, chemotherapeutic
  agents 4

toxicity, radiation 5
translocation 65
transverse myelitis 168
treatment plan 2
triretinoin 69
trisomy 99
tumor
– control dose50 (TCD 50) 79
– development 5
– growth delay 79
– suppresor genes 59, 61, 320
– virology 56
tumors of the spinal cord see spinal
  cord
Turcot's syndrome 361
Turner's Syndrome 10

ulcerative colitis 360
ultraviolet light 9
ureterosigmoidoscopy 361
urinary tract, radiation related normal tissue effects 36

vascular lesions 244
vasculopathy, late 138
vasoactive intestinal peptide
  (VIP) 176
veno-occlusive disease 35, 110
vessels, large 30
vincristine 4, 256
visceral larva migrans 321
visual pathway gliomas see gliomas
von Hippel-Lindau Disease 10
von Hippel-Lindau syndrome 244
von Recklingshausen's disease 7

white matter abnormality, delayed
  diffuse 137
Wilms' tumor 1, 5, 10, 16, 17, 18,
  32, 81, 251–262, 379
– clinical presentation 252
– diagnostic evaluation 252
– geographic and ethnic variation 8
– molecular biologic studies 251
– National Wilms' Tumor
  Study 254
– pathology 254
– patterns of spread 252
– radiation therapy 257
– staging system 254
– surgery 252
– treatment 255
– – bilateral Wilms' tumor 256
– – outcome 258–260
– whole abdomen
  radiotherapy 261

xerostomia 22

List of Contributors

K.KIAN ANG, M.D., Ph.D.
Professor and Deputy Chairman
Department of Radiation Oncology
M.D. Anderson Cancer Center
1515 Holcombe Blvd.
Houston, TX 77030
USA

JAMES A. BELLI, M.D.
Professor and John Sealy Centennial Chair
Department of Radiation Oncology
The University of Texas Medical Branch
Galveston, TX 77550-2780
USA

AMY LOUISE BILLET, M.D.
Pediatric Oncology
Dana Farber Cancer Institute
Harvard Medical School
44 Binney Street
Boston, MA 02115
USA

J. ROBERT CASSADY, M.D.
Professor and Head
Department of Radiation Oncology
The University of Arizona
Health Sciences Center
1501 North Campbell Ave.
Tucson, AZ 85724
USA

SARAH S. DONALDSON, M.D.
Professor of Radiation Oncology
Department of Radiation Oncology, Room A-083
Stanford University School of Medicine
Stanford, CA 94305
USA

PATRICIA J. EIFEL, M.D.
Associate Professor
Department of Clinical Radiotherapy
The University of Texas
M.D. Anderson Cancer Center
1515 Holcombe Blvd.
Houston, TX 77030
USA

RICHARD G. EVANS, Ph.D., M.D.
Professor and Chairman
Department of Radiation Oncology
University of Kansas Medical Center
3901 Rainbow Blvd.
Kansas City, KS 66103
USA

K. WILLIAM HARTER, M.D.
Associate Professor and Vice Chairman
Department of Radiation Oncology
Georgetown University Medical Center
Vincent T. Lombardi Cancer Center
3800 Reservoir Rd. NW
Washington, DC 20007
USA

JOHN J. HUTTER, M.D., Ph.D.
Associate Professor
Department of Pediatrics
Arizona Health Sciences Center
University of Arizona
1501 N. Campbell Ave.
Tucson, AZ 85724
USA

LARRY E. KUN, M.D.
Chairman, Department of Radiation Oncology
St. Jude Children's Research Hospital
332 North Lauderdale, P.O. Box 318
Memphis, TN 38101-0318
USA

ROBERT B. MARCUS, Jr., M.D.
Professor of Radiation Oncology and Pediatrics
University of Florida College of Medicine
Department of Radiation Oncology
University of Florida Health Science Center
P.O. Box 100385
Gainesville, FL 32610-0385
USA

KENNETH L. MCCLAIN, M.D., Ph.D.
Associate Professor, Department of Pediatrics
Baylor College of Medicine
Texas Children's Hospital
6621 Fannin Street MC 3-3320
Houston, TX 77030-2399
USA

PAUL S. MELTZER, M.D., Ph.D.
Head, Section of Molecular Genetics
Laboratory of Cancer Genetics
National Center for Human Genome Research
9000 Rockville Pike/Bldg 49 Rm 4A10
Bethesda, MD 20892
USA

NANCY PRICE MENDENHALL, M.D.
Professor and Chair
Department of Radiation Oncology
University of Florida
Health Science Center
P.O. Box 100385
Gainsville, FL 32610-0385
USA

STEPHEN E. SALLAN, M.D.
Clinical Director
Pediatric Oncology
Dana Farber Cancer Institute
Harvard Medical School
44 Binney Street
Boston, MA 02115
USA

BALDASSARRE STEA, M.D., Ph.D.
Associate Professor
Department of Radiation Oncology
University of Arizona Health Sciences Center
1501 North Campbell Avenue
Tucson, AZ 85724
USA

PATRICK S. SWIFT, M.D.
Assistant Professor
Department of Radiation Oncology
University of California San Francisco
Long Hospital, Room L-75
Parnassus Avenue
San Francisco, CA 94143-0226
USA

ALBERT J. VAN DER KOGEL, Ph.D.
Professor of Experimental Radiotherapy
Institute of Radiotherapy
University of Nijmegen
Geert Grooteplein 32
P.O. Box 9101
6500 HB Nijmegen
The Netherlands

EMMANUEL VAN DER SCHUEREN, M.D.
Professor and Head, Department of Radiotherapy
Academisch Zuikenhuis
St. Rafael's Kliniek
Kapucijnenvoer
3000 Leuven
Belgium

MOODY D. WHARAM, JR., M.D.
Professor
Division of Radiation Oncology
Johns Hopkins Oncology Center
600 N. Wolfe Street
Baltimore, MD 21287
USA

Titles in the series already published

Lung Cancer
Edited by C. W. SCARANTINO

Innovations in Radiation Oncology
Edited by H. R. WITHERS and L. J. PETERS

Radiation Therapy of Head and Neck Cancer
Edited by G. E. LARAMORE

Gastrointestinal Cancer - Radiation Therapy
Edited by R. R. DOBELBOWER, Jr.

Radiation Exposure and Occupational Risks
Edited by E. SCHERER, C. STREFFER, and K.-R. TROTT

Radiation Therapy of Benign Diseases –
A Clinical Guide
Edited by S. E. ORDER and S. S. DONALDSON

Innovations in Diagnostic Imaging
Edited by J. H. ANDERSON

Interventional Radiation Therapy Techniques –
Brachytherapy
Edited by R. SAUER

Radiopathology of Organs and Tissues
Edited by E. SCHERER, C. STREFFER, and K.-R. TROTT

Concomitant Continuous Infusion Chemotherapy
and Radiation
Edited by M. ROTMAN and C. J. ROSENTHAL

Radiology of the Upper Urinary Tract
Edited by E. K. LANG

Intraoperative Radiotherapy –
Clinical Experiences and Results
Edited by F. A. CALVO, M. SANTOS, and L. W. BRADY

The Thymus – Diagnostic Imaging, Functions,
and Pathologic Anatomy
Edited by E. WALTER, E. WILLICH, and W. R. WEBB

Radiotherapy of Intraocular and Orbital Tumors
Edited by W. E. ALBERTI and R. H. SAGERMAN

Interstitial and Intracavitary Thermoradiotherapy
Edited by M. H. SEEGENSCHMIEDT and R. SAUER

Interventional Neuroradiology
Edited by A. VALAVANIS

Non-Disseminated Breast Cancer
Controversial Issues in Management
Edited by G. H. FLETCHER and S. H. LEVITT

Current Topics in Clinical Radiobiology of Tumors
Edited by H.-P. BECK-BORNHOLDT

Practical Approaches to Cancer Invasion and
Metastastes:
A Compendium of Radiation Oncologists'
Responses to 40 Histories
Edited by A. R. KAGAN with the assistance of
R. J. STECKEL

Radiology of the Pancreas
Edited by A. L. BAERT, co-edited by G. DELORME